Contemporary Health Policy

Contemporary
Health Policy

Beaufort B. Longest, Jr.

AUPHA
HAP

Health Administration Press, Chicago, Illinois
AUPHA Press, Washington, DC

04   03   02   01   00   5   4   3   2   1

The paper used in this publication meets the minimum requirements of American National Standard for Information Sciences—Permanence of Paper for Printed Library Materials, ANSW Z39.48-1984.⊗™

Library of Congress Cataloging-in-Publication Data

Longest, Beaufort B.
    Contemporary health policy / Beaufort B. Longest, Jr.
      p. cm.
    Includes bibliographical references and index.
    ISBN 1-56793-139-1 (alk. paper)
    1. Medical policy—United States.   I. Title.
  RA395.A3 L659   2000
  362.1'0973—dc21   00-058102

Health Administration Press
A division of the Foundation
  of the American College of
  Healthcare Executives
One North Franklin Street
Chicago, IL 60606
(312) 424-2800

Association of University Programs
  in Health Administration
1911 North Fort Meyer Drive
Suite 503
Arlington, VA 22209
(703) 524-5500

For Carolyn

" . . . where could I find again a face whose every
feature, even every wrinkle, is a reminder of the
greatest and sweetest memories of my life?"

Karl Marx

Contents

Part III   **The Contemporary American Healthcare System**

Acknowledgments

I want to thank the authors of, as well as the publishers who hold the copyrights to, the works reprinted in this book. The authors' efforts and the publishers' permission to include the works have made this anthology possible. In addition, appreciation is also extended to several organizations whose grants supported the original work incorporated herein: the Association of Schools of Public Health, the Centers for Disease Control and Prevention, The Commonwealth Fund, the Hopkins Population Center, the NICHD, The Pew Charitable Trusts, The Robert Wood Johnson Foundation, and the Russell Sage Foundation.

I am indebted to Herbert S. Rosenkranz, Ph.D., Interim Dean of the Graduate School of Public Health at the University of Pittsburgh, and to Arthur S. Levine, M.D., Senior Vice Chancellor for Health Sciences at the University of Pittsburgh, for establishing an environment conducive to scholarly endeavors by faculty members. I also thank Denise Thrower and Linda Kalcevic for their able assistance in this project.

Finally, I thank the staff at Health Administration Press for their professional competence in bringing this anthology to fruition.

Introduction to
the Readings

In *Health Policymaking in the United States* (Longest 1998), for which this anthology of contemporary readings is a useful companion, I define health policy as the collection of authoritative decisions made within government that pertain to health and to the pursuit of health. As such, health policy occupies an important place in American life, reflecting not only the high priority that many give to their personal health and to that of the people they care about, but also the increasing significance of the pursuit of health to the nation's economy. The definition of health policy, as well as the vital relationship of health policy to health, is considered more fully in Chapter 1 of this book.

The two-fold purpose of this anthology is: (1) to provide those who have an interest in health policy with a set of contemporary readings that are organized so that, collectively, they present a clear picture of the direct role health policy plays in the pursuit of health and in the health of the people in the United States; and (2) to provide an overview of some of the key contemporary health policy issues facing the nation. The first purpose is pursued in Part I, Relationships Between Health Policy and Health. The second purpose is pursued in Part II, Key Contemporary Health Policy Issues. The third part of this anthology includes background readings on The Contemporary American Healthcare System. The readings in each part are briefly outlined below.

PART I, RELATIONSHIPS BETWEEN
HEALTH POLICY AND HEALTH

The unifying theme of the readings in this part is that health policy plays a direct and formative role in the health of the American people. In reading 1, "Health and Health Policy," a framework is provided for appreciating the vital role health policy plays in health and in healthcare. This reading emphasizes that health, whether of individuals or populations, is a function of several determinants (i.e., genetic endowments; physical, sociocultural, and economic environments; lifestyles and behaviors; and health services), and that health policy directly affects these determinants and, thus, health.

In reading 2, "Medicare's Social Contract," Stuart Butler, Theda Skocpol, Robert M. Ball, and E. J. Dionne provide their perspectives on the nature of the

1

nation's most substantial health policy, Medicare, and emphasize the special role it plays in the health of so many elderly or disabled citizens. Medicare spends about $230 billion annually for healthcare services for its approximately 40 million beneficiaries.

In reading 3, "Rules of the Game: How Public Policy Affects Local Health Care Markets," Loel S. Solomon explores the effect of public policy on health systems. Based on a large tracking study, he reports on site visits in 12 communities which show that health policy is a potent force in shaping health systems by establishing "rules of the game" for private and public actors.

The extraordinary sensitivity of events in the world of healthcare delivery often seen in response to changes in health policy is illustrated clearly in reading 4, "Do Different Funding Mechanisms Produce Different Results? The Implications of Family Planning for Fiscal Federalism" by Deborah R. McFarlane and Kenneth J. Meier. This reading illustrates the "cause and effect" relationship vital to a full understanding of the role of health policy in the nation's pursuit of health.

The relationships between health policy and health insurance—in this case, insurance coverage of working families of low and moderate incomes—is clearly illustrated in reading 5, "Sliding-Scale Premium Health Insurance Programs: Four States' Experiences." The analysis traces the effect of higher out-of-pocket premium shares on participation rates in the four states studied.

To conclude Part I, Pamela A. Paul-Shaheen shows in reading 6, "The States and Health Care Reform: The Road Traveled and Lessons Learned from Seven that Took the Lead," that the cause and effect relationship between health policy, healthcare, and health can move in either direction. She describes the efforts of seven states to undertake significant policy initiatives to reform their healthcare systems: changes in the healthcare marketplace causing changes in health policy. She argues that the dominant reason for these states to undertake such difficult policy changes is that their healthcare costs to fund such items as health insurance for state employees, their share of Medicaid costs, and public health programs have risen at rates that concern officials. She then describes the changes undertaken in the seven states examined and considers some of their effect (or lack thereof) on healthcare delivery: changes in health policy causing changes in the healthcare marketplace.

PART II, KEY CONTEMPORARY HEALTH POLICY ISSUES

The overall purpose of the set of readings in Part II is to identify and elucidate some of the key contemporary health policy issues. The readings included are by no means a comprehensive set of important health policy issues; rather, they are intended to reflect some of the most important and visible issues facing the nation today.

Reflecting both the present magnitude of the role of the Medicare program in healthcare and health, as well as the growing—and eventually, unavoidable—crisis in the program's funding, the first two readings in this section pertain to this vital health policy, a policy that will occupy a central place in the health policy agenda for the forseeable future. In reading 7, "The Political Economy of Medicare," Bruce C. Vladeck reminds us of how inextricably Medicare policy is embedded in the nation's larger policymaking process and political system. He talks of Medicare as redistributive politics, Medicare as special-interest politics, and Medicare as distributive politics. Any one of these features makes reform of this massive policy difficult: together they form a formidable obstacle indeed!

In reading 8, "A Framework for Considering Medicare Payment Policy Issues," the Medicare Payment Advisory Commission (MedPAC), an independent federal body that advises the U.S. Congress on issues affecting the Medicare program (more information on the commission can be found at www.medpac.gov), outlines the issues regarding Medicare's payment policies that must be addressed in the coming years. MedPAC reminds readers that Medicare's payment policies determine the amounts providers will be paid for covered services and supplies used by program beneficiaries. Furthermore, if beneficiaries are to have access to necessary care, these payment policies must work well for thousands of products and services that are furnished by a multitude of providers—healthcare professionals, facilities, suppliers, and healthcare organizations—in hundreds of market areas nationwide.

In reading 9, "The Dilemmas of Incrementalism: Logical and Political Constraints in the Design of Health Insurance Reforms," Thomas R. Oliver simultaneously provides a comprehensive review of the main options of government in regulating private insurance and an explanation of why significant reforms in this area are very difficult to achieve.

With the 1999 publication of *To Err Is Human: Building a Safer Health System*, the Institute of Medicine has ensured a high place on the policy agenda for efforts to minimize medical mistakes. Chapter 7 from this volume, "Setting Performance Standards and Expectations for Patient Safety," is included as reading 10. It contains a discussion of the current approaches—private and public—to setting performance standards and suggests the magnitude of the policy challenges that lie ahead for federal and state policymakers regarding this important issue.

Offering a related perspective on this issue, Bryan A. Liang in reading 11, "Error in Medicine: Legal Impediments to U.S. Reform," outlines some of the major challenges of effective policy development in this important area.

He argues that, in addition to the technical challenges inherent in establishing effective practices to reduce human error in medicine, a set of legal impediments must be addressed before a safer health system can be built.

One important aspect of safety in healthcare is the qualifications of the healthcare workforce. In reading 12, "Strengthening Consumer Protection: Priorities for Health Care Workforce Regulation," Leonard J. Finocchio, Catherine M. Dower, Noelle T. Blick, Christine M. Gragnola, and the Taskforce on Health Care Workforce Regulation of the Pew Health Professions Commission focus on state-based professional regulation. They make specific recommendations to ensure a suitable workforce into the twenty-first century regarding professional regulatory boards, continuing competence of the workforce, and scopes of practice authority.

Addressing a related but different issue, in reading 13, "The Changing Nature of Health Professions Education," John Naughton takes a broad look at the education of health professionals, including the policies that have financed so much of this endeavor. He emphasizes that a policy challenge remains to develop workable future financing strategies.

In reading 14, "Litigation and Public Health Policy Making: The Case of Tobacco Control," Peter D. Jacobson and Kenneth E. Warner address the fundamental issue of how policy should be made regarding the use of tobacco products in the society. They also consider the roles of the market, the legislative and executive branches of government, and the courts in the development of appropriate public policy around this issue.

Constance A. Nathanson, in reading 15, "Social Movements as Catalysts for Policy Change: The Case of Smoking and Guns," uses two serious threats to health in American society to assess the ways in which the social movements that have been built up around tobacco control and gun control have influenced policy. In doing so, she provides excellent histories of policy development related to these two important health issues and a glimpse of what remains to be done as these threats continue to be challenged through changes in public policy.

In reading 16, "Genetic Privacy and Confidentiality: Why They Are So Hard to Protect," Mark A. Rothstein delineates some of the extraordinary complexity of protecting genetic privacy and confidentiality. He notes that the issue cannot be solved by a single procedural law and that policy steps taken thus far, as well as those proposed, tend to be "misguided, simplistic, and ineffective."

Fred J. Hellinger, in reading 17, "Antitrust Enforcement in the Healthcare Industry: The Expanding Scope of State Activity," describes the evolution of state antitrust policy that seeks to immunize collaborative activities in the healthcare industry from federal and state antitrust prosecution. This issue has taken on increasing importance as the extent and complexity of organizational integration within the healthcare industry has increased.

PART III, THE CONTEMPORARY
AMERICAN HEALTHCARE SYSTEM

The purpose of Part III is to provide the reader with some background information about the American healthcare system, especially focusing on the policy challenges inherent in a trillion-dollar sector of the economy that touches everyone in one way or another. The four readings are taken from a remarkable series of articles first published in the *New England Journal of Medicine* in 1999.

In reading 18, "Expenditures," John K. Iglehart points out that "inspite of all the money spent for medical care, education, and research, no one—whether patient, provider, or purchaser—seems satisfied with the status quo." In reading 19, "Health Insurance Coverage," Robert Kuttner traces the slow erosion of health insurance coverage in America, forecasting a continued decline in coverage, "unless there is a dramatic change in national policy." In reading 20, "Medicare," and reading 21, "Medicaid," John K. Iglehart reviews the status of these two vital health policies. The Medicare and Medicaid programs were the heart of historic legislation enacted in 1965 as key building blocks in President Lyndon Johnson's Great Society. From their common origin, however, they have diverged dramatically, primarily because Medicare has been a largely successful experiment in social insurance, while Medicaid has suffered most of the problems inherent in all of this nation's welfare policies. As Iglehart notes in "Medicaid," "the United States remains the only industrialized nation that has never settled on a social policy that, however policymakers choose to accomplish it, offers a basic set of healthcare benefits to all residents regardless of their ability to pay—certainly a regrettable failure in a nation blessed with so many resources."

REFERENCE

Longest, B. B., Jr. 1998. *Health Policymaking in the United States*, 2nd ed. Chicago: Health Administration Press.

Part I

Relationships Between Health Policy and Health

1 | Health and Health Policy

Beaufort B. Longest, Jr.

Health and its pursuit are tightly interwoven into the social and economic fabric of the United States. Health plays a direct and very important role not only in the physical and psychological well-being of the American people, but increasingly in their economic circumstances as well. Thus, it should be to no one's surprise that health receives considerable attention from the federal and state governments. This book is about the intricate process that public policymakers use as one means to influence the pursuit of health. Attention is focused primarily on the process at the federal level, although much of what is said applies at the state level as well.

In this chapter, some basic and underpinning definitions and concepts are established. In the next chapter, a general model of the public policymaking process is outlined and briefly described. The various interconnected parts of the model are then used as the means to organize subsequent chapters. The exploration of the policymaking process begins defining health and health policy and considering their relationship to each other.

HEALTH DEFINED

Although health is a universally important concept, its definition is far from universally agreed upon. Health can be thought about in negative or positive terms and narrowly or broadly (see Figure 1.1). Thought of negatively, health is viewed as the minimization, if not the absence, of some variable, as in the absence of infection or the shrinking of a tumor. At the extreme negative end of the conceptualization of health, it is thought of as the complete absence of disease or dysfunction.

In contrast, thought of more positive health can be viewed as a state in which variables are maximized. For example, viewing health positively and broadly,

Reprinted from Beaufort B. Longest, Jr., *Health Policymaking in the United States*, 2nd edition, pp. 1–30 (Chicago, 1999), with permission, AUPHA/Health Administration Press.

FIGURE 1.1

Dimensions of Conceptualizing Health

Positively

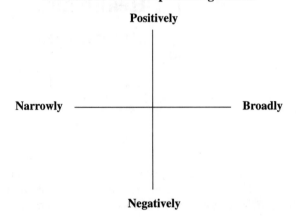

Negatively

the World Health Organization (1948) defines it as the "state of complete physical, mental, and social well-being, and not merely the absence of disease or injury." A more contemporary conceptualization, one which also incorporates a positive and broad perspective, views health as a state in which the biological and clinical indicators of organ function are maximized and in which physical, mental, and role functioning in everyday life are also maximized (Brook and McGlynn 1991).

The way in which health is conceptualized or defined in any society is important because it reflects the society's values regarding health and how far the society might be willing to go in aiding or supporting the pursuit of health among its members. For example, a society that defines health in negative, narrow terms might choose to intervene only in life-threatening traumas and illnesses. Conversely, a society that broadly defines health in positive terms might obligate itself to pursue a variety of significant interventions to help its members attain desired levels of health. Generally, negative and narrow conceptualizations of health lead to interventions that focus on correcting or reducing an undesirable state. Positive and broad conceptualizations of health, on the other hand, stimulate proactive interventions aimed at many variables in the quest for health.

The enormous range of possible targets for intervention in the pursuit of health in any society is illustrated by the fact that health in human beings is a function of many variables, which can be grouped under the headings of several *health determinants*. These health determinants include, for individuals or a population of individuals, their genetic endowments; the physical, sociocultural, and economic environments in which they live; their lifestyles and behaviors; and the health services that they utilize (Blum 1983; Evans, Barer, and Marmor 1994).

In any consideration of health, whether of individuals or of populations, it is important to remember that people are not all alike. They vary along many dimensions, including their health and their health-related needs. The citizenry of the United States is a remarkably diverse montage of people. Although not capturing the full richness of their diversity, nor all of the variation in their health and health-related needs, two demographic variables bear significantly on the health of the American people: the changing age structure of the population and its racial and ethnic diversity.

In 1990, about 32 million Americans were over the age of 65, and 13.5 million of them were over 75 years of age. By 2000, about 35.2 million will be over 65, with about 16.7 million of them over 75. Two decades after that, in 2020, these numbers will increase to 52.7 million and 21 million (Burner, Waldo, and McKusick 1992). These demographic changes are important in thinking about health and its pursuit because older people consume relatively more health services, and their health-related needs differ in significant ways from those of younger people. One such difference is the greater likelihood that older people will consume long-term care services and community-based services intended to help them cope with various limitations in the activities of daily living.

Advancing age can mean increased fragility and susceptibility to acute health problems such as injuries resulting from falls or infections, and to chronic health problems such as emphysema or cirrhosis. Cardiovascular disease, cancer, diabetes, and osteoarthritis will remain serious health problems for elderly people well into the twenty-first century. Especially devastating can be the combination of acute and chronic health problems with cognitive impairments such as Alzheimer's disease that may occur with advancing age.

Although the view of the United States as a great melting pot of people and cultures was always more myth than reality, two groups now challenge this view in fundamental ways. African Americans and (especially) Latinos represent growing parts of the population. Both groups are currently underserved disproportionately for health services, and both groups are underrepresented in all of the health professions.

African Americans have long faced fewer opportunities for education, employment, health services, and long, healthy lives than the numerically predominant European Americans (Hacker 1992; Ayanian 1993). For some of the same reasons, and for a variety of others, including language, geographic concentration, and cultural preferences, many Latinos are also unlikely to become well-integrated into the nation's dominant culture.

Although the nation's population is diverse, with differences in health status, health-related needs, and access to the benefits of the services of the healthcare system, the dominant culture does reflect a rather homogeneous set of values that directly affects the basic approach to health in the United States. To a very great extent, American society places a high value on individual autonomy, self-determination, and personal privacy, and maintains a widespread, although not universal, commitment to justice for all members of society. Other characteristics of the core society that significantly influence the pursuit of health include a deep-seated faith in the potential of technological rescue and, although it may be beginning to change, a long-standing desire to prolong life, with scant regard for the costs of doing so. These values help shape the private- and public-sector efforts related to health, including the elaboration of public policies related to health and its pursuit.

HEALTH POLICY DEFINED

In view of the obvious desirability of a healthy population, and of the important role that the quest for health plays in the nation's economy—Americans spent more than $1 trillion in pursuit of health in 1997, and this could rise to $1.5 trillion by 2002 (Thorpe 1997)—it is not surprising that government, at all levels, is keenly interested in health and its pursuit. This interest is reflected vividly in the diverse activities that occur within the expansive forum of public policymaking and in the resulting public policies that relate to health.

Public policies are authoritative decisions that are made in the legislative, executive, or judicial branches of government. These decisions are intended to direct or influence the actions, behaviors, or decisions of others. The word *authoritative* is crucial in this definition. It means decisions made within the three branches of government—at any level of government—that are within the legitimate purview of those who make the decisions. These can be legislators, executives of government, or judges in their official roles and capacities.

When public policies—or authoritative decisions—pertain to health or influence the pursuit of health, they become *health policies*. Generally, health policies affect or influence groups or classes of individuals (such as physicians, the poor, the elderly, or children) or types or categories of organizations (such as medical schools, managed care organizations, integrated health services delivery systems, medical technology producers, or employers).

In the United States, health policies—as well as other types of public policies pertaining to defense, education, transportation, or communication, for example—are made within a dynamic public *policymaking process*. This process, which is modeled in Chapter 2, involves many interactive participants in several interconnected phases of activities. Health policies are established at federal, state, and local levels of government, although usually for different purposes. At any given time, the entire set of health-related policies or authoritative decisions, made at any level of government, can be said to constitute that level's *health policy*.

Policies made through the *public* policymaking process are distinguished from policies made in the *private* sector. Although it is beyond the scope of this book to discuss private-sector health policies in any depth, authoritative decisions made in the private sector by such decision makers as executives of managed care organizations about such issues as their product lines, pricing, and marketing strategies, for example, are policies. By definition, these are authoritative decisions intended to influence the actions, decisions, or behaviors of others. Similarly, such organizations as the Joint Commission on Accreditation of Healthcare Organizations (JCAHO), a private accrediting body for health-related organizations (http://www.jcaho.org), and the National Committee for Quality Assurance (NCQA), a private organization involved in assessing and reporting on the quality of managed care plans (http://www.ncqa.org), make authoritative decisions assigning criteria to use in their reviews of healthcare organizations and managed care plans. These also are private-sector health policies.

The focus of this book is limited to the public policymaking process and the public-sector health policies that result. But there are indeed private-sector health policies, and they also play a vitally important role in the ways society pursues health. The rich and complex blend of public- and private-sector policies and actions that shape the American pursuit of health reflect the extraordinary reluctance of Americans to yield control of the healthcare system to government. In part, this illustrates a unique feature of the American psyche. Perhaps Morone (1990, 1) captures it best when he says:

> At the heart of American politics lies a dread and a yearning. The dread is notorious. Americans fear public power as a threat to liberty. Their government is weak and fragmented, designed to prevent action more easily than to produce it. The yearning is an alternative faith in direct, communal democracy. Even after the loose collection of agrarian colonies had evolved into a dense industrial society, the urge remained: the people would, somehow, put aside their government and rule themselves directly.

In no aspect of American life is this "dread and yearning" more visible or relevant than in regard to health and health policy. Despite a substantive role for government in health affairs (more fully explored in subsequent chapters), most of the resources used in the pursuit of health in the United States are controlled by the private sector. Even when government is directly involved in healthcare, with some exceptions such as the Department of Veterans Affairs Health Administration (http://www.va.gov), it focuses on finding ways to ensure broader access to those health services that are provided predominantly through the private sector and financed through the uniquely American mix of both public and private payments for these services.

FORMS OF HEALTH POLICIES

Health policies take one of several basic forms. Some policies are the decisions made by legislators that are codified in the statutory language of enacted legislation. Others are the rules and regulations established to implement legislation or to operate government and its various programs. Still others are judicial decisions related to health. Examples of health policies include:

- the 1965 federal public law (P.L. 89-97)* that established the Medicare and Medicaid programs;
- an executive order regarding operation of federally funded health centers;
- a court's ruling that an integrated delivery system's acquisition of yet another hospital violates federal antitrust laws;
- a state government's procedures for licensing physicians;
- a county health department's procedures for inspecting restaurants; and
- a city government's ordinance banning smoking in public places within the city.

Thus, health policies may take any of several specific forms.

Laws

Laws enacted at any level of government are policies. Laws that are health policies include such examples as the 1983 federal Amendments to the Social Security Act (P.L. 98-21), which authorized the prospective payment system (PPS) for reimbursing hospitals for Medicare beneficiaries and state laws that govern the licensure of health-related practitioners and institutions. Laws, when they are "more or less freestanding legislative enactments aimed to achieve specific objectives" (Brown 1992, 21), are sometimes called programs. The Medicare program is a federal-level example. An example at the state level can be found in the certificate-of-need (CON) programs through which many states seek to influence capital expansion in their healthcare systems.

Rules/Regulations

Another form policies can take are the rules or regulations established to guide the implementation of laws. Such rules, made in the executive branch of government by the organizations and agencies responsible for implementing

---

*Federal public laws are given a number that designates both the enacting Congress and the sequence in which the law was enacted. P.L. 89-97, for example, means that this law was enacted by the 89th Congress and was the 97th law passed by this Congress.

laws, are also policies. The rules associated with the implementation of complex laws routinely fill hundreds and sometimes thousands of pages. Rulemaking is an important and highly proscribed activity in the larger policymaking process and will be discussed in detail later, especially in Chapter 4.

Operational Decisions

When organizations or agencies in the executive branch of a government, regardless of level, implement laws, they invariably must make many operational decisions as implementation proceeds. These decisions, which are different from the formal rules that also influence implementation, are also policies. For example, in implementing the Water Quality Improvement Act (P.L. 91-224), the several federal agencies with implementation responsibilities establish operational protocols and procedures that help them deal with those affected by the provisions of this law. These protocols and procedures, because they are authoritative decisions, are a form of policies. Frequently, the best way to distinguish between rules and operational decisions is that rules are intended to be more permanent. As a practical matter, the distinction is not very important. Both rules and operational decisions made within the context of implementing public laws, because they are authoritative decisions intended to influence the behaviors, decisions, and actions of others, are themselves public policies.

Judicial Decisions

Judicial decisions are another form of policies. An example is the U. S. Supreme Court's reversal in 1988 of the earlier decision of the U. S. Court of Appeals for the Ninth Circuit in the *Patrick v. Burget* case. The decision in this case, which involved the relationship between peer review of professional activities and antitrust liability, is a policy by the foregoing definition because the reversal is an authoritative decision that has the effect of directing or influencing the actions, behaviors, or decisions of others. As is often the case with judicial decisions, this one disrupted an established pattern of prior decisions and behaviors. Similarly, an opinion issued in 1992 by a U.S. Department of Health and Human Services (DHHS) administrative law judge stating that a hospital was in violation of the Rehabilitation Act Amendments of 1974 (P.L. 93-516) when it prohibited a HIV-positive staff pharmacist from preparing intravenous solutions is also a policy (Lumsdon 1992).

Macro Policies

A final form health policies can take—a form that is really a matter of scale more than anything else—is macro policies. Macro policies, which are broad and expansive, help shape a society's pursuit of health in fundamental ways.

The United States has a few health-related macro policies, such as its Medicare program or its regulation of pharmaceuticals. However, other advanced nations, Canada and Great Britain most notably, have much more expansive macro policies that govern their approaches to the pursuit of health almost entirely. In the United States, reflecting the preferences of the majority of its citizens, government chooses a more incremental, or piecemeal, approach to its health policy. The net result is a very large number of policies, but few of them dealing with the pursuit of health in any broad or expansive way. All of the various forms of health policies fit into one of two basis categories—allocative or regulatory.

CATEGORIES OF HEALTH POLICIES

In capitalist economies, such as that of the United States, the presumption is that private markets best determine the production and consumption of goods and services, including health services. In such economies, government generally intrudes with policies only when private markets fail to achieve desired public objectives. The most credible arguments for policy intervention in the nation's domestic activities begin with the identification of situations in which markets are not functioning properly.

The health sector is especially prone to situations in which markets do not function very well. Theoretically perfect (i.e., freely competitive) markets, which do not exist in reality but which provide a standard against which real markets can be assessed, require that:

- Buyers and sellers have sufficient information to make informed decisions.
- A large number of buyers and sellers participate.
- More sellers can easily enter the market.
- Each seller's products or services are satisfactory substitutes for those of their competitors.
- The quantity of products or services available in the market does not swing the balance of power toward either buyers or sellers.

The markets for health services in the United States violate these under-pinnings of competitive markets in a number of ways. The complexity of health services reduces the ability of consumers to make informed decisions without guidance from the sellers or from other advisers. The entry of sellers in health services markets is heavily regulated, and widespread insurance coverage affects the decisions of both buyers and sellers in these markets. These and other factors mean that the markets for health services frequently do not function competitively, thus quite literally inviting policy intervention.

Furthermore, the potential for private markets, on their own, to fail to meet public objectives related to health and its pursuit in the society is not limited to the production and consumption of health services. For example, markets, on their own, might not stimulate the conduct of enough socially desirable medical research or the education of enough physicians or nurses without the stimulus of policies that subsidize certain costs associated with these ends. These and many similar situations in which markets do not lead to desired outcomes provide the philosophical basis for establishing public policies to correct market-related problems or shortcomings. The nature of the problems or shortcomings of the market that health policies are intended to overcome or ameliorate help shape the policies in a direct way. Based on their basic natures and purposes, health policies fit broadly into allocative or regulatory categories, although the potential for overlap between the two categories is considerable.

Allocative Policies

Allocative policies are designed to provide net benefits to some distinct group or class of individuals or organizations, at the expense of others, in order to ensure that public objectives are met. Such policies are in essence subsidies through which policymakers seek to alter demand for or supplies of particular products and services or to guarantee access to products and services for certain people. For example, on the basis that without subsidies to medical schools markets would undersupply the preparation of physicians, government has heavily subsidized the medical education system. Similarly, because markets would undersupply hospitals in sparsely populated regions or low-income areas, government subsidized the construction of hospitals for many years.

Other subsidies have been used to ensure that certain people have access to health services. The most obvious examples of such policies are the Medicare and Medicaid programs. Note 1 contains brief overviews of these programs; additional information can be found on the Internet by following the health policy links at the Electronic Policy Network's web site (http://www.epn.org) and at the Health Care Financing Administration's (HCFA) web site (http://www.hcfa.gov). In addition, federal funding to support access to health services for Native Americans, veterans, and migrant farmworkers, and state funding for mental institutions are other examples of allocative policies that are intended to assist individuals in gaining access to needed services. People sometimes think of subsidies as reserved for people on the basis of their impoverishment. However, subsidies such as those inherent in much of the financial support for medical education, the Medicare program (the benefits of which are not based primarily on the financial need of the recipients), and the exclusion from taxable income of employer-provided health insurance benefits illustrate that poverty is not necessary to receive subsidies available through the allocative category of health policies.

Regulatory Policies

Policies designed to influence the actions, behaviors, and decisions of others through directive approaches are regulatory policies. In a variety of ways, all levels of government seek to influence the actions, behaviors, and decisions of others through regulatory policies. As with allocative policies, government establishes regulatory policies for the purpose of ensuring that public objectives are met. There are five basic categories of regulatory health policies:

- market-entry restrictions;
- rate or price-setting controls on health service providers;
- quality controls on the provision of health services;
- market-preserving controls; and
- social regulation.

The first four of these are variations of economic regulation; the fifth seeks to achieve such socially desired ends as safe workplaces, nondiscriminatory provision of health services, and reduction in the negative externalities (side effects) that can be associated with the production or consumption of products and services (Bice 1988; Williams and Torrens 1993).

Market-entry restricting regulations include those through which health-related practitioners and organizations are licensed. CON programs, through which approval for new capital projects by health services providers must be obtained from the state before the projects can be developed, are also market-entry restricting regulations.

A common example of price regulation is government's control of the retail prices charged by public utilities, such as those selling natural gas or electricity. Some aspects of the pursuit of health are also subject to price regulations. A price regulation with enormous impact is the federal government's control of the rates at which it reimburses hospitals for care provided to Medicare patients under the PPS and its establishment of a fee schedule for reimbursing physicians who care for Medicare patients.

A third class of regulations are those intended to ensure that health services providers adhere to acceptable levels of quality in the services they provide and that producers of health-related products such as imaging equipment and pharmaceuticals meet safety and efficacy standards. The federal Food and Drug Administration (FDA) (http://www.fda.gov) is charged to ensure that new pharmaceuticals meet safety and efficacy standards. In addition, the Medical Devices Amendments (P.L. 94-295) to the Food, Drug and Cosmetic Act (P.L. 75-717) placed all medical devices under a comprehensive regulatory framework administered by the FDA.

Because the markets for health services do not behave in truly competitive ways, government intervenes in these markets by establishing and enforcing rules of conduct for market participants. These rules of conduct form a fourth class of regulation, market-preserving controls. Antitrust laws, such as the Sherman Antitrust Act, the Clayton Act, and the Robinson-Patman Act, which are intended to maintain conditions that permit markets to work well and fairly, are good examples of this type of regulation.

The United States is entering a new era in regard to market-preserving regulations in the health sector as it moves toward higher levels of managed care. Managed care stimulates the development of integrated delivery networks of health services providers that can compete with each other for pools of insured people within a framework that encourages cost-conscious decision making by consumers (Coddington, Moore, and Fischer 1996; Shortell et al. 1996). If managed care is to work well, it will likely require the elaboration of many new market-preserving regulations. Already, for example, regulations pertaining to the inclusion of publicly sponsored Medicare and Medicaid beneficiaries in managed care systems have become necessary.

The four classes of regulations outlined above are all variations of economic regulation. The primary purpose of social regulation, the fifth class of regulation, is to achieve such socially desirable outcomes as workplace safety and fair employment practices and to reduce such socially undesirable outcomes as environmental pollution or the spread of sexually transmitted diseases. Social regulation usually has economic impact, but the impact is secondary to the primary purposes of the regulations. Federal and state laws pertaining to en-vironmental protection, disposal of medical wastes, childhood immunization requirements, and the mandatory reporting of communicable diseases are but a few obvious examples of social regulations at work in the pursuit of health.

Whether public policies take the form of laws, rules and regulations, judicial decisions, or macro policies, they are always established within the context of a complex public policymaking process. Both allocative and regulatory policies are made within the process, and the activities and mechanisms used to create both categories of policies are essentially identical. A comprehensive model of this process, which applies to any level of government, is presented in Chapter 2. Before examining the model, however, it will be useful to consider the ways that health policies affect health and its pursuit. There is, in fact, a direct and crucially important connection between health policies and health, which makes an understanding of the health policymaking process all the more important.

THE CONNECTION BETWEEN HEALTH POLICIES AND HEALTH

From government's perspective, the central purpose of health policy is to en-hance health or to facilitate its pursuit by the citizenry. Of course, it is possible for other purposes to be served through specific health policies, including providing economic advantages to certain individuals and organizations. But the defining purpose of health policy, so far as government is concerned, is to support the people in their quest for health.

The mechanism of this support is conceptually straightforward. Policies are connected to health—that is, they have their impact on health—through an intervening variable, health determinants. The health determinants, in turn, directly influence health as follows:

Health Policies ⟐ Health Determinants ⟐ Health

As noted above, the determinants of health, whether applied to individuals or populations of people, include their genetic endowments; the physical, sociocultural, and economic environments in which they live; their lifestyles and behaviors; and the health services available for use in their pursuit of health.

Thus, when considering the relationship between health policy and health, especially with regard to ways in which health policy can affect health, it is necessary to consider the role of health policy in:

- environmental conditions, including physical, sociocultural, and economic environments under which people live;
- behavioral choices that people make and the role that genetics plays in their health; and
- health services available to people and their access to these services.

Health policies have significant effects on each of these three determinants of health. The nature of these effects is explored more fully in the next sections.

HEALTH POLICIES AND THE ENVIRONMENT

When people are asked about what they think contributes to their health, they respond that the quality of their health services is a very important contributor. But, they also list clean air, safe neighborhoods, and well-paying jobs (Louis Harris and Associates 1996). People think their environments contribute to their health status, and they are right. When people are exposed to harmful agents such as asbestos, excessive noise, ionizing radiation, or toxic chemicals, their health is directly affected. Dangerous exposure possibilities pervade the physical environments of many people. Some of the exposure is through agents such as synthetic compounds that are introduced into the environment as by-products of technological growth and development. Some exposure is through wastes that result from the manufacture, use, and disposal of a vast range of products. And some of the exposure is through naturally occurring agents such as carcinogenic ultraviolet radiation from the sun or naturally occurring radon gas in the soil.

Often, the hazardous effects of naturally occurring agents are exacerbated by their combination with agents introduced by human activities. For example, before its ban, the widespread use of Freon in air-conditioning systems and of chlorofluorocarbons (CFCs) in aerosolized products reduced the protective ozone layer in earth's upper atmosphere, allowing an increased level of ultraviolet radiation from the sun to strike the planet's inhabitants. Similarly, exposure to naturally occurring radon gas appears to act synergistically with cigarette smoke as a carcinogenic hazard.

The health effects of exposure to hazardous agents, whether they are introduced into the environment or occur naturally, is increasingly well understood. Air, polluted by a number of agents, has a direct, measurable effect on such diseases as asthma, emphysema, and lung cancer, and it aggravates cardiovascular disease. Asbestos, which can still be found in buildings constructed prior to its ban, causes pulmonary disease. Lead-based paint, when ingested, causes permanent neurological defects in infants and young children. This paint is still found in older buildings and is especially concentrated in poorer urban communities.

In what he terms its "environmental tradition," Thompson (1981) points out that government has been involved in a variety of efforts to exorcise environmental health hazards through public policies. Examples of such federal policies include the Clean Air Act (P.L. 88-206), the Flammable Fabrics Act (P.L. 90-189), the Occupational Health and Safety Act (P.L. 91-596), the Consumer Product Safety Act (P.L. 92-573), the Noise Control Act (P.L. 92-574), and the Safe Drinking Water Act (P.L. 93-523).

In addition to their physical environments, the sociocultural and economic environments in which people live also play important roles in their health. Chronic unemployment, the absence of a supportive family structure, poverty, homelessness, substance abuse, violence, and despair affect the health of people as surely and dramatically as harmful viruses or carcinogens.

People who live in poverty experience measurably worse health status (i.e., more frequent and more severe health problems) than people who are more affluent. Consequently, African Americans, Latinos, and Native Americans, who are disproportionately represented below the poverty line, experience worse health status than the white majority (Klerman 1992). The poor also obtain their health services in a different manner than the more affluent. Instead of receiving care that is coordinated, continuing, and comprehensive, the poor are far more likely to receive a patchwork of services, often provided by public hospitals and local health departments. In addition, poor people are more often treated episodically, with one provider intervening in one episode of illness and another provider handling the next episode.

The impact of economic conditions on the health of the poor is especially dramatic for children. Impoverished children have double the rates of low birth weight and more than double the rates of conditions that limit school activity compared to other children (Starfield 1992). These children are more likely to become ill and to have more serious illnesses than other children because of their increased exposure to harmful environments, inadequate preventive services, and limited access to health services.

Economic constraints are only part of a larger set of difficulties that unevenly affect people in their quests for health. Living in an inner city or a rural setting often increases the challenge of finding health services because the availability of providers is not adequate in many of these locations. Lack of or inadequate information about health and health services is a significant disadvantage— one compounded by language barriers, functional illiteracy, or marginal mental retardation. Even cultural backgrounds and ties, especially among many Native Americans, Latinos, and Asian immigrants, for all the support they can provide, sometimes also create a formidable barrier between people and the mainline healthcare system.

Health policies that mitigate the negative influences of physical, sociocultural, and economic environments on health or that take advantage of their positive potential for affecting health are important aspects of any society's ability to help its members achieve higher levels of health. But there are other determinants of health as well. They provide additional avenues to improved health.

HEALTH POLICIES AND HUMAN BEHAVIOR AND GENETICS

As Rene Dubos observed decades ago, "To ward off disease or recover health, men [as well as women and children] as a rule find it easier to depend on the healers than to attempt the more difficult task of living wisely" (1959, 110). The price of this attitude is partially reflected in the causes of death in the United States. Ranked from highest to lowest, and with the order remaining stable for many years, the leading causes are heart disease, cancer, stroke, accidents, chronic obstructive pulmonary disease (COPD), diabetes, suicide, liver diseases, and acquired immunodeficiency syndrome (AIDS).

Underlying these causes of death are a set of behavioral choices—including choices about the use of tobacco and alcohol, diet and exercise, illicit drug use, sexual behavior, and violence—as well as genetic predispositions that help explain the pattern. Furthermore, underlying the behavioral factors and choices are such root factors as stress, depression, anger, hopelessness, and emptiness, which are exacerbated by economic and social conditions. Lifestyles and behaviors are reflected in the diseases that kill and debilitate Americans. Changes in lifestyles and behaviors can change the pattern.

The death rate from heart disease, for example, has declined dramatically in recent decades. Although aggressive early treatment has played a role in reducing this death rate, better control of several behavioral risk factors, including cigarette smoking, elevated blood pressure, elevated levels of cholesterol, diet and exercise, and stress reduction, explain much of this improvement. Even with this impressive improvement, however, heart disease remains the most common cause of death and will continue to be an important cause for the foreseeable future. Cancer death rates continue to grow, with much of the increase attributable to lung cancer, a type of cancer that is strongly correlated with behavior. Deaths from accidents and suicides are also obviously affected by behaviors, as are those from liver cirrhosis and AIDS.

Even in the face of the direct relationships between particular behaviors and certain deadly diseases, policymakers have been reluctant to impose penalties for behaviors that lead to illness and death or to provide overt rewards for the avoidance or modification of such behaviors. Instead, health policy interventions in diseases that are behaviorally caused or exacerbated have favored increased funding for research into the behaviors or increased efforts to influence behavior through education. Venturing beyond these actions into the domains of individual choice and liberty rights has been carefully avoided. It is clear, however, that the impacts of human behavior and genetics on health are potentially productive avenues for increased and perhaps different policy interventions in the future.

HEALTH POLICIES AND HEALTH SERVICES

Another important determinant of health is the availability of and access to health services, which are any of a host of activities that maintain or improve health or that prevent decrements of health. Health services can be preventive, acute, chronic, restorative, or palliative in nature. The production and distribution of health services require a vast set of resources—including money, people, and technology—that health policies heavily influence. Health services are provided through the healthcare system, which is composed of the organizations that transform these resources into health services and distribute them to consumers.

Health policies have a major bearing on the nature of the health services available to people through their impact on the resources required to produce the services, as well as on the healthcare system through which the services are organized, delivered, and paid for. Some of the key aspects of these relationships are now examined, beginning with the relationship between monetary resources and the pursuit of health.

Money

As shown in Figure 1.2, national health expenditures, both in dollars and as a percentage of the nation's gross domestic product (GDP), are expected

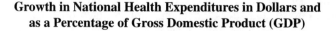

FIGURE 1.2

**Growth in National Health Expenditures in Dollars and
as a Percentage of Gross Domestic Product (GDP)**

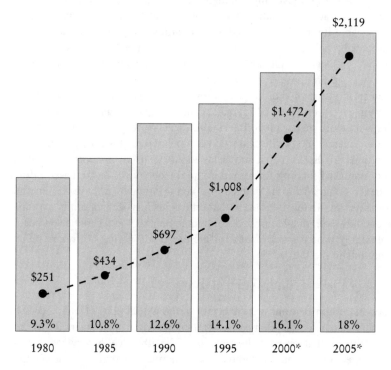

■   Health expenditures as percentage of GDP

- ● - National healthcare expenditures (in billions)

  *   Projected

Source: Congressional Budget Office 1996

to continue their steep rise into the future, approaching $1.5 trillion by the turn of the century. As can be seen in Figure 1.3, as a proportion of the total expenditures, private sources are declining while public sources (federal and state combined) are increasing.

The United States spends more on health than does any other country (Schieber, Poullier, and Greenwald 1992), in large part because of some significant variations in policies that affect health services. For example, other

FIGURE 1.3

National Health Expenditures by Source of Funds

| | | As a Percentage of Total Expenditures | | |
| | | Government | | |
Year	Private	Federal	State and Local	Total
1965	75.3%	11.6%	13.2%	100%
1980	58.1	28.7	13.3	100
1985	59.7	28.4	11.9	100
1990	58.9	28.1	13.0	100
1993	56.1	31.7	12.1	100
1995	54.8	33.2	12.0	100
2000*	52.3	35.8	11.8	100
2005*	49.6	38.8	11.6	100

Source: Prospective Payment Assessment Commission, *1996 Annual Report to Congress*, from Congressional Budget Office data.
*Projected

countries have been far more likely to adopt policies such as global budgets for their healthcare systems, or to impose restrictive limitations on the supplies of health services.

The implications of the level of health expenditures and their rate of increase over the past several decades, as well as projections of future increases, are significant. The increasing health expenditures, in part, reflect higher prices. These higher prices have reduced many people's access to health services by making it more difficult for them to purchase either the services or the insurance needed to cover those services. The increases in health expenditures also have absorbed much of the growth of workers' real compensation over the past two decades, helping to explain why their cash wages have hardly grown at all during this period as employers spent more and more for health insurance benefits.

Because federal and state governments now pay for so much healthcare, rising health expenditures have put substantial pressures on their budgets. As health expenditures consume a growing portion of government resources, it becomes more difficult for government to support other priorities such as education, other social programs, or tax relief.

People

The talents and abilities of a large and diverse workforce constitute another of the basic resources used to provide health services. These human resources are directly affected by health policies. More than 10 million health-related workers in the United States today represent about 11 percent of the nonagricultural workforce. They have been the fastest growing group of American workers over recent years (O'Neil 1993a). There are about 600,000 active physicians; 1.7 million registered nurses (RNs); 172,000 pharmacists; 140,000 active dentists; and more than 3 million allied health workers in more than 200 distinct disciplinary groups such as clinical laboratory technology, dental hygiene, dietetics, medical records administration, occupational therapy, physical therapy, radiologic technology, respiratory therapy, and speech-language pathology/audiology to name but a few (O'Neil 1993b).

The nature of the significant impact of health policies on health-related human resources can be seen in the fact that the number of physicians has doubled in the past 30 years, largely in response to federal policies intended to increase their supply. For example, the Health Professions Educational Assistance Act of 1963 (P.L. 88-129) and its amendments of 1965, 1968, and 1971 helped to double the capacity of the medical schools in the United States by the early 1990s. Now, however, the attention of policymakers is turned to concerns about the perceived oversupply of physicians and about the inadequate proportion who practice in the primary care specialties of general practice, family practice, general internal medicine, and general pediatrics.

Technology

A third type of resources used in providing health services, and upon which health policies have significant impact, is health-related technology. Broadly defined, technology is the application of science to the pursuit of health. Technological advances result in better drugs, devices, and procedures used in providing health services. Technology has had a major effect on the pursuit of health in America. It has meant that many diseases have been eradicated, and diagnoses and treatment for others have been greatly improved. In fact, diseases that once were not even diagnosed are now routinely and effectively treated. Advancing technology has brought medical science to the brink of understanding disease at the molecular level and intervening in diseases at the genetic level.

However, as technology has advanced, societal expectations regarding the possible contributions of technology to the pursuit of health have risen, sometimes unrealistically. In addition, the costs of health services have risen as the new technology is utilized and paid for. One paradox of advancing health-related technology is that, even as people live longer because of these advances, they then may need and utilize additional health services. As a result, the net effect is to drive up health expenditures both for the new technology and for other services made possible by extended life.

The United States produces and consumes more, and spends far more for, health-related technology than any other nation; it has provided technology with a uniquely favorable economic and political environment. As a result, health-related technology is widely and readily available to the citizens of the United States.

Funding for the research and development (R&D) that leads to new technology is an important way in which health policy affects the pursuit of health, although the private sector also pays for a great deal of the R&D that leads to new health-related technology. The United States has a long history of support for the development of health-related technology through policies that directly support biomedical research and that encourage private investment in such research. From a total of about $300 in 1887, the National Institutes of Health (NIH) (http://www.nih.gov) now has an annual budget of more than $12 billion. In addition, encouraged by government policies that permit firms to recoup their investments in research and development, private industry spends even more than the NIH on biomedical R&D (National Institutes of Health 1997). Another way in which health policy affects technology is through the application of regulatory policies, such as those promulgated by the Food and Drug Administration (FDA) as a means of ensuring technology's safety and efficacy.

Healthcare System

In addition to its impact on the various monetary, human, and technological resources that are used in providing health services, health policy also has significant impacts on the healthcare system that uses these resources to organize and deliver the services. Although there are few guarantees for the future, there is abundant evidence that the American healthcare system has been developed under extraordinarily favorable public policies. For example, enactment in 1946 of the Hospital Survey and Construction Act (P.L. 79-725) placed Congress squarely in support of expanded availability of health services and improved facilities. This legislation, known as the Hill-Burton Act after its authors, provided funds for hospital construction and marked the beginning of a decades-long program of extensive federal developmental subsidies aimed at increasing the availability of health services.

Another important aspect of the development of the healthcare system— again one supported and facilitated by public policy—has been the expansion of health insurance coverage. Beginning during World War II, when wages were frozen, health insurance and other benefits in lieu of wages became very attractive features of the American workplace. Encouraged by policies that excluded these fringe benefits from income or Social Security taxes and by a Supreme Court ruling that employee benefits, including health insurance, could be legitimately included in the collective bargaining process, employer-provided health insurance benefits grew rapidly in the middle decades of the twentieth century (Health Insurance Association of America 1992).

Beyond private-sector growth in health insurance coverage came the passage in 1965 of the Medicare and Medicaid legislation, providing more access to mainstream health services for the aged and many of the poor through publicly subsidized health insurance. With enactment of these programs, fully 85 percent of the American population had some form of health insurance.

Although public policies have been extremely important factors in the development of the American healthcare system, this system has emerged in the context of a market economy. Thus, much about it has been shaped by the market forces of supply and demand and by the related decisions and actions of the buyers and sellers in this marketplace. The combination of these market forces and public policies have shaped a complex and dynamic healthcare system. Key aspects of the system and its evolution can be readily traced.

To start with the present for a moment, fundamental changes in the organization and delivery of health services are sweeping across the United States. A new structural paradigm for the organization and provision of health services is emerging—in fact, it is well under way in its development (Shortell et al. 1996; Zelman 1996). The new healthcare system paradigm features a shift from a fragmented, compartmentalized past to a future characterized by much higher levels of integration among the organizations involved in producing and delivering health services.

The essence of the structural changes occurring in the healthcare system involve the movement of the organizations involved in the system from their past state of relatively fragmented independence from each other and arm's-length interdependence with each other to a future in which they are highly integrated. This shift is actually a continuum of activity rather than an abrupt change, although the pace of the shift has gained momentum in recent years. The continuum exhibits three rather distinct phases, as depicted in Figure 1.4.

In Phase I, which is the period prior to the 1970s, organizations in the healthcare system remained almost exclusively independent of each other. Fueled by the unfettering of post–World War II consumer demand for more health services and by federal policies such as the Hill-Burton program of hospital construction and generous federal support for medical education and biomedical research, the nation experienced an extraordinary proliferation of health-related organizations during the 1950s and 1960s. But importantly, in part reflecting strongly held preferences for independence and autonomy among the leaders of most of these organizations—Ummel (1997, 13) characterizes this phenomenon as a "deeply rooted fixation on autonomy"—the organizations remained essentially independent of each other except for their arm's-length transactions and economic exchanges.

FIGURE 1.4

The Changing Structure of American Healthcare: Fragmentation to Integration

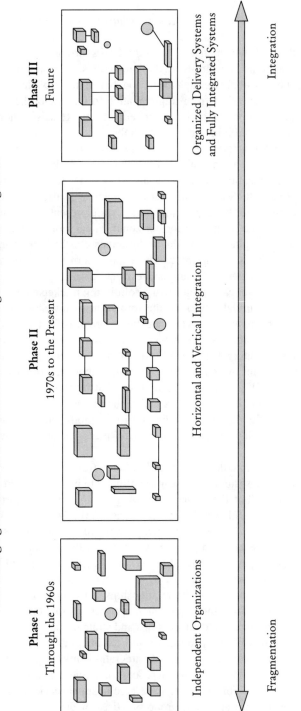

In Phase II, which encompasses the 1970s through the present, some previously autonomous health-related organizations, very slowly and cautiously at first but increasingly through the period, began to establish formal links among themselves. The shift from fragmentation to integration has been under way throughout this period, although movement was exclusively horizontal initially and only later did it include vertical links.

Horizontal integration, which links similar components (hospital to hospital or physician to physician), was the first form of integration among health-related organizations, in part because it is easier to accomplish than vertical integration, which links different components. It also emerged first because the incentives for horizontal integration were present before those for vertical integration. The incentives for horizontal integration, in which hospitals link with other hospitals or in which physicians cluster into group practices, for example, include opportunities for economies of scale in operations, sharing scarce management and support services, garnering greater political clout, building stronger capital bases, and solidifying marketshares.

Hospitals, initially through the formation of investor-owned horizontally integrated hospital systems and later by the growth of not-for-profit horizontally integrated hospital systems, have shown a significant propensity for horizontal integration (Starkweather 1981). In 1995, about 300 horizontally integrated hospital systems owned, leased, or managed about half of the nation's hospitals (Dowling 1995). There are predictions that by the turn of the century only about 5 percent of all hospitals will remain independent (Savage et al. 1997). Horizontal integration is not limited to hospitals, however. Nursing homes, HMOs, physician groups, pharmacies, hospices, and others have also integrated horizontally.

During this middle phase in the evolution from fragmentation to integration, the healthcare system's landscape continued to include numerous independent organizations but there was a growing complement of horizontally linked groups of essentially similar organizations. The horizontal integration occurring in this phase involved both ownership arrangements and less restrictive contractual arrangements encompassing a variety of partnerships and strategic alliances among participating organizations (Kaluzny, Zuckerman, and Ricketts 1995). However, the common thread in all forms of horizontal integration is that it changes the nature of the relationships between and among participating organizations. They move past mere market transactions with each other to relationships in which their missions and strategies are more closely linked.

Late in this phase, patterns of vertical integration also began to emerge. Technically, the vertical form of integration links organizations that are at different stages of the production process of delivering patient care (Conrad and Dowling 1990). For example, acute care hospital services can be linked with home health care agencies, group practices of physicians, and rehabilitative services organizations. Vertical integration can move forward or backward. A large health services delivery system, for example, can integrate backward by linking to a medical supply company from which it will obtain needed supplies at favorable prices. In forward integration, the same large delivery system can move forward toward the customer by integrating with a physician group practice to link the flow of the practice's patients to the system.

The incentives for vertical integration are more complicated than those for horizontal integration. Vertical integration is best understood in the context of what it replaces: a fragmented, compartmentalized state in which health-related organizations are predominantly independent of each other or are formally linked only to groups of similar organizations through horizontal integration. Driven by the emergence of managed care and its demands for more and better coordination of patient care along the spectrum of health services, vertical integration expanded in the late 1980s. This potent pressure for vertical integration continues apace.

Managed care has become the dominant template for providing and financing health services in the United States. More than 130 million citizens are now enrolled in some form of managed care, half of all physicians participate in managed care plans, about three-fourths of hospitals have managed care contracts, and the vast majority of employers offer their employees managed care plans (Fubini and Antonelli 1997). Vertical integration, because it links components that are involved in different aspects of patient care services, was and remains crucial for managed care to have an opportunity to realize efficiencies in the provision of these services.

Although there is still extreme diversity in the forms of integration and wide geographic differences in the pace and extent of integration, the shift is markedly toward more integration among health-related organizations. Eventually, the unfolding pattern of integration may lead to an overall American healthcare system that largely comprises sets of integrated organizations called "organized delivery systems" with each of these being "a network of organizations that provides or arranges to provide a coordinated continuum of services to a defined population and is willing to be held clinically and fiscally accountable for the outcomes and the health status of the population served" (Shortell et al. 1996, 7).

Even beyond the level of integration inherent in organized delivery systems, future health services may be organized and delivered through even more extensively integrated systems and networks in which providers, spanning the full continuum of health services, are integrated with health plans or insurers and perhaps with suppliers to form entities that tie together extensively many categories of organizations involved in the pursuit of health. Although limited in number, and still somewhat limited in scope, some more fully integrated systems have already begun to form (KPMG Peat Marwick LLP 1996). The jury is still very much out on the question of the wisdom for all parties in the integration of insurers and health plans with organized delivery systems. Nevertheless, these more fully integrated systems or networks of organizations, which can provide an extensive and coordinated continuum of health services to enrolled populations, may be the future of the nation's decreasingly fragmented approach to its pursuit of health.

Already, the early stages of development of such extensively integrated systems or networks are apparent. Some are being built by integrated provider organizations either buying, establishing, or contracting with health plans or insurance organizations, or alternatively by plans creating their own provider networks, usually through selective contracting. Some of the resulting entities are more virtual than real. They are being constructed through the use of strategic alliances and contractual arrangements as well as the more traditional ownership arrangements.

The existence of large numbers of organized delivery systems and, perhaps, even more fully integrated systems and networks will define Phase III of the healthcare system's continuing evolution from fragmentation to integration (see Figure 1.4). Although just how far the emerging pattern of integration will eventually extend is still an open question, it is clear in the late 1990s that the healthcare system's structural revolution is being driven toward more and more integration among organizations by very powerful market forces, which are supported by such health policies as those that permit Medicare and Medicaid participants to enroll in managed care programs.

The combined market and policy pressures driving the shift in the healthcare system include continuing pressure to contain healthcare costs, growing pressure for higher levels of quality, more cohesion among employers regarding their interests in and sense of urgency about reducing their health benefit expenditures, and the prevalence and continuing growth of managed care for both privately insured and publicly sponsored consumers. These forces show no signs of abatement and will very likely continue to exert pressure for more integration among organizations within the healthcare system into the foreseeable future.

The future healthcare system, in many respects, will be shaped by health policy, as has the past and present system. Market forces will certainly also continue to exert their influence. Health in America is pursued within a market-driven economy. However, public policy will also play an important role. For example, changes in health policy have the potential to remove some of the remaining barriers to continued development of integration, such as antitrust-based prohibitions against some forms of integration and overly restrictive personnel licensure and certification policies. The future of the healthcare system also depends, in part, on the elaboration of health policies that actively promote or facilitate the formation of systems such as policies that permit capitated payments that cover all components of care provided by vertically integrated systems or that permit and encourage coordinated benefit packages or promote group practice formation (Shortell et al. 1996).

THE IMPORTANCE OF POLITICAL COMPETENCE IN THE PURSUIT OF HEALTH

As the preceding discussion about the connection between health policy and health illustrates, there is a powerful link between policy and health. The link is formed through the relationship of policy to the various determinants of health, each of which is affected, sometimes dramatically, by health policy. Anyone professionally involved in the pursuit of health through any of these determinants has a vested interest in understanding the health policymaking process. Such an understanding is the first step in developing a higher degree of political competence. This, in turn, supports the ability to assess the impact of public policies on one's domain of interest or responsibility and the ability to exert influence in the public policymaking process (Longest 1997).

Increasingly, political competence is important to anyone who wishes to be effectively involved in the nation's pursuit of health. Within the context of the political marketplace, where public policymaking occurs, many participants seek to further their objectives by influencing the outcomes of this process. Political competence is an imperative ingredient for success in this arena. This competence entails knowing how and where to exert influence. It is also based on a thorough knowledge of the complex process through which public policies are formulated, implemented, and modified.

Politically competent people can become involved in this process at many points. For example, in the formulation phase of public policymaking they might become involved in setting the policy agenda by helping define the problems that policies might address; by participating in the development of possible solutions to the problems; or by helping to create the political circumstances necessary to turn the ideas for solving problems into actual policies (Kingdon 1995). Politically competent people also know how to participate effectively in the actual drafting of legislative proposals or in providing testimony at the hearings in which legislation is developed. They also can influence health policy in the implementation phase of the process by focusing on the rulemaking that helps guide the implementation of policies. Such involvement routinely includes providing formal comment on proposed rules or providing ideas and comments to task forces and commissions established by rulemaking agencies as a means to obtain advice on their work.

The point is that an adequate degree of political competence is a necessary condition for effectively participating in the policymaking process and, through this participation, exerting some influence on the shape of future health policies. This competence is built upon an understanding of the public policymaking process, which is modeled in the next chapter and discussed in depth in subsequent chapters.

Summary

Health can be usefully conceptualized as the maximization of the biological and clinical indicators of organ function and the maximization of physical, mental, and role functioning in everyday life (Brook and McGlynn 1991). Thinking of health in this way emphasizes the need to address many variables, or health determinants, if health is to be affected: the physical, sociocultural, and economic environments in which people live; their lifestyles, behaviors, and genetics; and the type, quality, and timing of health services that people receive.

Health policies are defined as authoritative decisions made within government that are intended to direct or influence the actions, behaviors, or decisions of others pertaining to health and its determinants. These policies are the principal means through which a developed society helps shape the pursuit of health by its members. These decisions can take the form of laws, rules and operational decisions made in the context of implementing laws, and judicial decisions. Policies can be allocative or regulatory in nature.

No matter which determinants of health such policies are intended to affect, and no matter what their form, all health policies are made within the context of a rather well-understood, although complex, process. The process is described in the next chapter, and details are provided in subsequent chapters. A thorough understanding of this process provides a foundation upon which to build political competence.

Note

1. Medicare, the principal social health insurance program in the United States, was enacted into law as Title XVIII of the Social Security Act (P.L. 89-97) on July 30, 1965. Medicare, a federally administered program, is the nation's single largest health insurer. It covers more than 38 million Americans, roughly 14 percent of the population, for a variety of hospital, physician, and other health services at an annual cost in 1997 of approximately $220 billion. Program beneficiaries include virtually all of those over the age of 65 as well as disabled individuals who are entitled to Social Security benefits and people with end-stage renal disease.

The Medicare program includes two parts, A and B. Part A covers inpatient hospital care, very limited nursing home services, and home health services. Part A is paid for through a payroll tax of 2.9 percent, which is split evenly between the employee and employer. Part B covers physician services, physician-ordered supplies and equipment, and certain ambulatory services such as hospital outpatient visits. Part B is voluntary, although about 97 percent of Part A beneficiaries choose to enroll in Part B, and is paid for by a combination of enrollee monthly premiums ($43.80 in 1997) and by general tax revenues.

Because Medicare does not cover all of the health expenses of the elderly, most of them also have private supplemental, or Medigap, health insurance plans. In the 1990s, there has been a pronounced shift of the Medicare population into managed care programs, especially into health maintenance organizations (HMOs). Although only about 14 percent of Medicare beneficiaries are currently enrolled in managed care plans, the number is growing rapidly.

Medicaid, enacted along with Medicare, as Title XIX of the Social Security Act (P.L. 89-97), is an important part of the federal-state social welfare structure. It provides health insurance coverage for preventive, acute, and long-term care for some of the nation's poorer citizens. This program covers about 35 million people, or about 13 percent of the population, at an annual cost in 1997 of about $158 billion. The program's costs are covered by a combination of state funds and federal subsidies to the states depending on the per capita income in each state. In return for the subsidy, the states administer their Medicaid programs, but do so under broad federal guidelines regarding the scope of services to be covered, the level of payments to healthcare services providers, and eligibility requirements for coverage under the program.

Medicaid expenditures are among the fastest-growing components of most state budgets. As a result, in 1997 a total of 42 states have received waivers of certain federal Medicaid rules so that they can require at least some of their Medicaid program beneficiaries to enroll in managed care plans in an attempt to slow the rate of growth in program expenditures.

REFERENCES

Ayanian, J. Z. 1993. "Heart Disease in Black and White." *New England Journal of Medicine* 329 (9): 656–58.

Bice, T. W. 1988. "Health Services Planning and Regulation." In *Introduction to Health Services*, 3d ed., edited by S. J. Williams and P.R. Torrens, 373–405. New York: John Wiley & Sons.

Blum, H. K. 1983. *Expanding Health Care Horizons: From a General Systems Concept of Health to a National Health Policy*, 2d ed. Oakland, CA: Third Party Publishing Company.

Brook, R. H., and E. A. McGlynn. 1991. "Maintaining Quality of Care." In *Health Services Research: Key to Health Policy*, edited by E. Ginzberg, 784–817. Cambridge, MA: Harvard University Press.

Brown, L. D. 1992. "Political Evolution of Federal Health Care Regulation." *Health Affairs* 11 (4): 17–37.

Burner, S. T., D. R. Waldo, and D. R. McKusick. 1992. "National Health Expenditures Projections Through 2030." *Health Care Financing Review* 14 (1): 1–29.

Coddington, D. C., K. D. Moore, and E. A. Fischer. 1996. *Making Integrated Health Care Work*. Englewood, CO: Center for Research in Ambulatory Health Care Administration.

Conrad, D. A., and W. L. Dowling. 1990. "Vertical Integration in Health Services: Theory and Managerial Implications," *Health Care Management Review* 15 (4): 9–22.

Dowling, W. L. 1995. "Strategic Alliances as a Structure for Integrated Delivery Systems." In *Partners for the Dance: Forming Strategic Alliances in Health Care*, edited by A. D. Kaluzny, H. S. Zuckerman, and T. C. Ricketts, III, 139–75. Chicago: Health Administration Press.

Dubos, R. 1959. *The Mirage of Health*. New York: Harper.

Evans, R. G., M. L. Barer, and T. R. Marmor. 1994. *Why Are Some People Healthy and Others Not? The Determinants of Health of Populations*. New York: Aldine De Gruyter.

Fubini, S., and V. Antonelli. 1997. "1997 Health Care Industry Outlook," *Healthcare Trends Report* 11 (7): 1–20.

Hacker, A. 1992. *Two Nations: Black and White, Separate, Hostile, Unequal*. New York: Macmillan.

Health Insurance Association of America. 1992. *Source Book of Health Insurance Data*. Washington, DC: The Association.

Kaluzny, A. D., H. S. Zuckerman, and T. C. Ricketts, III (eds.). 1995. *Partners for the Dance: Forming Strategic Alliances in Health Care*. Chicago: Health Administration Press.

Kingdon, J. W. 1995. *Agendas, Alternatives, and Public Policies*, 2nd ed. New York: HarperCollins College Publishers.

Klerman, L. V. 1992. "Nonfinancial Barriers to the Receipt of Medical Care." *The Future of Children* 2 (2): 171–85.

KPMG Peat Marwick LLP. 1996. *Integrated Patient Care: Managing Health Care Costs, Maximizing Health Care Value and Quality*.

Longest, B. B., Jr. 1997. *Seeking Strategic Advantage Through Health Policy Analysis*. Chicago: Health Administration Press.

Louis Harris & Associates. 1996. *Getting Involved Survey*.

Lumsdon, K. 1992. "HIV-Positive Health Care Workers Pose Legal, Safety Challenges for Hospitals." *Hospitals* 66 (18): 24–32.

Morone, J. A. 1990. *The Democratic Wish: Popular Participation and the Limits of American Government*. New York: Basic Books.

National Institutes of Health. 1997. *NIH Data Book*. Washington, DC: National Institutes of Health.

O'Neil, E. H. 1993a. "Academic Health Centers Must Begin Reforms Now." *The Chronicle of Higher Education* (September 8): A48.

———. 1993b. *Health Professions Education for the Future: Schools in Service to the Nation*. San Francisco: Pew Health Professions Commission.

Savage, G. T., R. L. Taylor, T. M. Rotarius, and J. A. Buesseler. 1997. "Governance of Integrated Delivery Systems/Networks: A Stakeholder Approach." *Health Care Management Review* 22 (7): 7–20.

Schieber, G. J., J. P. Poullier, and L. M. Greenwald. 1992. "U.S. Health Expenditure Performance: An International Comparison and Data Update." *Health Care Financing Review* 13 (4): 1–87.

Shortell, S. M., R. R. Gillies, D. A. Anderson, K. M. Erickson, and J. B. Mitchell.

1996. *Remaking Health Care in America: Building Organized Delivery Systems.* San Francisco: Jossey-Bass Publishers.

Starfield, B. 1992. "Child and Adolescent Health Status Measures." *The Future of Children* 2 (2): 25–39.

Starkweather, D. B. 1981. *Hospital Mergers in the Making.* Chicago: Health Administration Press.

Thompson, F. J. 1981. *Health Policy and the Bureaucracy: Politics and Implementation.* Cambridge, MA: Institute of Technology Press.

Thorpe, K. E. 1997. *Changes in the Growth in Health Care Spending: Implications for Consumers.* Washington, DC: The National Coalition on Health Care.

Ummel, S. L. 1997. "Pursuing the Elusive Integrated Delivery Network." *Healthcare Forum Journal* 40 (2): 13–19.

Williams, S. J., and P. R. Torrens. 1993. "Influencing, Regulating, and Monitoring the Health Care System." In *Introduction to Health Services*, 4th ed., edited by S. J. Williams and P. R. Torrens, 377–96. Albany, NY: Delmar Publishers Inc.

World Health Organization. 1948. "Constitution of the World Health Organization, 1948." In *Basic Documents*, 15th ed. Geneva, Switzerland: World Health Organization.

Zelman, W. A. 1996. *The Changing Health Care Marketplace: Private Ventures, Public Interests.* San Francisco: Jossey-Bass Publishers.

| # Medicare's Social Contract

Stuart Butler,
Theda Skocpol,
Robert M. Ball,
and E. J. Dionne

Several authors in this chapter address the Medicare social contract created between the federal government and the program beneficiaries more than thirty years ago. Although the authors agree on the significance of the contract to discussions of Medicare reform, they disagree on whether specific changes would preserve or destroy the program.

THE CONTRACT AND MEDICARE REFORM
Stuart Butler

When the Medicare system was created in the mid-1960s, the social contract generally promised to provide the elderly with medical services that were similar to those enjoyed by the typical worker and to do so at reasonable cost to the elderly and to society. What the United States achieved in trying to fulfill the contract was, unfortunately, badly flawed. Medicare was a compromise that reflected the politics of the Vietnam War and Johnson administration years. Now the system is frozen in time according to the politics of thirty years ago.

Medicare has a mandatory social insurance component, principally to pay for hospital care (and other institutional care and home health care), that is funded by a payroll system. In addition, it has a heavily subsidized system of voluntary insurance run by the government. This covers and subsidizes physicians' and other nonhospital services without regard to the income of the people receiving the services. So, the arrangement in place is a hybrid and not one a policymaker would initially think of to carry out the contract.

Reprinted from Reischauer, Butler, and Lave (eds.), *Medicare: Preparing for the Challenges of the 21st Century*, pp. 15–41 (Washington, D.C., 1998), with permission, National Academy of Social Insurance, Brookings Institution Press.

First, the system promised specific benefits irrespective of cost. The cost was going to be paid mostly by society. Unlike Social Security, which promised specific levels of income, Medicare promised specific benefits. Second, Medicare used central planning to deliver services at a cost affordable to patients and society. This meant using administered prices, regulation, and centralization to try to bring about the contract itself at reasonable cost. Third, the system was not means tested, although a person's payroll taxes were linked to his income. The subsidy for the delivery of hospital services and the voluntary physician payments were and remain not linked to income. Fourth, no limit was placed on the total financial exposure of the patients, the elderly themselves.

The problems that have arisen as a result of the way Medicare was designed are now demanding to be addressed. The one that attracts the most attention in Washington during the budget cycle is that the program has chronic financial problems that are related both to the public's perception of it and to the means established to discharge the social contract.

Most people have the notion that Medicare is a true social insurance program, that whether one is rich or poor, one has paid for the benefits. Therefore, any attempt to adjust premium costs, such as raising those paid by the very affluent, leads to righteous indignation among people who feel that they are merely getting back what they paid. Anybody who knows anything about the finances of the program knows, of course, that it is not true social insurance, but a large segment of the population that is not poor resists changing it.

But government, with the means currently used to fulfill the social contract, is failing to deliver. The quality and quantity of benefits are more similar to those of private plans in the 1960s than those of the 1990s. Medicare does not cover people for the cost of pharmaceuticals out of hospital. Surgery is covered, but drugs used during recovery at home are not. A surgical patient has to buy medigap coverage or pay for the necessary drugs himself. Finally, there is no true catastrophic coverage.

Moreover, Medicare no longer effectively protects society from high costs. Not only is there no effective means of making sure that costs to the elderly are reasonable, but the funding of part B has also given unlimited exposure to the ordinary taxpayer in order to provide heavy subsidies to people who, in many cases, do not need it.

If one looks fairly at the problems, it is not unreasonable to say, "Maybe we should start reevaluating the system." Are there better ways to achieve the contract and provide a better program for the elderly? This does not mean destroying the system and the social contract itself. This means improving Medicare.

One of the basic flaws is centralization. Central planning and its price controls and regulations did not work in Soviet agriculture, and they do not work in Medicare. The program has used price controls, or administered pricing, since its inception in an attempt to keep costs down. Policymakers had hoped this would not lead to distortions and inefficiency, but that is exactly what has happened. So more and more controls have been added, which means more and more intrusion and more and more cheating by care providers. The providers always have better computers and experts to figure out ways of using the system than the Health Care Finance Administration has computers and experts to stop them. There is a continuous cat-and-mouse game in which the providers always seem to win and the taxpayers always seem to lose.

Another feature of this highly centralized administered agreement is the barriers encountered in trying to make any fundamental changes in the price structure. Those who would change the program must mount an enormous campaign over many years and obtain statutes in Congress by taking on all the lobbyists to effect a change that a corporation and its union can agree on in one Friday afternoon meeting. That is the result of a system that is centralized, one that the Congress of the United States is essentially designing every detail of and running. It necessarily follows that it is extremely difficult to make any reasonable adjustment of the system.

The system of benefits is inefficient for the same reason. Every change is resisted by those who believe they would lose something. So it is extremely difficult to make even the most subtle and reasonable change to allow Medicare to catch up with the private sector. And that is why, when people go into Medicare, in many ways they feel they are entering a time warp and why it is so difficult to introduce reasonable changes to improve the program.

In considering all this, it becomes clear that America needs a public debate to figure out ways, first of all, to reaffirm the original social contract itself, but then to look at more effective ways of fulfilling it.

I believe the social contract today should assure the elderly and the disabled that they will have a modern health care system, including modern benefits, comparable to that available to the rest of the population. We should deliver health care at an affordable cost to all the elderly, rich or poor, and at a reasonable cost to society. That should be our contract.

Two broad steps must be taken to bring about that result. First, the social contract needs to be much clearer to people and must recognize the deficiencies of the past thirty years. This means looking very carefully at the distinction between a subsidized system and a true social insurance system. If under the current arrangements we were to try to turn Medicare into a true social insurance system paid for by working people through payroll taxes, we would need staggering increases in taxes. Alternatively, we could give up on any kind of payroll payment and no longer consider Medicare a social insurance program. The federal government could simply pay for it out of general revenue without regard to any kind of control on costs. But this solution would create another staggering problem.

The right approach would be to redefine the contract by explicitly stating that Medicare should be partly a social insurance program, which guarantees people specific benefits, and partly a true means-tested subsidy program. This means we might want to consider not doing away with the distinction between part A and part B, as some people suggest. To do so would add to the problems of making any change and confuse the public even further about what kind of program Medicare really is. As an alternative, part A could be turned into a true, fully funded social insurance program. It could be made more comprehensive in the services it provides, but the extent of public financial support could be made leaner through higher deductibles, higher copayments, and so forth. At the same time, part B could be turned into a true means-tested program assigned to give people financial help if they need it to deal with the out-of-pocket expenses associated with a redefined and restructured part A.

In other words, through part A, an elderly person in America would have much more comprehensive benefits with higher deductibles and copayments. But through part B, a poorer elderly person would be heavily supported to pay for the out-of-pocket costs that he or she could incur. Wealthy people would get very little, if anything, in part B support. It seems to me that this proposal would lead to public recognition that the current system is not equitable.

A second broad change that needs to be made is to alter the locus of control of the system's finances. Right now, central control means that Washington determines what payments should be made. Washington also determines what is good value for the money. But we should move toward allowing the elderly to take the financial value of their Medicare benefits and obtain a plan or coverage in some other way than through the traditional program or an HMO. This would constitute an important step in recognizing that it is the enrollees themselves who should be the arbiters of value. They should have the right to get the benefits that they need rather than those determined by Congress and the lobbyists. Taking this step would give incentives to providers to satisfy the beneficiaries rather than the latest rule from HCFA.

The National Academy of Social Insurance is currently engaged in this kind of rethinking, exploring these and other directions for change. There are many possible models to look at, and they are being examined in the various study groups.

One system that I have found very attractive is the Federal Employees Health Benefits Program. Whether one agrees with the FEHBP or not, it certainly suggests a very different structure for the way government could function: a revised Medicare system. The FEHBP model, like others we are looking at, would encourage the government to increase and improve the kind of information it provides to people, focusing much more on making options available. Instead of trying to micromanage pricing throughout the entire industry, an FEHBP-type Medicare would require the government to focus on allowing new services and options, providing better information, and carefully structuring a market in which to make decisions.

We may be at a stage in the debate over the future of Medicare where we can actually begin to have some thoughtful discussion about what kinds of changes can work and what they would mean. Americans need to have that if we are going to have a system that is modern and can actually fulfill the promised social contract.

PUNDITS, PEOPLE, AND MEDICARE REFORM
Theda Skocpol

The 1995–96 election cycle brought to national attention Medicare and its problems and revealed the chasm that separates elite and popular opinion about this crucial part of modern U.S. social provision. Pundits and people are not on the same wavelength, which could have dire consequences for the future of American democracy as well as for the shape and extent of the nation's commitment to decent health care for the elderly.

Contrary to the near consensus that grips Washington policy analysts, most Americans are not ready to have experts and politicians whom they profoundly distrust fundamentally restructure a cherished health security program on which they or their loved ones greatly depend. Most Americans do not want to give up a national commitment to fund a consistent set of health services with maximum choice of providers in favor of a leap into a world of more paperwork, more bureaucracy, increasing complexity and unpredictable costs for individuals, and much more anxiety for the elderly and their relatives. The pundits are ready to move from defined benefits to fixed and shrinking public contributions, but most of the people do not want to go along.

Bill Clinton trounced Bob Dole with nearly half the popular vote in 1996 while congressional Democrats also gained significant ground. The turnaround for Democrats was striking in that they had been left for dead after the Republican triumphs two years earlier. In large part, Democrats did well in 1996 because less economically privileged voters came back to the polls, looking to the president and other Democrats to defend "M2E2," that is Medicare, Medicaid, federal commitments to education, and national environmental regulations.[1] President Clinton may have pronounced big government dead in January 1996, but he rode America's biggest and best-loved public programs—Medicare above all—to his second-term victory. An immediate postelection poll found continuing majority support for universal health coverage and concluded that most of the American public "is focused on protecting Medicare from cuts, not on entitlement reform."[2]

Voters hardly had time to get home from the polls before editorialists and advocacy groups declared that the election was an endorsement for a "dynamic center" determined to undertake far-reaching entitlement reforms.[3] President Clinton was urged to be "courageous," to "rise above partisanship" by appointing a bipartisan commission led by experts to fundamentally restructure Social Security and Medicare. Clinton, the pundits declared, should avoid short-term fixes and instead undertake major restructurings, even more breathtaking in scope and departure from the status quo than his failed health reform effort of 1993–94.

Medicare is the prime object of structural reformist zeal. Crisis fever is harder to whip up about Social Security because its trust fund is, after all, currently in surplus; Social Security's problems will grow gradually only after 2012, and immediate modest adjustments could fend off the projected trouble. But Medicare part A has been declared near bankruptcy, meaning that some serious decisions about benefits or finances or both *do* need to be made very soon. Immediate difficulties in the program open the door wide for those who want the president and Congress also to address the projected rapid increases in Medicare spending that will accompany the aging of the baby boom generation. Since its inception as a program that catered to doctors and private insurance companies, Medicare has become part of the overall rapid increase in U.S. health spending; and it sticks out as a huge part of federal spending during an era of budget-balancing politics. In short, all sorts of crises and problematic trends converge to make demands for an immediate drastic Medicare overhaul plausible in elite circles.

Without going into the details of clashing plans for structural reform, it is clear that responsible experts and pundits (translation: conservatives and centrists, not "irresponsible" liberals) are focusing on plans to transform Medicare from a promise of predictable payment for a defined package of health services for each elderly person into a shrinking public contribution to part of the variable amounts individuals would need to pay for decent health coverage. There are also schemes for (more or less forcibly) injecting new kinds of so-called choices into each individual's situation: not just the choice of service providers (fee for service or an HMO) that already exists in Medicare, but also choices about how to spend a fixed voucher on one of hundreds of private insurance plans or perhaps even a choice between medical savings accounts and payments toward more complete coverage. The existing system of fairly open personal flexibility to connect to many doctors would be compromised or abolished in the schemes for structural reform that are currently fashionable.

Much of this book focuses on the details of alternative reform schemes, with arguments about the advantages and dangers of each. I will not burden readers with my opinions on every alternative. But I cannot resist saying that given the realities of U.S. politics and public administration, all the schemes for defined contribution reforms are likely to make inequalities of income worse and hamper the elderly's access to decent care. No matter how well designed on paper, all the schemes would end up allowing the better-off elderly and the momentarily healthier to separate themselves from increasingly inadequate provisions for the less-well-off and the sicker. The contemplated structural reforms in Medicare would promote what Robert Reich calls the "secession of the affluent" from shared public social provision. And there will be gender as well as class effects, because women tend to live longer. Even a well-off woman like me does not look forward to living to be a post-eighty-five-year-old subject to any of the plans for structural reform that are being bruited about. As the cartoon goes:

> Doctor to older patient: "I've got good news and bad news!"
> Patient: "What's the good news?"
> Doctor: "You're going to outlive Medicare!"
> Patient: "What's the bad news?"
> Doctor: "You're going to outlive Medicare!"[4]

Joking aside, my message is directed at all those clashing experts, everyone vying for a place on that Commission to End Medicare As We Know It. My message is, look before you leap. Trained (in most cases) as economists, health care experts are accustomed to arguing in terms of static technical design and rational claims about cost efficiency. But historically grounded moral understandings are much more important for other citizens. And institutional realities are much more relevant for predicting what will actually occur as plans meet politics, as proposals are eviscerated and reworked amidst congressional and interest-group maneuvers over reforming Medicare. Remember Ira Magaziner and his friends? They did not pay much attention to history, institutions, and predictable political processes when they drew up their ideal health care plan for the Clinton administration to lay before Congress. We all know what happened next.[5]

Consider the big picture of historically evolved public understandings about Medicare. Today Medicare has become a potential albatross for Social Security because Medicare's problems could end up dragging a much healthier Social Security system into a donnybrook over radical restructuring. But a little over thirty years ago, Medicare complemented a popular Social Security system. Medicare delivered much needed additional protections to retirees eligible for Social Security. More important, Social Security's main institutional feature—payroll tax financing and benefits delivered to former workers and their families without demeaning or intrusive means tests—provided a solid basis on which to build Medicare. Although Medicare was certainly more institutionally complex, reform advocates in the 1960s could argue that the program would work like Social Security. Most Americans heard that message, and liked it very much.[6]

From early in our nation's history, successful American social policies have shared certain basic features.[7] From public schools and Civil War benefits in the nineteenth century, through early twentieth-century programs for mothers and children, and on to Social Security, the GI bill, and Medicare, effective and politically popular U.S. social programs have embodied a recognizable moral rationale and encompassed broad constituencies. The best have promised supports for individuals in return for service to the larger community. And they have delivered benefits without means tests to individuals and families across lines of class, race, and place. Social Security and Medicare are both very much part of this tradition, offering substantial and honorable help to retired people who are understood to have contributed to the nation through lifetimes of work.

We need to realize that the social transaction here is much more than an individualistic investment of payroll taxes to buy pensions or services in the future. People believe that there is a morally grounded contract between families and the nation; they see eventual retirement benefits as something they earn through work, not just by virtue of making tax payments. Professional and managerial elites may have lost sight of popular moral understandings in recent years because most highly educated and powerful people do not look forward to retirement at all. But the bulk of American working people are not doing thrilling or self-fulfilling jobs. They are more likely to see their lives as a moral story with deserved rewards coming at the end.[8] People work hard, often in jobs that are neither well paid nor very secure, and they raise their children and cooperate with their neighbors. At the end of a lifetime of such socially responsible contributions lies a secure and dignified retirement, primarily anchored for most people in Social Security and Medicare.

As a poster in the 1930s put it, "Old Age Should Be the Harvest of a Fruitful Life," and most Americans still fervently believe this.[9] Perhaps all the more so today, in the wake of two decades of hard times for less privileged workers and families.[10] When people hear elites telling them that their hard-earned retirement protections may not be there, they profoundly resent and fear the message. Ordinary Americans feel betrayed by the thought that the federal government and the nation's leaders may break the social contract they have tried to live by and want to grow old by.

For more than a decade now, antigovernment conservatives have been pursuing a grand strategy to undermine Americans faith in Social Security and Medicare, carrying out plans such as the one Stuart Butler and Peter Germanis outlined in the early 1980s article, "Achieving a Leninist Strategy."[11] This remarkable piece outlined tactics for undermining Americans' faith in public social insurance and preparing the ground for eventual individualistic and market-oriented privatization. Of course, there have been many parts to the overall assault that opponents of social insurance have mounted. One key part has been an effort to shake the faith of young people, especially affluent young people, that systems such as Medicare and Social Security are sound enough to be there for them in the future. Conservatives have talked incessantly about generational warfare, deploying economic projections and statistics sorted out by age cohorts. Conservatives in American politics are very good at getting their polemic messages broadly disseminated, so the generational assaults on Social Security and Medicare have spread much further than just to the readers of highbrow publications.

Efforts to undermine popular faith in social insurance have made some headway. Today, younger Americans are no longer sure that those protections will exist when they get old. But in another sense, generational warfare arguments have not worked well. Younger Americans remain just as supportive of generous social provision for the elderly as do the elderly themselves, indeed sometimes more so.[12] In real life, people are connected to one another as parents and children, grandparents and grandchildren.[13] Folks just do not think like "generational accounting" economists. Most American adults, especially adult women, report being in weekly or daily touch with their mothers.[14] Particularly among women, America's generations are not really socioculturally separated, let alone at war.

There is a perfectly understandable social dynamic behind the growing gender gap in American politics, especially about attitudes toward social programs such as Medicare. When an elderly woman starts worrying about "the government messing with her Medicare," the first person to hear about it is her daughter. And her daughter is very likely to listen closely, because she knows very well that if anything happens to the personal expense or quality of her mother's health care, it will not be Pete Peterson or Newt Gingrich who will have to take "more personal responsibility." She knows that *she* is the one who will have to do more to help her mother, perhaps taking money from a hard-pressed family budget or sparing precious hours amidst the pressures of her overcrowded days. After two hours getting everyone out the door in the morning, followed by eight hours at the office and several hours of housework and helping the children with their homework at night, our putative adult woman knows she can then look forward to talking with her mother about how to keep her beloved doctor or pay extra money to the right specialist. After a decade or so of doing all this, that same woman could look forward to a retirement full of hassles with whatever the Washington elites have dreamed up for her, too, instead of Medicare. She could anticipate worrying about which HMO to join, or wondering whether her voucher will pay for decent health care. Revisions of popular health programs like Medicare (and Medicaid) are, in short, not just issues for the elderly. They are family issues. Consequently, women of all ages will be paying close attention and worrying a lot about who is planning what for Medicare.

To get back to the big picture, there are good moral and social reasons why millions of Americans say that they are not very enthusiastic about big structural changes in Medicare. For all of its shortcomings people have come to trust and rely on Medicare as we know it. They like its predictable benefits and the choice of health care providers it allows. They do not see the sharp generational trade-offs that the privatizers posit. Nor do they care for the argument—now routine at places like the Brookings Institution—that elderly Americans have to be "brought into the same system" of health care delivery and financing as everyone else. Working-aged Americans of modest means know that many of them do not have health coverage or else have to pay more and more for increasingly niggardly and bureaucratically inflexible forms of care. Most people want better than that for their parents—and for themselves, too, when they make it to the promised land of retirement.

Experts, of course, believe that most Americans are childish about trade-offs, that they refuse to acknowledge national budget problems and do not want to pay taxes for a cherished program that is doomed by demography and medical technology. Maybe there is some truth in such views of the great unwashed. But it is also true that Americans have been fairly consistent, and not so irrational, in what they tell pollsters and their elected leaders.[15] Most Americans want the federal budget balanced but would prefer do it slowly if that is necessary to sustain Medicare. Most people argue for making cuts in payments to doctors and hospitals first. And most would consider raising taxes and premiums on very well off employees and beneficiaries. Americans have also made it clear that they would like to see cutbacks in government programs besides Medicare and Social Security.

Pundits routinely editorialize that America cannot abide an expanding proportion of its public expenditures devoted to the elderly (the implication is that old people are a waste, not a good investment). But average citizens apparently do not see things this way. Most seem willing to have more spent on the elderly as the country grays. And why is it so unthinkable that the United States might spend a growing proportion of its tax resources on our parents and grandparents (rather than, say, on corporate subsidies and B-1 bombers)? Understandably, congressional representatives and institutional elites want substantial tax monies channeled into manipulable programs rather than automatic entitlements. Meanwhile, though, most Americans might be very happy with a federal government that concentrates on well-understood social insurance programs that deliver a modicum of security with dignity to millions of families.

In the final analysis, maybe American elites just do not want to hear what a majority of their fellow citizens are saying, particularly about programs such as Medicare and Social Security.[16] Elites think they know what is best and are determined to forge ahead with structural reforms that may end up hurting and disillusioning millions of their fellow citizens. At a time when citizen distrust of the federal government is at an all-time high, policy experts, editorialists, and other pundits are urging the president and Congress to undertake radical transformations in Medicare, changes very much at odds with historically evolved moral understandings and different from the incremental steps that most voters have said they prefer.

With his eye on the editorial pages and his ear to the think-tank ground, President Clinton may soon take the plunge into commission-mandated structural reform. Maybe Congress will even manage to process recommended structural changes in Medicare, writing lots of subsidies for the health services and insurance industries into the details of the bills as they pass through committees. I hope not. Given today's bitter partisan divisions, I even tend to doubt it. (Sometimes gridlock is a good thing.) But all of this could happen, because the pundit consensus is so strong and elected politicians have so many incentives to slash the federal budget and avoid taxes while devising new subsidies for businesses.

But if top-down attempts at structural transformations of Medicare are made during the next several years, whatever finally spews forth from the congressional process is not likely to be good for average and less privileged Americans. Structural transformations proposed of by a commission and disposed of by Congress as we know it could be even worse for American democracy than for people's health care. Citizens who already believe there is little to like and trust about Washington may end up with their worst fears confirmed. This seems almost certain to be the result if experts and pundits insist on going forward with radical proposals for Medicare restructuring that head in directions most of the American people do not want to go.

So I say to all of the experts, for the sake of American democracy (not to mention for the good of old ladies, past and future), think carefully about institutional legacies, social morality, and political realities. Do not concentrate just on ideal plans and the technical details of reform proposals. Keep the health of American democracy in mind as you proceed, lest you leap too rashly into the brave new world of radically restructuring a program that most of your fellow citizens view as a keystone of the nation's social contract and a cherished support for their own life stories. Find gradual ways to adjust our shared and dignified Medicare program for the future. And if you must bring all Americans into the same system of health care and insurance, consider improving and universalizing coverage for working-aged families rather than reducing coverage for our retired grandparents.

NOTES

1. Ruy Teixeira, "Who Rejoined the Democrats? Understanding the 1996 Election Results," Economic Policy Institute, Washington, November 1996.

2. "The Popular Mandate of 1996: The Voter Concerns That Decided the Election and That Will Shape the Future Agenda," Greenberg Research and CAF, Washington, November 12, 1996.

3. Details in Harold Meyerson, "Dead Center," *American Prospect,* no. 30 (January–February 1997), pp. 60–67.

4. This cartoon appears in Marilyn Moon, *Medicare Now and in the Future,* 2d ed. (Washington: Urban Institute Press. 1996), p. xvii.

5. See Theda Skocpol, *Boomerang: Clinton's Health Security Effort and the Turn against Government in U.S. Politics* (Norton, 1996).

6. Theodore R. Marmor, *The Politics of Medicare* (Chicago: Aldine, 1973); and Lawrence R. Jacobs, *The Health of Nations: Public Opinion and the Making of American and British Health Policy* (Cornell University Press, 1993), chap. 9.

7. For background, see Theda Skocpol, *Protecting Soldiers and Mothers: The Political Origins of Social Policy in the United States* (Harvard University Press, 1992); and Skocpol, *Social Policies in the United States: Future Possibilities in Historical Perspective* (Princeton University Press, 1995).

8. See the splendid research on the views of non-college-educated working people in Stanley B. Greenberg, *The Economy Project* (Washington: Greenberg Research, 1996).

9. The poster is cited in the *New York Times,* January 19, 1997, p. C1.

10. Sheldon Danziger and Peter Gottschalk, *America Unequal* (Harvard University Press, 1995).

11. Stuart Butler and Peter Germanis, "Achieving a Leninist Strategy," *Cato Journal,* vol. 3 (Fall 1983), pp. 547–61.

12. This finding appears again and again in opinion studies, including Fay Lomax Cook and Edith J. Barrett, *Support for the American Welfare State* (Columbia University Press, 1992).

13. Eric R. Kingson, Barbara A. Hirshorn, and John M. Cornman, *Ties That Bind: The Interdependence of Generations* (Cabin John, Md.: Seven Locks Press, 1986): and Vern L. Bengston and Robert A. Harootyan, *Intergenerational Linkages: Hidden Connections in American Society* (Springer Publishing, 1994).

14. Leora Lawton, Merril Silverstein, and Vern L. Bengston, "Solidarity between Generations in Families," in Bengston and Harootyan, *Intergenerational Linkages,* pp. 26–27.

15. In addition to "Popular Mandate of 1996," see Robert J. Blendon and others, "The Public's View of the Future of Medicare," *Journal of the American Medical Association,* vol. 274 (November 1995), pp. 1645–48.

16. The thesis that elites are not listening is elaborated and documented in Lawrence R. Jacobs and Robert Y. Shapiro, "The Politicization of Public Opinion," prepared for a forthcoming Brookings Institution—Russell Sage Foundation book edited by Margaret Weir.

REFLECTIONS ON HOW MEDICARE CAME ABOUT
Robert M. Ball

To help readers understand how this rather strange collection of legal provisions and administrative choices called Medicare came about requires me to try to recapture the times and the goals of those of us who put it together and, in my case, had the responsibility for administering it during its first seven years.[1]

Much can be explained by our reliance on the guiding hand of pragmatism, what we could get Congress to agree to—what could pass—and in administration what would work. As critics might say, our decisions were frequently the triumph of opportunism over principle. And there is truth in this observation, although on some points there was a stubborn defense of principle that at times seemed to threaten the very operation of the program. For example, we took the view that for hospitals, principally southern hospitals, simply to submit plans for desegregation would not be enough to qualify them for the Medicare program, although "plans" had been considered enough in the case of schools. Instead, just months before Medicare was to start paying for hospital services and while hundreds of hospitals were not yet certified, the program had a thousand inspectors in the field, visiting hospitals to make sure that blacks and whites were being assigned to semiprivate rooms without regard to race. And remember, these were older people who had lived their lifetimes in rigid segregation. The *New York Times* suggested that the Johnson administration ought to make up its mind. Did it want to supply medical care services in the South or did it want hospital integration? The administration, it was argued, clearly could not have both. But in fact we did get both, just about everywhere.

There were a few holdouts, particularly in a chain of religious hospitals in the South. But to an extent pragmatism came to the program's aid here too. It paid for "emergency services" in unapproved hospitals if they were substantially closer to the patient at the time of the emergency than any other hospital. (And for a time, we were not too strict about the definition of an emergency.) No one died from lack of care because of the insistence on integration, or at least no one made that case. Perhaps here is a principle of successful public administration: Go as far as you can in the right direction from the beginning without causing a stalemate, but be prepared to tighten up later. Reimburse HMOs 95 percent of the cost of providing services on a fee-for-service basis, for example, but if with experience that proves to be too much, turn the screws a bit.

Although integrating hospitals principally illustrates devotion to principle, there was, as I have said, pragmatism too. Medicare legislation had marched up the Hill and back again several times before it passed. Votes were always close.

Some of this material appeared first in "What Medicare Architects Had in Mind," *Health Affairs* (Winter 1995), p. 62.

The American Medical Association (AMA) was strongly opposed to the idea and had at least the superficial support of all parts of the medical enterprise, except the nurses, and the strong support of the insurance industry and most of the business community. When at last the legislation was in the Senate under circumstances in which passage seemed very likely—Lyndon Johnson had just been elected overwhelmingly to a new term—the application of the recently passed civil rights law to Medicare's hospitals was on the minds of most southern senators. They, and the administration, needed at all costs to avoid an explicit vote on the matter. So the only legislative history that we had to rely on for the drive against segregation was a colloquy on the Senate floor when Senator Abraham Ribicoff replied to a question that "Yes, title VI would, of course, apply." That was it. No debate, no newspaper story, nothing.

Pragmatism appeared in the shape of the program itself. Why, with no experience with a federal health insurance program, did the United States choose to start a program with the elderly, from any rational viewpoint the most unlikely initial group? The administration did not know how to run a health insurance program, so why did it decide to begin with the most difficult possible group? The elderly were by far the most costly group: admissions would be more frequent and stays would be longer than those of other age groups, the patients would have multiple illnesses, and after expensive treatment, they would, nevertheless, frequently die. Even when cured they were not a very good investment in terms of years of life ahead.

As a society if America was going to start with a given age group, it would seem to have made much more sense to start with children or perhaps mothers and children. They did not need expensive care very often, and the investment would make a difference for a lifetime ahead. So why not children? Why the elderly? Only one reason. Politically, the administration had the best chance with them. It is important at this stage of the story to remember that those who advocated Medicare wanted something more. The AMA was right. This was to be the entering wedge for a universal health plan. Those of us who were active at the time are still astounded that more than thirty years later only the disabled have been added to the program. We had hoped that long before now the feasibility and desirability of a universal system would have been demonstrated and it would be in operation.

Medicare came about because the advocates of universal health insurance were discouraged. The idea of a universal program had never made much progress in the United States. Ironically, national health insurance was advocated in 1916 by the leaders of the AMA, who were favorably impressed by the systems that had been established in Germany (1883), Britain (1911), and later in several other countries. Equally ironic was that much of the American labor movement in 1916 was opposed. Samuel Gompers, president of the American Federation of Labor, preferred collective bargaining to political solutions and feared that if workers began leaning on government, they might feel less need for unions.

These positions were soon reversed. By 1920 the AMA was firmly established in opposition to government health insurance. The unions, however, eventually went all out in favor of a government plan and indeed provided the backbone of its support. These two powerful groups became the main antagonists, first over national health insurance and then over the much more modest recommendations for Medicare.

President Franklin Roosevelt did not support national health insurance at the time of the 1934 recommendations of the Committee on Economic Security, and it was not included with the recommendations that formed the basis for the Social Security Act in 1935. He feared, probably correctly, that because health insurance had such strong opposition from physicians and others, if it were included in his program for economic security, he might lose the entire program. In later years he often commented favorably on universal health coverage, but he never offered or endorsed a national health insurance plan. He called for social insurance from the cradle to the grave, and in his 1944 State of the Union message, looking to the nation's postwar needs and goals, he proposed an Economic Bill of Rights that included the "right to adequate medical care and the opportunity to achieve and enjoy good health." But occasional rhetorical sorties aside, he was content to let the Social Security Board push for national health insurance without adding his personal endorsement.

President Harry Truman specifically advocated a national health insurance plan. His power to get any domestic legislation passed, however, was weak, both while he was filling out Roosevelt's fourth term and after he had surprised everyone but himself by getting elected on his own in 1948. Facing Republicans in control of both houses of Congress, he had no chance of getting universal compulsory health insurance enacted, a situation that everyone but the AMA seemed to understand.

The AMA's opposition approached hysteria. For the first time, members were assessed special dues, which were used to fight health insurance. The organization created a $3.5 million war chest—very big money for the time—with which it conducted a campaign of vituperation against the advocates of national health insurance. It also exerted strict discipline over the few of its members who took an "unethical" position favoring the government program. This was a warm-up for later campaigns against Medicare.

Even before the AMA launched its attack, however, the Truman administration had given up on universal health insurance and was casting about for something less ambitious that might have a better chance. That is how Medicare was born—as a fallback. It was publicly advocated for the first time by a government spokesman when Oscar Ewing, head of the Federal Security Agency (now, after several reincarnations, the Department of Health and Human Services), unveiled it on February 27, 1952. The idea was to cover all Social Security beneficiaries: the elderly, widows, and orphans (persons with disabilities were not yet under Social Security). Social Security was part of the Federal Security Agency, and we had worked up the plan for Ewing.

Initially, it went nowhere. President Truman never specifically endorsed the shift from support of universal health insurance to the limited Medicare program, but even if he had, he would not have been able to get Congress to consider it. He was within months of the end of his term. And Adlai Stevenson was soon to be overwhelmingly defeated for the presidency by Dwight D. Eisenhower.

The design of Medicare, which was taking shape in an unsympathetic political climate, was based entirely on a strategy of acceptability: What sort of program would be most difficult for opponents to attack and most likely to pick up critical support? Later modification to include just the elderly rather than all Social Security beneficiaries and to cover them only for hospitalization had the same motivation. By the time John F. Kennedy campaigned on the issue in 1960, we had decided that even trying to provide coverage for inpatient surgery was a mistake. If physician services were left out entirely, we reasoned, the AMA's opposition would have less standing. By that time it was clear that the elderly had the most political appeal and potentially the most muscle. We wanted to get something going, and this seemed a politically plausible first step.

The elderly were an appealing group to cover first in part because they were so ill suited for coverage under voluntary private insurance. They used on average more than twice as many hospital days as younger people but had only about half as much income. Private insurers, who set premiums to cover current costs, had to charge them much more, and the elderly could not afford the charges. Group health insurance, then as today, was mostly for the employed and was just not available to the retired elderly. The result of all this was that somewhat less than half of the elderly had any kind of health insurance, and what they had was almost always inadequate, often paying only so much per day for hospitalizations of limited duration. So the need was not hard to prove, nor was it difficult to prove that voluntary individual insurance was not only not meeting the need, but that it really could not meet the need.

Our principles were pragmatic and goals were limited. We did not propose a program to reform the health care delivery system. We proposed assuring the same level of care for the elderly as was then enjoyed by paying and insured patients; otherwise, we did not intend to disrupt the status quo. Had we advocated anything else, it never would have received serious consideration. Thus the bill we wrote followed the principles of reimbursement that hospitals all over the country had worked out with the Blue Cross system. Government would be unobtrusive. Hospitals would be allowed to nominate an intermediary to do the actual bill payments and to be the contact point with hospitals. The carrot was that hospital bills that had previously gone unpaid because many of the elderly had no money would now be paid.

What the hospitals worked out with Blue Cross was retroactive cost reimbursement. Hospitals had an even better deal with the commercial insurance companies, which based their reimbursement on hospital charges that were ordinarily higher than costs. But at that time we had no plans for prospective payment or even prospective budgeting. By and large, our stance was not to rock the boat and to pay full costs, not intervening very much in how hospitals, at least the better ones, conducted their business.

We intended to bring the elderly, and under Medicaid the poor, the same standard of treatment as paying patients received. At that time amenities for the poor were very few, and the aged, who were mostly poor, were usually treated in hospital wards where their care was often left to interns and medical students. Indeed, one of organized medicine's objections to Medicare and Medicaid was that these programs would close off their main sources of teaching material. (Of course, that did not come to pass. After the Medicare legislation became law, it soon became evident that elderly patients in the program would happily cooperate with student caregivers under proper supervision.)

We believed that to make all of this happen, Medicare had to pay its own way and pay fully. We opposed shifting costs to other payers, and we avoided discounts beyond what the program's contractors might have secured for their own insured population. We pursued a careful, minute accounting for the costs of treatment for the elderly because the rule was to pay for them but for no one else. The program would not pay a share of a hospital's bad debts because it paid fully for its patients, but it would pay a share of teaching costs because everyone ultimately benefited from that. The program would allow a somewhat higher reimbursement rate for nursing the elderly on the theory that it took longer, but it insisted on lower per diem costs because of the longer stays of the elderly and the concentration of hospital costs in the first few days after admission.

One early frustration was the chaotic state of accounting in many if not most hospitals. They shared an unbusinesslike approach to management that was common at the time to many church-run and other nonprofit organizations. Nevertheless, we continued to believe that it was possible to set up systems that would produce good data on what it cost to take care of just the elderly.

As policymakers we did not try for more than we could accomplish. The program accepted the quality standard for hospitals as certified by the private Joint Commission on the Accreditation of Hospitals, as long as the hospital also had a utilization review committee and met the civil rights standard. We set up somewhat less stringent quality standards for other hospitals, mostly smaller ones, and contracted with state public health agencies for their inspection. This limited approach brought most hospitals into the program and gradually improved their quality. But we bent where we had to. For example, one of the requirements was that there be a trained nurse on duty at all times, and a little hospital in Johnson City, Texas, did not have one for some shifts. However, with Lyndon Johnson president, I could not conceive of not certifying the one hospital in Johnson City, so we stretched the requirement. We held that if a physician was on duty when there was no nurse, we would assume that the physician could perform the same duties as a nurse. That is not really true, but we stretched it.

It was important that the program start up smoothly. We worked with the hospitals and physicians and considered all shades of opinion in getting advice before we issued rules. At one time, nine informal working groups were discussing the interpretation of various provisions of the program. Each group had representatives of just about all the forces in American medicine. Many of these people would not have come into the same room together before the Medicare legislation passed. The groups were made up of fifteen or twenty people: experts from the universities, representatives from the AMA, specialty medical organizations, group practice prepayment plans (which were then anathema to organized medicine), and labor unions and consumer groups, all working with the government and doing their best to come forward with the most desirable interpretations of this new law. They did not always try for agreement, but each group gave us their best advice after discussing the matter with each other. And I really mean that. To a remarkable degree, opponents as well as supporters tried hard to be helpful.

It is a long way from legislation to a going program. We consulted very widely, and in setting up the regulations worked finally with a legislatively required advisory body that was also broadly representative of diverse interests and opinions. Although we could obviously not decide in the end in favor of all the varying positions, just about everybody came through the process feeling they had had their day in court. Thus, actual administration of the program began with widespread support among the hospitals, physicians, and the public.

Establishing the program went off, really, without a hitch, although there were some hectic moments just before the deadline for beginning to provide services. A couple of weeks, or maybe somewhat more, before the program was to go into effect, for some reason the president got nervous. When the president is nervous, the cabinet officer under him gets nervous. That made me nervous because I was just one step below that and in charge.

The president was worried that people who were eligible had been saving up for years all their handicaps and illnesses—everything that was wrong with them—and on the day the program opened there were going to be lines around the block at every hospital because just about everyone older than 65 was going to be seeking services. But a 20 percent increase in the use of hospital beds by the elderly would have amounted to only a 5 percent increase in the total number of people in the hospitals. And the program was to begin in July, when hospital occupancy is lowest. So until the president stirred things up, we felt pretty comfortable. An increase of 20 percent for the elderly seemed an adequate allowance.

Nationally, we believed, there were plenty of hospital beds. But it is true that the best hospitals frequently are near their capacities even in July. So, we got out the maps. There was a pin on the map representing every major hospital in the country. Helicopters were standing by to move people to where there were vacancies. Public health hospitals, veterans hospitals, and army hospitals all across the country were alerted to be ready to handle emergency cases. And then absolutely nothing happened. There was no line anywhere. Medicare had a very smooth start.

The principle of our mostly accepting the current situation and gradually tightening up later is also illustrated in the initiation of Medicare part B, covering physician services. For part B there was no civil rights or utilization review requirement. The program was explicitly based on a private insurance plan, an Aetna plan for federal workers under the Federal Employees Health Benefits Program. It was to be voluntary: not paid-up insurance but insurance financed by a current premium with half paid by the elderly who elected coverage and half by the federal government.

Part B had been added to the administration's hospital insurance plan at the last moment by Wilbur Mills, chairman of the House Ways and Means Committee, who wanted part of the plan to follow the principles advocated by some of the congressional Republicans. The government subsidy, now controversial, was an unavoidable result of making part B voluntary. Without it, rates based on the average cost of all of the elderly would have been unattractive to the younger group of elderly persons, but if the rates were varied by age, the premiums would have been prohibitive for those older than 80.

We had spent many years perfecting the legislation covering hospitals, but we had only one weekend in which to try to adapt the private Aetna plan to a government-run plan. There were no quality standards in the Aetna plan and no cost controls other than a vague stipulation that services had to be "medically required." Reimbursement was to be a "reasonable" charge determined by the customary charges of the particular physician and the prevailing charges in the locality for similar services. We had considerable concern about such a plan but decided that it was better than not covering physician services at all and that this was our only chance. So the administration supported it. We also had a naive faith that when we had more experience with the program, we could get reasonable changes made in the law.

With a government program, sooner or later, public policy concerns such as cost and quality move front and center. These concerns caused the program to become a leader in the health insurance field. After-the-fact reimbursement for hospital costs clearly was a flawed policy, and within a couple of years other government officials and I were calling for some form of prospective payment. When Medicare finally adopted the diagnosis-related group (DRG) system in 1983, it was an important advance for all who reimbursed for hospital care. The principle of setting in advance a rate for a given diagnostic group gave hospitals a huge incentive to keep costs down as compared with the previous system of reimbursing them case by case for whatever "reasonable costs" were received. This change, applied to all age levels by many plans, made the lengths of stay in U.S. hospitals the shortest in the world.

Similarly, we knew from the beginning that we needed some kind of fee schedule in part B, but we had to struggle with the term "reasonable," defined as "customary and prevailing," all through the early years. When Medicare finally adopted the resource-based relative value scale (RBRVS) in 1992, it was again pioneering a technique that helped other insurers. After Medicare adopted physician reimbursement standards based on the resources required to deliver the service and related the relative cost of one service to another, the method was widely adopted. The unit underlying the comparison of one service to another could be set generally at any level desired, but the relationship among services could stay the same and the level of the unit negotiated. It is doubtful that this method would have been feasible before Medicare did the necessary research and adopted the system. Other contributions to health insurance were the program's insistence on more careful administration by contractors than they were used to and better accounting by hospitals.

But to return to the early steps of implementing the program, we were greatly aided by the tremendous build-up of excitement among elderly people and their sons and daughters. After the long fight, there was great enthusiasm. I remember talking to maybe 15,000 people in Detroit, and you could feel the excitement in that group of older people who were being told for the first time about the start-up of Medicare.

Part B was voluntary, and we had to sign people up for it. We sent out punch card applications to all the addresses that we had for people 65 and older. We had, of course, addresses for Social Security beneficiaries, people in private retirement plans, welfare beneficiaries, and anybody who had paid income tax. We sent applications out to almost everybody—hospital and nursing home patients too—then followed with other efforts to emphasize the need to sign up by a specified date: the sides of post office delivery trucks carried the deadline for signing up. Forest rangers looked for hermits in the woods. Everybody participated.

The program was immensely popular. One of the punch card applications came back from a man who was afraid that we might misunderstand his intentions. You could check yes or no on the application, but he wanted to be sure and had cut the no right out of the card. It did not work very well in the punch card equipment, but we managed.

As I said, there was no intention of reforming the nation's health care system. The intention was to put Medicare patients in an equal position with those already covered under private insurance or those who could pay their own way. In fact, the law forbade us to interfere in any way with the practice of medicine or the administration of hospitals. But it became clear that the original direction in the law had to be interpreted liberally. There was no way the program could be administered without some interference with the practice of medicine and the operation of hospitals. But the language in the law shows the extreme of the hands-off policy the program started with.

Medicare has done well what it was designed to do. Because of the program, hundreds of millions of older people and their children have been better off. Not only has the cost of medical bills been made bearable, but lives have been saved and the quality of life of the elderly has been greatly improved. Medicare has made available modern medical techniques—cataract removal, artificial hip transplants, cardiac bypasses—that otherwise might have been affordable only for the affluent. Medicare also has undoubtedly contributed to longevity: the United States (with Japan) leads the world in the expected remaining length of life for those who have reached age 65. In its present form, however, Medicare is clearly not prepared to cope with the huge increase in the number of beneficiaries that will take place beginning about 2010. To keep the program solvent and viable, changes will have to be made.

It is as true now as it was thirty years ago that the Medicare program is needed to give the elderly the same health care under the same conditions as is available to insured younger patients. Now, as then, most group insurance is furnished through employment, and individual insurance is simply too expensive for an age group (and those with disabilities who are also now included in the program) that needs much more health care and, on average, has lower incomes than do younger employed persons. For elderly persons and for the family members who otherwise would be saddled with their medical bills, Medicare continues to be—often literally—a lifesaver.

But it is a lifesaver itself in need of saving. Once a leader in providing health care, the program has fallen behind. First of all, Medicare's benefit package is considerably less comprehensive than packages offered by the better employer plans. In any long-range reform, the package should be improved, particularly by including a stop-loss provision to protect beneficiaries and their families against catastrophic costs and by adding drug coverage and more prevention services. Medicare also needs to take the lead once again in developing important cost-reduction techniques that can be followed in private plans, as it did with the invention of DRGs and the RBRVS.

I have one other thought. I do not know exactly what the next steps in cost control should be, but I find very promising the proposals Robert Reischauer and others have been working on that would set the value of a government-paid-for voucher at the average offer of bids to supply the Medicare package of services in a given geographical area. And I want to confess a major mistake we made. If there is a way to correct this mistake, it might make a difference. We had no idea that the Medicare cost-sharing provisions—the copayments and the deductible—would be canceled out by the growth of a medigap industry. We thought that the bills Medicare left uncovered were mostly too small to justify the administrative costs of supplementary insurance programs. Maybe they are, but a major industry of Medicare supplementation has developed nevertheless, and Medicare is paying a heavy price as private insurance rests on top of the basic Medicare coverage. The result is that neither the patient nor the physician on behalf of the patient has an incentive to think twice about the cost of a procedure. Somehow, we must get private insurers to share the costs they have created for Medicare by nullifying the copayments and deductibles, and somehow we must get the patients and physicians to agree that costs make a difference. With all its problems, managed care does help keep physicians aware of costs. In addition, are there well-constructed experiments to be performed on applying the hospital DRG-type approach to other services? How can we put back together some of the services that have been unbundled?

It is clear, I think, from the Medicare experience that in such a program everything depends on the human factor, on how patients, physicians, hospital administrators, insurers, and others behave. The program is not a mechanical model but a system that has all the messiness that arises when human beings are called on to run complicated, interrelated institutions that depend on human behavior. We should not be discouraged about further extensions of health insurance, but neither should we expect a smooth-running, purring machine. As Mark Twain said, "Man was made at the end of the week when God was tired."

NOTE

1.   Some of the details in the following discussion are indebted to Peter A. Corning, *The Evolution of Medicare from Idea to Law,* research report 29 (Office of Research and Statistics, Social Security Administration, 1969); Richard Harris, *A Sacred Trust* (New American Library, 1966); and Social Security Administration, bound volumes of the Social Security Act and its amendments.

SOCIAL INSURANCE COMMENTARY
E. J. Dionne

Social insurance is, to my mind, one of the most brilliant creations of a century of democratic (small "d") politics. It is an idea rooted in socialist, and arguably biblical, thought that saved capitalism. Social insurance arises from the understanding that competitive market economies do not distribute their fruits equally and that competitive economies sometimes break down. Competition has benefits and costs, and both are shared unequally.

Social insurance was a wise admission on the part of supporters of competitive economies that citizens would take the risk such economies require only if they were provided with a degree of security, especially against old age, unemployment, the sudden death of a spouse, and the vicissitudes of health. Risk is tolerable, even desirable, as long as every one of life's risks does not become an all-or-nothing game. This is especially true when one's family, not simply one's self, is put at risk. The power of the social insurance idea rests on a respect for individualism, not on a utopian and mistaken view of what radical individualism can accomplish.

In 1910 in *Social Insurance,* Henry Rogers Seeger, a Columbia University economist, wrote,

> Up to a certain point, it is moral and commendable for each to look after his own interests and the interest of those dependent upon him. It is a mistake to think that self interest in this sense is synonymous with selfishness. Adam Smith's assertion that "it is usually by pursuing our interests with due consideration to the interest of others that we contribute most to the common well being," is true of the ordinary man in the ordinary situation. But along with our individual interests, which can best be cared for by individual enterprise, industry, and forethought, there are other interests that call for a collective and cooperative action.

Seeger then described risks that we now have forms of social insurance for: industrial accidents, illness, premature death, unemployment, and the like. He concluded, "By . . . the means of cooperative action and the creation of social insurance, and by these means only, in my opinion, can we hope to raise the whole mass of wage earners to higher standards of efficiency and earnings and to more intelligent appreciation of all of life's possibilities." He turned out to be right. That is why we embarked on a system of social insurance.

Franklin D. Roosevelt said it even better. In a 1938 radio address on the third anniversary of the Social Security Act, he observed that the first in American history to seek governmental protection were not the poor and lowly but the rich and strong. They sought protective laws to give security to property owners, industrialists, merchants, and bankers. He did not blame the wealthy for seeking these protections. Instead, he saw that workers, too, sought protections as they became more articulate through organization.

> Strength or skill of arm or brain did not guarantee a man a job. It does not guarantee him a roof. It did not guarantee him the ability to provide for those dependent upon him or to take care of himself when he was too old to work. . . . Long before the economic blight of the Depression descended on the nation, millions of our people were living in wastelands of want and fear. Men and women too old and infirm to work either depended on those who had but little to share or spent their remaining years within the walls of a poorhouse. . . . Because it has become increasingly difficult for individuals to build their own security single handed, government must now step in and help them lay the foundation stones just as government in the past has helped lay the foundations of business and industry. We must face the fact that in this country we have a rich man's security and a poor man's security and that the government owes equal obligations to both. National security is not a half-and-half matter. It is all or none.

The United States has been remarkably successful because it followed the path laid down by Seeger and Roosevelt. Other industrial economies did the same. In many cases they did more than we did in the sphere of social insurance. We have established throughout the industrial democracies what Walter Russell Meade has called "the social democratic bargain," a marriage between market economies preached by capitalists and worker protections preached by socialists. Most economic decisions remain in private hands, but national governments use the tools at their disposal, notably taxing and spending. You are not supposed to talk about these anymore. But it was spending to take the edge off economic downturns that hastened the return to prosperity.

Labor laws guaranteed workers the right to organize, which boosted their share of economic largess. Government helped citizens of modest means secure housing, educate their children, and have a decent retirement. That social democratic bargain has been a good deal. It was possible because market economies delivered the goods and national governments had the power to tax, spend, and regulate pretty much as they and their electorates chose.

I would argue that the political unhappiness we are experiencing now in the United States and in many countries of Western Europe is not primarily the result of scandal; it is not primarily the result of negative advertising; and it is not the product of politicians being mean to one another. Politicians have long been mean to one another. Instead, it is the result of the weakening of the social democratic bargain and of the social insurance state.

This bargain is under siege from many directions. The global economy puts new competitive pressures on both businesses and governments to trim benefits that had once been taken for granted. In the welfare states of western Europe, this pressure is largely on public benefits. In the United States, we have an intensive system of private benefits in the form of company-provided health insurance and pensions. As we debate our public social insurance benefits, these basic private social benefits are being eroded. The proportion of workers without health insurance is growing. And the proportion of workers with pension plans involving substantial assured contributions from their employers is shrinking.

A second factor weakening the social democratic bargain is the decrease in the proportion of workers who are unionized. This is especially pronounced here and in Great Britain. A third factor is aging populations, accompanied by rising health care costs, which are putting great pressures on social insurance programs for health care in every country in the West. Finally, a technological economy that puts a high premium on skills and education seems to be widening economic inequalities. This produces a paradox. Growing inequalities create new dissatisfactions with government and taxation, while at the same time putting more pressure on government to rectify the imbalances.

In the most pessimistic light, the social insurance state faces a profound political contradiction. On the one hand, we have steadily increasing demands on government precisely because the social democratic bargain is breaking down. On the other hand, we have increasing mistrust of government, which makes it difficult to expand the social insurance state where necessary, particularly in providing health care. I am an optimist, so I do not accept this pessimistic view. I believe that the idea of social insurance is becoming more popular again precisely because the underlying reasons for its existence are becoming more explicit.

The basic idea behind social security, the need for collective provision against certain forms of insecurity, remains deeply and broadly popular despite the rise of the ideology of privatization. Advocates of privatization keep running into the stubborn fact that most Americans broadly like Social Security because it works and because it accords with their values.

The original idea of the Social Security Act could have been proposed by new Democrats no less than old Democrats, and a lot of Republicans. If there was ever a program designed to help those who "work hard and play by the rules," to use the president's phrase, this is it. If there was ever a program designed to offer a "hand up, not a handout," surely Social Security and other provisions of the social insurance state meet that criterion.

Some believe that the strongest danger facing America is financial insolvency in these programs. Others talk about a low savings rate. Still others emphasize the dangers of big government. But I believe the biggest danger is that we will forget why we have social insurance, and why its preservation is necessary not only to a civilized society but also to the very market economy that has provided us with so much wealth.

The programs of the social insurance state, especially Medicare and Social Security, loom very large on the balance sheets of government. As the baby boomers march inexorably toward old age and retirement, the costs will loom larger still. Nevertheless, fixing the social insurance state is very possible and within our reach. Saving it is absolutely necessary. Social insurance is the basic insurance policy Americans have for social stability, a modicum of social justice, and a society in which risks are taken freely and energetically because there is some protection against catastrophe and social breakdown.

Few business people I know would cut their expenses by canceling their fire insurance. Social insurance is the cost of doing business for a society that seeks to remain dynamic and inventive as well as just and fair. We need to rediscover the power of this idea and its value to us all.

3 | Rules of the Game: How Public Policy Affects Local Health Care Markets

Loel S. Solomon

The tumultuous pace of health system change is driven, in large measure, by private-sector actions such as the vote of a community hospital board to affiliate with a national hospital chain or the decision of a large employer to move its employees into managed care plans. Given the headline-grabbing nature of these changes, it is easy to lose sight of the critical role that public policy plays in shaping health system change.

This paper explores the impact of public policy on local health care systems in a representative sample of twelve U.S. communities being monitored as part of the Community Tracking Study, conducted by the Center for Studying Health System Change and sponsored by the Robert Wood Johnson Foundation (RWJF).[1] The first round of site visits conducted between May 1996 and January 1997 revealed wide variation in the mix of policies in effect in particular health care markets. It also underlined considerable differences in the way state and local officials implement similar policies and identified unique political cultures and interest-group dynamics. Although this high degree of cross-site variation makes it difficult to generalize across communities, several overarching themes emerge.

Reprinted from *Health Affairs*, 17, no. 4 (July/August 1998): 140–48. Copyright 1998. The People-to-People Health Foundation, Inc. All rights reserved. Used with permission.

This paper was presented at "Dynamics of Health System Change: Lessons Learned from Twelve Communities," a conference conducted by the Center for Studying Health System Change, 22 September 1997, in Washington, D.C.

THEMES

First, the Community Tracking Study reinforces findings from previous studies that public policy is a major force that influences health system change.[2] Public policy establishes the underlying "rules of the game" that circumscribe the behavior of actors in local markets. These rules also influence national and regional entities' decisions to enter or exit local markets. As a result, rules of the game are critical to establishing the baseline against which to measure health system change.

Second, a general trend in U.S. health policy toward deregulation is counter-balanced by a wide range of policies aimed at curbing the perceived excesses of the market. The balance that policymakers appear to be striking—reliance on market forces for cost control and a willingness to use public policy to mitigate the negative consequences of those forces— confirms an important trend identified by the RWJF's 1995 Community Snapshots Study.[3]

Third, players in local health care markets are more likely to emphasize policy change over background rules of the game as a major factor influencing strategic decisions. This suggests that established rules may have a different type of impact on health care decision making than recent or anticipated changes in public policy may have; we were not able to fully explore this hypothesis in this study.

Finally, impending change in the policy environment alters market dynamics in important ways, regardless of whether the policy is ever enacted or enforced. For instance, in several markets local providers have forged various kinds of affiliations in anticipation of the implementation of major policy shifts such as the introduction of Medicaid managed care programs and deregulation of hospital rate setting.

This paper focuses on select areas of public policy that have a major influence on health system change across Community Tracking sites and also high-lights important emerging areas of health policy. These areas include Medicaid managed care; Medicare risk contracting; regulation of private managed care plans; regulation of provider organizations through certificate-of-need (CON) licensure and hospital rate setting; and oversight of nonprofit hospitals' and health plans' conversions to for-profit status.[4]

MEDICAID MANAGED CARE

State and local policymakers in most of the study communities struggle to resolve two opposing policy objectives: to hold down the rapidly rising costs of their Medicaid programs and to extend health insurance to growing numbers of uninsured residents. Some of the more ambitious changes in Medicaid include

(1) managed care programs that require or encourage beneficiaries to enroll in Medicaid health maintenance organizations (HMOs); and (2) programs that subsidize the purchase of Medicaid coverage for families with incomes just above the Medicaid eligibility limit.[5]

Only five of the twelve Community Tracking sites had mandatory Medicaid managed care programs in operation during the study period; several others have received federal approval to move forward with such programs. By contrast, most study communities have voluntary managed care programs in place, although enrollment is often quite low. A handful of states also have moved forward with significant Medicaid access expansions for near-poor children, spurred in large part by new federal funds available for such programs. The major effects of Medicaid policy on health system change are discussed below.

MEDICAID CAN STIMULATE MANAGED CARE IN LOCAL MARKETS

In some of the study communities Medicaid managed care programs have driven change in the broader health care system by creating both a hospitable environment for managed care and an imperative for the development of novel risk-bearing delivery systems. Phoenix offers a striking example. Arizona established the nation's first mandatory Medicaid managed care program in 1982. Respondents reported that over the intervening years the Medicaid program stimulated the growth of managed care in Phoenix by encouraging hospitals and physicians to organize themselves into integrated delivery systems so that they could receive Medicaid payments from the state. Indeed, five of the seven Medicaid managed care plans offered in Phoenix at the time of our visit were sponsored by providers. Respondents also reported that the Arizona Health Care Cost Containment System (AHCCCS, Arizona's Medicaid equivalent) increased providers' comfort and familiarity with managed care, making them less resistant to contracting with HMOs for their private-pay and Medicare patients.

Even in markets with voluntary Medicaid managed care programs, such as Miami, Syracuse, and Boston, local Medicaid providers are forging alliances with other providers in the community and developing an organizational capacity to manage risk. These relationships help local providers to establish credible, state-approved managed care plans by demonstrating that they can manage patients along the continuum of care.

In a few study communities Medicaid also represents the leading edge in the market's move to global capitation. For instance, respondents in Seattle reported that physicians participating in the state's Medicaid program prefer capitation to fee-for-service, in large part because of the generous capitation rates historically offered by that program. However, enthusiasm for global capitation, both in Seattle and elsewhere, is reportedly starting to diminish as those rates are lowered.

COMPETITION FOR MEDICAID PATIENTS IS INTENSIFYING

Respondents reported that expanded choice offered to beneficiaries by Medicaid managed care also can result in reduced patient volume and a consequent drop in Medicaid revenues for traditional Medicaid providers.[6] These reports come from areas such as Miami, where Medicaid managed care plans are a well-established presence, as well as areas such as Little Rock, where Medicaid managed care has been slow to arrive. Traditional Medicaid providers reported that this loss of patient volume increases their financial vulnerability. However, intensified competition for Medicaid patients also creates an incentive for these providers to organize into networks or to align with larger systems. Providers reported that together they are less likely to be excluded from selective Medicaid managed care networks.

DECLINING MEDICAID REVENUES IMPERIL INDIGENT CARE

Respondents reported that declines in Medicaid revenues have significant financial implications for indigent care providers, since many of those providers rely on Medicaid revenue to subsidize the cost of treating uninsured and underinsured patients. Recent events in Indianapolis are emblematic of these interactions. In 1994 the state cut physician payment rates nearly in half and cut hospital payments by a lesser amount. Those reductions reportedly contributed to a budget shortfall at several area clinics. In response, one clinic system instituted a temporary limit on the number of new uninsured patients treated, citing the cut in payment rates coupled with a decline in projected Medicaid patient volume. Informants reported that reductions in Medicaid revenue have limited providers' ability to continue funding indigent care in several other study communities, including Orange County (California), Seattle, Miami, and Newark. Providers that have few other payers from whom they can generate cross-subsidies felt the effects most dramatically.

MEDICARE RISK CONTRACTING

Respondents identified Medicare payment rules for HMOs as having a major influence on local health system change. Under Medicare risk contracting, Medicare HMOs are paid on the basis of the average fee-for-service costs incurred by Medicare beneficiaries in a county. Because average fee-for-service costs vary considerably from site to site, Medicare HMO payment rules historically have encouraged Medicare HMOs in areas with high Medicare fee-for-service costs such as Miami and Orange County and discouraged Medicare HMOs in relatively low cost areas such as Greenville and Syracuse.[7]

MEDICARE LURES HEALTH PLAN CHAINS TO LOCAL MARKETS

In several Community Tracking sites with large Medicare populations and/or high Medicare payment rates, the Medicare risk program has attracted regional or national HMOs to the local market. Even in sites with low-to-moderate levels of Medicare HMO penetration, such as Little Rock and Cleveland, respondents reported that the prospect of significant growth in this area has helped to lure regional and national plans, including United Healthcare, Aetna, and Anthem. Out-of-area plans can change the nature of competition. In Seattle, for instance, respondents reported that PacifiCare, the nation's largest Medicare HMO chain, introduced a zero-premium product in 1996—an offer that others, including the dominant local player, Group Health Cooperative of Puget Sound, were forced to match.

MEDICARE RULES CAN SPUR COMMERCIAL HMO ENROLLMENT

In a number of Community Tracking sites, including Phoenix and Miami, respondents reported that Medicare managed care plans have led to increased levels of HMO enrollment among privately insured nonelderly populations. This "spillover" effect is driven largely by the Health Care Financing Administration's (HCFA's) fifty-fifty rule, which requires Medicare HMOs to enroll one privately sponsored enrollee for every Medicare beneficiary. Faced with this requirement, Medicare HMOs have had to expand their commercial business to continue enrolling new Medicare beneficiaries. In addition, in some markets where intense competition for private patients holds down private HMO premiums, respondents reported that Medicare HMOs use profits generated from their Medicare business to cross-subsidize commercial premiums.

NEW RISK-CONTRACTING RULES MAY ALTER THESE DYNAMICS

New Medicare rules enacted as part of the Balanced Budget Act of 1997 may have a large influence on both the entry of outside plans into local markets and the magnitude of the spillover effect.[8] With the introduction of payment rates that reflect a blend of national and local rates, HMO payments are expected to fall in high-cost communities that have witnessed the greatest amount of Medicare HMO activity to date and rise in low-cost areas where Medicare HMO growth has been comparatively slow.[9] Meanwhile, elimination of the fifty-fifty rule might lead to the expansion of Medicare HMOs in highly competitive managed care markets, since the ability of a plan to expand its Medicare business will no longer depend on its success in marketing to privately insured persons. At the same time, to the extent that the fifty-fifty rule has helped to drive commercial HMO penetration, this rule change can be expected to have a slight moderating influence on levels of HMO penetration among the nonelderly.

STATE REGULATION OF MANAGED CARE

Laws restricting the practices of managed care plans are highly visible and controversial in most study communities. Although a few states with Community Tracking sites, such as New York and New Jersey, recently enacted comprehensive managed care laws, most states have regulated managed care plans in a more piecemeal fashion, frequently in response to perceived abuses in the managed care industry brought to light by news reports or highly publicized lawsuits. Common managed care regulations in such states include bans on "gag rules" that restrict the ability of doctors to tell patients about alternative courses of treatment: minimum postpartum stay requirements; direct access to obstetrician/gynecologists; "prudent layperson" standards for coverage of emergency room visits; and restrictions on the ability of HMOs to require enrollees to use network pharmacists.

MANY RESTRICTIONS HAVE A LIMITED IMPACT
ON CARE DELIVERY

Despite the considerable attention generated by proposals to regulate managed care, most restrictions enacted in states we studied appear to have had only a minor impact on local health care systems. Such rules tend to address specific medical conditions or populations (for example, postpartum stays) or highly controversial issues that have little influence on how most HMOs do business (for example, gag rules). By contrast, Community Tracking states generally have avoided rules that affect the key mechanisms HMOs use to control costs, such as selective contracting with providers and financial incentives for physicians.

In the few Community Tracking sites whose states enacted more far-reaching rules during the study period, such rules have tended to be vitiated by subsequent policy actions. For instance, between 1995 and 1996 several states enacted "any-willing-provider" statutes that restrict plans' ability to selectively contract with providers. Interest groups in Indiana reportedly secured an exemption for HMOs; regulations implementing the state's any-willing-provider statute now ironically apply only to preferred provider arrangements and traditional indemnity plans. The Washington State legislature repealed the chief provisions of its any-willing-provider statute along with other key elements of that state's comprehensive reform bill. Finally, a sweeping any-willing-provider law was struck down by a U.S. district court judge in Arkansas as violating the Employee Retirement Income Security Act (ERISA), the federal pension law.[10]

NETWORKS AND "DOWNSTREAM RISK" ARE EMERGING ISSUES

Regulation of provider-sponsored networks (PSNs) is an emerging issue in many study communities. Sponsors of these networks contend that HMO-licensing rules requiring them to set aside reserves to protect enrollees against insolvencies create an insurmountable barrier to entry and are unnecessary since providers can "work off" unexpected claims costs. Policies that regulate PSNs differently than traditional HMOs inherently favor some players over others; this generates a high level of interest-group politics where these policies have been proposed.

To date, only two states with Community Tracking sites, New York and Ohio, have established such laws.[11] In Ohio new PSNs are required to set aside $200,000 less than other types of managed care plans are.[12] In New York new rules give regulators the authority to modify HMO solvency standards for PSNs based on a number of factors, including the level of risk sharing among participating providers and the plans' reinsurance arrangements.[13] In addition, the recently enacted federal budget law allows PSNs to be offered to the Medicare population and exempts such plans from state financial solvency rules in cases where those rules are judged to be a barrier to entry.[14] These new rules are likely to stimulate the development of PSNs, thereby forcing the issue of how these entities should be regulated onto the legislative and regulatory agendas in many more states.

A related issue concerns regulation of "downstream risk"—capitated payments and other forms of risk-based reimbursement passed on to provider groups by HMOs. Many Community Tracking states regulate these arrangements indirectly through solvency and quality standards imposed on the HMOs with which provider groups contract. Other states have established alternative HMO licensure requirements for providers accepting downstream risk for medical services they do not provide directly. In California, for instance, state law requires provider groups accepting global capitation to secure a limited HMO license that applies most quality and solvency requirements while waiving standards determined to be irrelevant to provider-sponsored entities, such as marketing rules and service-area requirements.[15] These provisions can have important market consequences. For instance, respondents in Orange County reported that limited HMO licensure has lowered the regulatory hurdle for providers seeking global capitation arrangements.

REGULATION OF PROVIDERS

State and local governments historically have implemented a wide array of policies regulating health care providers, including (1) CON laws, which establish a review process for providers seeking to build new facilities or offer certain services or procedures; and (2) hospital rate-setting systems, which set the prices facilities can charge for inpatient care. Cost control is the primary but not the exclusive goal of both types of policies.

The major trend in both of these policy areas is toward deregulation. Since the 1986 repeal of the federal statute mandating state CON programs, more than a dozen states, including four of the twelve states with Community Tracking sites, have repealed their CON laws or allowed those laws to sunset.[16] Rate-setting laws have been affected even more dramatically by deregulation: Laws have been repealed or allowed to sunset in each of the four study states that had such programs.

PROVIDERS USE REGULATION TO PURSUE COMPETITIVE ADVANTAGE

In several of the Community Tracking sites providers use their CON licenses to achieve competitive advantage. In Greenville, for instance, the largest hospital in the area has adroitly leveraged its monopoly over open-heart surgeries to secure managed care contracts that name the system as the exclusive hospital provider. CON programs also can affect market dynamics by increasing the market value of institutions that have been awarded CON licenses. In Newark, for example, the state's largest hospital system cited a local hospital's CON licenses for pediatrics and open-heart surgery as key factors in its recent decision to acquire that institution.

Hospital rate regulation also has affected the competitive balance in local markets, principally at the health plan level. By disallowing plans other than HMOs from negotiating hospital rates in New York and Massachusetts, state rate-setting laws have effectively precluded the development of viable preferred provider organization (PPO) markets in those states. Without the ability to secure hospital discounts, PPOs historically have been unable to distinguish themselves in those marketplaces.

MARKET RELATIONSHIPS CHANGE WITH DEREGULATION

Significant changes in market relationships and competitive strategies appear to take place in communities where CON and rate-setting laws have recently been repealed or where such actions are anticipated. In Syracuse, for instance, many respondents noted that a historical culture of cooperation and collaboration in the hospital sector is yielding to increased competition as providers prepare for a new era without hospital rate setting. In anticipation of the change, hospitals initiated various physician/hospital affiliations to secure referrals and maintain volume. In Boston and Newark a number of mergers and other types of affiliation agreements were consummated following repeal of their states' rate-setting laws, although respondents identified several additional factors driving these affiliation decisions.

DEREGULATION AFFECTS INDIGENT CARE

Indigent care programs and hospital rate-setting systems are closely linked in states that have implemented such systems. Historically, rate-setting programs have included both surcharges used to fund uncompensated care pools as well as a variety of mechanisms for channeling those funds to charity-care providers. Because of these linkages, respondents reported that the demise of rate-setting laws has posed difficult questions about whether and how communities will pay for indigent care in the future. In Newark, for example, deregulation of the state's rate-setting system eliminated the principal funding mechanism for indigent care—a 19 percent surcharge on hospital bills.[17] At the same time, insurers in Newark have used their newly won ability to negotiate discounted hospital rates, driving down hospital margins. Newark's safety-net hospitals have found it difficult to survive in this new environment. One of these hospitals closed in early 1997 with a $50 million debt attributed to the institution's loss of funding for indigent care. Other inner-city hospitals in Newark were reported to be vulnerable as well, with several recently announcing layoffs, reductions in beds, and cuts in major service lines.

Recent deregulation of hospital rates in Massachusetts and New York also has led to concerns about indigent care. In both of those states, however, a combination of public policy and market forces appears to have forestalled a major breach in the safety net, at least for now.

REGULATION AND OVERSIGHT OF NOT-FOR-PROFIT CONVERSIONS

The increasing pace of conversions of non-profit hospitals and health plans to for-profit status is leading to heightened oversight and regulation in several study communities. In at least two states, Massachusetts and California, conversion policy is set forth in guidelines issued by the state attorneys general.[18] The central goal of these guidelines is to protect the public's investment in nonprofit entities conferred through tax exemptions and other forms of public finance. Consequently, the major policy issues addressed by these rules are (1) how converting assets should be valued; (2) who gets the money from the sale of charitable assets and for what ends; (3) processes for disclosing the terms of these transactions and for securing public input; and (4) assurances that unprofitable services such as trauma care, emergency room services, and care for the uninsured will be maintained.

Courts often play an active role in the shaping of conversion policy because of the ambiguous nature of most state laws specifying who owns nonprofit corporations, a deficiency that frequently results in litigation.[19] In some states with Community Tracking sites high-profile conversions also have stimulated increased legislative activity to clarify the law and increase public oversight over such transactions. Since mid-1996 no fewer than five states with Community Tracking sites have passed new laws regulating such transactions.[20]

PUBLIC OFFICIALS CAN CHANGE THE TERMS OF PRIVATE TRANSACTIONS OR BLOCK THEM OUTRIGHT

Intervention by public officials can alter the terms of these transactions, often in significant ways. For instance, according to one account of the conversion of Health Net, a California HMO, regulatory intervention resulted in a final valuation equal to three times the initial proposal as well as an 80 percent equity interest in the plan's converted for-profit business. The cash and stock were used to endow a grant-making charity (the California Wellness Foundation) with assets that are now worth $800–$900 million.[21] Explicit valuation guidelines are likely to have a more systematic impact on the terms of conversions, although respondents reported that their impact has not yet been sufficiently tested.

Regulators in a number of the study communities also have used the courts or their own administrative authority to block the conversion of nonprofit entities outright. Importantly, these actions have slowed the entry of outside players into local health care markets. In Lansing a state judge effectively blocked Columbia/HCA's attempt to acquire Michigan Capital Medical Center through a proposed joint venture that would have transferred 50 percent of the nonprofit's assets to Columbia/HCA along with effective control over several key corporate functions.[22] According to informants, Columbia/HCA's proposal heightened concerns about the market entrance of an "outsider" and stimulated a plan proposed by the United Auto Workers and several area purchasers to play a more active role in the community's hospital sector.

In a second case that generated national attention, Ohio's attorney general successfully sued to prevent a joint venture between Columbia/HCA and Blue Cross and Blue Shield of Ohio, which would have established a for-profit subsidiary holding 85 percent of the health plan's assets.[23] In contrast, policymakers in Ohio have not blocked the acquisition of several hospitals in the Cleveland area by Columbia/HCA and Primary Health Systems, another investor-owned hospital chain.

ISSUES TO TRACK

The Community Tracking study sheds light on the important role of public policy in shaping health system change. Although deregulation is a dominant theme in several policy areas such as provider rate setting and CON programs, policymakers appear willing to assert a more active public policy role in other areas, such as the regulation of managed care plans and oversight of nonprofit conversions. Evidence from this study suggests that health policy is likely to reflect a constantly shifting blend of these approaches, with policymakers relying primarily on market forces to control health care costs but resorting to regulation to mitigate harms perceived to result from these forces.

Several areas of health policy merit continued monitoring as policymakers endeavor to strike this balance. First, many states with Community Tracking sites are at a critical juncture with respect to regulation of managed care. Will policymakers stop with enactment of high-visibility/low-impact regulations such as prohibition of gag rules and postpartum-stay standards, or will they push for more aggressive regulations that could cause premiums to increase? State policymakers also will have to make decisions about how to regulate downstream risk and novel organizational forms such as provider-sponsored networks. The federal government's embrace of PSNs for Medicare enrollees can only be expected to speed the pace of state-level policy development in this area.

Continued efforts to control public-sector health spending also will have a major impact on health system change. Recent changes in the way Medicare calculates HMO payment rates can be expected to have important implications for the growth of managed care in the Community Tracking sites, while changes in Medicare reimbursement rates for providers will have a direct impact on hospitals' bottom lines. States' efforts to control Medicaid spending through managed care also warrant close attention, given the number of states with Community Tracking sites that will be implementing such programs over the next several years.

Finally, policy executed over the next few years will be critical to the continued financial viability of indigent care providers and access to care for the growing numbers of uninsured and underinsured Americans. A number of the states we studied, including Massachusetts, Arkansas, and Florida, are undertaking major initiatives to provide insurance coverage to uninsured children. These initiatives, bolstered by new federal dollars available for state-run children's health insurance programs, are likely to ease the strain on the health care safety net. It is unclear, however, how these initiatives will fare against the adverse effects of other policy changes, falling rates of employer-sponsored insurance, and increasing discounts demanded by public and private payers—forces that are likely to pose a continued threat to indigent care providers and the patients they serve.

NOTES

1.   The design of the Community Tracking Study is described in P. Kemper et al., "The Design of the Community Tracking Study: A Longitudinal Study of Health System Change and Its Effect on People," *Inquiry* (Summer 1996): 195–206. The twelve metropolitan statistical areas that are part of the Community Tracking Study are Boston, Massachusetts; Cleveland, Ohio; Greenville, South Carolina; Indianapolis, Indiana; Lansing, Michigan; Little Rock, Arkansas; Miami, Florida; Newark, New Jersey; Orange County, California; Phoenix, Arizona; Seattle, Washington; and Syracuse, New York. For descriptions of the communities and site visit methods, see L. Kohn et al., eds., *Health System Change in Twelve Communities* (Washington: Center for Studying Health System Change, 1997).

2.   See, for instance. A. Katz and J. Thompson, "The Role of Public Policy in Health Care Market Change," *Health Affairs* (Summer 1996): 77–91; P. Starr, *The Social Transformation of American Medicine* (New York: Basic Books, 1982); and J. Robinson and H. Luft, "Competition, Regulation, and Hospital Costs: 1982 to 1986," *Journal of the American Medical Association* (11 June 1988): 2676–2682.

3.   Katz and Thompson, "The Role of Public Policy in Health Care Market Change," 90; and P.B. Ginsburg, "The RWJF Community Snapshots Study: Introduction and Overview," *Health Affairs* (Summer 1996): 7–20.

4.   Indigent care policy and other policies relating specifically to care for the poor are discussed in detail in a Lewin Group paper: R. Feldman and R. Baxter, "The Impact of Health System Change on Traditional Providers of Care to the Poor" (forthcoming).

5.   These programs implemented at the discretion of the states are distinguished here from early implementation of federally mandated increases in the federal poverty level for children and pregnant women who are categorically eligible for Medicaid.

6.   R.J. Baxter and R.E. Mechanic, "The Status of Local Health Care Safety Nets," *Health Affairs* (July/August 1997): 7–23.

7.   W.P. Welch, "Improving Medicare Payments to HMOs: Urban Core versus Suburban Ring," *Inquiry* (Spring 1989): 62–71.

8.   *Balanced Budget Act of 1997*, HR. 2015,105th Cong.,1st sess. (1997), sec. 5001.

9.   "New Medicare HMO Rates: One Plan's Ceiling Is Another Plan's Floor," *Medicine and Health*, 15 September 1997, 1.

10.   "Update: Any Willing Provider," *State Health Notes*, 3 April 1997, 3.

11.   National Association of Insurance Commissioners, "Draft White Paper on State Regulation of Risk-Bearing Entities" (Washington: NAIC, December 1996).

12.   Ty Pine, Ohio State Department of Insurance. personal communication, 16 September 1997.

13.   A.B. 11330, sec. 4408, "Financial Requirements for Integrated Delivery Systems," New York State Department of Insurance (Undated draft).

14.   *Balanced Budget Act of 1997*, H.R 2015, sec. 5001.

15.   Lewin Group, *State Regulatory Experience with Provider Sponsored Organizations: Final Paper* (Prepared for the U.S. Department of Health and Human Services,

Office of the Assistant Secretary for Planning and Evaluation, HHS Contract no. 100-93-0012, 11 June 1997), C-3.

16. Health Policy Tracking Service, Intergovernmental Health Policy Project, National Conference of State Legislatures. Washington. D.C., October 1996.

17. That reform followed a federal judge's ruling, later overturned, that the surcharge violated the Employee Retirement Income Security Act (ERISA). See J. Cantor, "Health Care Unreform: The New Jersey Approach, *Journal of the American Medical Association* (22/29 December 1993): 2968.

18. California Department of Justice, Office of the Attorney General, *Review Protocol: Ownership or Control Transfers of Nonprofit Health Facilities* (Corporations Code Sections 5914 et seq.) (Sacramento, undated); and Office of the Attorney General, Commonwealth of Massachusetts, *For-Profit Conversions and Acquisition of Non-Profits: Attorney General Issues and Procedures* (Boston, 30 October 1995).

19. D. Shriber, "State Experience in Regulating a Changing Health Care System," *Health Affairs* (March/April 1997): 49–50.

20. S. 1288 (Arizona), enacted 7 April 1997; H. 1826 (Indiana), enacted 13 May 1997; H. 242 (Ohio), enacted 6 May 1997; S. 5227 (Washington), enacted 13 May 1997; and A.B. 3101 (California), enacted 30 September1996.

21. J. Bell et al., "The Preservation of Charitable Health Care Assets," *Health Affairs* (March/April 1997): 126.

22. R. Tomsho, "Columbia/HCA Move into Michigan Blocked by Judge," *Wall Street Journal*, 9 September 1996, B8.

23. Shriber, "State Experience in Regulating a Changing Health Care System," 63.

4 | # Do Different Funding Mechanisms Produce Different Results? The Implications of Family Planning for Fiscal Federalism

**Deborah R. McFarlane
and Kenneth J. Meier**

Fiscal federalism is again on the national agenda. The 104th Congress, marking the first Republican control of both houses in forty years, provided the most recent impetus. Immediately following the 1994 election, some Republican governors and pivotal House members discussed replacing more than three hundred federal assistance programs worth $125 billion per year with block grants to the states (Katz 1995a). These proposals dwarfed even the most sweeping changes that Ronald Reagan entertained in 1981.

Federal block grants are lump sums that the federal government gives to subnational governments, usually the states. Block grants allow state and local governments to choose how to spend their federal money within broad areas (e.g., maternal and child health, social services, community development). In the past, block grants often have been formed by combining several categorical grants. Unlike block grants, federal categorical grants are awarded for particular

Reprinted from *Journal of Health Politics, Policy and Law*, 23, no. 3 (June 1998): 423–54. Copyright 1998. Duke University Press. All rights reserved. Reprinted with permission.

programs. Categorical grants specify the purpose of the aid and how funds are to be used. Over the years, Congress has enacted many categorical grant programs to address geographic and socioeconomic inequities in particular services.

How federal aid is to be structured is a controversial subject. Block grant proponents argue that states and other subnational governments should determine their own needs and priorities (Brandt 1981; Williamson 1990). Moreover, block grants may provide administrative savings (G. Peterson et al. 1986). However, critics point out that under block grants, service needs in the states often remain unmet. States' political preferences often influence their allocation of federal block grants more so than their actual needs (Henig 1985). Administrative savings from consolidating categorical grants have also not been demonstrated (U.S. GAO 1984).

This time, block grants had a new twist (Katz 1995c). Congress considered not only consolidating federal categorical grants to the states, but also converting federal entitlement programs to block grants.[1] Entitlement programs provide benefits to anyone meeting their qualification criteria (Fraley 1995). When President Clinton signed the Temporary Assistance for Needy Families (TANF) Act into law on 22 August 1996, a block grant replaced Aid to Families with Dependent Children (AFDC), "the nation's main cash welfare program and several related programs" (Katz 1996: 2192). Turning a federal entitlement program into a block grant was unprecedented (Katz 1996). Both Congress and the National Governors' Association, however, proposed this change not only for welfare but also for the Medicaid program (Pear 1996; MacPherson 1995).

Medicaid is the largest intergovernmental entitlement, accounting for more than 40 percent of all federal outlays to the states (ACIR 1995). With its huge cost increases and "a constituency with relatively little clout," the Medicaid program has been an obvious budget target (A Range of Budget Targets 1995). At a mere $17 billion in 1995, federal outlays for welfare (family support) were eclipsed by the $88.4 billion Medicaid program. Nevertheless, welfare is even less popular than Medicaid (Schlesinger and Lee 1993), so Medicaid emerged mostly unscathed, while AFDC was altered profoundly.[2]

Currently, the new welfare block grant program is being implemented. Eventually, budgetary pressures on the federal government will force Congress to address the structure of Medicaid as well as that of other entitlement programs. The purpose of this article is to examine whether changing the grant mechanisms will make a difference. In other words, are certain grant mechanisms more effective than others? Will program impacts change if different grant mechanisms are used?

We approach these questions in several ways. First, we establish a context by providing a brief history of federal assistance to subnational governments. Second, we review empirical and theoretical literature relevant to the impact of different types of federal aid. Third, we describe a federal policy—family planning—funded by four statutes that employ three different types of grants. Fourth, we recount the empirical research that has been conducted on family planning impacts. Fifth, we develop hypotheses about differential program impacts. Sixth, we use a pooled time series analysis to partition out the respective impacts of each grant program. Seventh, and finally, we examine the implications of our findings for family planning, health policy, and fiscal federalism.

A BRIEF HISTORY OF FEDERAL AID

GROWTH OF GRANTS AND EXPENDITURES (1960–1995)

Federal aid to subnational governments is largely a phenomenon of the second half of the twentieth century. In 1950, federal aid totaled about $2.23 billion annually and funded fifty-two separate programs. By fiscal 1981, outlays for intergovernmental grants were $54.0 billion, with 540 intergovernmental grants. The Reagan devolution reduced the number of grants to 404; by 1984, however, the total outlays of $90.8 billion already exceeded the 1981 expenditure levels. By fiscal 1995, the number of intergovernmental grants had risen to 633 with outlays totaling $225.7 billion (ACIR 1995).

Even considering inflation, tremendous growth has occurred in intergovernmental grants. From 1975 to 1995, federal expenditures (in real dollars) for intergovernmental grants increased nearly 80 percent. Most of that growth emanated from the entitlement programs (ACIR 1995). Over the last thirty years this growth has contributed to the debate about the structure of federal aid (Conlan 1984, 1988; A Range of Budget Targets 1995).

DEBATING THE STRUCTURE OF FEDERAL AID (1967–1996)

Johnson Administration

During the 1960s, federal expenditures for intergovernmental programs nearly tripled, while the number of grants increased by 258 percent. Recognizing the administrative problems resulting from the rapid expansion of federal programs during the post–World War II period (especially from 1964 to 1968), Johnson initiated a number of grant consolidations (Conlan 1984).

Nixon Administration

Under the auspices of his New Federalism, Nixon also supported grant consolidation. The president favored block grants, not only for managerial streamlining, but also for partisan and ideological reasons. By consolidating categorical grants into block grants, Nixon hoped to reduce the influence of the so-called iron triangles, the Washington-based interest groups and their congressional and bureaucratic allies who advocated for and presumably benefited from individual categorical grants (Conlan 1984).

Nixon's proposals met with limited success. Only two block grants were enacted during his five-year presidency—the Comprehensive Employment Training Act (CETA) and Community Development Block Grants (CDBG). Both grants *increased* federal spending, partly to finance "hold harmless" provisions, which were enacted to protect former categorical recipients from loss of funds (Conlan 1984). Another block grant program—title XX of the Social Security Act—was designed by the Nixon administration, but was not enacted until 1975. Title XX, the Social Services Block Grant, did not consolidate categorical grants per se. Instead, this block grant put a ceiling on federal social services grant spending and gave states more discretion in using those funds (Derthick 1975). No other federal block grants were enacted during the 1970s.

Reagan Administration

Dramatic changes in intergovernmental aid occurred in the early 1980s. In 1981, the Reagan administration was able to consolidate seventy-seven categorical grants into nine block grants. In this process, sixty-two other programs were terminated. This time, "hold harmless" provisions were not considered. Retrenchment was very much a goal of grant consolidation, along with devolving programmatic and fiscal responsibilities to the states (Nathan and Dolittle 1987). Overall, these grant consolidations reduced 1981 categorical grant funding levels by 9 percent, although reductions for individual health programs ranged from 17 to 45 percent (Peterson 1984). At the time, the 1981 block grant consolidations were the largest in American history (Benda and Levine 1988).

In spite of this upheaval, neither the structure nor the expenditure patterns of intergovernmental grants was permanently altered. During the remainder of the 1980s and early 1990s, the number of categorical grants increased again. By 1991, there were more categorical grants (384) than in 1981 (361). There was a net increase of only three block grants from 1982 to 1995. In terms of outlays, however, entitlements became increasingly dominant (ACIR 1995).

Medicaid Growth

The most prominent increase in federal grant outlays to subnational governments occurred in the Medicaid program. To put this program into historical perspective, Medicaid costs in 1975 represented only 14 percent of total federal grant outlays. By 1995, 39 percent of total federal grant outlays went to support the Medicaid program (ACIR 1995).

Another way to look at the magnitude of Medicaid is to examine the percentage of state spending. In 1994, Medicaid accounted for 19.4 percent of state spending, nearly double the 10.2 percent of 1987 (Fraley 1995: 1637). Indeed, state costs for Medicaid were a major factor in putting health care reform on the national agenda in 1993 and 1994 (ACIR 1993). Of course, agenda setting and policy enactment are not the same (Kingdon 1984, 1995), and the demise of federal health care reform and its etiology have been amply documented (Skocpol 1995; Steinmo and Watts 1995). What is germane here is that without a major intervention, such as national health insurance, Medicaid costs have continued to increase rapidly.

The 104th Congress

The Republican majority came to Washington intent on keeping its "Contract with America," which included balancing the budget. That, of course, meant budget cuts. Initially, federal programs in eight areas were considered, encompassing 336 federal programs worth about $125 billion per year. As the deliberations continued, four types of assistance remained on the active agenda: cash welfare (mainly AFDC), child welfare, child care, and food and nutrition (Katz 1995b). Except for the food stamp program, which was strongly backed by the agricultural industry (Leone 1995), each of the other three programs was converted to a block grant during the 104th Congress.

PRIOR RESEARCH ON THE EFFECTS OF FEDERAL AID

Even within the context of the dynamic history of intergovernmental transfers, the budgetary cuts proposed by the 104th Congress were enormous. Although many of the proposals were not enacted, the structural changes passed into law were unprecedented. Few argue that services will not be decreased as a result of budgetary cuts alone, but do the structural changes themselves portend massive shifts in the impact of public programs?

In order to address this question, we turn to both empirical and theoretical literature. Empirical studies of Reagan's federalism document state behavior during massive shifts in intergovernmental transfers. In political science, the Mazmanian and Sabatier model of policy implementation posits that program impacts are actually a function of policy construction. In public finance economics, the Gramlich typology of intergovernmental aid focuses on a single characteristic of distributive public policy and indicates that different grant forms produce different outputs.

STUDIES OF REAGAN'S FEDERALISM

Descriptive studies of another dramatic shift in the structure of federal aid, Reagan's new federalism, did not address program impacts. These studies did document reductions in program outputs, namely, expenditures. Federal budget cuts fell disproportionately upon the poor and most states did not replace those dollars (G. E. Peterson et al. 1986; Nathan and Dolittle 1987; U.S. GAO 1984; Custis 1988). Using an econometric model, one study of education policy during this period projected that merely moving federal funds from categorical to block grants would reduce the total amount spent for public education (Craig and Inman 1982).

SABATIER AND MAZMANIAN'S POLICY IMPLEMENTATION MODEL

The policy implementation literature from political science arose in response to the alleged failures of federal enactments passed from the mid-1960s to the early 1970s. What began as many disparate case studies of different policy areas culminated in the development of models of the implementation process in general. Among these important efforts were Van Meter and Van Horn (1975), Barduch (1977), and Berman (1978). Each of these contributed to the development of the widely cited and applied Mazmanian and Sabatier implementation framework (1981, 1983, 1989).

This model does consider factors that affect program impacts. Indeed, Mazmanian and Sabatier hypothesize that both program outputs and outcomes are functions of policy construction (Mazmanian and Sabatier 1981, 1983, 1989). More specifically, a policy's *coherence* is directly related to the likelihood that statutory goals will be achieved (McFarlane 1989). The seven conditions for statutory coherence include the following: (1) precise and clearly ranked objectives; (2) the incorporation of adequate causal theory; (3) sufficient financial resources for implementing organizations; (4) hierarchical integration within and among implementing organizations (meaning few veto points in the implementation process, as well as sanctions or inducements to overcome resistance); (5) favorable decision rules for implementing organizations; (6) the commitment of implementing agencies and officials; and (7) opportunities for formal participation by supporters of statutory objectives.

More than twenty-five empirical assessments have used portions of the Mazmanian and Sabatier framework (1989: 292), but only three have addressed the statutory coherence hypothesis directly (Sabatier and Klosterman 1981; McFarlane 1989; Meier and McFarlane 1996). The findings of each study supported the statutory coherence hypothesis, including the most recent work, which extended the analysis to policy impacts. How policies are constructed affects program impacts.

GRAMLICH'S TYPOLOGY OF INTERGOVERNMENTAL GRANTS

In his seminal review of intergovernmental grants, Gramlich focuses upon a single characteristic of distributive public policy—the grant form used to allocate

TABLE 4.1

Intergovernmental Grant Mechanisms

Grants	Mechanism	Process	Empirical Results	Examples
Type A	Open-ended, matching	Alters the relative prices of designated public services.	Usually less additional spending than size of the grant.	AFDC, Medicaid
Type B	Closed-ended, unconditional assistance	Changes income of subnational community.	Some tax reduction and some expenditure increase, less than for Type A.	Revenue-sharing, some block grants
Type C	Closed-ended, conditional	Requires expenditures for certain goods or services.	Local spending roughly equal to size of grant.	Title X of the PHS

Source: Gramlich 1977.

funding. From the field of public finance economics, Gramlich's typology of grants discusses the differential performance of intergovernmental transfers. He divided federal aid into three types of grants: Type A, Type B, and Type C. Type A grants are open-ended matching grants that alter the relative prices faced by lower levels of government. Medicaid is an example. Type B grants are closed-ended, nonrestrictive grants to lower levels of government (e.g., revenue sharing and block grants). Type C grants are closed-ended, categorical grants (Gramlich 1977).[3]

Gramlich summarized the empirical findings about expenditures under each type of grant. Open-ended federal matching grants (Type A) usually result in somewhat less spending than the size of the grant. Type B grants stimulate more local spending, but the expenditure increase for Type B grants is less than for open-ended matching grants (see Table 4.1). Typically, the federal government establishes rather tight controls over the way Type C grant money can be spent, so it is not surprising that categorical grants stimulate subnational spending roughly equal to the grant amount (Gramlich 1977).

In summary, empirical research has shown that functional spending— that is, expenditures for specific program areas—varies by the type of intergovernmental grant. Gramlich encouraged researchers to extend their work on the outputs (e.g., expenditures) of federal grants to include the outcomes of such programs. To date, no one has undertaken that challenge. This study is an effort to fill that gap.

TABLE 4.2

Federal Statutes Authorizing Funds for Family Planning Services, Grant Characteristics, and Administrative Mechanisms, by Grant Type (Gramlich)

Statute	Grant Characteristics and Administrative Mechanisms	Grant Type (Gramlich)
Maternal and Child Health, title V, Social Security Act	Closed-ended, formula grants matched by the states. Administered by state health departments.	Type B
Family Planning and Population, title X, Public Health Service Act	Categorical legislation with project grants. May or may not be administered by a state agency.	Type C
Medicaid, title XIX, Social Security act	Reimbursement of providers for services rendered to eligible clients. Must be administered by a state agency.	Type A
Social Services, title XX, Social Security Act	Block grant to state agency, usually state welfare department. Allocation based on state's population size.	Type B

FEDERAL FAMILY PLANNING POLICIES

Four statutes, representing three types of grant mechanisms, authorized most of the federal funds for publicly supported family planning services during fiscal years 1982–1994: title V of the Social Security Act, title X of the Public Health Service Act, title XIX of the Social Security Act, and title XX of the Social Security Act (see Table 4.2). Each statute provides funding to all fifty states, but not all states use monies from each of the grants for family planning services (see Table 4.3).

TITLE V OF THE SOCIAL SECURITY ACT

Title V is a block grant program (Type B), which uses a formula to award maternal and child health monies to state health departments. States with poorer health indicators (e.g., numbers of low-income children) receive proportionately more title V money than states where maternal and child health status is better (U.S. Department of Health and Human Services Public Health Service 1997). States have to match federal title V allocations: for every $3 contributed by the federal government, the states must match it with $4. States are not required to spend title V monies for family planning nor does title V define what services are included in family planning.

TABLE 4.3

Number of States Using Specific Sources of Federal Funding

Year	Title V	Title X	Title XIX	Title XX
1982	37	50	43	28
1983	39	50	47	25
1985	36	50	43	21
1987	32	50	49	19
1990	35	50	47	15
1992	34	50	46	16
1994	36	50	45	16

Source. 1982 expenditures (AGI 1983); 1983 expenditures (Gold and Nestor 1985); 1985 expenditures (Gold and Macias 1986); 1987 expenditures (Gold and Guardado 1988); 1990 expenditures (Gold and Daley 1991); 1992 expenditures (Daley and Gold 1993); 1994 expenditures (Sollom et al. 1996).

TITLE X OF THE PUBLIC HEALTH SERVICE ACT

Title X is a categorical program (Type C), emanating from the Population Research and Family Planning Act of 1970 (see Table 4.4). Title X is earmarked to fund *only* family planning services. The regional offices of the U.S. Public Health Service award grants directly to projects that either provide or subcontract for services. By accepting these funds, title X grantees agree to adhere to strict guidelines regarding the provision and breadth of family planning services. Unlike the other three federal grant programs, title X does not mandate that a state agency has to be the grantee, though state agencies are not excluded from seeking these funds. In thirty-five states, the state health department is the title X grantee.[4]

TITLE XIX OF THE SOCIAL SECURITY ACT

The Medicaid program is a federal-state venture to provide health services to certain categories of the poor (Type A). Title XIX mandates state agency administration, which is the welfare department in most states. Medicaid reimburses providers for services rendered to eligible persons. Unlike the other federal sources of family planning funding, there is no federal ceiling on Medicaid. The federal government simply reimburses the state for a proportion of the amount that it spends. Not surprisingly, the Medicaid program was the only one of the four federal statutes that actually increased its family planning expenditures throughout the past decade. Across the states, there is no uniform definition for federal family planning services.

TABLE 4.4

**Federal Expenditures for Family Planning Services by
Source of Funding (Dollars in Millions) and Percentage
Contribution to Federal Outlays (FY 1982–1994)**

Source of Funding	*Fiscal Year*[1]						
	1982	*1983*	*1985*	*1987*	*1990*	*1992*	*1994*
Title V	16.6	19.1	23.1	31.0	27.1	29.3	34.1
(state administered MCH block grants)	(6%)	(7%)	(7%)	(9%)	(7%)	(6%)	(6%)
Title X	118.1	117.1	133.5	130.7	111.8	110.4	151.1
(federally administered categorical family planning grant)	(43%)	(41%)	(40%)	(39%)	(31%)	(23%)	(27%)
Title XIX[2]	94.2	108.8	137.1	137.8	190.0	319.2	332.4
(state administered Medicaid program)	(34%)	(38%)	(41%)	(41%)	(52%)	(65%)	(60%)
Title XX[3]	46.2	37.9	40.1	35.3	34.3	29.8	33.6
(state administered social services block grant)	(17%)	(13%)	(12%)	(11%)	(9%)	(6%)	(6%)
TOTAL	275.1	282.9	333.8	334.8	363.2	488.7	553.6

Source. 1982 expenditures (AGI 1983); 1983 expenditures (Gold and Nestor 1985); 1985 expenditures (Gold and Macias 1986); 1987 expenditures (Gold and Guardado 1988); 1990 expenditures (Gold and Daley 1991); 1992 expenditures (Daley and Gold 1993); 1994 expenditures (Sollom, Gold, and Saul 1996).
Note. Due to rounding, the percentages in this table may not add up to 100.
[1]Expenditure data were not collected for FY 1984, 1986, 1988, 1989, 1991, or 1993.
[2]Expenditures for contraceptive services only.
[3]Expenditures for medical services only.

TITLE XX OF THE SOCIAL SECURITY ACT

The social services block grant funds (Type B) of title XX are allocated to the states on the basis of population. Unlike the Medicaid program, there is a national ceiling on title XX funds. By statute, state welfare or social service departments administer title XX funds. States have great discretion here and may choose to spend these monies for any type of social service, including family planning. In 1994, only sixteen states spent title XX monies for family planning, accounting for 6 percent of all federal family planning expenditures (see Table 4.4). This situation contrasts greatly with state title XX spending in 1981, when there was a favorable federal match for title XX expenditures for family planning. At that point, thirty-four states spent title XX funds for family planning services, accounting for 19 percent of the federal family planning effort (McFarlane and Meier 1993).

EMPIRICAL RESEARCH ON FAMILY PLANNING IMPACTS

The benefits of family planning are well known. Family planning services assist people in planning their fertility. By decreasing unintended pregnancies, family planning services can reduce the number of abortions and unwanted births. Family planning services also contribute to improved maternal and child health (Institute of Medicine 1995; Meier and McFarlane 1994).

Various studies have evaluated the impact of publicly funded family planning services. Using 1969–70 data, Cutright and Jaffe (1976) concluded that the U.S. family planning program reduced the fertility of low-income women by helping them prevent unwanted and mistimed births. In an analysis of 1980 data, Anderson and Cope (1987) documented that public family planning programs actually lower fertility in areas where they operate. Grossman and Jacobowitz (1981) and, subsequently, Corman and Grossman (1985) reported that organized family planning services reduced both infant and neonatal mortality rates.

Forrest and Singh performed cost-benefit analyses for the United States as a whole (1990a) and for California in particular (1990b). Their studies showed that for every dollar of public funds spent to provide contraceptive services, an average of $4.40 was saved in public sector costs. The savings were more in states that have relatively generous health and social service benefits. For example, the comparable savings from funding a dollar of family planning services in California was $7.70.

These studies did not look at public sector savings by source of funding. The researchers did not consider whether different sources of funding might yield different cost-benefit ratios. That savings may differ by source of funding is suggested by a 1989 study (Radecki and Bernstein), conducted in Los Angeles, showing that family planning services funded by Medicaid were almost twice as expensive as those provided by publicly supported family planning clinics. A high proportion of the Medicaid services were delivered by private physicians; presumably, almost all of the publicly supported family planning clinics had at least some title X money.

Meier and McFarlane (1994) analyzed the public health benefits from funding family planning and abortion services from 1982 to 1988. They assessed *how much* public expenditures for family planning and abortion improved maternal and child health, including unwanted fertility. Among their findings were that states that had higher total public expenditures for family planning had significantly fewer abortions, low-birthweight babies, births with late or no prenatal care, infant deaths, and neonatal deaths. Subsidized family planning services, on the other hand, did not affect the teen birthrates or the percentage of premature babies. The differential impact of various funding sources was not assessed in this work. A more recent study did show that a dollar expenditure on family planning by title X had more impact on maternal and child health during 1982–1988 than did a dollar spent by a combination of the other sources of public family planning funds (Meier and McFarlane 1996).

While these findings are reassuring to advocates of family planning, they do not provide sufficient guidance to policy makers involved in the legislative process. Family planning is funded by four different federal statutes, each of which goes through a separate authorization process and is administered by a separate federal agency. To date, no published study has examined whether the different grant mechanisms that fund family planning services produce the same impacts (Institute of Medicine 1995: 219). This study addresses that question and uses the Gramlich typology to develop specific hypotheses about the performance of family planning grants.

HYPOTHESES

Because it is a categorical program, we expect that title X is the most effective federal family planning statute in terms of producing desired impacts. We also expect that title XIX, an entitlement program or a Type A grant, is more effective than the block grants, titles V and XX, in producing fertility and health benefits.

METHODS AND MATERIALS

DEPENDENT VARIABLES

Unintended Pregnancies

Annual state data on unintended pregnancies do not exist; however, an increase in unintended pregnancies affects two measures for which data are available— the birthrate and the induced abortion rate.[5] We believe that these are valid proxies. Over half of unintended pregnancies result in induced abortions (Forrest 1994),[6] and 44 percent of all births in the United States are the result of unintended pregnancies (Institute of Medicine 1995). The measures are the birthrate (number of births per 1,000 population) and the abortion rate (number of abortions per 1,000 women ages fifteen to forty-four).[7]

Maternal and Child Health

We used a single indicator of maternal and child health—infant mortality. Both the social science and biomedical literatures have documented that infant mortality is an important indicator of a population's health status and well-being (Singh and Yu 1995). The infant mortality rate is the number of deaths among

TABLE 4.5

Descriptive Statistics

Variable	Mean	Standard Deviation
Family Planning		
Title X	.58	.19
Title XIX	.59	.46
Titles V and XX	.22	.22
State Funding	.27	.38
Dependent Variables		
Birth Rate	15.92	2.11
Abortion Rate	22.25	9.73
Infant Mortality	10.07	1.65
Control Variables		
Population		
Black	9.53	9.14
Hispanic	5.11	7.26
Catholic	18.68	13.28
Income (in $1000)	14.39	3.42
Female Labor Participation	56.08	4.87
Abortion Facilities	27.71	27.71
Funded Abortion Rate	1.39	3.00

infants less than one year of age per 1,000 live births in that year.[8] The means and standard deviations for all variables are shown in Table 4.5.

Family planning programs have the potential to reduce infant mortality rates in several ways. Women whose pregnancies are planned are more likely to receive adequate prenatal care than women experiencing unplanned pregnancies (Institute of Medicine 1995; Joyce and Grossman 1990; Weller, Eberstein, and Bailey 1987; Marsiglio and Mott 1988). Women with unintentional conceptions are more likely to smoke and to drink during pregnancy (Institute of Medicine 1995). Smoking, in particular,[9] is a risk factor for low birthweight and infant mortality (Shiano and Behrman 1995). Clearly, less prenatal care, along with other behavioral risk factors associated with unintended pregnancies, should increase infant mortality rates.

INDEPENDENT VARIABLES

Family Planning Funds

As discussed earlier, four sources of federal funds may be used for publicly subsidized family planning services in the states. Title X provides funding through categorical grants (Type C) that can be used only for family planning.

Titles V (Maternal and Child Health) and XX (Social Services) are block grants (Type B). Title XIX is the Medicaid program (Type A).

The best source of data for family planning funds is the Alan Guttmacher Institute (AGI), but the institute does not collect data for every year. Because title X funds are specifically earmarked for family planning, an alternative source of annual data is available. Total title X funds per state for each year were taken from the U.S. Domestic Programs Database (Bickers and Stein 1994). We relied on the AGI data for 1982–1991 for the other sources of federal funding. Where data were missing, we called the state agencies responsible for title X implementation. In most cases, we had to follow-up with calls to other state agencies, such as the state welfare department or the state health department. If the state agencies did not know the amounts of specific annual expenditures, or when follow-up was unsuccessful, we interpolated to estimate missing data. Except for a few cases where the states themselves provided data, we interpolated for missing years. These expenditure data were converted to per-capita expenditures in 1982 constant dollars.[10] Since our concern was the relative impact of the various types of grant programs, we included per-capita measures of title X (Type C), title XIX (Type A), and the combined total for title V and title XX (Type B). Because some states also appropriate money for family planning expenditures, we included state funds as a separate category.

Control Variables

Unintended pregnancy rates as well as infant health are obviously influenced by a variety of forces besides family planning efforts. In order to get a precise estimate of the impact of the individual family planning policies, some effort must be made to control for these other forces. Perhaps the most important single influence on both unintended fertility and infant health is poverty.

Race and poverty are intertwined in the United States. About 14.5 percent of the U.S. population lives in poverty. The racial breakdown is that 11.6 percent of whites, 33.3 percent of blacks, and 29.3 percent of Hispanics live in poverty (U.S. Bureau of the Census 1994: Table 730). The racial composition of a state's population can affect the dependent variables in several ways. Overall, nonwhite women experience higher fertility rates than do white women (U.S. Bureau of the Census 1994: Table 92). "Consistent with the higher rates of unintended pregnancy among women in poverty, unintended pregnancy is much more common among black than among white women" (Institute of Medicine 1995: 33). Black women are less likely to receive adequate prenatal care (Sable et al. 1990; National Center for Health Statistics 1993). Not surprisingly, the percentage of children born into poverty is higher among nonwhite women. In addition, the abortion rate among nonwhite women is 2.7 times higher than among white women (Henshaw 1992). Because of these relationships, measures of the percentage of population that is black and Latino are included in the model.[11]

More direct measures of poverty can also be used. Female labor force participation is related to a wide variety of improvements in maternal and child health (Meier and McFarlane 1994; Medoff 1988). Similarly, per-capita income is a relatively direct measure of state wealth. Both variables are included as controls in the model.[12]

Religion can have an indirect effect on pregnancy rates as well as on maternal and child health. However, accessing annual information by state about religion is difficult; only for Catholicism is such information available. The Catholic Church is officially opposed to the use of artificial birth control. Although Catholics are just as likely as non-Catholics to use modern contraceptives (Goldscheider and Mosher 1991), the presence of Catholics in a state signifies at least monetary support for the Catholic Church. The Catholic Church supports a well-organized, national pro-life or antiabortion effort that works in every diocese and congressional district. For the most part, this effort does not distinguish family planning from abortion; the Catholic church is opposed to both (McKeegan 1992). Hence, our measure is the percentage of the state population that is Catholic (Garand, Monroe, and Meyer 1991).

Birthrates, abortion rates, and even maternal and child health are affected by poor women's access to abortion (Meier and McFarlane 1994). Several states fund all or most abortions for Medicaid-eligible women; other states rarely fund any abortions for low-income women except in the most extreme circumstances. We include a funded abortion measure that is the ratio of publicly funded abortions in a state per 1,000 women aged fifteen to forty-four.[13]

A final control included in the model is geographic access to abortion. Our measure is the number of abortion facilities in a state. Shelton, Brann, and Schultz (1976) found that the further a woman must travel in order to obtain an abortion, the less likely she is to get one. Wide variations in the provision of abortion services have been observed for various localities. A survey published in 1990 by the Alan Guttmacher Institute indicated that over 30 percent of women of reproductive age live in counties with no abortion provider (Henshaw and Van Vort 1990: 106). Because of this variation and the expected positive relationship between the number of providers and the rate of abortions, a variable that measures the percent of a state's population living in counties with large providers of abortion (facilities where four hundred or more abortions are performed per year) was included as a control variable.

ANALYSIS

The analysis is a pooled time series of all U.S. states from 1982 to 1991. Each dependent variable was examined as the result of the seven control variables, as well as per-capita family planning spending by title X, title XIX, state programs, and the combined total of title V and title XX. Pooled time series designs permit researchers to assess relationships across both time and states. A pooled time series design, however, is often plagued by major problems of autocorrelation and heteroscedasticity (Hsiao 1986; Judge et al. 1985; Pindyck and Rubinfeld 1991; Stimson 1985). Although the current data set is cross-sectionally dominant, preliminary analysis revealed that first-order autocorrelation was the major problem. This problem dictated that all models would be estimated using generalized least squares–autoregressive moving average models without forced homoscedasticity. After the initial estimation of these models, residuals were examined to determine if significant fixed effects were omitted from the model. As would be expected, in many cases individual states deviated greatly from the model. To control for such influences, a series of state-dummy variables was incorporated into the equations.[14] In the case of abortion rates, the number of fixed effects was so large that we estimated the model with an error components procedure (Judge et al. 1985).

FINDINGS

The impact of family planning expenditures on pregnancies (birthrates and abortions) is shown in Table 4.6. Because all family planning measures are in dollars per capita, the relative impact of the family planning programs can be compared directly. We do not interpret the coefficients for the control variables here because we were concerned with the impact of family planning funds rather than with the determinants of fertility or maternal and child health.

Table 4.6 shows that every dollar spent by title X in a state is associated with a decline of .594 births per 1,000 population. This impact is much larger than the size of the impact for other family planning funds. Title XIX has an impact of –.215 and titles V and XX have an impact of –.317. State expenditures have an unexpected positive relationship with birthrates because state expenditures are highly skewed. Most state expenditures are in a few states with relatively high birthrates.

The equation for abortion rates shows a much different impact. Only title X and title XIX have significant impacts. The results are consistent with the hypotheses. The impact of title X on the state abortion rate is nearly three times the impact of title XIX. Finally, the infant mortality results show a somewhat more balanced impact. A one-dollar increase in title X expenditures is associated with a .544 drop in the infant mortality rate. This impact is larger than that for state funds (–.445), title V and XX (–.417), and title XIX (–.315).

Overall our first hypothesis is consistently confirmed. Title X expenditures from the categorical grant program are associated with the largest declines in

TABLE 4.6

The Impact of Family Planning Programs on Birthrates, Abortion Rates, and Infant Mortality

Independent Variables	Dependent Variables		
	Birthrate	*Abortion Rate*	*Infant Mortality*
Family Planning Funding			
TitleX	−.594	−3.162	−.544
	(2.19)	(2.13)	(1.88)
Title XIX	−.215	−1.128	−.315
	(2.96)	(3.27)	(2.29)
Titles V and XX	−.317	.089	−.417
	(2.20)	(.07)	(2.29)
State Funds	.258	−.467	−.445
	(2.72)	(.90)	(3.77)
Control Variables			
Black Population	.021	.096	.127
	(2.89)	(1.43)	(20.99)
Latino Population	.147	.212	−.006
	(16.59)	(2.67)	(.90)
Catholic Population	−.025	.005	−.006
	(4.75)	(.10)	(1.14)
Income (in $1000s)	−.016	−.104	−.189
	(1.10)	(1.40)	(11.90)
Percent Females in Labor Force	.023	−.148	−.045
	(1.98)	(1.98)	(4.14)
Abortion Facilities	−.003	.237	.047
	(1.09)	(8.57)	(1.91)
Abortion Funding Rate	−.039	.082	.002
	(1.84)	(.81)	(.10)
Buse R-Square	.64	.26	.67
Adjusted R-Square	.62	.24	.66
Rho	.62	.80	.34
Houseman Specification Test	2.64	2.54	1.06

Notes. Coefficients are unstandardized regression coefficients. T-scores are listed in parentheses. Fixed effects controls: Birthrate—Alaska, Florida, Hawaii, Idaho, Louisiana, North Dakota, South Dakota, Utah, West Virginia, and Wyoming. Infant mortality—Alaska, Arkansas, Delaware, Illinois, South Dakota, and Utah. Abortion rate estimated with error components.

birthrates, abortion rates, and infant mortality rates. Our second hypothesis receives somewhat mixed confirmation. Title XIX consistently has a significant negative relationship with birthrates, abortion rates, and infant mortality rates; it is the only program other than title X that does. Title XIX does not, however, consistently have the second strongest impact; only for abortion rates is that the case. Overall, however, the conclusion must be that title XIX is the second most effective program. Finally, even the block grants, titles V and XX, are associated with positive health improvements in birthrates and infant mortality—the association is not as strong as those for title X, but is positive nonetheless.

DISCUSSION AND CONCLUSION

The results of this analysis have implications for both policy and theory. Clearly, they are important for family planning policy; moreover, they can inform broader health policy and fiscal federalism generally. By supporting our hypotheses, these findings corroborate Gramlich's observations about intergovernmental aid and extend empirical tests to program impacts.

Our study supports the view that public family planning funds reduce unintended fertility, and it demonstrates that these funds contribute to increased infant survival in the states. Additionally, we have shown the size of these impacts—that is, how much family planning affects infant health and unintended fertility. Our most striking results, however, are the differential impacts of the various federal family planning policies.

For every measure of maternal and child health or unintended fertility that we examined, title X, the categorical program, was far more cost effective than were each of the other federal authorizations or state appropriations. We also found that the expenditure of a Medicaid dollar for family planning usually had a greater impact than did an outlay of a dollar from the block grants.

Program impacts do vary by grant mechanism, and those differences are consistent with our hypotheses. The most cost-effective way to fund family planning services that reduce the number of unintended pregnancies and promote infant health is through the categorical grant mechanism. The second best alternative is probably to use the Type A grant—in this case, the Medicaid program.[15] Although block grant expenditures for family planning certainly produce benefits, they are the least cost-effective of the three grant types.

GRANT TYPES AND STATUTORY COHERENCE

These findings also corroborate the statutory coherence hypothesis from the Mazmanian and Sabatier model of policy implementation. In an earlier study, we derived measures from Mazmanian and Sabatier's seven prescriptive criteria

TABLE 4.7

Statutory Coherence Scores and Grant Types for Titles V, X, XIX, and XX

	Title V	Title X	Title XIX	Title XX
(1) Precision and Clear Ranking	0000	1100	0000	0000
Total	0	.50	0	0
(2) Validity of Causal Theory	0	1	1	0
(4) Decision Rules	0	1	1	1
(6) Official Commitment	0	1	0	0
(7) Formal Access	0	1	0	0
Total	0	4.5	2	1
Grant Type	B	C	A	B

for effective policies (i.e., statutory coherence). From those measures, we calculated statutory coherence scores for each of the four federal family planning statutes. In the interim, we have modified those measures slightly. The modified statutory coherence scores are shown in Table 4.7.

The statutory coherence hypothesis would have predicted our findings about the impacts of different grant types. Title X, which employs the most cost-effective grant mechanism, also has the highest statutory coherence score. Similarly, title XIX, the second most cost effective, has the second highest statutory coherence score. Are the three different grant categories and statutory coherence measuring the same phenomena? To a large extent, the answer is affirmative. For example, categorical grants are more likely than Type A and Type B grants to have clear mandates and monitoring requirements, both of which are elements of statutory coherence. Block grants, by definition, usually have the least statutory prescription embedded in their authorizations. In general, statutory coherence provides more detail about the inner workings of a program, although the type of grant mechanism may be the single most important variable. In other health policy areas, statutory coherence criteria could be used to measure the characteristics of different policies that employ the same grant mechanisms. With better measures, these statutory coherence scores eventually may be used to predict the magnitude of differences in outputs and impacts.

TITLE X: COST EFFECTIVENESS AND POLITICS

The direction of these findings will not surprise those who are familiar with public family planning programs. Although there are no national service cost data, the Radecki and Bernstein study (1989) did show that Medicaid family planning services were twice as expensive as those delivered by clinics subsidized by title X. At half the price, a title X dollar could certainly produce a greater impact. Furthermore, as we discussed earlier, when a title X grantee has other funding sources for family planning, title X guidelines prevail. This rule magnifies the impact of title X.

Title X is the most efficient and effective way to fund family planning services, yet its relative importance has diminished over the years. In 1982, title X accounted for 43 percent of all federal expenditures for family planning, while the same proportion was 27 percent for fiscal year 1994. Medicaid's proportion of federal family planning funding increased from 34 percent to 60 percent during the same period. The blocks (titles V and XX) moved from 23 percent of total federal family planning expenditures to 12 percent. Obviously, the federal government is not employing the most cost-effective mechanism to fund family planning services.

This trend, of course, is the result of politics, not policy analysis. During the 1980s, with a conservative presidency greatly influenced by the Christian coalition (McKeegan 1992), title X simply was not allowed to expand so that it could cover the needs of low-income women and keep up with inflation (McFarlane and Meier 1993). In fact, title X began the decade with a 25 percent cut, as a result of Reagan's retrenchment efforts.

Throughout the decade and the early 1990s, antiabortion activists argued that title X, abortion, and Planned Parenthood of America were related.[16] Although many members of Congress were skeptical, they also feared the power of the antiabortion movement and the Christian coalition. As a result, title X has not been reauthorized since 1985.

IMPLICATIONS FOR HEALTH POLICY

While these findings are important for family planning, they also provide insights for health policy more generally. First, these results affirm the efficacy of government. Second, these findings show that not all policy instruments are equally cost effective. Finally, our research illustrates the utility of good outcomes measures and reliable data.

Our study shows that public policies can improve the health status of populations. Indeed, government programs can "make a difference." Moreover, the methodology exists for measuring the size of those impacts. Ideally, health policies should have clear objectives so that researchers know which outcomes to measure and constituents know what to expect. We recognize that policy analysis and politics may lead to different policies. Nevertheless, we argue that documenting policy impacts promotes the potential for accountability in health policy.

Not all types of health policies perform equally well. This study shows that the most tightly constructed policy that employed the categorical grant mechanism was the most cost effective. Next in line was the entitlement program, Medicaid, which was authorized by a statute with more prescriptive criteria (i.e., statutory coherence) than the block grants. Our findings imply that advocates should work diligently to ensure that Medicaid is not replaced by block grants, even if Medicaid is capped at the national level.

The link between program outputs (services produced) and program impacts (health status) is not as well documented for many health services as it is for family planning (Donabedian 1992; Ellwood 1988; Evidence-Based Medicine Working Group 1992). Moreover, the capacity for collecting national health data has diminished over the last fifteen years (Norwood 1995). However, researchers and even political necessity may eventually persuade policy makers that clear objectives tracked by reliable data measuring outputs and outcomes are well worth the effort and expense. Part of this data collection effort must also include more accurate accounting for specific health services.

The finding that the categorical program is the most cost-effective family planning policy may present a dilemma for health policy makers. Does this result imply that publicly financed health care delivery should become more fragmented? First of all, this type of study needs to be replicated for other health policies so that the findings are more generalizable. Second, a distinction between funding mechanisms and health care delivery systems needs to be made. Specialized and accountable funding is not necessarily incompatible with comprehensive health care delivery. For example, title X actually promotes the delivery of integrated health services that are funded by different sources.

IMPLICATIONS FOR FISCAL FEDERALISM

This study has important implications for fiscal federalism—that is, the distribution of resources and responsibilities among the national, state, and local governments. The type of grant mechanism that the national government uses to allocate funds to subnational governments does affect the impact of federal programs. Our findings show that categorical programs are the most cost effective, followed by entitlements and then block grants.

The policy implications of our findings and the actions of the 104th Congress contradict one another. The 104th Congress converted entitlements into block grants and has been reluctant to initiate the use of categorical grants. Perhaps the most notable feat of this Congress was to convert the federal welfare program (AFDC) to a block grant (TANF).

Based on our findings and on other reported literature, we can make certain predictions for the nation's welfare system. One of the immediate results will be that the states and the national government will save money in welfare costs.

As in the Reagan years, states are unlikely to substitute their own dollars for federal cuts in the welfare program (Nathan and Dolittle 1987; G. E. Peterson et al. 1986). Not all states will react the same way, so there may be more variation in state welfare benefits. In terms of state variation in benefits, a countervailing force is the so-called race to the bottom, where contiguous states try not to provide more generous benefits than their neighbors, believing that otherwise they might become welfare magnets (Scheve, Peterson, and Rom 1996). With either scenario, poor women and children will receive fewer benefits overall, so that ultimately the positive benefits from welfare (e.g., shelter, food, and medical care)[17] will decrease. However, without good national data, which block grant programs seldom produce, we will be less capable of substantiating the impacts or even the outputs of welfare than we can now.

Some states are using the welfare block grants to experiment with new methods of service delivery. Using block grant funds, some states are even contracting with private corporations to operate their welfare programs (Bernstein 1996). We hearken back to the importance of the *adequacy of causal theory* variable in Mazmanian and Sabatier's policy implementation model (1989). Although fixed price contracts may be financially attractive in the immediate future, their long-term impacts are unknown. These private arrangements are not modest demonstration projects, but large-scale experiments risking real human costs. And the long-term impacts of reducing the social safety net may be very expensive.

Our skepticism about the new welfare law reflects observations from other scholars of American federalism. Both Thomas Anton (1989) and Paul Peterson, Barry Rabe, and Kenneth Wong (1986) have argued that the federal government should be responsible for redistributive policies. Peterson (1995) points out that for all their ability to work with business leaders to enhance community prosperity, state and local governments have difficulty meeting the needs of the poor and needy. Without a strong national presence exemplified by tightly constructed federal statutes and categorical grants, federalism can lead to great regional inequities. Moreover, the need for establishing cooperative relationships among governments (e.g., national and state) can lead to great inefficiency. This point was also made by Mazmanian and Sabatier when they encouraged policy makers to minimize hierarchical integration.

By showing differences in the cost effectiveness of different grant types, our findings substantiate inefficiencies in federalism. However, federal programs are the products of a political system (Anton 1989: 232). That is not to say that policy analysis does not inform and influence public decision making, but there are many other factors that influence policy making as well. For example, Clinton's decision to convert welfare to a block grant program, but not to do so with the much more costly Medicaid, was political (Gilens 1996; Rubin 1995).

The political climate of the 104th Congress precluded many policymakers from publicly acknowledging that unintended pregnancy is one of the primary reasons that so many women and children need welfare benefits and Medicaid. In other words, missing from this discussion was what lands many women and children on welfare in the first place. Within five years of the birth of their first child, nearly 77 percent of unmarried adolescent mothers become welfare recipients (Katz 1995c). Ironically, a proven way to reduce welfare costs—increasing funding for family planning and abortion—was not on the active agenda of the 104th Congress.

REFERENCES

Advisory Commission on Intergovernmental Relations (ACIR). 1993. *Characteristics of Federal Grant-in-Aid Programs to State and Local Governments: Grants Funded FY 1993.* Washington, DC: U.S. Advisory Commission on Intergovernmental Relations.

———. 1995. *Characteristics of Federal Grant-in-Aid Programs to State and Local Governments: Grants Funded FY 1995.* Washington, DC: U.S. Advisory Commission on Intergovernmental Relations.

Alan Guttmacher Institute (AGI). 1983. *Current Functioning and Future Priorities in Family Planning Services Delivery.* New York: Alan Guttmacher Institute.

Anderson, J. E., and L. G. Cope. 1987. The Impact of Family Planning Program Activity upon Fertility. *Family Planning Perspectives* 19:152–157.

Anton, T. J. 1989. *American Federalism and Public Policy: How the System Works.* Philadelphia: Temple University Press.

A Range of Budget Targets. 1995. *Congressional Quarterly* 53(5): 353.

Barduch, B. 1977. *The Implementation Game.* Cambridge: MIT Press.

Benda, P M., and C. H. Levine. 1988. Reagan and the Bureaucracy: The Bequest, the Promise, and the Legacy. In *The Reagan Legacy: Promise and Performance,* ed. C. 0. Jones. Chatham, NJ: Chatham House.

Berman, P. 1978. The Study of Macro- and Microimplementation. *Public Policy* 26:157–184.

Bernstein, N. 1996. Giant Companies Entering Race to Run State Welfare Programs. *New York Times,* 15 September, pp. A1, A26.

Bickers, K., and R. M. Stein. 1994. *Codebook: U.S. Domestic Assistance Programs Database.* Ann Arbor, MI: University of Michigan Inter-University Center for Political and Social Research.

Brandt, E. N., Jr. 1981. Block Grants and the Resurgence of Federalism. *Public Health Reports* 96:495–497.

Conlan, T. 1984. The Politics of Federal Block Grants. *Political Science Quarterly* 99(2):247–270.

———. 1988. *New Federalism: Intergovernmental Reform from Nixon to Reagan.* Washington, DC: Brookings Institution.

Corman, H., and M. Grossman. 1985. Determinants of Neonatal Mortality Rates in the U.S. *Journal of Health Economics* 4:213–236.

Craig, S. G., and R. P. Inman. 1982. Federal Aid and Public Education: An Empirical Look at the New Fiscal Federalism. *Review of Economics and Statistics* 64(4): 541–552.

Custis, V. R. 1988. *Blocking Maternal and Child Health Funds: An Analysis of Services and State Expenditures.* Master's thesis, College of Public Health, University of Oklahoma.

Cutright, P, and F. S. Jaffe. 1976. Family Planning Program Effects on the Fertility of Low-Income Women. *Family Planning Perspectives* 8: 100–110.

Daley, D., and R. B. Gold. 1993. Public Funding for Contraceptive, Sterilization, and Abortion Services, Fiscal Year 1992. *Family Planning Perspectives* 25: 244.

Derthick, M. 1975. *Uncontrollable Social Spending for Social Service Grants.* Washington, DC: Brookings Institution.

Donabedian, A. 1992. Role of Outcomes Research in Quality Assessment and Assurance. *Quality Review Bulletin* 18(11): 356–360.

Ellwood, P M. 1988. Outcomes Management: A Technology of Patient Experience [Shattuck Lecture]. *New England Journal of Medicine* 318(23): 1549–1556.

Evidence-Based Medicine Working Group. 1992. Evidence-Based Medicine: A New Approach to Teaching the Practice of Medicine. *Journal of the American Medical Association* 268(17):2420–2425.

Forrest, J. D. 1994. Epidemiology of Unintended Pregnancy and Contraceptive Use. *American Journal of Obstetrics and Gynecology* 170:1485–1488.

Forrest, J. D., and S. Singh. 1990a. Public Sector Savings Resulting from Expenditures for Contraceptive Services. *Family Planning Perspectives* 22:6–15.

———. 1990b. The Impact of Public-Sector Expenditures for Contraceptive Services in California. *Family Planning Perspectives* 22:161–168.

Fraley, C. 1995. States Guard Their Borders as Medicaid Talks Begin. *Congressional Quarterly* 53(23): 1637–1642.

Garand, J. C., P. A. Monroe, and G. Meyer. 1991. Does the Welfare State Increase Divorce Rates in the American States? Paper presented at the annual meeting of the Southern Political Science Association, Tampa, Florida, November.

Gilens, M. 1996. "Race Coding" and White Opposition to Welfare. *American Political Science Review* 90(3):593–604.

Gold, R. B. 1990. *Abortion and Women's Health: A Turning Point for America?* New York: Alan Guttmacher Institute.

Gold, R. B., and D. Daley. 1991. Public Funding of Contraceptive, Sterilization, and Abortion Services, Fiscal Year 1990. *Family Planning Perspectives* 23:204–211.

Gold, R. B., and S. Guardado. 1988. Public Funding of Family Planning, Sterilization, and Abortion Services, 1987. *Family Planning Perspectives* 20:228–233.

Gold, R. B., and J. Macias. 1986. Public Funding of Contraceptive, Sterilization, and Abortion Services, 1985. *Family Planning Perspectives* 18:259–264.

Gold, R. B., and B. Nestor. 1985. Public Funding of Contraceptive, Sterilization, and Abortion Services, 1983. *Family Planning Perspectives* 17:25–30.

Goldscheider, C., and W. D. Mosher. 1991. Patterns of Contraceptive Use in the United States: Importance of Religious Factors. *Studies in Family Planning* 22:102–115.

Gramlich, E. M. 1977. Intergovernmental Grants: A Review of the Empirical Literature. In *The Political Economy of Fiscal Federalism,* ed. W. E. Oates. Lexington, MA: Lexington.

Grossman, M., and S. Jacobowitz. 1981. Variations in Infant Mortality Rates among Counties of the U.S.: The Roles of Public Policies and Programs. *Demography* 18:695–713.

Henig, J. R. 1985. *Public Policy and Federalism.* New York: St. Martin's.

Henshaw, S. K. 1992. Abortion Trends in 1987 and 1988: Age and Race. *Family Planning Perspectives* 23:85–86.

Henshaw, S. K., and J. Van Vort. 1988. *Abortion Services in the United States, Each State and Metropolitan Area, 1984–1985.* New York: Alan Guttmacher Institute.

———. 1990. Abortion Services in the United States, 1987–1988. *Family Planning Perspectives* 22:102–108.

———. 1994. Abortion Services in the United States, 1991 and 1992. *Family Planning Perspectives* 26:105.

Hsiao, C. 1986. *Analysis of Panel Data.* New York: Cambridge University Press.

Institute of Medicine. 1985. *Preventing Low Birthweight.* Washington, DC: National Academy.

———. 1988. *Prenatal Care: Reaching Mothers, Reaching Infants.* Washington, DC: National Academy.

———. 1995. *The Best Intentions: Unintended Pregnancy and the Well-Being of Children and Families.* Washington, DC: National Academy.

Joyce, T. J., and M. Grossman. 1990. Pregnancy Wantedness and the Early Initiation of Prenatal Care. *Demography* 27:1–17.

Judge, G. G., W. E. Griffiths, R. C. Hill, H. Lutkepohl, and T. Lee. 1985. *The Theory and Practice of Econometrics.* New York: Wiley.

Katz, J. L. 1995a. Members Pushing to Retain Welfare System Control. *Congressional Quarterly* 53(4):280–283.

———. 1995b. Key Members Seek to Expand State Role in Welfare Plan. *Congressional Quarterly* 53(31):159–162.

———. 1995c. New Welfare Overhaul Plan Expected to Clear Panel. *Congressional Quarterly* 53(6):459.

———. 1996. After 60 Years, Most Control Is Passing to States. *Congressional Quarterly* 54(31):2190–2196.

Kingdon, J. W. 1984. *Agendas, Alternatives, and Public Policies.* Boston: Little, Brown.

———. 1995. *Agendas, Alternatives, and Public Policies.* 2d ed. New York: Harper-Collins.

Leone, R. C. 1995. Foreword. In *The Price of Federalism,* by P E. Peterson. Washington, DC: Brookings Institution.

MacPherson, P. 1995. Medicare, Medicaid on Table for Possible Cuts. *Congressional Quarterly* 53(6):458.

Marsiglio, W., and F. L. Mott. 1988. Does Wanting to Become Pregnant with a First Child Affect Subsequent Maternal Behaviors and Infant Birthweight? *Journal of Marriage and the Family* 50:1023–1036.

Mazmanian, D. A., and P. A. Sabatier. 1981. *Effective Policy Implementation.* Lexington, MA: D. C. Heath.

———. 1983. *Implementation and Public Policy.* Glenview, IL: Scott Foresman.

———. 1989. *Implementation and Public Policy: With a New Postscript.* Lanham, MD: University Press of America.

McFarlane, D. R. 1989. Testing the Statutory Coherence Hypothesis: The Implementation of Federal Family Planning Policy in the States. *Administration and Society* 20:395–422.

McFarlane, D. R., and K. J. Meier. 1993. Restructuring Federalism: The Impact of Reagan Policies on the Family Planning Program. *Journal of Health Politics, Policy and Law* 18(4):821–850.

McKeegan, M. 1992. *Abortion Politics: Mutiny in the Ranks of the Right.* New York: Free Press.

Medoff, M. H. 1988. An Economic Analysis of the Demand for Abortions. *Economic Inquiry* 26:353–359.

Meier, K. J., and D. R. McFarlane. 1994. State Family Planning and Abortion Expenditures: Their Effect on Health. *American Journal of Public Health* 84(9): 1468–1472.

———. 1996. Assessing the Impact of Statutory Coherence: The Case of Family Planning. *Journal of Public Policy* 15:281–298.

Nathan, R. P, and F. C. Dolittle. 1987. *Reagan and the States.* Princeton, NJ: Princeton University Press.

National Center for Health Statistics. 1993. Advance Report of Final Natality Statistics, 1991. *Monthly Vital Statistics Report* 42 (3, Suppl.): 40–41.

———. 1982–1991. *Vital Statistics of the United States.*

Nestor, B., and R. B. Gold. 1984. Public Funding of Contraceptive, Sterilization, and Abortion Services, 1982. *Family Planning Perspectives* 16:128–133.

Norwood, J. L. 1995. *Organizing to Count: Change in the Federal Statistical System.* Lanham, MD: University Press of America.

Pear, R. 1996. What Welfare Research? *New York Times,* 15 September, p. E4.

Peterson, G. E. 1984. Federalism and the States: An Experiment in Decentralization. In *The Reagan Record: An Assessment of America's Changing Domestic Priorities,* ed. J. L. Palmer and I. V. Sawhill. Washington, DC: Urban Institute.

Peterson, G. E., R. R. Bovbjerg, B. A. Davis, W. G. Davis, E. C. Durman, and T. A. Gallo. 1986. *The Reagan Block Grants: What Have We Learned?* Washington, DC: Urban Institute.

Peterson, P. E. 1995. *The Price of Federalism.* Washington, DC: Brookings Institution.

Peterson, P. E., B. G. Rabe, and K. K. Wong. 1986. *When Federalism Works.* Washington, DC: Brookings Institution.

Pindyck, R. S., and D. L. Rubinfeld. 1991. *Econometric Models and Econometric Forecasts.* New York: McGraw-Hill.

Radecki, S. E., and G. S. Bernstein. 1989. Use of Clinic versus Private Family Planning Care by Low-Income Women: Access, Cost, and Patient Satisfaction. *American Journal of Public Health* 79:692–697.

Rubin, A. J. 1995. GOP Walking Into a "Hornets' Nest" . . . As It Takes Aim at Health Programs. *Congressional Quarterly* 53(16): 1112–1113.

Sabatier, PA., and B. J. Klosterman. 1981. A Comparative Analysis of Policy Implementation under Different Statutory Regimes: The San Francisco Bay Conservation Development Commission 1965–1972. In *Effective Policy Implementation,* ed. D. A. Mazmanian and P A. Sabatier. Lexington, MA: D. C. Heath.

Sable, M. R., J. W. Stockbauer, W. F. Schramm, and G. H. Land. 1990. Differentiating the Barriers to Adequate Prenatal Care in Missouri, 1987–88. *Public Health Reports* 105:549–555.

Scheve, K. F., P E. Peterson, and M. C. Rom. 1996. State Welfare Policy: A Race to the Bottom. Cambridge: Harvard University, Center for American Political Studies. Occasional Paper no. 96-1, February.

Schlesinger, M., and T. Lee. 1993. Is Health Care Different? Popular Support of Federal Health and Social Policies. *Journal of Health Politics, Policy and Law* 18(3): 551–628.

Shelton, J., E. A. Brann, and K. F. Schultz. 1976. Abortion Utilization: Does Travel Distance Matter? *Family Planning Perspectives* 8:260–262.

Shiano, P. H., and R. E. Behrman. 1995. Low Birthweight: Analysis and Recommendations. *The Future of Children* 5(1):4–18.

Singh, G. K., and S. M. Yu. 1995. Infant Mortality in the United States: Trends, Differentials, and Projections. *American Journal of Public Health* 85:957–964.

Skocpol, T. 1995. The Aftermath of Defeat. *Journal of Health Politics, Policy and Law* 20(2):485–489.

Sollom, T., R. B. Gold, and R. Saul. 1996. Public Funding for Contraceptive Services, Sterilizations, and Abortion Services, 1994. *Family Planning Perspectives* 28:166–173.

Steinmo, S., and J. Watts. 1995. It's the Institutions, Stupid! Why Comprehensive National Health Insurance Always Fails in America. *Journal of Health Politics, Policy and Law* 20(2):329–372.

Stimson, J. 1985. Regression in Space and Time: A Statistical Essay. *American Journal of Political Science* 29:914–947.

U.S. Bureau of the Census. 1982–1991. *Census of Population* and annual state updates. Washington, DC: Government Printing Office.

———. 1994. *Statistical Abstract of the United States: 1994.* 114th ed. Washington, DC: Government Printing Office.

U.S. Department of Health and Human Services Public Health Service. 1997. *Understanding Title V of the Social Security Act: A Guide to the Provisions of Federal Maternal and Child Health Legislation after the Enactment of the Omnibus Reconciliation Act (OBRA) of 1989 (PL 101-239)* Rockville, MD: Health Resources and Services Administration Maternal and Child Health Bureau (DHHS Publication no. MCH 92-5).

U.S. General Accounting Office (U.S. GAO). 1984. *Maternal and Child Health Block Grant: Program Changes Emerging under State Administration. Report to the Congress by the Comptroller General of the United States.* Washington, DC: U.S. General Accounting Office.

Van Meter, D., and C. Van Horn. 1975. The Policy Implementation Process: A Conceptual Framework. *Administration and Society* 6 (February):445–488.

Weller, R. B., I. W. Eberstein, and M. Bailey. 1987. Pregnancy Wantedness and Maternal Behavior during Pregnancy. *Demography* 24:407–412.

Williamson, R. S. 1990. *Reagan's Federalism: His Efforts to Decentralize Government.* Lanham, MD: University Press of America.

NOTES

1.   Note that this classification is different from that used by the Advisory Commission on Intergovernmental Relations (ACIR), which categorizes grants into *categorical* and *block grants*. In the ACIR schema, categorical grants provide aid for specific, narrowly defined activities, while block grants are for broad, functional areas where the funds may be used at the recipients' (e.g., states') discretion (ACIR 1995). The ACIR definition of a block grant is the same as that used in this article, although in practice, many block grants have some loosely construed requirements for both state and beneficiaries.

ACIR breaks categorical grants into *formula-based* and *project* grants. According to ACIR, a formula grant is distributed by a legislative or administrative formula. In terms of usage in this article, the formula-based grants are called *entitlements* and the project grants are called categorical grants.

2.   Medicaid, unlike welfare, also benefits health care providers. These other beneficiaries and the large Medicaid costs of the elderly may explain why welfare was blocked but Medicaid was not.

3.   Gramlich's typology differs from the categorization of grants used by ACIR (see n. 1). Although we use ACIR data in this article, we employ Gramlich's typology. At times, we also refer to Type A grants as *entitlements*.

4.   The consolidation of categorical grants occurred during the early years of the Reagan Administration. In 1981, for example, only twenty-four state health departments were title X grantees.

5.   We use the total birthrate rather than birthrates by age groups as our dependent variable. Meier and McFarlane (1994) found that teen birthrates were not affected by family planning expenditures. If family planning funding affects birthrates in any age group, however, it should also show up in the birthrate for all age groups.

6.   The Forrest analysis did not include miscarriages because "the number of preg-

nancies ending in miscarriage is not well established and because there is no information on the distribution by intention status" (Institute of Medicine 1995: 25). The proportion attributed to each outcome changes of course when the incidence of miscarriage is estimated. About 12 percent of pregnancies end in miscarriage (Gold 1990: 11).

7. Data on total state births were taken from the National Center for Health Statistics, *Vital Statistics of the United States* annual (1982–1991). Population data were taken from the U.S. Bureau of the Census, *Census of Population*, and their annual updates. Except for the years 1983, 1986, 1989, and 1990, all abortion data were obtained from the Alan Guttmacher Institute (Henshaw and Van Vort 1988, 1990, 1994). To provide estimates for other years an interpolation procedure similar to that of Meier and McFarlane (1994) was used; these estimated data can be obtained from the authors.

8. All data are from the National Center for Health Statistics, *Vital Statistics of the United States* annual (1982–1991). Other measures were considered. However, data measuring known risk factors for infant mortality, such as late prenatal care (Institute of Medicine 1988) and low birthweight (Institute of Medicine 1985) were not available for the last three years of the study due to the lag time in the publication of national vital statistics. Similarly, state-level data measuring neonatal mortality, a major component of infant mortality, were not available. These factors are all related to infant mortality, so infant mortality is probably the best overall indicator of child health.

9. "Cigarette smoking is the single largest modifiable risk factor for low birthweight and infant mortality. It accounts for up to 20 percent of all low birthweight. Smoking retards fetal growth. On average, babies born to smokers weigh about one-half pound less than babies born to nonsmokers" (Shiano and Behrman 1995: 11).

10. Title X data are available for every year (Bickers and Stein 1994). Other family planning data are from the Alan Guttmacher Institute's periodical, *Family Planning Perspectives*; for 1992, see Daley and Gold 1993; for 1990, see Gold and Daley 1991; for 1987, see Gold and Guardado 1988; for 1985, see Gold and Macias 1986; for 1983, see Gold and Nestor 1985; and for 1982, see Nestor and Gold 1984. We interpolated data for the missing years by averaging data from the year before and the year after. For example, the 1984 estimate was done with 1983 and 1985 data.

11. Data are from the U.S. Bureau of the Census's *Statistical Abstract of the United States* for various years (1983–1992). For the Latino population, individual years had to be interpolated from the 1980 and 1990 census data.

12. Data are from the U.S. Bureau of the Census' *Statistical Abstract of the United States* for various years (1983–1992).

13. In 1982, fifteen states funded abortions: Alaska, California, Colorado, Connecticut, Hawaii, Maryland, Massachusetts, Michigan, New Jersey, New York, North Carolina, Oregon, Pennsylvania, Washington, and West Virginia (Nestor and Gold 1984). AGI did not collect expenditure data in 1984. In 1985, the same fifteen states funded abortions for low-income women (Gold and Macias, 1986). In 1987, fourteen states (Colorado stopped that year) funded abortions for low-income women (Gold and Guardado 1988). AGI did not collect expenditure data for 1988 and 1989 (Gold and Daley 1991). AGI also did not collect expenditure data for 1991. In 1992, the same thirteen states as in 1990 funded abortions for low-income women (Daley and Gold 1993). AGI did not collect expenditure data for 1993. In 1994, fifteen states (with the addition of Idaho and West Virginia) officially funded abortions for low-income women (Sollom, Gold, and Saul 1996).

14.   We ran the Hausman specification test to compare the fixed effects models to random effects models. In each case, the insignificant result suggests that the fixed effects model is the appropriate one. The dummy variables, as expected, have a substantial impact on the fit of the regression line and reduce the degree of autocorrelation. Their inclusion does not have much impact on the coefficients that indicate the impact of family planning. If anything, the introduction of state effects appears to reduce the size of the family planning coefficients; the result is a conservative estimate of the impact compared to the ordinary least squares estimates.

15.   Because Medicaid is an insurance program, its impact in a state will depend on the cost and quality of care delivered by the amalgamation of Medicaid providers.

16.   In fact, title X has forbidden the use of its funds for abortion since 1970 when it was first enacted. During the 1980s, the national office of Planned Parenthood Federation of America (PPFA) became a vocal advocate for freedom of choice in the abortion debate. Because many PPFA affiliates were title X grantees, the antiabortion movement tried to link all Planned Parenthood activities to abortion.

17.   Although food stamps and Medicaid are not directly tied to welfare, welfare eligibility is often linked to receipt of these benefits.

5 | Sliding-Scale Premium Health Insurance Programs: Four States' Experiences

**Leighton Ku and
Teresa A. Coughlin**

An important goal for the nation has been to reduce the number of uninsured Americans, particularly those in working-class families. One major policy option is helping lower-income families purchase insurance by offering government subsidies. The 1997 creation of the Children's Health Insurance Program (CHIP) signals the nation's continuing commitment to expand coverage using public programs. Earlier in the decade, many states began initiatives to offer insurance coverage to families whose incomes were above the traditional limits of eligibility for programs like Medicaid. These initiatives included state-funded health insurance programs like Washington's Basic Health Plan and Minnesota's MinnesotaCare, as well as Medicaid Section 1115 demonstration projects like Tennessee's TennCare or Hawaii's QUEST (Wooldridge et al. 1996; Coughlin et al. 1997; Nichols et al. 1997; Lipson and Schrodel 1996; Diehr et al. 1996; Call et al. 1997). These programs required that some participants pay premiums on a sliding-scale basis. The enabling legislation for CHIP also let states require that enrollees pay a modest share of the premiums for CHIP coverage.

Reprinted with permission from *Inquiry*, 36, no. 4 (Winter 1999/2000): 471–80. © 1999. Blue Cross and Blue Shield Association and Blue Cross and Blue Shield of the Rochester Area. The Robert Wood Johnson Foundation provided support for this research.

In contrast, Medicaid is free to participants. Since the greatest numbers of uninsured people are in working households of low to moderate income (Hoffman 1998), initiatives to expand coverage to people with incomes above the poverty level have led to the question of whether the recipients should bear responsibility for paying a share of the cost of insurance.

Policy discussions about cost sharing raise many issues. Proponents note that sliding-scale premiums target subsidies toward lower-income people and provide less governmental assistance to those with more income. Some believe that cost sharing promotes personal responsibility and eases some of the political and social stigma associated with Medicaid. Premium sharing makes the government assistance more like private health insurance, in which cost sharing is the norm, and may serve as a better bridge between public and private health insurance. Similarly, requiring people to pay part of the premiums might reduce "crowd out," a practice in which some people drop private coverage to take advantage of the free (or less expensive) public benefits (Cutler and Gruber 1997; Call et al. 1997; Dubay and Kenney 1996, 1997). Finally, cost sharing reduces governmental outlays, because beneficiaries shoulder some of the expenses and participation tends to be lower.

However, requiring that beneficiaries pay part of the premium also has disadvantages. Most important, this cost sharing reduces participation among the target population. Many families may choose to use their income to pay for food, rent, clothing or other goods rather than buy health insurance. Some families, especially those below the poverty level, may lack the discretionary income to buy insurance, no matter how cheap. Premiums can lead to adverse selection, because sicker people may be more likely to buy in than the healthy. This problem may be exacerbated if people choose to pay premiums in the months when they need medical care, but not when they are healthy.[1] The net result is that people covered might have higher-than-average medical needs, leading to higher medical expenditures per beneficiary. However, an early study of Washington's Basic Health Plan failed to find evidence of adverse selection (Diehr et al. 1993). Lastly, premiums increase programs' administrative complexity, requiring a billing system and development of policies on handling delayed payment or nonpayment of premiums.

Because states did not charge premiums until recently, there has been little information about how cost-sharing programs are designed or administered, or how they affect participants. To understand these programs, we interviewed state officials and reviewed state documents and data, including the premium schedules and participation counts. This paper reviews a number of the issues concerning sliding-scale premium schedules and the experience of four states—Hawaii, Minnesota, Tennessee, and Washington—that initiated such programs. We focus on policies and experiences in 1995, although we briefly discuss programmatic changes since that time. First, we provide a brief background on each of these four state programs. Next, we discuss how they structured their premium programs. We then provide some preliminary analyses of participation rates and the relationship of price and participation. We conclude by discussing the policy implications of our findings.

WHAT HAPPENED IN THE FOUR STATES?

Four states served as laboratories for understanding how sliding-scale premiums work for low- to middle-income families. Hawaii, Minnesota, Tennessee, and Washington developed relatively large, subsidized insurance programs in the early 1990s. Each had ambitious goals to reduce the number of uninsured people and each wanted to cover uninsured working families. At the same time, state policymakers felt it was appropriate to require that higher-income participants contribute to the cost of insurance. As a result, the states designed cost-sharing systems, including sliding-scale premiums charged to beneficiaries. An additional element in these states' reforms was the development of managed care systems. Hawaii, Tennessee, and Washington required that participants join capitated managed care plans, and Minnesota required joining a health plan in 1996.

While they all were state-initiated, the programs' origins varied. Washington and Minnesota began programs using only state funds. While this meant that they had more flexibility, it also meant that budgets and benefit packages were tighter. Tennessee's and Hawaii's programs were funded jointly by the state and the federal governments as Section 1115 Medicaid demonstration programs. Thus, the federal government needed to approve the policies and some Medicaid legislative requirements still applied. Tennessee's TennCare and Hawaii's QUEST had broad, Medicaid-like benefit packages and were barred from charging premiums to those who were previously eligible for Medicaid.

TENNCARE

In January 1994, Tennessee implemented one of the most expansive subsidized insurance programs in the nation. Initially, all uninsured people, if they were uninsured on a given date before application, were eligible to join, but subsidies were available only for those with family incomes up to 400% of the poverty level. While TennCare was free to those below poverty, premiums gradually rose above that level. TennCare recipients with incomes above poverty also were subject to deductibles and copayments. Because of budget constraints, TennCare stopped enrolling new uninsured people in January 1995. It continued to enroll people covered under regular Medicaid eligibility rules and those who were uninsurable due to special medical conditions. The uninsured people already participating in TennCare were grandfathered and continued to get insurance. In 1997, the program was reopened to displaced workers and children under the state's CHIP.

In the beginning, Tennessee's program had some serious administrative weaknesses. Because of its mail application system, applicants usually did not know how much they owed until *after* they were enrolled. Further, the state failed to send out premium billing notices for six months and did not send another billing notice until December 1994. When participants finally received billing notices for back-owed premiums, many were unable or unwilling to pay. The state dropped more than 60,000 participants for nonpayment during 1995, while thousands of others covered their debts by paying under an installment plan.

QUEST

Hawaii's program began in August 1994. It served nondisabled, nonelderly people who had incomes up to 300% of the poverty level and were not covered by the state's employer-mandated private health insurance. In 1994, people with incomes between 133% and 300% of poverty paid sliding-scale premiums and were subject to nominal copayments. Due to fiscal problems and a class action lawsuit, Hawaii undertook a series of changes to reduce caseloads and spending.[2] In 1995, the state raised recipients' share of premiums. In 1996, it imposed an assets test, charged full premiums to those above 100% of poverty and imposed a limited moratorium on enrolling new applicants. In 1997, QUEST eligibility was limited to those with incomes below poverty (except for pregnant women and infants with family incomes up to 185% of poverty and children ages 1 to 5 with incomes up to 133% of poverty).

BASIC HEALTH PLAN (BHP)

Washington began its BHP in 1989 as a pilot program that was administratively separate from Medicaid. Under the program, adults and children had different rules. For example, in 1995, children who were enrolled in BHP and had family incomes below 200% of poverty were counted under a Section 1902(r)(2) amendment, were eligible for federal match payments under Medicaid, and received the broad Medicaid benefits package. By contrast, adults had a more restricted benefits package that was closer to private insurance than Medicaid (e.g., no prescription drug coverage, deductibles for hospital stays). Sliding-scale premiums applied to adults at all income ranges; those with no income were charged $10 per month for an individual or $20 for a family.[3] The premium subsidies declined to zero for people with incomes above 200% of poverty, although people with higher incomes could enroll. In early 1996, the state reduced premium levels in a successful attempt to boost participation. Later in 1996, the state capped the number of adults admitted because the program reached its funding limits.

MINNESOTACARE

In 1992, Minnesota created its subsidized insurance program, MinnesotaCare. It served uninsured families with incomes below 275% of poverty, as well as single adults and childless families with low incomes (up to 135% of poverty in 1996). Participants had to have been uninsured at least four months before applying and could not have had access to employer-paid (i.e., employer pays more than half the premium) insurance within the previous 18 months. Like BHP, it had a narrower benefit package (e.g., a deductible and $10,000 limit for inpatient care) than Medicaid and was administered separately. Premiums were based on a sliding scale, except that children in families with incomes under 150% of poverty (who were not otherwise Medicaid eligible) paid a flat $4 per month. Premiums were charged for adults with incomes above the maximum Medicaid income eligibility level. In 1995, MinnesotaCare operated as a fee-for-service insurance program, but it shifted to capitated managed care the next year. In 1996, benefits for pregnant women and children under age two with incomes below 275% of poverty, and other Medicaid-eligible people (e.g., 11-year-olds under 100% of poverty) who chose MinnesotaCare, became eligible for federal financial matching under a Section 1115 demonstration program.

HOW WERE THE PREMIUMS STRUCTURED?

A key aspect to subsidized premium programs is the design of the premium schedule. All four states created premium structures that were progressive from no income to 200% of poverty; that is, the price (as a percentage of family income) rose for those with higher incomes. Each state charged full premiums to families at the top end of the income range. Thus, prices were quite high at the top of the income range—more than 5% of family income. Tables 5.1, 5.2, 5.3, and 5.4 provide data about the premium levels in 1995 for a single adult and for a family of four.

There were some interesting differences in how states structured their programs. Minnesota and Washington charged small amounts even to those with incomes below the poverty line (e.g., a family with no income would pay $12 per month in Minnesota or $20 in Washington), while those below poverty in Tennessee and Hawaii were not charged anything. Minnesota and Hawaii capped eligibility to those with incomes below 275% or 300% of poverty, respectively, while people with incomes beyond the subsidy limit could enroll in TennCare or BHP, but had to pay full premiums.

States also varied in the relative price of premiums for individuals and families. Minnesota and Washington had similar or lower prices for families

TABLE 5.1

Premium Levels for Participants in Hawaii QUEST, Early 1995

| Income as % of Poverty | Individual Premium Share | | | Family of Four Premium Share | | |
	Monthly Payment ($)	% of Full Premium[a]	% of Income	Monthly Payment ($)	% of Full Premium[a]	% of Income
0%	0	0	0	0	0	0
50%	0	0	0	0	0	0
100%	0	0	0	0	0	0
150%	13	7	1.4	53	7	2.8
200%	38	20	3.0	150	20	6.0
250%	113	60	7.2	451	60	14.3
300%	188	100	10.1	752	100	19.8
350%	Not eligible	Not eligible	Not eligible	Not eligible	Not eligible	Not eligible
400%	Not eligible	Not eligible	Not eligible	Not eligible	Not eligible	Not eligible

*Note:*No cost sharing at or below 133% of poverty or for pregnant women and children under 185% of poverty.
[a]Assumes a premium of $188 per person, single or family. Every additional person is added at the rate of a single person, up to a family size of five. The premium shares are based on the percentage of poverty, but the actual costs vary with the island and the plan selected by the client, includes medical and dental costs.

(measured as a percentage of family income) than for single adults.[4] To do this, both states provided higher subsidies (as a percentage of the full premium) for families than individuals. In contrast, Tennessee and Hawaii used similar subsidies for individuals and families, expressed as a percentage of the full premium; the net effect was that families paid a larger share of family income than individuals. In Hawaii, higher-income families could owe as much as 20% of family income at the upper range of income. To keep relative premium levels similar for families and individuals, states need to offer higher subsidy rates for families.[5]

The programs varied in how they calculated the amount beneficiaries were charged. MinnesotaCare's fee-for-service premium was fixed and TennCare set the capitation rates for all plans. Thus, the out-of-pocket premium schedules were uniform for people with equivalent incomes. In comparison, Hawaii and Washington paid health plans different prices and provided percentage-based subsidies. Thus, there was a modest incentive to pick a less expensive plan. For example, if a person who owed a 20% premium share could choose two plans that differed in full premiums by $10, that person would have to pay $2 more to get the higher-cost plan. Neither state used a defined contribution approach, which sets a fixed-dollar subsidy at a given poverty level and makes

TABLE 5.2

Premium Levels for Participants in MinnesotaCare, Late 1995

Income as % of Poverty	Individual Premium Share			Family of Four Premium Share		
	Monthly Payment ($)	*% of Full Premium*[a]	*% of Income*	*Monthly Payment ($)*	*% of Full Premium*[a]	*% of Income*
0%	4	4	Not applicable	12	4	Not applicable
50%	5	5	1.6	12	4	1.9
100%	14	13	2.2	29	9	2.3
150%[a]	Not eligible	Not eligible	Not eligible	72	23	3.8
200%[a]	Not eligible	Not eligible	Not eligible	149	48	5.9
250%[a]	Not eligible	Not eligible	Not eligible	278	89	8.8
300%	Not eligible	Not eligible	Not eligible	Not eligible	Not eligible	Not eligible
350%	Not eligible	Not eligible	Not eligible	Not eligible	Not eligible	Not eligible
400%	Not eligible	Not eligible	Not eligible	Not eligible	Not eligible	Not eligible

Note: MinnesotaCare is a state-funded program with a limited benefit package. Under a 1902(r)(2) rule, children and pregnant women can be enrolled in MinnesotaCare and also be covered by Medicaid.
[a]Income eligibility up to 275% of poverty for families with children or up to 135% for childless adults. Individual members of families with children may join, in which case they pay premiums equal to 3.9% of income at 150% of poverty, 5.9% of income at 200% of poverty, and 6.7% of income at 250% of poverty. Families do not pay for more than three members. Assumes full premiums of $104 per month for an individual and $312 for a family of four.

the beneficiary responsible for any difference between the full premium and the fixed subsidy.

Although this paper focuses on the 1995 experiences of the four states, there were changes in premium schedules over time. Two states purposefully used premiums as a caseload management tool, with mixed success. Hawaii initially increased premiums in order to reduce QUEST participation levels. Preliminary data indicate that the caseloads did not change noticeably until the state made much stricter changes in eligibility (e.g., imposing a moratorium on new cases and adding an assets test). On the other hand, Washington state was concerned that BHP had low participation, and greatly reduced BHP premiums in early 1996. Participation in the program roughly doubled after the prices were lowered.

WHAT WERE PARTICIPATION RATES?

The share of the premium that people must pay may affect participation levels and, consequently, determine the extent to which public subsidy programs

TABLE 5.3

Premium Levels for Participants in TennCare, Early 1995

Income as % of Poverty	Individual Premium Share			Family of Four Premium Share		
	Monthly Payment ($)	% of Full Premium[a]	% of Income	Monthly Payment ($)	% of Full Premium[a]	% of Income
0%	0	0	0	0	0	0
50%	0	0	0	0	0	0
100%	3	2	.4	7	2	.5
150%	11	8	1.2	27	8	1.4
200%	55	40	4.4	137	40	5.4
250%	74	54	4.7	184	54	5.8
300%	95	70	5.1	238	70	6.3
350%	109	80	5.0	273	80	6.2
400%	137	100	5.5	342	100	6.8

[a]The premiums for those at or above 200% of poverty are based on the "low deductible" option. Using the "high deductible" option would lead to lower premiums, but higher deductibles. There are no copayments for those below poverty or Medicaid eligibles. Between 101% and 199% of poverty, the copayments range from 2% to 8% and are set at 10% above 200% of poverty. Assumes full premiums are $137 per month for one person and $342 for a family of four.

achieve their goals of lowering the number of uninsured people. Premium shares are relevant to program budgeting, since they may affect both the number of people participating and the amount of government subsidy per participant. In this section, we estimate 1995 program participation rates for three of the four states.

We used the following strategy to estimate participation rates. Each state provided data about the number of participants at varying income levels in 1995, which corresponded to differing premium levels paid by beneficiaries. We excluded data from Tennessee because it appeared that many of those who joined TennCare did not know how much they would pay when they signed up and, because of billing problems, many never paid their premiums anyway.[6] Thus, the TennCare experience did not always reflect people's willingness to buy coverage.

We estimated the size of the eligible population in each state by using a merged three-year sample of the 1991–1993 Current Population Surveys (CPS). The CPS data were edited to adjust for Medicaid undercounts using the Urban Institute's TRIM2 microsimulation model (Winterbottom, Liska, and Obermaier 1995). We estimated the number of uninsured people in each state in income cohorts, where each cohort is defined by a range of 25 percentage points of the federal poverty level (i.e., 101% to 125%, 126% to 150%, etc.).

TABLE 5.4

Premium Levels for Participants in the
Washington Basic Health Plan (BHP), Late 1995

Income as % of Poverty	Individual Premium Share			Family of Four Premium Share		
	Monthly Payment ($) a	*% of Full Premium[b]*	*% of Income*	*Monthly Payment ($)[a]*	*% of Full Premium[b]*	*% of Income*
0%	10	8	Not applicable	20	5	Not applicable
50%	10	8	3.2	20	5	3.2
100%	23	19	3.7	46	11	3.6
150%	52	44	5.6	104	25	5.5
200%	123	104	9.9	246	59	9.7
250%	123	104	7.9	246	59	7.8
300%	123	104	6.6	246	59	6.5
350%	123	104	5.6	246	59	5.6
400%	123	104	4.9	246	59	4.9

Note: BHP is a state program with a limited benefit package, although children may participate in BHP Plus, which is under Medicaid.
[a]Includes a minimum of $10 per individual and $20 per family. Also, for those at or above 200% of poverty, includes a $5 per person administrative fee, which adds another 4%.
[b]Actual premiums vary by plan, although consistent premium shares are used. Assumes monthly premiums of $118 for single adults and $419 for family of four. Because of Medicaid tie-in, children under 18 under 200% of poverty are not charged premiums.

We "aged" these estimates forward to 1995 levels. Using state administrative data on the number of participants as numerators, and CPS estimates of the eligible population as denominators, we computed participation rates in each income cohort. Finally, we computed the median monthly cost of premiums for two people in a two-person family (an adult and a child) to represent the premiums paid in each income bracket (Ku and Coughlin 1997). A two-person family corresponds to typical insurance units in the programs and includes a higher- (adult) and lower- (child) cost beneficiary.

The estimates for the three states are summarized in Table 5.5 and shown graphically in Figure 5.1. Within each state, the general relationship showed—as expected—that participation fell as the amount that people had to pay rose. The figure shows a curve that summarizes the relationship of premiums as a percentage of family income and participation rates for the three states, pooled together. The method of estimating this relationship is shown in the notes section.[7] We chose to pool the data for the three states because there was a very limited number of observations and because pooling reduces the impact of sampling error in any given observation or in any given state.

FIGURE 5.1

**Estimated Level of Participation, Based
on Premium Levels in Three States, 1995**

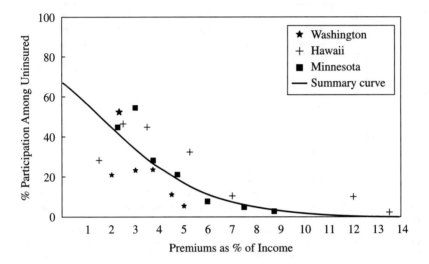

The summary curve helps illustrate the general relationship of price and participation. Three insights also can be drawn from the summary curve (and also hold true for each state individually). First, average participation rates fall as the relative price (premium share as a percentage of income) rises. Second, even when the premium share is relatively high, a few people still participate. Third, if we extrapolate the curve, it is apparent that many eligible people will not participate even when programs are free.

More specifically, the summary curve estimates that raising premium shares from 1% to 3% of family income decreases expected participation rates from about 57% to 35% among the uninsured. When the premium is 5% of income, participation is about 18%. This model suggests that a useful way to analyze the effect of cost sharing is by measuring the premium share as a percentage of family income.

The data suggest that participation levels were somewhat lower in Washington state than Minnesota or Hawaii. As mentioned earlier, Washington officials also were concerned about poor participation, and lowered premiums to increase participation in 1996. The reason for Washington's lower participation rate in 1995 is not clear, but we can offer a few possible explanations. BHP offered a limited benefit package, which might have been less attractive than a richer

TABLE 5.5

**Premium Levels and Estimated
Participation Rates by Poverty Range, 1995**

Income Range as % of Poverty	Median Premium for Two as % of Income	Estimated Participation as % of Uninsured
Hawaii QUEST—early 1995		
133–149%	1.4	42
150–174%	2.4	47
175–199%	3.5	45
200–224%	5.3	33
225–249%	6.9	11
250–274%	11.9	10
275–300%	13.6	3
MinnesotaCare—late 1995		
100–124%	2.3	45
125–149%	3.1	55
150–174%	3.8	29
175–199%	4.8	21
200–224%	5.9	8
225–249%	7.4	5
250–275%	8.8	3
Washington BHP—late 1995		
25–49%	3.2	32
50–74%	1.9	21
75–99%	3.1	33
100–124%	3.0	24
125–149%	3.7	24
150–174%	4.4	11
175–200%	5.1	6

Medicaid-type benefit. On the other hand, MinnesotaCare's benefits also were limited, but that program had higher participation. BHP required that families with incomes below poverty pay premiums, but MinnesotaCare did so as well. It appeared that each of the three programs had a lot of publicity and outreach, but it is possible that public awareness was lower in Washington, although this is hard to measure. A host of other factors, such as the employment, cultural, or health care environment in each state also may affect participation rates.[8] We were not able to control for these factors in this analysis.

This simple and preliminary analysis indicates the general relationship of premium share to income and participation rates. Many important issues that might affect participation remain unresolved. For example, is participation higher in states with more generous benefit packages? How do operational factors, such as outreach or ease of application, affect participation rates? More research is needed to answer these questions.

DISCUSSION

The experiences of Hawaii, Minnesota, Tennessee, and Washington demonstrate that sliding-scale premium programs for low-income individuals and families are feasible. There are some administrative complexities, however. Implementing such a system requires that states carefully design premium share schedules, establish administrative policies for problems such as what to do when people do not pay their premiums, and arrange for either the state agency or health plans to administer bill collection.

More recent interest in premiums has been fueled by the creation of CHIP programs. Federal legislation lets states charge premiums or copayments, particularly when the CHIP programs are independent of Medicaid. For example, children in families with incomes above 150% of poverty cannot bear total costs greater than 5% of family income. Preliminary information indicates that the actual CHIP premiums tend to be very low (e.g., $5 to $10 per child per month) and generally have just one or two levels (Riley and Pernice 1998). While we believe that the experiences reported here are relevant to CHIP programs, they are not identical. Most important, CHIP programs are only for children, while the programs in the four study states were for adults as well as children. It is possible that the willingness to buy insurance differs for situations in which only children or the whole family are covered.

States likely will continue to test ways to expand health insurance coverage using subsidy programs for working-class families. The experience of these four states illustrates the possibilities and limitations of such programs. However, these findings are not generalizable to all possible subsidy arrangements: they reflect a handful of states with specific types of programs. Another commonly mentioned policy option is subsidizing the purchase of private insurance using tax credits or vouchers. This option poses a different set of operational and conceptual issues and the findings of this study are not applicable.

In designing and implementing subsidized insurance programs, there is an inherent tension between the goals of lowering governmental cost or encouraging personal responsibility (leading to higher premium shares) and maximizing participation (leading to lower premium shares). The data from these states suggests that, while many low-income people would pay premiums to purchase subsidized health insurance, their willingness to pay is limited. If, for example, the government subsidizes half the full cost of insurance for a family of four with an income of 200% of poverty, the family's out-of-pocket price still would be relatively high (about 7% of income). This study suggests that few, perhaps less than 10% of the uninsured, would participate if they had to pay 7% of their income for health insurance. Surveys consistently show that a major reason that people lack health insurance is because they say they cannot afford it (Thorpe and Florence 1999). It seems likely that future efforts to expand insurance coverage will require premium sharing by some beneficiaries. In designing and implementing these new initiatives, policymakers need to be careful in balancing budget resources with the goal of reducing the number of uninsured people.

NOTES

The authors are grateful to officials in Hawaii, Minnesota, Tennessee, and Washington for providing information about their programs. A number of colleagues provided useful assistance or advice about this paper, including (in alphabetical order): Linda Blumberg, John Holahan, Bethany Kessler, Sharon Long. Shruti Rajan, Tim Waidman, Sean Williams, and Steve Zuckerman. Anonymous reviewers and Kathy Swartz, the journal editor, also provided helpful advice. All opinions are those of the authors and should not be viewed as positions of the Urban Institute or the Robert Wood Johnson Foundation.

1. Programs can create some safeguards to minimize the extent of drop-out/drop-in. For example, if people voluntarily drop out of MinnesotaCare or are terminated for nonpayment of premiums, they are barred from re-entering the program for four months, with certain hardship exceptions. This is intended to prevent adverse selection.

2. The plaintiffs' attorney argued that since QUEST was only for nondisabled people, those with disabilities faced more restrictive eligibility criteria. They sought relief under the Americans with Disabilities Act. In light of the lawsuit and the state's fiscal problems, Hawaii made QUEST income eligibility much tighter.

3. Children under 200% of poverty and a few others are not charged premiums.

4. The family cost in Washington was lower than for a single adult, because children under 200% of poverty were free due to their Medicaid status.

5. A key reason for this discrepancy is that there are different economies of scale used in poverty measures and the pricing of insurance premiums. For example, poverty scales assume that a four-person family needs twice as much income as one person, while insurance costs for a four-person family are typically about three times as high as for a single adult.

6. Even so, participation rates for TennCare were similar to the other three programs'.

7. To generate the summary curve shown in Figure 5.1, we used a grouped logit model (Greene 1990) of the form:

$$\text{in } [p_i/(1 - p_i)] = \beta + \beta X_i + \epsilon_i$$

where p_i is the participation rate for a given income poverty "cohort" in a state, X_i is the premium level and other related income measures, βs are estimated coefficients and ϵ_i is the error term. Weights were based on the number of people in each income bracket, normalized to average 1.0. There are 21 observations, shown in Table 5.2, each

Main and Alternative Models of the Relationship of Premiums and Participation Rates in Hawaii, Minnesota, and Washington, 1995

	Model 1 (Main Model)		Model 2		Model 3		Model 4		Model 5		Model 6	
	Coefficient	t	Coefficient	t	Coefficient	t	Coefficient	t	Coefficient	t	Coefficient	t
Using premiums as % of income												
Intercept	.7239	1.803	.4633	1.054	−.3678	−.293						
Premiums as % of income	−.4555	−4.056	−.6353	−3.642	−.3343	−.727						
Income as % of poverty			.0065	1.329	.0105	1.394						
Interaction premium and income					−.0015	−.709						
Adjusted R-squared	.436		.458		.442							
Using premiums in $ per month												
Intercept							−.1444	−.581	−1.0356	−1.720	−.8381	−1.404
Premiums in $							−.0161	−3.314	−.0294	−3.091	−.1002	−2.080
Income as % of property									.0108	1.612	.0192	2.240
Interaction premium and income											.0002	1.498
Adjusted R-squared							.333		.384		.425	

Note: Dependent variable: in $[p/(1 - p)]$ where p = probability of participation among the uninsured.

representing hundreds or thousands of people in each state who fall into a given income cohort. Because the range of eligibility differs in each state, the number of cohorts and income range represented varied from state to state.

We tested alternative model specifications including income (as a percentage of poverty), premiums expressed in dollar terms (rather than as a percentage of poverty) and interactions of income and premiums (Appendix Table). We included income terms and interactions of premiums and income in light of the concern that insurance might be a superior good and those with higher incomes are more willing to purchase it. The estimated models yielded consistent results that, as expected, higher premiums are associated with lower participation rates. In models that included income, income generally was not significant at a .05 level, but the non-significant trend suggested that higher incomes were associated with greater participation. The interactions of premium levels and income were not significant, but that is not surprising given the limited sample sizes. The simplest model (model 1), which used premiums as a percentage of income as the only independent variable, explained just about as much variance as the model which also included income. Addition of more variables did not substantially improve model fit or modify the coefficient for premiums. The curve shown in Figure 5.1 is based on the simple model 1.

We also estimated the models under a different approach, using bootstrap resampling methods with random resampling of the 21 cases with replacement to create 50 bootstrap data sets. We used the 50 data sets to examine the possibility that the model may be biased because the underlying population parameters are not normally distributed or that extreme values in one or two observations may skew results (Mooney and Duval 1993: Veall 1998). The bootstrap coefficients were quite similar to the single model and the standard errors were marginally larger, suggesting that bias was minimal. For example, the single model estimates that participation with a premium share at 1% of income would be 57%, while the pooled bootstrap estimate is 55%, virtually the same.

We acknowledge that this analysis is simplistic and is sharply limited by data availability. A better data set would include large representative surveys of low-income people in each state, measuring program participation, income and premiums paid, as well as factors that also might affect the demand for insurance, including health status, family composition, employment status, and perceptions of the program, including awareness of the insurance program, ease of application, and perceived generosity of benefits. However, we are unaware of a better data set for this purpose.

8.   Lastly, the difference might be an artifact of sampling error. Because of limited sample sizes in the CPS (even using a three-year merged file), there is uncertainty in the estimates of the denominators. In this event, the apparently low participation rates in Washington may be caused by random noise and might have been found in one of the other two states if different samples were drawn.

REFERENCES

Call, K., N. Lurie, Y. Jonk, R. Feldman, and M. Finch. 1997. Who Is Still Uninsured in Minnesota: Lessons from State Reform Efforts. *Journal of the American Medical Association* 278(14):1191–1195.

Coughlin, T., S. Rajan, S. Zuckerman, and J. Marsteller. 1997. *Health Policy for Low-Income People in Minnesota.* Assessing the New Federalism. Washington. D.C.: Urban Institute.

Cutler, D., and J. Gruber. 1997. Medicaid and Private Insurance: Evidence and Implications. *Health Affairs* 16(1): 194–200.

Diehr, P., C. Madden, A. Cheadle, et al. 1996. Will Uninsured People Volunteer for Voluntary Health Insurance? Experience from Washington State. *American Journal of Public Health* 86(4):529–532.

Diehr, P., C. Madden, D. Martin, et al. 1993. Who Enrolled in a State Program for the Uninsured: Was There Adverse Selection? *Medical Care* 31:1093–1105.

Dubay, L., and G. Kenney. 1996. The Effects of Medicaid Expansions on Insurance Coverage of Children. *Future of Children* 6(1):152–161.

———. 1997. Did Medicaid Expansions for Pregnant Women Crowd Out Private Coverage? *Health Affairs* 16(1): 185–193.

Greene, W. 1990. *Econometric Analysis.* New York: Macmillan.

Hoffman, C. 1998. *The Uninsured in America: A Chart Book.* Washington, D.C.: Kaiser Commission on Medicaid and the Uninsured.

Ku, L., and T. Coughlin. 1997. The Use of Sliding Scale Premiums in Subsidized Insurance Programs. Working paper. The Urban Institute, Washington, D.C.

Lipson, D., and S. Schrodel. 1996. *State Subsidized Insurance Programs for Low-Income People.* Washington, D.C.: Alpha Center.

Mooney, C., and R. Duval. 1993. *Bootstrapping: A Non-parametric Approach to Statistical Inference.* Newbury Park, Calif.: Sage Publications.

Nichols, L., L. Ku, S. Norton, and S. Wall. 1997. *Health Policy for Low-Income People in Washington.* Assessing the New Federalism. Washington, D.C.: Urban Institute.

Riley, T., and C. Pernice. 1998. *How Are States Implementing Childrens Health Insurance Plans?: An Analysis and Summary of State Plans Submitted to the Health Care Financing Administration, second edition.* Portland, Maine: National Academy for State Health Policy.

Thorpe, K. E., and C. S. Florence. 1999. Why Are Workers Uninsured? Employer-Sponsored Health Insurance in 1997. *Health Affairs* 18(2):213–218.

Veall, M. 1998. Applications of the Bootstrap in Econometrics and Economic Statistics. In *Handbook of Applied Economic Statistics,* A. Ullah and D. Giles, eds. New York: Marcel Dekker, Inc.

Winterbottom, C., D. Liska, and K. Obermaier. 1995. *State-Level Data Book on Health Financing and Access, second edition.* Washington, D.C.: Urban Institute.

Wooldridge, J., L. Ku, T. Coughlin, et al. 1996. *Implementing State Health Care Reform: What Have We Learned from the First Year?* The first annual report of the Evaluation of Health Reform in Five States. Princeton, N.J.: Mathematica Policy Research, Inc.

6

The States and Health Care Reform: The Road Traveled and Lessons Learned from Seven that Took the Lead

Pamela A. Paul-Shaheen

We can make dust or eat dust.[1]

Over the last decade, an arena of major policy activity for states has been health care reform. Given the complexity of this issue and the acrimony surrounding the most recent federal debate on this topic, why, one might ask, would states even want to tackle "the eight-hundred-pound gorilla"?[2] Although numerous reasons have been cited, one appears to dominate—escalating health care costs. Costs are of particular concern to states because they are major purchasers of health care services and, on average, 20 percent of a state's budget goes to fund health care programs (U.S. General Accounting Office 1992: 15). The dollars appropriated finance all (or a major portion) of the health insurance purchased for state employees and retirees, finance and/or provide health services to prisoners and other eligible groups such as education personnel, fund a broad

Reprinted from *Journal of Health Politics, Policy and Law*, 23, no. 2 (April 1998):319–61. Copyright 1998. Duke University Press. All rights reserved. Reprinted with permission.

range of public health programs, and provide funds to pay a portion of the cost of indigent care.

This investment in health care—coupled with the constitutional requirement for a balanced budget and the need to respond to both the requirements and the constraints imposed by federal statutes (Medicaid and ERISA, the Employee Retirement Income Security Act of 1974, come specifically to mind)—has placed enormous pressure on states to find innovative new ways to reduce rising health care costs; this need has pushed them to undertake new reform efforts, while at the same time they try to preserve (if not expand) access to health care for the under- and uninsured. In essence, states are pressured from all sides. As Deborah Stone observed: "From above, the federal government mandates states to provide more benefits to more people while cutting its own contributions to state revenues. From below, the cities and counties come to states for fiscal relief as their uncompensated care bill grows. And from within, the business community complains to state government about the escalating costs of insurance or the inability to obtain employee coverage at all" (1992: 2).

In every state, legislation has been introduced to address various aspects of the problem and to accomplish a wide range of health policy objectives. These include regulating insurance practices for underwriting and rate-setting in the small group insurance market; providing state-subsidized insurance programs and creating risk pools for specific uninsured groups; providing tax credits or other incentives to encourage the purchase of insurance coverage; moving populations underwritten by state governments into managed care arrangements; changing health care delivery system financing and provision of care arrangements; establishing global budgets and imposing risk sharing; establishing IRAs (individual retirement accounts) for medical care; and most recently, implementing new health care purchasing arrangements designed to empower health care consumers and purchasers in the insurance marketplace, that is, enacting managed competition strategies (Ladenheim 1993).

As of January 1995, seven states (Florida, Hawaii, Massachusetts, Minnesota, Oregon, Vermont, and Washington) had progressed the furthest in enacting comprehensive statutes designed both to move toward providing universal coverage to state residents and to slow the growth in health care costs. As these states struggled to enact these reforms, numerous researchers chronicled one or more of their efforts to further our understanding of the dynamics of state health policy reform (Ascuaga 1992; Bergthold 1988; Brown 1991, 1993a; Crittenden 1993; Goldberger 1990; Kronick 1990; Leichter 1993; and Neubauer 1993). Building on these case study analyses, I attempt to extend this work by using a multistate analysis to answer the following question: "In looking at these seven states, what were the common challenges faced by each, and was there a set of common factors evident that facilitated their enacting these major reform bills?"

The approach involved analyzing select characteristics of the seven states and of the reform process to determine which among them made a contribution. Unfortunately, time and resource constraints precluded comparing these seven with other states that had also attempted but failed to enact such reforms, to determine whether or not similar attributes were present. Thus, the observations and conclusions presented must be seen as preliminary. It is my hope that publication of this article will encourage other researchers interested in state health policy to initiate such comparisons. Additional work in this area is clearly needed to enhance our understanding of the conditions necessary to accomplish and sustain comprehensive state health care reform and to determine whether states can perform this task adequately. Such analyses are even more imperative today given the public's dissatisfaction with federal reform efforts, the current fiscal environment, and the interest on the part of Congress in devolving more responsibility to states and localities.

To address the key question of interest, three approaches were used. First, the literature on state health care reform was reviewed. Second, key individuals involved in the health care reform process were identified and interviewed to augment the information available in the literature. Their names and the roles they played are noted in Table 6.1. Their comments, insights, and enthusiasm were invaluable and the richness of these findings is, in great part, a reflection of their collective contribution. Third, a series of "maps" were prepared that depict the road to reform traveled by each of the states, as described by the literature and those interviewed. The maps identified the key starting point for each state's reform effort and traced the subsequent policy activity undertaken that contributed to their achievement of the intended policy goals.[3]

ENACTING COMPREHENSIVE HEALTH REFORM: EMERGING LESSONS

From the literature reviewed, interviews conducted, and maps created, a series of lessons emerged about the reform effort in those seven states. Some lessons identified and discussed here, including the use of crisis to create "windows of opportunity," the expanding role of the bureaucracy, and the destabilizing influence of new interest groups, have also been identified by others as important contributors to reform (see Kingdon 1984; Morone 1994; Baumgartner and Jones 1993). Other lessons—the key role of entrepreneurs and others in the reform process, the emergence of large-scale reform from a series of smaller initiatives, the role that elections, the media, and the public can play in determining the course of reform, and the unique influence of the single-payer option—are new observations emerging from this analysis. In all, nine lessons were identified. For purposes of the discussion that follows, they are clustered in two major categories. The first encompasses those lessons that

TABLE 6.1

State Officials Providing Background

FLORIDA

Michael Abrams   Member, Health Subcommittee of the House Health Care and Insurance Committee; Chair, House Finance and Tax Committee

Gary J. Clarke   Deputy Assistant Secretary for Health Planning and Regulation, Florida Department of Health and Rehabilitative Services; Deputy Director, Health Program Office, Florida Department of Health and Rehabilitative Services; Director, Florida Medicaid Program, Florida Department of Health and Rehabilitative Services

Ralph Glatfelter   Executive Director, Florida League of Hospitals

Joan Glickman   Aid to Senator Forman

Mike Hanson   Staff Director, House Health Care Committee

Carl Homer   Vice President for Public Policy, Blue Cross and Blue Shield of Florida

Sharon Jacobs   Staff Director, House Insurance Committee; Bureau Chief, MEDAC-CESS, Agency for Health Care Administration

Ree Sailors   Senior Policy Analyst, Task Force on Competition and Consumer Choice (1982); Member, Task Force on Private Sector Health Care Responsibilities (1989); President and CEO, Florida Health Access

HAWAII

Henry Foley, Ph.D.   Director of Behavioral Services, Hawaii Department of Health; Faculty, University of Hawaii Medical School; Director, Ke Ola O Hawaii, Inc.

John C. Lewin, M.D.   Director, Hawaii Department of Health

Deane Neubauer, Ph.D.   Professor of Political Science, University of Hawaii; Facilitator, Governor's Blue Ribbon Panel on Health Care (1990)

James Shon   Chair, House Health Committee

Peter A. Sybinsky, Ph.D.   Administrative Assistant to the Director, Hawaii Department of Health; Deputy Director, Hawaii Department of Health

Nadao Yoshinaga   Chair, Senate Ways & Means Committee

Albert H. Yuen   Administrative Vice President, Hawaii Medical Services Administration

MASSACHUSETTS

John Crosier   Executive Director and President, Massachusetts Business Roundtable

Michael S. Dukakis   Governor of Massachusetts

Catherine Dunham   Director, Governor's Office of Human Resources

David MacKenzie   Director of Policy, Senate Ways & Means Committee

John McDonough   Member, Joint Committee on Health Care

Susan Sherry   Director, Massachusetts Health Action Alliance; Executive Director, Health Care for All

Steven Tringale   Intern, Joint House & Senate Health Care Committee; Staff, Joint House & Senate Health Care Committee; Staff, Massachusetts Rate Setting Commission; Vice President, Life Insurance Association of Massachusetts; Division President, Seniors, Blue Cross and Blue Shield of Massachusetts

continued

TABLE 6.1 *continued*

MINNESOTA

Linda Berglin   Chair, Senate Health and Human Services Committee

Lee Greenfield   Chair, Human Services Finance Division of House Appropriations

Luanne Nyberg   Director, Children's Defense Fund—Minnesota

Mary Jo O'Brien   Director, Legislative Relations, Minnesota Medical Association; Deputy Commissioner, Minnesota Department of Health; Commissioner, Minnesota Department of Health

Paul Ogren   Chair, House Health Committee Chair, House Taxation Committee

Michael Scandrett   Senate Counsel; Lead Staff for the Gang of Seven; Executive Director, Minnesota HealthCare Commission

OREGON

Bruce Bishop   Kaiser Permanente; Oregon Hospital Association

Michael McCracken   House Member, Legislative Emergency Board; Staff Director, Commission on Health Care (1988); Administrator, Senate Committee on Health Insurance and Bioethics; Consultant, Oregon Health Decisions; Legislative Liaison, Oregon Medical Association

Ellen Pinney   Director, Oregon Health Action Campaign

Robert Shoemaker   Legal Counsel, Multnomah County Medical Society; Chair, Senate Committee on Health Insurance and Bioethics (1989–1995); Core Faculty, Forum for State Health Policy Leadership, GWU

VERMONT

Paul Wallace-Brodeur   Executive Director, Health Policy Corporation; Executive Director, Health Policy Council; Vermont Health Care Authority

Hamilton Davis   Chair, Hospital Data Counsel; Special Counsel to the Governor for Health Policy; Member, House Health and Welfare Committee; Associate Research Professor, University of Vermont, College of Medicine

Paul Harrington   Chair, House Commerce Committee; Member, the Vermont Health Care Authority Board

Jeanne Keller   President, Vermont Employers Health Alliance

Karen Meyer   Executive Director, Vermont State Medical Society

WASHINGTON

Bob Crittenden, M.D.   Research Analyst, House Health Committee; Associate Executive Director, Washington Health Care Project Commission; Special Assistant to the Governor for Health; Faculty, School of Medicine, University of Washington

Susan Crystal   Director, Democratic Policy Office, House of Representatives; Special Assistant to the Governor for Health Policy

Leo Greenawalt   President, Washington State Hospital Association

William Hagens   Senior Research Analyst, House Health Care Committee

Featherstone Reid   Staff Counsel, Senate Ways and Means Committee; Senior Staff Counsel, Senate Democratic Caucus

Don Sloma   Staff Coordinator, Senate Health and Long Term Care Committee

Margaret Stanley   President, Health Plus HMO; Administrator, Washington Health Care Authority reaffirm the conventional wisdom from other studies of state and national health care reform efforts. The second category encompasses new lessons that emerge from this analysis of state efforts to enact and sustain comprehensive health care reform. I hope that this work helps extend our understanding of the complex dynamics that contribute to catalyzing and sustaining these reform efforts. These categories and their related lessons are identified below and discussed in detail in the text that follows.

Category 1. Lessons Reinforcing Our Current Understanding of State Health Reform

1. The perception of a crisis serves as a powerful catalyst for political action, creating the window of opportunity for policy change.
2. The emergence of new interest groups destabilizes the existing policy monopoly and enhances the opportunity for reform.
3. The highly technical nature of the health care reform process creates expanded opportunities for bureaucratic influence.

Category 2. Lessons Extending Our Understanding of State Health Reform

4. "Timing" is a major influence in the reform process.
5. The state's reform process is a continuum—comprehensive reforms are the product of earlier, smaller steps that serve as building blocks.
6. Entrepreneurship is an essential component of the reform equation. Comprehensive reform requires individuals with vision, pragmatism, and dedication to guide the way.
7. The attention of the media and public opinion helps keep the issue on the policy agenda.
8. Comprehensive health care reform efforts are initiated by the Democratic side of the aisle.
9. The single-payer option is the paper tiger of health care reform.

CATEGORY 1

LESSON 1. "CRISIS" AS CATALYST

Important in these reform efforts were the periodic windows of opportunity that opened along the way. According to Kingdon (1984), such windows occur when a long-standing condition reemerges as a problem, when a solution deemed to address the problem is developed and available for adoption, when a political or environmental change enhances the timing for policy change, and when the constraints are not severe enough to preclude action. Without exception, the key "crisis" that served as the rallying cry for comprehensive state reform in these seven states was escalating health care costs.[4] Those advocating for reform found early on that framing the issue as a cost "crisis"—for the middle class, the government, and/or the business community—significantly increased the likelihood that political inertia could be overcome and policy action advanced. The cost "crisis," however, was never one-dimensional. In Florida, it arose in the context of the concentration of the state's uncompensated care burden in select public hospitals. In Washington State, the "crisis" occurred when Blue Cross officials informed the governor and the legislature that the state employees' health insurance fund had a $40 million deficit. In Massachusetts, it emerged from the business coalition's concern over cost shifting, and in Oregon, the "crisis" came in the form of the media's coverage of the death of Coby Howard, a seven-year-old transplant candidate, following the elimination of transplant coverage from the state's Medicaid program.

While escalating health care costs initially catalyzed the debate, that issue was quickly joined with the issue of access as policy makers, struggling to solve the cost problem, realized that the two were inextricably linked. In Massachusetts, for example, Nelson Gifford, chair of the Massachusetts Business Roundtable Healthcare Coalition, quickly came to realize that in order to reduce the burden of the cost of uncompensated care on corporations offering health care coverage, an effort would have to be undertaken to address the cost-shifting problem. That would require finding other options to cover those who were not insured.

Thus, although the major driver of change in a majority of the seven states was the compelling need to address a health care cost crisis, access also became part of the reform equation, given the relationship between the two. As such, the solutions adopted by these states reflect broad attempts to address both issues. Most important, it was the joining of these issues that enhanced the political legitimacy of health care reform. Up to this point, health care reform was most often characterized as an issue of the political left and discussed in terms of expanded access. Political conservatives realized that to control costs they would have to address access, which allowed the two issues to be put on the table simultaneously, and thus significantly expanded the political constituency for state health care reform.[5] It was the convergence of these factors that greatly facilitated the opportunity for policy enactment.

LESSON 2. THE ROLE OF SPECIAL INTERESTS

The politics of health care has been particularly subject to interest group pressure because it has been historically dominated by one of the most prestigious and lucrative professions in America—physicians. As Morone noted: "A single pattern dominated American health politics for most of the twentieth century:

public power was ceded to the medical professions. Health care providers acted as trustees of health care policy" (1990: 254). This dominance supported the continuation of health care policies favorable to the medical profession and contributed to the states' inability to enact other than incremental changes in existing law through the 1970s and early 1980s.[6] By the mid-1980s, however, physician dominance had been severely eroded in these states for several reasons. First, the physician lobby was joined by other health care groups who actively began to represent their interests in the legislative process. Most important, these groups were often subdivided into a number of factions with differentiated interests and points of view on the question of how the health care crisis should be addressed. Often, the result was that representatives of the public health community, nursing, and the other allied health professions espoused one policy agenda, hospitals and physicians espoused another, and HMOs and insurers espoused a third, thus eliminating the opportunity for these interests to collectively demonstrate a united front. Second, as will be discussed in more detail later, other stakeholder groups organized and entered the policy dialogue and began advocating change. Finally, in some states, the cost crisis and its impact on the states' budgets grew too problematic for the executive and legislative branches to ignore. Here, the budget problem was perceived to be so great that legislators were able to muster the internal resolve necessary to "do something," despite significant provider opposition.

This is not to say that provider stakeholder groups did not retain a powerful role in the process—in several of these reform states, they were the key set of stakeholder interest groups to be reckoned with. However, where they faced no heavy counter stakeholder opposition, there ultimately came a time in the reform process when the pressure for reform was so great that continued opposition on their part would only lead to their organizations being viewed as obstructionist, or worse yet, to their being shut out of the reform dialogue altogether. Thus, by the time major reform legislation was adopted, it was ultimately done with a majority of the health care stakeholder groups supporting the reform effort.[7]

In these reform states, the strongest counterweight to the health care lobby was the business coalition. During the past two decades, business coalitions focused on health care issues have rapidly emerged as business has tried to respond to the impact of escalating health care costs on their bottom line and as business leaders have become angered by what they view as a lack of discipline and rationality in the health care system (Bergthold 1990). As a 1970 *Fortune Magazine* article wryly noted: "Our present system of medical care is not a system at all. The majority of physicians constitute an army of pushcart vendors in an age of supermarkets" (cited in Martin 1993).

The entry of business changed both the dynamics and the nature of the health care reform debate in these states. First and foremost, it provided a rationale for Republicans to become active participants. Whereas Republican legislators may have been reluctant to advocate health care reform, given their historical alignment with providers, there now was another powerful constituency traditionally aligned with Republican interests urging them to do so. Second, business interests were viewed as being a significant concern in these states and business leaders were seen as possessing the political clout necessary to deliver key votes. Their political clout, coupled with their initial comfort in pursuing a reform agenda encompassing both market-based and government-mandated initiatives targeted at controlling costs, made them a formidable force in the legislative deliberations on health care reform.[8]

Consumer coalitions were also represented in these reform efforts. The experience of these seven states, however, suggests that their influence varied considerably. In many cases, their presence was considered highly suspect by other stakeholder groups. As Massachusetts's David MacKenzie, director of Policy for the Senate Ways and Means Committee observed, "They were viewed by other interests as bringing lots of 'demands' to the table but no 'votes.' " Even so, Massachusetts's Catherine Dunham, director of the Governor's Office of Human Resources, noted "they often did play an important role, serving as a 'conscience' in the debate, articulating the problems experienced by consumers seeking insurance or care and providing evidence of the impact of various reform options on them."

Consumer advocates were most influential in reform efforts in Massachusetts, Minnesota, Oregon, and Vermont. Three factors appeared to contribute to their success. First, in these states, these groups' membership was more organized and active and could be effectively mobilized to write letters, call legislators, appear in demonstrations, work to represent their issues with the media, and/or testify at legislative hearings. Second, they had paid staff, which meant the group's representatives were available to actively participate in the many meetings and hearings during which the legislation was developed. Third, in some cases, powerful executive or legislative sponsors created a place for them at the reform table, making sure their issues got on the agenda as part of the policy debate. Such was the case in Massachusetts where Health Care for All— a coalition of consumer advocates working initially on Medicare and Medicaid access issues—became a player in the Massachusetts health care reform effort because of the Dukakis administration's interest in their concerns. As a result, they were given statutory representation on the Study Commission for Health Care Financing and Delivery Reform when it was established in 1985, and their influence carried over into the legislative process when Senator Pat McGovern (D), a key sponsor of the reform legislation, expressed support for their issues and sought input from them in the reform negotiations.[9]

What is clear from the reform efforts of these seven states is that the fractionalization of the health lobby into subunits with competing interests and the concurrent rise of the business and consumer coalitions contributed significantly to destabilize the existing policy monopoly controlled primarily by physicians, hospitals, and insurers and to the opportunity to enact substantive health care reform legislation in each of these states. This pattern is one noted by Baumgartner and Jones (1993) whose research suggests that the opportunity for sweeping change in policy often emerges during a period when the existing structure of special interests supporting the status quo is significantly altered, as was clearly the case here. Their future influence and the relative position of these stakeholder groups in this process continue to evolve as state policy makers reassess the role they can play and the political currency they bring to the table.

LESSON 3. THE EXPANSION OF BUREAUCRATIC INFLUENCE

With our collective emphasis on free enterprise and individualism, American culture has generally cast the bureaucracy in an unfavorable light (Thompson 1981). Yet one of the most striking elements of the reform efforts in these seven states is the role the bureaucracy played and/or the expansion of bureaucratic responsibility as a result of the statutory changes made. As Minnesota's Mary Jo O'Brien (then Deputy Commissioner of Minnesota's Department of Health) observed, "We have to find a new name for the bureaucracy, something more neutral, like 'infrastructure'—some term that connotes both capacity and competence, given that the term 'bureaucracy' is now a negative label—because these institutions are critical to advancing our policy goals in achieving health reform." Reforming the health care system proved a highly complex task, given that the subject area is both broad in scope and highly technical. Morone (1994) argues that the emerging politics of American health care policy increasingly operates with the language, methodology, and mind-set of bureaucratic actors. This was clearly the case with these seven states.

Early on, state policy makers came to realize that to accomplish meaningful reform and not just marginal change, they needed health care reform from a system-wide perspective, a focus which, in many cases, led to major statutory changes in how health care was to be financed, regulated, and monitored. In Minnesota, for example, the major provisions of Minnesota's HealthRight legislation contained several new cost containment strategies, provided for health insurance reform, expanded access to the uninsured, addressed select rural health care issues, and provided for new data collection and research efforts. Washington State's Health Services Act established certified health plans and health purchasing cooperatives, a state regulatory commission, and insurance premium caps; provided for a system of individual and employer mandates—combined with state subsidies—to create nearly universal coverage statewide, enhanced public health services, and provided for malpractice reform. Florida's Health Care and Insurance Reform Act established a voluntary managed competition model for health care reform in the state, created community health purchasing alliances, and reformed the small group insurance market. In a majority of cases, implementing these new mandates fell to the states' health bureaucracy.

Additionally, the bills containing these provisions were highly technical, with interdependent provisions, and often ran hundreds of pages in length. In many states, state agency representatives played key roles in developing major provisions of the bills. This was particularly true when (a) the scope of the legislation was both broad and ambitious, requiring that many statutory changes and/or additions be embodied in the bill(s), and when (b) the bureaucracy was seen by the governor's office and legislature as a credible resource. Jean Thorne, director of the Office of Medical Assistance Programs for Oregon's Department of Human Resources, Minnesota's Mary Jo O'Brien, and Margaret Stanley, administrator for the Washington Health Care Authority, all remember spending "hundreds of hours" identifying issues, researching alternatives, drafting language, and managing the politics of the process.

States also sought to facilitate reform by reorganizing the state agencies involved and/or by creating new institutions and empowering them with new responsibilities. Many of these new agencies were created to allow the governor and the legislature to get things done at a faster pace than would have been possible if these functions had been vested in existing organizations with their own agendas and internal cultures. Observed then-director of the Hawaii Department of Health, John Lewin, M.D., "In some cases, you need to create a new agency to promote change. It [statutory creation] also allows you to vest the agency with sufficient resources and authority. The alternative is to have sufficient time to change the internal culture of existing agencies, and, odds are, that it is a less likely outcome." Examples of states where reform efforts elected this option include Minnesota and Florida. For MinnesotaCare, the Minnesota HealthRight Act of 1992 created a Health Care Commission and several new committees to complete reports and studies and make recommendations on a variety of topics, ranging from devising a plan providing universal health coverage for all Minnesotans to making recommendations on the appropriate dissemination of technology throughout the state (Yawn, Jacott, and Yawn 1993). In Florida the Health Care Reform Act of 1992 created the Agency for Health Care Administration; State Representative C. Fred Jones intended to get the attention of the health care industry. To accomplish this, the legislation empowered the agency to conduct a broad range of functions, including purchasing, planning, policy analysis, and regulation.

Interestingly, in select states, these new entities have become the *key* focal point for new policy recommendations. Thus, as reforms are implemented, these new organizations begin to set the institutional agenda for future change. As experience in these states has unfolded, it reflects what appears to be an emerging cycle in the expansion of bureaucratic influence in state health care reform—one wherein commissions and task forces (often with bureaucratic representatives) initially establish policy frameworks; governors and legislators then translate these policy frameworks into legislation (often with agency assistance); the legislation, as adopted, creates new administrative roles and new bureaucratic organizations, which subsequently become influential in the development of additional policies.

CATEGORY 2

LESSON 4. TIMING IS EVERYTHING

In show business, it is often said that timing is everything. This observation also appears to apply to state health care reform as well. As Washington State's Sue Crystal (special assistant to the governor for health policy) observed, "After the election, there was a 'harmonic convergence.' We had before us a 105-day session, a new governor and insurance commissioner, Democratic control of both houses, strong health committee chairs, and a supportive leadership—we were ready!"

Timing, as it turns out, has many dimensions. In several cases, the reality of deadlines—particularly the close of a legislative calendar—added impetus to the process. This was particularly true in states that operate on a short legislative calendar, such as Vermont, Oregon, and Washington State. In these cases, policy supporters often felt pressured to complete actions before the close of an official legislative session, lest they lose momentum, short-circuiting the opportunity for enacting reforms in a later session.

The timing of state elections was also influential. In Minnesota and Washington, statewide elections actually became public referenda on the health care reform effort. Public support at the time was high, and as Minnesota's Michael Scandrett (then legislative staffer to the house-senate reform group) noted, "The political winds of the times indicated the public wanted the state to take action." Thus, according to state Representative Lee Greenfield (D), "Incumbents who supported reforms were seen in a favorable light by their constituents because they were working to solve a problem of concern to the electorate."[10] In other states, state elections had a negative effect—as the defeat of Chiles's Florida Health Security Proposal in 1994 made clear. The proposal, considered a key plank in the administration's reform platform, went down to defeat when the Florida Senate, divided evenly among Democrats and Republicans, voted 20 to 20 on the measure. Noted Gary Clarke, former director of the Florida Medicaid Program, "That session no one [in the Republican camp] wanted to enact Florida Health Security because no one wanted to give Chiles a 'platform' to run on for governor" (1991).[11]

The timing of national events also played a role. In Massachusetts the presidential bid of Michael Dukakis was key to the enactment of the Massachusetts Health Security Act. According to Catherine Dunham, "As Michael Dukakis's star rose in the presidential primaries, it allowed the Democrats in Massachusetts to rally together so that Massachusetts could be the first state after Hawaii [to achieve reform] and the best:" Observed state Representative John McDonough (D): "Some in Massachusetts felt the bill would never have been enacted if Dukakis had not been running for president. House members did not want to mess up Dukakis's presidential aspirations." Dukakis himself put it this way: "The presidential campaign also played an important role. I started making real progress in the early primaries. I talked a lot about our efforts in Massachusetts. I think there was a genuine sense of excitement about the campaign and about the leadership role that Massachusetts had taken on a whole host of important issues during the previous three to four years: welfare reform, urban revitalization, child care policy, plant closing notification, and many more. Unemployment in the state had dropped to below three percent. Universal health care was, in a sense, the crown jewel of a remarkably creative period in the state's political history, and the presidential campaign helped to crystallize that feeling in a very special way."

In Oregon, national events proved to have more negative consequences as Oregon's interface with the timing of national events led to unanticipated delays in securing a key federal Medicaid waiver required to implement a major provision of the state's Basic Health Services Act. Here the delays resulted principally from the presidential election of 1992. The state's initial waiver request had been forwarded to the Health Care Finance Administration in 1991, and according to Jean Thorne, state officials hoped that it would be quickly approved. Not so, as the waiver was not secured from the federal government until March 1993. In the interim, according to Jean, the Oregon waiver became "the political hot potato," with which neither the outgoing Bush administration nor the incoming Clinton administration wanted to deal, much to the frustration of Oregon's public officials. Such was the case in each of these seven states. Timing was critical in these states in another way that was noted previously by Sue Crystal of Washington State. For in each of these states, a series of factors had come to the fore. In each, the issues of rising health care cost and limited access achieved heightened public attention. In each, an entrepreneur or entrepreneurs emerged, willing to serve as a catalyst for and broker in the political process; new stakeholders identified health care as an issue and became engaged in the policy debate; legislative leaders gave their tacit approval to undertaking such an effort; the public appeared supportive; and a key task force or commission had also developed a blueprint for action. Thus it was through the "harmonic convergence" of these factors that a window of opportunity was opened and the stage set for comprehensive reform.[12]

LESSON 5. THE HEALTH CARE REFORM CONTINUUM

One common characteristic of these seven states is that the major reforms enacted, when mapped to create a "road to reform," are part of a longer continuum of change marked along the way by the enactment of other pieces of legislation interspersed with the work of the task forces and commissions. In Washington State, for example, those interviewed traced the history of the comprehensive Washington Health Services Act of 1993 back to the establishment of the Governor's Commission on Public Cost Containment in 1982, which was intended to review all state government expenditures in health, and which the 1993 act incorporates as a key provision. The Basic Health Plan was established in 1987 to make low-cost health insurance available to the working uninsured. In both Minnesota and Vermont, crucial early steps on the road to reform were the successful enactment of legislation to expand access to health care for children (i.e., Minnesota's Children's Health Plan in 1987 and Vermont's Dr. Dynasaur Program in 1989). Early precursors in Massachusetts and Florida were the enactment of statutes in 1976 and 1979, respectively, to collect and report on health care costs; these statutes ultimately provided evidence of the cost "crisis" used to enact the later legislation. These building block approaches, according to Margaret Stanley, "facilitated political consensus because they [the reforms] built upon a set of decisions previously committed to." Thus, the broader reforms that followed were often viewed by state policy makers as having been based on the lessons learned and commitments made as part of actions previously taken—in other words, extensions of old, more familiar initiatives.

This incrementalism, however, should not lead readers to assume that the reform laws enacted in these states made only minor changes in their existing health care systems, for this is not the case. In each of these states, sweeping changes were made in how health care was to be delivered, regulated, and financed (Oliver and Paul-Shaheen 1997). As such, the evolutionary process of health care policymaking evidenced in these states appears to reflect the "punctuated equilibrium model" of policy change posited by Baumgartner and Jones (1993). According to their model, policy making in a particular arena (in this case, health care) is marked by periods of relative stability during which only minor incremental modifications are made, followed by periods of rapid, dramatic, and nonincremental change.[13] In their analysis, key factors contributing to the opportunity to make major policy changes include changes in public mood, the perceived salience of the issue, the emergence of a window of opportunity, the efforts of policy entrepreneurs, and changes in the power and influence of key stakeholder groups; all of these, as discussed later in this article, occurred in these seven states.

Another distinguishing characteristic of the major reforms enacted by these seven states is that they were all highly individualized pieces of legislation. Although many of these acts share a common framework (for example, provisions to expand access to care), the statutory provisions enacted were highly individualized and, in each state, built upon earlier efforts that had proven successful.[14] This pattern may emanate from the fact that, as Rose (1993) points out, "policy makers are inheritors before they are choosers. As a condition of taking office, they swear to uphold the laws and programs their predecessors have set in place" (78). This research supports the hypothesis that policy choices elected at one point also constrain and shape the policy options considered later, because they create "lock-in effects" through the organizational patterns they support and the social and political relationships they establish among the key stakeholder groups involved (Pierson 1992). These internal constraints appear to severely limit the degree to which any one state can adopt wholesale models of reform either developed in other states or offered in the national marketplace of ideas. Thus, in a policy arena as complicated as health care reform, states do not appear to serve as pure "laboratories" (i.e., as testing substantive new approaches), but rather take existing approaches and tailor them to meet their individual needs.

The reform continuum in each state also reflects another point of commonality—the blend of legislative enactment with education and consensus-building among key stakeholders—for in all seven states, legislative enactment was interspersed with the work of special task forces and study commissions. Although establishing such groups is often viewed as a way to kill a proposal, in these seven states these entities served several critical functions. First, as noted by Brown (1993b), they created a mechanism whereby a wide range of key actors—both legislators and others of diverse partisan, ideological, regional, and economic orientations—were educated together about the complexities of health care reform. They provided an environment where people learned to work together to develop a common mission, and most important, to gain a sense of trust. As Margaret Stanley (administrator of the Health Care Authority for Washington State) observed, "This approach enhanced the opportunity for legislative enactment because many of the key stakeholders supported the effort based upon the philosophy of the approach, which evolved out of the past history of the group's working together in an atmosphere of mutual respect." Second, they fostered the process of member "enlightenment," whereby information gathered informed the debate and altered perceptions of the seriousness of the problems, the relative importance of different causes, and/or enhanced understanding of the effects of the major policy options being considered (Sabatier 1991).

Task force members were often drawn from the state's health policy community. Members of such communities—state bureaucrats, executive and legislative personnel, interest group leaders, researchers, and specialist reporters—

possess a knowledge of the subject area, have a professional stake in the reform process, and because of their expertise and influence, an ability to shape the policy options—not only in the short term, but also in the long term (Sabatier 1991). Establishing periodic task forces and commissions creates additional opportunities for dialogue among these individuals. Through such dialogues, incentives develop for finding accommodation, that is, common ground (Simon 1979). Through the process of negotiation, compromise, and consensus building, the deals were struck, with each deal satisfying enough of the stakeholder participants' expectations such that they were willing to support the recommendations, believing that they are not going to get a better deal elsewhere. The recommendations emanating from these groups also often served as a core framework for the reform legislation that was ultimately adopted. Such was the case in Florida where the Health Care Access Act of 1984 incorporated many of the recommendations issued by the Competition and Consumer Choice Task Force, which had conducted its deliberations in 1982, and in Washington State, where the key recommendations of the Washington Health Care Commission[15] and the Washington Health Care Authority[16] were incorporated in the Washington Health Services Act. This approach is evident in the other states as well.

Somewhat unexpectedly, these task forces and commissions also provided a unique opportunity for participants to explore the relative roles and responsibilities of government and the private sector in health care reform. According to Minnesota's commissioner of health at the time, Mary Jo O'Brien, "they provided an environment in which the appropriate role of government in health care reform could be explored, discussed, and agreed to." In several cases, this expanded understanding contributed to the enactment of reform language under which state government was able to consolidate related health care functions and take on a broader range of responsibilities.[17]

Finally, representatives of these commissions and task forces often became the primary stakeholders advocating the policy changes reflected in the major reform bills during the legislative debate, as well as serving as the institutional memory for implementing the legislation following enactment. In sum, these groups played critical roles in all stages of the reform process.

LESSON 6. THE ESSENCE OF ENTREPRENEURSHIP

A major factor in achieving policy reform in each of the seven states, without exception, was effective leadership. Although it was true that the circumstances had to be "ripe" for action to occur, the critical matching of problems and solutions was most often the result of the drive and imagination of a gifted leader (or leaders). In each state, this leadership was provided by key individuals who served as "entrepreneurs," guiding the reform process to a successful conclusion. Entrepreneurship is the process of introducing innovation to society, and although it is traditionally associated with private business, entrepreneurship applies to the public sector as well. In the health policy arena, entrepreneurship encompasses the process of combining policy innovation—fashioning new goals, procedures, organizations, or programs in the public sector to address salient problems with political acumen—with the ability to successfully fashion a guide to policy strategy through the legislative process (Oliver 1991). A defining characteristic of political entrepreneurs, much like that of a business entrepreneur, is their willingness to invest their resources—time, energy, reputation, and sometimes money—in the hope of a future return. Their challenge is to design a proposal, or to shepherd the development of a proposal, with sufficiently acceptable provisions that it will attract ample support for enactment (Bardach 1972). According to Peterson (1992), to successfully accomplish this change, entrepreneurs have to address four key tasks, all of which were reflected in the experiences of these seven states. First, they must identify the target problems that need to be addressed. Second, they must identify and promote broadly recognized options for addressing these problems. Third, they must identify and market effective strategies for advancing the reform agenda, and, fourth, they must enlist coalitions of supporters, both in and out of government, as advocates for the reform effort.

In these seven states, individuals in both the private and public sectors served as entrepreneurs in the reform effort, and in only one state—Oregon—was a single individual identified as having solely played that role. That individual was John Kitzhaber (D), a physician then serving as senate president. In three states, governors were widely credited as playing the entrepreneurship role—Michael Dukakis in Massachusetts, Lawton Chiles in Florida, and Howard Dean in Vermont—but each of these individuals had strong complements in the house, senate, or private sector. In some instances, governors found themselves "leading" the reform effort after much of the groundwork had been laid initially by others in the legislature or in the private sector. Massachusetts serves as a good example. According to those interviewed, the initial catalytic figure in the Massachusetts reform effort was a visionary businessman named Nelson Gifford. Gifford, president of Dennison Manufacturing Corporation, came into the policy debate in 1982. As chair of the politically powerful Massachusetts Business Roundtable's Health Care Coalition, Gifford saw the problem from a variety of different perspectives, given that he simultaneously served as a hospital trustee, a member of the board of directors of the John Hancock Insurance Company, and as vice chairman of the board of Tufts University—a prestigious academic institution with a major medical school. Gifford was viewed as conceptually and intellectually ahead of his peers, and he and the members of the Health Care Coalition played a powerful role in developing and enacting many of the policies leading up to the Massachusetts Health Security Act. In 1985, his stewardship was joined with that of the Dukakis administration, and in 1987, their network was expanded to include Senator Pat McGovern, the powerful Chair of the Joint Ways and Means Committee, who according to Steven Tringale (Massachusetts Office of Insurance and Rate Regulation), "knew she was at a unique point in time—provided with an opportunity that might never come again." It was the leadership triumvirate of Gifford, Dukakis, and McGovern that gave the Massachusetts Health Security Act a fighting chance in the state's legislature.

In several states, the reform effort was predominantly driven by legislators. In Minnesota, the original Minnesota Health Care Plan (known as House File 2, or HF2) was crafted initially by three legislators; Senator Linda Berglin (D), and Representatives Paul Ogren (D) and Lee Greenfield. House File 2 passed both the house and senate, but was vetoed by the governor. Following the veto, Paul Ogren entered into a series of exploratory discussions with Representative Dave Gruenes, a key Republican leader and member of an appropriations subcommittee. According to Ogren, Representative Gruenes had independently concluded that without system-wide reform, Minnesota would not be able to control health care costs, an issue of concern to the business community—one of Gruenes' major constituencies.[18] Through these exploratory conversations, sufficient common ground was found to bring others into the dialogue, and the "Gang of Seven"—the group of seven legislators most responsible for "entrepreneuring" the enactment of Minnesota HealthRight—was born. As a Republican member of the Gang put it, "We realized that we needed each other; they had the votes and we had the veto!" (Leichter 1993).

Much has been made, in recent years, of the qualities that characterize entrepreneurial American business leaders.[19] Many such qualities can also be applied to the policy entrepreneurs who led the health care reform effort in their respective states. Several other distinguishing characteristics common to these individuals also deserve particular mention. First, they had a *passion* for change. Whether this passion arose out of an interest in developing a dialogue on the inequities of the current health care system to explore the question of what people are entitled to in a democracy (Senator Kitzhaber, Oregon); out of an interest in enfranchising citizens to enable them to get the services they needed (Senator James McDermott, D-Washington State); out of a need (after the bombing of Pearl Harbor) to prove that individuals of Japanese descent could be loyal Americans (Senator Nadao Yoshinaga, D-Hawaii); out of an interest in completing the last plank in the New Deal (Representative Ogren, Minnesota); or out of the opportunity to combine personal commitment with political opportunity (Governors Dukakis, D-MA, and Chiles, D-FL); the passion was there, giving these individuals the drive and commitment needed to see the process through.

Second, these individuals were political pragmatists. They did not hold a rigid position on *how* reform should be accomplished, since they always remained conscious of the fact that a policy "success" is defined first and foremost in terms of affirmative votes, and is defined only secondarily in terms of its substance. The primary concern of those involved was to engineer a set of politically viable reforms, not to champion an intellectually coherent product. Thus, the resulting reform packages reflect a weaving together of a range of ideas, incorporating provisions that blended competitive and regulatory strategies, provided benefits to both specific groups and the general population, and relied both on tried and untried methods and on institutions (Oliver and Paul-Shaheen 1997).

This approach reinforces the distinction noted by Peterson (1992) between "policy entrepreneurs" (those who promote ideas for policy innovation), and "politics entrepreneurs" (those who seize opportunities for policy innovation). According to Peterson, "effective politics entrepreneurs grasp *when* the occasion for innovation is politically at hand, but also determine *what* policy alternatives are advantaged and then communicate both aspects persuasively to other responsible political actors" (8). An observation made by David MacKenzie about his former boss, Massachusetts senator McGovern, epitomizes this characteristic. "Senator McGovern was a very practical politician—although compassionate, she was only interested in working on legislation that would pay off and would never elect to be a legislative kamikaze."

Third, with rare exception, people serving in this capacity held key positions of power. Some, such as Chiles, Dean, Dukakis, and Michael Lowry, were chief executives in their respective states. Others occupied critical leadership positions in the legislature. Kitzhaber, for example, was president of the Oregon Senate; Senator McDermott chaired the Washington State Senate's Ways and Means Committee; Senator McGovern was Chair of the Senate Ways and Means Committee of the Massachusetts Legislature; Representative Michael Abrams (D) chaired the Finance and Tax Committee of the Florida House; and Representative Ogren chaired the Minnesota House Taxation Committee. As Ogren observed, "Dollars drive policy. I have far more influence over health care policy and legislative votes here than I ever would chairing the Health Policy Committee." Thus, by virtue of the key positions they held, these individuals commanded power and influence and the ability to garner votes in the legislative process.

Fourth, they understood the health care issues involved in the debate. In some instances, such as that of Minnesota's Senator Berglin, a key member of the Gang of Seven, this knowledge had been gained through years of serving on the key legislative committees that dealt with health issues. Here, they often picked an issue or issues in which to specialize and then worked over several legislative sessions demonstrating increasing competence (Weissert 1991). Oftentimes, this on-the-job learning was complemented by also having served on special state task forces and commissions. Serving in these capacities provided policy makers with additional opportunities to gain greater insight into the problems besetting the health care system and the policy options available for solving them. Some others, such as Senator John Kitzhaber, M.D., came from a health care background[20] that put them ahead of the game in terms of understanding the issues involved. For all, command of the issues was an important tool in the legislative debate. As Florida's Abrams observed, "Very few people in the legislature know anything about health care; it is a very dense topic. Command of the subject matter gives you great influence in the process—others will look to you for guidance on how to vote. Also, it [knowledge] allows you to effectively counter the influence of certain lobbyists."

Fifth, those playing the entrepreneurial role were masters of the political process. They understood how the policy game was played and what was required to win. They also knew how to manipulate the process to achieve their objectives. The activities of the Minnesota Gang of Seven (G-7) serve as a prime example. Because they were pressed for time, the G-7 introduced the Minnesota HealthRight Bill simultaneously in several house and senate committees. This approach, according to Representative Greenfield, was highly unusual and subsequently resulted in MinnesotaCare having its own unique legislative calendar. Additionally, the construction of the bill's elements took place behind closed doors; that is, the G-7 group operated without allowing in the press or special interest groups.[21] Hearings on the bill were also conducted simultaneously in many committees, and in select instances, no amendments were allowed. Observed Greenfield, "Someone from the Gang of Seven always attended these hearings to provide testimony and answer questions. The legislation was on such a fast track that in some cases, legislators were voting on sections of the bill that were still in the process of being written." Finally, the entire process, from introduction to enactment, was completed within six weeks—quite a record, given the scope and breadth of the legislation.

In sum, five core characteristics exhibited by the entrepreneurs operating in these states—passion, pragmatism, power, political savvy, and knowledge of the issues and process—combined to create a powerful force for change that served as a key counterweight, both to the structural inertia built into the legislative process itself and to the influence of special interest groups opposed to health care reform.

In the policy formulation process, leaders never act alone, and policy entrepreneurship in every state was also facilitated by individuals who served in critical supporting roles. Although often they were not as much in the limelight, these supporting actors were critical for assuring enactment. As Minnesota's Mary Jo O'Brien observed, "there are individuals in the process who are the 'ultimate insiders'; they are the ones who carefully follow the process and preside over all the details; they often provide guidance and direction without visibility; and they serve as go-betweens and information gatherers and are often the 'glue' that keeps the process going."

A wide variety of individuals played these supporting roles, and the group often included members of the state's bureaucracy and/or key legislative and governors' staff members.[22] Mary Jo O'Brien played this role in Minnesota, as did Jean Thorne in Oregon, and Don Sloma (staff coordinator, Senate Health and Long-Term Care Committee) and Bill Hagens (senior research analyst, House Health Care Committee), in Washington State. These individuals and others in similar capacities in these reform states spent significant amounts of time engaged in the policy debate. They were often called upon to provide background research on the issues, to review information provided by various state agencies, to negotiate with various stakeholder and constituent groups, and in several instances, they were primarily responsible for drafting the legislation. For example, David MacKenzie, working closely with his boss, Massachusetts senator McGovern, became one of the principal architects of the Massachusetts Health Security Act. As one of his many activities, MacKenzie codeveloped an econometric model for estimating the cost in Massachusetts of expanding coverage to the uninsured. According to MacKenzie, the model "had the largest spreadsheet anyone in the legislature had ever seen." In all cases, these individuals were called upon to bring both political acumen and technical expertise to the process to ensure that the evolving legislation, along with doing some good, did no unintended harm. Such expertise was particularly critical given the expansive nature of the legislation and the intricacies involved in making it work.

Members of key interest groups also served as supporting actors. Their efforts were most noteworthy in Florida and Washington State. In Florida, individuals representing Associated Industries of Florida, the Florida League of Hospitals, the Florida Medical Association, seven insurance companies, and Blue Cross-Blue Shield of Florida formed a lobbying group that was highly instrumental in working out the final compromise on the Health Care Reform Act of 1992.[23] In Washington State in 1982, Leo Greenawalt, president of the Washington State Hospital Association, and Gail Warden, then president of Group Health Cooperative of Puget Sound, established and financed the Committee for Affordable Health Care. Composed of key representatives of the business and health sectors, the committee was intended to educate policy makers and the public on the problems of the uninsured and the negative incentives built into the existing health care system. According to Greenawalt, "the intent of the group was to make sure that any health reforms that were enacted in Washington State addressed the problems of the health system as a whole and not just the uncompensated care problem in isolation." The group worked over a ten-year period to increase public awareness, educate policy makers about the scope of the problem, and explore policy options; the group operated behind the scenes to influence policy outcomes. Throughout the state, "the affordables" became recognized as an integral part of the reform tapestry. Washington State's Robert Crittenden, M.D., on the faculty at the University of Washington, summarized their influence this way: "The group has become the discussion club on health issues. They are important because they are composed of a set of power elites, and, although they are very selective in the causes they take on, when they get active, they bring both political muscle and resources to the table."

Supporting actors worked behind the scenes to blend policy and politics into a viable piece of legislation. In some instances, their involvement was limited but essential. In others, their role was more protracted with their involvement extending over a longer period of time.[24] In some cases, these individuals moved from the role of supporting actor to the role of policy entrepreneur as the state's health care reform process evolved.

Together, the individuals serving as policy entrepreneurs and supporting actors became what Sabatier (1986) calls an advocacy coalition—a group composed of politicians, agency officials, interest group leaders, and intellectuals who share a set of normative and casual beliefs on core policy issues. Working as consensus advocacy coalitions, they fashioned the reform framework over time, served to promote its adoption, and became the institutional memory for its implementation. By working together, policy entrepreneurs and supporting actors—organized as advocacy coalitions—were able to catalyze and sustain the reform effort. Without their involvement, these major reforms would not have been possible.

A key contributor to the success of the coalition in every reform state was the strategic support of house and senate leadership (and the governor, when that individual was not actively involved as an entrepreneur in the process). The support of these individuals—the major gatekeepers of the states' policy agenda—was critical for moving the process forward. In Minnesota, for example, Speaker of the House Dee Long (D), according to Representative Lee Greenfield, was "the person who sanctioned the Gang of Seven and gave us our head." Greenfield also identified Roger Moore (D), senate majority leader, as playing a crucial role; so did the governor, who was actively involved in recruiting Republican votes in the senate, where the Democratic majority was much smaller. In Washington State, Senate Majority Leader Marc Gasper (D) and Speaker of the House Brian Ebersole (D) provided critical political cover for the effort, signaling to the membership that their interest was in having the effort move forward. According to Massachusetts representative John McDonough, Charles Flarity's role was absolutely critical to the success of the reform effort. Flarity (D), then house majority leader, played the key role in the house in garnering the needed votes for passage. Noted McDonough, "the original vote for the bill was 77 to 75. If one vote had changed, it would have killed the bill." Similar observations were made by individuals interviewed from the other reform states; all emphasized the critical support provided by leadership that sustained the effort once a window of opportunity opened.

LESSON 7. THE MEDIA AND PUBLIC OPINION

Most of us, including policy makers, get information about public issues from newspapers, magazines, radio, and television. Additionally, when policy makers want to disseminate ideas about public issues, they hold press conferences, distribute press releases, leak information, and give speeches designed to receive press coverage (Linsky 1988). Thus, the media have become an important communication link between policy makers and the public. They also play an important role in moving issues onto the public policy agenda and in framing the ways those issues are handled. As noted earlier, health care was historically dominated by the medical community, that for years operated as a policy monopoly. Their domination was supported by the fact that the subject matter of health policy is highly technical and complex— as Massachusetts representative McDonough observed, "The topic does not readily lend itself to the thirty-second radio or television sound bite." Such dominance was also supported by the fact that health professionals historically have been considered by the public as the most legitimate decision makers. Because of this, the public willingly ceded decision-making authority in this policy arena to health professionals, and as such, they defined the issues that were placed on the policy agenda. This situation supported the perpetration of a policy monopoly. The monopoly began to break down with the emergence of new stakeholder groups—purchasers and consumers—calling for change, the emergence of new entrepreneurs hoping to move their initiatives onto the state's policy agenda, and the reemergence of the problem as redefined by these groups in the media. Members of the Dukakis administration, for example, worked to provide the press with stories to ensure that health reform took on a human face. Catherine Dunham remembers spending from 5:00 to 7:00 P.M. weekday evenings in telephone conversations with Richard Knox of the Boston *Globe*. The Dukakis administration purposefully focused on human interest stories describing the challenges faced by Massachusetts residents in their efforts to obtain needed health care services, as well as on details about the reform effort and how the administration's proposal would address these issues. This approach (designed to give the often dense and technical health material a human face) was undertaken to varying degrees and with varying levels of success in each of the seven states, in an effort to keep the media engaged. These efforts helped redefine the issues, and contributed to destabilizing the existing policy monopoly and increasing the opportunity for major policy change. The press assisted in keeping the issue before the public, and this, in turn, served as an additional impetus to the reform effort. As Baumgartner and Jones (1993) have noted, the media are important because public attention is a scarce resource, and the gatekeeping processes of the media are crucial in determining which issues receive public attention and which do not.

Utilizing the media effectively in the health care reform debate, however, presents some unique challenges, given the experiences of these seven states. One of these is the nature of the debate itself. As former Vermont state representative Hamilton Davis (D) (himself a former journalist) observed: "The subject [health care reform] is so dense that when reporters wander into these issues they get lost" (Davis 1994). Providing good coverage of a complex, technical subject such as health care reform appeared to have been beyond the ability or interest of some of the reporters involved. Despite these limitations, policy entrepreneurs in these states were often masterful in using the media to promote their policy agendas, especially when they could capitalize on the media's interest in conflict and/or human interest stories. Representative Ogren, a member of Minnesota's G-7 group, was well known for his selective conversations with members of the press. When negotiations in the G-7 group bogged down, Ogren would sometimes "chat" with the press, providing updates on how the negotiations were progressing, where problems were emerging, and who the recalcitrant legislative parties were. According to Minnesota's Scandrett, "Paul knew full well when he did this that a story covering the contentious issue and naming names would often appear in the paper the following day. This strategy drove members of the G-7 crazy, and because they knew they might see their comments and concerns repeated in the press, they were more likely to stay at the negotiating table to iron out their differences." Discussion of the issue by the press served, in turn, as an impetus to the reform effort, encouraging legislators to take action because of the level of interest in the topic. Thus, the media played an important role in redefining the issue and in increasing public attention, both of which contributed to destabilizing the prevailing distribution of political advantage, thus promoting the politics of disequilibrium.

V. O. Key, Jr., defined public opinion as "those opinions held by private persons which government finds it prudent to heed" (1967: 14). Although policy research suggests a fairly strong correlation between important shifts in public opinion and changes in the general direction of public policy, its specific effects are far less certain (Sabatier 1991). Studies analyzing the impact of public opinion indicate that its influence is not reflected principally in terms of government compliance with specific demands (although this assertion is largely untested), but rather in terms of public opinion controlling the general ideological direction of state policy. Rather than demanding much, it sets the boundaries that rational politicians seek to learn and then heed (Erikson, Wright, and McIver 1993). In these seven states, evidence of public support for health care reform gained through polling appears to have been most influential in those states where a major statewide election coincided with the reform debate in the legislature. Here, where public opinion polls showed strong majority support for reform, the polls enhanced the salience of the issue in the legislative process, and where legislators may have been initially reluctant to vote for reform, their comfort level was raised when strong polling data confirmed support for their actions among the general public and their constituents. As Lee Greenfield observed, "It [polling] made it clear that the public wanted to address the problem and so the legislature felt it was getting support for its action." Thus, in these cases, supportive public opinion appears to have assisted in building a voting majority in the legislature for enactment, serving as a subtle counterweight to the pressure of select opposing interest groups. However, even in states where public opinion was highly supportive of the reform effort, voting for comprehensive reform was not easy. As Minnesota's Luanne Nyberg (director of the Children's Defense Fund) observed, "the final vote was extremely close and leadership had to hold the voting board open more than an hour so that the 'yes' votes could be rounded up. Even though it was a bipartisan effort, a lot of people were scared."

LESSON 8. COMPREHENSIVE HEALTH CARE REFORM IS INITIALLY A DEMOCRATIC AFFAIR

As one considers the political affiliations of the policy entrepreneurs involved, the predominance of Democrats among them is somewhat striking. If these seven states are predictors of what might happen in the other forty-three, comprehensive health care reform efforts (i.e., those involving *major* changes in state policy to address cost and access problems, and those proposing an expanded role for government in this regard) are initially spearheaded by Democrats. Additionally, the most sweeping reforms have been enacted in states with Democratic majorities in both the house and the senate, and (with one exception—Minnesota) in states where the chief executive was also a Democrat. This predominance of Democrats serving as spear carriers for comprehensive state health care reform efforts may be a function of the historical fact that the Democratic party has been more willing to develop broad social reforms that involve both the public and private sectors. It has also been more willing to expand the role and authority of the public sector to implement the policy agenda, and more willing to impose additional obligations on the private sector as a way of addressing key social problems. As such, the comprehensive nature of the reforms proposed in these states is more easily aligned with a Democratic reform agenda than with a Republican one. However, lest the reader assume that Republicans play only a minimal role in comprehensive state health reform efforts, one need only point out that the states that have been most successful in staying the implementation course are those where both Democrats and Republicans collaborated in developing the reform legislation that was enacted. In those states, although implementation has also been difficult, bipartisan support has had more of a stabilizing effect, allowing some reform elements to move forward as planned, while minimizing the elimination or modification of others. Thus, although comprehensive reform efforts are most often initiated by Democrats, progress in the reform implementation process benefits greatly from early and continuing bipartisan support.

LESSON 9. THE SINGLE-PAYER PHENOMENON IS THE PAPER TIGER OF HEALTH CARE REFORM

Both Brown (1993a) and Leichter (1993) have commented on the influence of single-payer proponents and the role single-payer legislation has played in the political process. Leichter has observed that "the Canadian system has replaced socialized medicine as the great attention-getting device in the health reform debate" (80). Conversations I had with state policy makers suggested that the role played by the single-payer issue was a subtle but illusory one. Its prime merit was its external effect—the impression it left on key interest groups—particularly the hospital and physician lobbies. As Hamilton Davis, a Vermont legislator, observed: "Although we never determined how real it was, it changed the character of the health care reform debate in Vermont." Minnesota's Michael Scandrett referred to it as the "demon lurking in the closet." Comments by other state policy players revealed similar perceptions. However, if put to the test, the single-payer proposal probably would have gone down to defeat. As David McKenzie observed, "The only way Massachusetts will have a Canadian health care system is if it secedes from the United States and becomes part of Canada."

Although not politically sustainable, the single-payer concept did retain great value in legislative negotiations, for it allowed the center of the debate to move farther left. Thus, the single-payer issue facilitated the adoption of more expansive changes because by comparison, they looked less onerous than those embodied in a single-payer bill. Additionally, the fear by those key stakeholder groups trying to influence the process, that the single-payer bill just might pass, kept them motivated to remain at the bargaining table to work out a better, less onerous solution.

Traveling Further Down the Road

As these seven states moved through 1995 and 1996, their reform agendas faced a number of challenges, and many shelved their most ambitious plans for health care reform and turned their attention to other policy matters. Massachusetts was an early bellwether; by mid-spring of 1994, the legislature had delayed implementing the employer "pay-or-play" mandate for the third time to August 1996, when the legislature passed some additional insurance coverage for children and senior citizens in exchange for repealing the employer mandate. In Vermont, on 11 May 1994, the legislature derailed Act 160, the state's most ambitious reform effort, by failing to enact either of the reform options developed by the Vermont Health Care Authority (as Act 160 had mandated), and by failing to enact any of the other alternatives put forth by either the governor or the legislature. According to former state representative Hamilton Davis, health care reform was "the victim of a cascade of failure—of nerve, of technical analysis, of political leadership—but most of all, a victim of sheer complexity and scope." In Washington State, lawmakers compromised on a scaled-back alternative, H1046, to avoid a complete repeal of the 1993 Washington Health Services Act. The compromise legislation eliminated the employer and individual mandates, the accompanying ERISA waiver request, the various controls on insurance rates, the requirement for a minimum benefit package, the requirement for a "pure" version of community rating, the health data requirements, and the premium cap; it also converted the Washington Health Services Commission to the Health Care Policy Board, a principally advisory entity with authority limited to approving applications for antitrust exemptions.

In Oregon, although the waiver to proceed with the Oregon Health Plan was granted in March 1993, because the state did not receive an ERISA waiver from Congress—as had been called for in the 1993 state reform act—the employer mandate was automatically repealed in January 1996. In his 1996 state of the state address, Governor Kitzhaber, the Oregon Health Plan's primary architect, indicated that he intended to reexamine the issue and would propose new legislation in 1997. In the interim, the Oregon Health Plan faced an additional $16.78 million in program cuts because of cost overruns and income shortfalls. In 1995, legislation was adopted in Minnesota that repealed the 1997 deadline for universal coverage, modified enacted insurance reforms, amended the rules governing integrated service networks, continued but reduced the MinnesotaCare expansions, and repealed the regulated all-payer option. In Florida, lawmakers initially put on hold Governor Chiles's Florida Health Security Act and the subsequent HCFA waiver received to implement it—an initiative that would have channeled Medicaid managed care savings into subsidies for insurance coverage for low-income residents after Congress signaled an interest in supporting the Medicaid program with block grants.

Several factors contributed to the major retrenchments among these seven states. First, many hit the roadblock posed by ERISA governing employer-sponsored pension and welfare plans. In enacting ERISA, Congress had two straightforward goals: (1) to ensure that workers counting on private pension and welfare benefits when they retired actually received them, and (2) to encourage employers to establish employee pension and welfare benefit plans. Buried in section 514(a) of the 208-page statute, however, is a clause that protects self-insured businesses by exempting them from state insurance regulations and premium taxes. Known as the preemption clause, the language has become the Achilles heel of many a state health care reform effort, because it insulates and protects self-insured employers from having to comply with many state health care reform activities that affect their group health plan. Since estimates indicate that employers of approximately two-thirds of the nation's work force are probably self-insured, this exemption poses big problems for states enacting reform strategies that rely on these employers.[25]

To date, only one state, Hawaii, has received a total ERISA exemption. The exemption, however, only covered the enactment of Hawaii's Prepaid Health Care Act, adopted in 1974, and under the provisions of the exemption, no substantive changes can be made in the legislation without seeking an additional congressional exemption from ERISA. As a result, Hawaii's Prepaid Health Care Program, according to Peter Sybinsky, former deputy director of Hawaii's Department of Health, "has been frozen in time." Efforts were made in Congress in 1994 to grant ERISA exemptions to four additional states, but they were unsuccessful, principally due to the active lobbying in opposition of self-insured employers and trade groups. In 1995, in a unanimous ruling on *Pataki v. Travelers,* the U.S. Supreme Court overturned two lower court rulings and upheld New York State's surcharges on hospital bills paid by commercial insurers and HMOs; this offered states some guidance on the limits of ERISA exemptions in such cases. The justices held that the surcharges, which were intended to spread the burden of providing indigent care, were not precluded by ERISA. As noted by Justice Souter, "ERISA was not meant to preempt basic rate regulation." The court, however, did not address the applicability of such surcharges to self-insured funds (National Health Lawyers News Report 1995). Although representatives from a group of states continue to push for changes in the law, the outlook for such efforts is clearly uncertain, particularly given the Republican majority in Congress and the continuing opposition of the business community.[26] If no relief is forthcoming, the ability of these states to vigorously pursue their reform agendas will be severely compromised.

State reform efforts were also stymied by the significant redistribution of power that occurred over the past several electoral cycles. As noted earlier, the principal drivers of state health reform have been Democrats, and comprehensive reforms have been enacted where Democratic majorities existed in both state houses and, with one exception, in the governor's office. During the last few election cycles, Republicans made major gains in Congress and state legislatures, and in capturing state governorships. Among these seven states, Republicans now hold two governorships (Massachusetts and Minnesota), reflect senate majorities in Florida and Vermont, and hold house majorities in Oregon and Washington State. Additionally, even where Democrats hold a majority in the house and/or senate, these bodies have become more conservative—

a reflection of the public mood. As Florida's Joan Glickman (aid to state Senator Howard Forman [D]) noted, "Although the Florida House currently has sixty-three Democratic members and fifty-seven Republicans, philosophically, however, it is a very conservative body." In some cases, these new incumbents campaigned on a platform of amending or repealing selected portions of the state's health care reform law.

The earliest example of this occurred in Massachusetts. The Massachusetts Health Security Act became law in 1988. During that period, the state was governed by a Democrat, Governor Michael Dukakis, and had relatively strong Democratic majorities in both houses. Following the 1990 statewide elections, William Weld (who as Republican candidate for governor campaigned for repeal of the Health Security Act) was elected, and although both houses remained Democratic, the Democrats were far less inclined to impose what were viewed as new economic burdens on business, given the state's strained economy.

Other states experiencing similar partisan shifts in their legislative or executive branches have similarly modified and scaled back their reform efforts or are poised to do so. According to Washington State's Don Sloma, "the 1994 election was viewed as a referendum on government-run health care." In its wake, bills were introduced in the house to repeal everything but the expansion of the basic health plan and small group insurance reforms. In the senate, proposals included repealing the employer mandate, modifying community rating, and eliminating the Health Services Commission, and as noted earlier, many of these "reforms" were enacted, prompting one reform advocate to observe: "The current situation here is somewhere between bleak and desperate." In most states, campaign rhetoric was turned into legislative action, further complicating an already complicated implementation process by creating high levels of uncertainty and redirecting time, energy, talent, and resources away from the tasks of implementation and toward the tasks of rewriting or defending the legislation.

Fallout from the national health care reform debate and the failure of the Clinton plan also impacted state health care reform efforts. Americans now were not sure comprehensive health care reform is a good idea—particularly if the "reform" may cost them more in higher taxes or increased insurance premiums, and may provide them with less in terms of benefits. Additionally, the public has become equally wary, thanks to Harry and Louise and other media hype, of reforms that involve an expanded role for government. These shifts in public sentiment have made it more difficult—if not impossible— to maintain political support for many of the reforms enacted in these seven states, particularly where these reforms have created a greatly expanded role for government.

Finally, these states faced an additional challenge—the fact that they initially succeeded. Once legislation has been enacted, the public and participating interest groups often feel that the problem is solved, causing their interest to wane. This can create difficulties in maintaining momentum during the implementation process. In commenting on the Minnesota implementation experience, former Representative Paul Ogren put it this way: "The will to act in Minnesota has been severely diminished. There's no longer a grassroots constituency out there advocating for reform. This is partly because they [the public] feel that the care is already out there and there is now a way to receive it. That is, most Minnesotans perceive that the 'deed is already done,' and they are just waiting for things to happen."

Even though these states face enormous challenges, and in some cases, have jettisoned major elements of their plans, we must also remember that some reform efforts are progressing, especially those that seek to expand access to health care coverage. For example, Massachusetts implemented key provisions of the Massachusetts Health Security Act; these provisions included the Commonhealth Program, the student mandate, expanded coverage for severely disabled children and adults, and an unemployment tax surcharge that pays the cost of coverage for unemployed, uninsured adults and their dependents. Reform efforts undertaken by Oregon to expand eligibility under the state's Medicaid program, by limiting coverage to a list of prioritized services, have resulted in an additional 100,000 individuals becoming eligible under the plan. In Florida, the Community Health Purchasing Alliances (CHPAs) are up and running, and over 2,000 state businesses have already purchased coverage through them. Thus, although there have been significant setbacks as these states try to implement their reform plans, some progress is being made— progress, without which, I would argue, the number of uninsured would be higher nationally than it is now, and climbing at a steeper pace.

Most important, in evaluating progress, one must take the long view. As noted earlier, progress is composed of a series of incremental steps and comes as part of an *evolutionary,* not a *revolutionary* process. Such a process can often involve two steps forward and one step back. But with each step, progress is made: services and eligibility are expanded and more people are educated about the dimensions of the health care crisis. This creates a more informed constituency, and gives the stakeholders in the policy dialogue additional opportunities to work together, develop trust, and find consensus—all necessary conditions for taking additional steps down the road to reform.

IMPLICATIONS FOR OTHER STATES

The focus of this research has been on describing the process of reform in these seven states to identify the lessons learned thus far. A question that yet remains is, "What are the implications of these findings for the other forty-three?" Based on this analysis, some initial observations can be made in response to that question. First, no state—because of certain environmental characteristics or previous innovative efforts—appears to have a unique lock on the health care reform process. Reform appears possible in small states as well as large, in rich states as well as poor, in rural as well as urban states, and in states without previous track records for innovation. This observation aside, there do, however, appear to be a series of necessary conditions that must be met in order to move a state forward on the road to health reform. First the timing must be right and a window of opportunity must open. That is, a brief period must emerge during which circumstances in the state are ripe for change. Whether the window is opened through a media event, such as the death of Coby Howard (Oregon); through an internal fiscal crisis (Washington State); through the organized pressure of the business community (Massachusetts); or through the combined interest of the governor and the legislature in having their state beat the national enactment of universal coverage (Hawaii)—such an opportunity must emerge in order to set the stage for further action.

However, no opportunity will be turned into action without policy entrepreneurship—the second essential condition. Whether these leaders emerge from the legislative process, as did Senator Kitzhaber (Oregon), Senator McGovern (Massachusetts), Representative McDermott (Washington State), and the Gang of Seven (Minnesota); from the governor's office as did Dean (Vermont), Dukakis (Massachusetts), and Chiles (Florida); from the executive branch as did Lewin (Hawaii); or from the private sector, such as Gifford (Massachusetts), they are essential for moving the process forward. These individuals must exhibit a passion for change, have an understanding of the issues involved, maintain a pragmatic outlook, and be willing to exercise the power of their positions in order to forge the deal. Without policy entrepreneurship, there is no reform.

Third, key interest groups must join with policy entrepreneurs and supporting actors and commit to the reform agenda to ensure its enactment. Whether they are there because of the pressure of the purchasing community, the state's negative fiscal condition, the fear that something worse (such as adoption of a single-payer system) will happen, or because they truly believe that the existing system is unsustainable and they must, in part, help craft an alternative, state health reform will not proceed if the major interest groups involved stonewall the process.

Fourth, the public must be viewed by elected officials as supporting comprehensive health care reform efforts. This is true even where all of the other factors strongly favor reform. Enacting a comprehensive health care reform agenda is difficult, at best, and will not be accomplished unless the governor and the legislature feel the public is solidly behind them so as not to punish[27] them in the next election. If public officials perceive that public support is lacking for such reform strategies, the odds favoring their enactment diminish considerably. If these conditions—*opportunity, entrepreneurship, stakeholder commitment, and public support*—are met, then it appears that a state can move forward in addressing aspects of its health care reform agenda. Where these are absent, such agendas may be stalemated.

A quick look at the existing political landscape across the states suggests to me that new comprehensive state reform efforts of the magnitude enacted by these seven states may be the exception rather than the rule for some time to come. Several factors influence this perception. First, as a result of the 1994 elections, Democratic influence (the driving force behind reform activities in these seven states) waned considerably, as Republicans achieved stunning electoral gains in state legislatures and governorships. Even where Democrats retained state majorities, their members have been far more conservative and far less inclined to support sweeping state health care reform efforts. Thus, the inclination of today's state leaders to become health care reform champions seems severely diminished. To apply an observation made earlier, no one wants to become a legislative kamikaze. Second, a majority of the states have imposed legislative term limits, an action that may have negative implications for health care reform, given the learning curve required for public officials to get up to speed on this issue. As was characteristic of these seven states, individuals emerging as health care reform policy entrepreneurs gained command of this challenging subject matter by participating in legislative committees and task forces—a learning process that occurred, in most cases, over a substantial period of time. Whether such learning can be condensed into a four-to-six-year period is questionable. Third, the change in public mood regarding comprehensive reform is also important, particularly now, when combined with the public's growing skepticism about the ability of government to develop appropriate solutions to address the problem. Given this situation, it is unlikely that additional states will pursue publicly supported comprehensive reform strategies in the near term. Finally, key interest groups, particularly providers and business— the most powerful of the three major stakeholder groups—are now aggressively pursuing health care reform in the private marketplace, an arena that allows them far more opportunity for flexibility.

However, lest one think the opportunity for comprehensive state health care reform is closed forever, it is important also to bear in mind that many of the systemic factors in the existing health care system that triggered the enactment of reforms in these seven states have yet to be addressed and will continue to contribute to rising health care costs and increasing numbers of uninsured persons.[28] These increases, in turn, may eventually put pressure on states to do something. Thus, whether the achievements of these seven states will be recorded as unique events in the history of federalism in the United States or as a prelude to more state activity, only time—and the emergence of another window of opportunity—will tell.

REFERENCES

Ascuaga, Camille. 1992. Universal Health Care in Massachusetts: Lessons for the Future. In *Health Policy Reform in America: Innovations from the States,* ed. Howard M. Leichter. New York: Sharpe.

Bardach, Eugene. 1972. *The Skill Factor in Politics: Repealing the Mental Commitment Laws in California.* Berkeley: University of California Press.

Baumgartner, Frank R., and Bryan D. Jones. 1993. *Agendas and Instability in American Politics.* Chicago: University of Chicago Press.

Bergthold, Linda A. 1988. Purchasing Power: Business and Health Policy Changes in Massachusetts. *Journal of Health Politics, Policy and Law* 13(3):425–451.

————. 1990. *Purchasing Power in Health: Business, the State, and Health Care Politics.* London: Rutgers University Press.

Brown, Lawrence D. 1991. The National Politics of Oregon's Plan. *Health Affairs* 10(2):28–51.

————.1993a. Dogmatic Slumbers: American Business and Health Policy. *Journal of Health Politics, Policy and Law* 18(2):339–357.

————. 1993b. Commissions, Clubs, and Consensus: Florida Reorganizes for Health Care Reform. *Health Affairs* 12(2):7–26.

Butler, Patricia A. 1994. *Roadblock to Reform: ERISA Implications for State Health Care Initiative.* Washington, DC: National Governors' Association.

Chirba-Martin, Mary Ann, and Troyen A. Brennan. 1994. The Critical Role of ERISA in State Health Reform. *Health Affairs* 13(2):142–156.

Clarke, Gary J. 1991. The Role of the States in the Delivery of Health Services. *American Journal of Public Health* 71(1):59–60.

Crittenden, Robert A. 1993. State Model: Washington. Managed Competition and Premium Caps in Washington State. *Health Affairs* 12(2):82–88.

Davis, Hamilton. 1994. What Went Wrong with Health Care Reform? Just About Everything. *College of Medicine Journal* (fall):2–4.

Drucker, Peter. 1982. *The Changing World of the Executive.* New York: New York Times Book Co.

————. 1985. *Innovation and Entrepreneurship.* New York: HarperCollins.

Erikson, Robert A., Gerald C. Wright, and John P. McIver. 1993. *Statehouse Democracy.* New York: Cambridge University Press.

Goldberger, Susan A. 1990. The Politics of Universal Access: The Massachusetts Health Security Act of 1988. *The Journal of Health Politics, Policy and Law* 15(4):857–885.

Key, Vladimir O., Jr. 1967. *Public Opinion and American Democracy.* New York: Knopf.

Kingdon, John W. 1984. *Agendas, Alternatives, and Public Policies.* Boston: Little, Brown.

Kronick, Richard 1990. The Slippery Slope of Health Care Finance: Business Interests and Hospital Reimbursement in Massachusetts. *Journal of Health Politics, Policy and Law* 15(4):887–913.

Ladenheim, Kala. 1993. Health Care Reform at the State Level. Paper prepared for the Intergovernmental Health Policy Project, 20 May.

Leichter, Howard M. 1993. State Model: Minnesota, the Trip from Acrimony to Accommodation. *Health Affairs* 12(2):48–58.

Linsky, Martin. 1988. *Impact: How the Press Affects Federal Policy Making.* New York: Norton.

Martin, Cathie Jo. 1993. Together Again: Business, Government, and the Quest for Cost Control. *Journal of Health Politics, Policy and Law* 18(2):359–393.

Morone, James A. 1990. *The Democratic Wish.* New York: Basic Books.

———. 1994. The Bureaucracy Empowered. *The Politics of Health Care Reform: Lessons from the Past, Prospects for the Future,* ed. James Morone and Gary Belkin. Durham, NC: Duke University Press.

National Health Lawyers News Report. 1995. 23(5), May.

Neubauer, Deane. 1993. State Model: Hawaii. A Pioneer in Health System Reform. *Health Affairs* 12(2):31–39.

Oliver, Thomas R. 1991. Ideas, Entrepreneurship, and the Politics of Health Care Reform. *Stanford Law and Policy Review* 3(1):160–180.

Oliver, Thomas R. and Pamela Paul-Shaheen. 1997. Translating Ideas into Actions: Entrepreneurial Leadership in State Health Care Reforms. *Journal of Health Politics, Policy and Law* 22(3):721–788.

Peters, Tom, and Nancy Austin. 1986. *A Passion for Excellence: The Leadership Difference.* New York: Wainer.

Peterson, Mark A. 1992. Leading Our Way to Health: Entrepreneurship and Leadership in the Health Care Reform Debate. Paper presented at the American Political Science Association Annual Meeting, Chicago, September.

Pierson, Paul. 1992. Policy Feedbacks and Political Change: Contrasting Reagan and Thatcher's Pension Reform Initiatives. *Studies in American Political Development* 6 (fall):359–390.

Rose, Richard. 1993. *Lesson Drawing in Public Policy.* Chatham, NJ: Chatham House.

Sabatier, Paul. 1986. Top-Down and Bottom-Up Models of Policy Implementation: A Critical Analysis and Suggested Synthesis. *Journal of Public Policy and Law* 6(1):21–48.

———. 1991. Toward Better Theories of the Policy Process. *Political Science and Politics* 24(2):144–156.

Simon, Herbert A. 1979. Rational Decision Making in Business Organization. *American Economic Review* 69(4):493–513.

Stone, Deborah A. 1992. State Innovation in Health Policy. Paper prepared for the Ford Foundation Conference on the Fundamental Questions of Innovation, held at Duke University, Durham, NC, July.

Thompson, Frank J. 1981. *Health Policy and the Bureaucracy: Politics and Implementation.* Cambridge: MIT Press.

Try, Try Again: What's Next for Health Care Reform? 1994. *Medicine and Health* 19 (September): 1–6.

U.S. General Accounting Office. 1992. *Access to Health Care: States Respond to the Growing Crisis.* Washington, DC: Government Printing Office.

Weissert, Carol S. 1991. Policy Entrepreneurs, Policy Opportunists, and Legislative Effectiveness. *American Politics Quarterly* 19(2):262–274.

Yawn, Barbara P., William F. Jacott, and Roy A. Yawn. 1993. MinnesotaCare (Health-Right) Myths and Miracles. *Journal of the American Medical Association* 269(4): 511–515.

NOTES

I thank Lawrence Brown, Brant Fries, John Griffith, Kenneth Warner, and Carol Weissert for their insights and comments on this manuscript, Mark Peterson for his guidance in framing the final version of this article, and most especially, Linda Collins for her dedication and administrative skill in seeing the manuscript through to completion. Unless otherwise indicated, all quotes in the article are from the author's interviews with the persons quoted.

1. Statement of Governor Lawton Chiles in challenging the Florida Legislature to make the issue of health care reform a priority. This and all other quotes are based on interviews by the author with government officials and staff members in all seven states.

2. This phrase was originally coined by C. Fred Jones, a member of the Florida House of Representatives, to describe the kind of organization he wanted to create in Florida to get the attention of the health care industry.

3. Readers interested in receiving copies of the state reform maps should contact the author at (517) 349-2628; (517) 349-2683 (fax); or cchmmphi@pilot.msu.edu (e-mail).

4. I place the word *crisis* in quotes deliberately for it was not the reality of the issue that counted, but rather its perception. In some states, health care cost increases, comparatively speaking, were less than dramatic. However, as noted in an old political adage: In politics, facts are negotiable.

5. Comments based on personal communication with H. Leichter.

6. A major reason for this is that consensual policy communities, particularly those dominated by extremely prestigious professional societies, such as physicians, are far more effective in fostering a positive public image of their issues and in insulating themselves from broad political concerns (see Baumgartner and Jones 1993).

7. A particularly striking example of this phenomenon was the influence of the health care lobby that occurred during the enactment of Florida's Health Care Access Act. According to state sources, the Health Care Reform Act of 1992 passed the senate (whose members were initially opposed) because of the work of the health care lobby (the "lobby" includes representatives from the Florida League of Hospitals, the Florida Medical Association, Blue Cross-Blue Shield, and other large insurers) that had committed to working with the business community to support the bill. When the bill initially went to the senate following house enactment, senators began amending it to death. When it looked as though the reform effort was about to unravel, representatives of the health care lobby began pulling senators aside to "educate" them on the merits of the house hill. As a result, the senate ultimately adopted the house version with no amendments. This group continues to operate, and according to Ralph Glatfelter, president of the Florida League of Hospitals, remains a powerful force in the Florida reform effort.

8.   However, although it was a critical factor in a majority of state reform efforts, the business lobby sometimes developed an Achilles heel—either in the form of membership conflicts or ideological differences. Membership conflicts most often occurred between major employers in the coalition and their small employer counterparts, or between ERISA exempt and non-ERISA exempt firms. Conflict often erupted when proposed reforms imposed additional employer burdens—most notably employer mandates—particularly where that burden fell on small business, a group historically exempt from providing health care. In Massachusetts, for example, the "pay-or-play" concept periodically caused major rifts to develop among the business constituency as the policy debate proceeded. As Massachusetts's Dunham observed, "as the legislative debate moved forward, small business started to 'decombust' all over the legislature." Ideology also served as an Achilles heel. Ideological conflicts most often surfaced when discussions focused on whether reforms should be regulatory or market-based, and on whether they should result in an expanded role for government. Here consensus became contentious when business representatives had difficulty determining which side of the debate they were on and why. Additionally, where their opposition was based on ideological grounds, they could often become intransigent. As the former president of the Massachusetts Business Roundtable, John Crosier wryly observed, "I can find good alternatives to counter opposition built on logic, but it is impossible to find good alternatives to counter arguments built on ideology."

9.   However, consumer stakeholder groups also suffered from their own unique drawbacks—their own Achilles heels—in the reform process. As Massachusetts' Susan Sherry (former director of Health Care For All) observed, "When this organization was formed in 1984, it really consisted only of a few people committed to the cause and a telephone number." This impeded the group's ability early on to bring constituent pressure to bear in the deliberations. Also, as noted earlier, these groups were often considered "lightweights" in the lobbying arena because very often they could not deliver many votes without working with other, more powerful groups. Thus, their efforts and interests were sometimes discounted by other stakeholders or policy entrepreneurs. Finally, schisms sometimes occurred between consumers focused on the single-payer approach as the "appropriate" solution and others in the organization who were committed to the same ends, but who were more pragmatic about the means of getting there. As Minnesota's Nyberg commented about another consumer coalition, "if you are not utterly 'pure' [i.e., supporting the single-payer method], you are seen [by them] as a 'sellout.' " Most important, once these groups begin to fractionate and infighting develops, their political clout drops precipitously.

10. Election influence was further heightened if incumbents felt that the statewide election might result in the new legislature being less supportive of health care reform than the existing one. Thus, on occasion, the timing of the election also helped solidify votes for the initiative.

11. Senate Republicans appeared to believe that public support for the measure was not strong enough to result in their being punished at the polls for their actions during the next election. Thus, achieving a *political* victory, that is, denying Chiles a major win to campaign on, became more important than achieving a *policy* victory, that is, enacting the legislation.

12. What should not be overlooked, however, is that in each state, with *each* legislative enactment along the road to reform, a policy window was required to open. Thus, timing and the availability of policy windows are critical parts of the evolution of policy in these seven states as they traveled the road to reform. As such, the enactment of

legislation to address the health care crisis appears partly a function of the serendipitous convergence of the aforementioned factors and partly a function of careful planning and political strategizing.

13. This observation is more fully discussed in an article by Oliver and Paul-Shaheen (1997).

14. According to Baumgartner and Jones (1993), stability is a function of two major devices: the existing structure of political institutions and the definition of the issues processed by those institutions.

15. The Washington Health Care Commission (WHCC) was composed of seventeen individuals and included consumer, purchaser, provider, and government representatives, as well as six legislative members. The commission had a small independent staff and was charged with making recommendations on access, cost containment, health services, and malpractice. It was initially chaired by Paul Redman, president of Washington Water and Power, and then by Richard Cooley, president of Seafirst Bank.

16. The Washington Health Care Authority's report covered every dollar on health care spent by state government and made recommendations on administrative consolidation, cost shifting, and service acquisition.

17. Such expansion is clearly evident in the reforms enacted by three states. The MinnesotaCare Act, for example, created a new health service delivery category—the integrated service network—and placed it under the supervision of the Commissioner of Health. It also established an all-payer system to regulate and monitor fees, utilization, and service quality, and established a global budget that set annual limits on the growth of health care costs. Washington State's Health Services Act established the Washington Health Care Authority, a new state agency responsible for consolidated state purchasing of health care benefits; Florida created an umbrella organization, the Agency for Health Care Administration, which integrated state government's health care purchasing policy and regulatory functions. The agency was given broad responsibility for assessing the state's health care problems, devising health care reform plans, and facilitating their enactment and implementation.

18. According to Luanne Nyberg of the Minnesota Children's Defense Fund, Gruenes was also concerned that Republicans could be hurt in the next election if they didn't "do something" to address health care concerns, given the defeat of HF2 by a Republican governor.

19. See Peters and Austin 1986 and Drucker 1982 and 1985.

20. Examples include Governor Howard Dean of Vermont, physician; Senator John Kitzhaber, physician and Oregon State Senate president; and Senator James McDermott, physician, former Chair of the Senate Ways and Means Committee, and a member of the Washington State Senate; John Lewin, physician and director of Hawaii's Department of Health; and Representative Ben Graber, physician and chair of the House Health Committee in the Florida Legislature.

21. According to Mary Jo O'Brien, the closed door approach should not be interpreted to mean that interest group concerns were not accounted for in the discussions. She and members of the Republican caucus met earlier in the summer with key stakeholder groups to get a sense of their issues and the options they would support for addressing them. These were reflected in the G-7 deliberations.

22.   Examples include Mike Hanson, Sharon Jacobs, and John Wilson in Florida; Michael Scandrett in Minnesota; Joe Alviani, Catherine Dunham, and David MacKenzie in Massachusetts; Mark Gibson and Michael McCracken in Oregon: and Sue Crystal, Jane Byer, Bill Hagens, and Don Sloma in Washington State.

23.   The group has stayed together, and with the addition of a member from the Florida Association of Life Underwriters, was also responsible for developing much of the language that became Florida's Health Care and Insurance Reform Act of 1993.

24.   Many of the individuals involved in health care reform have been involved throughout the process, although in many cases, they have played different roles. One example illustrates this point. Steven Tringale, an individual who figured prominently in the Massachusetts reform effort, first got involved in 1976 when he served as an intern for the Joint Legislative Health Care Committee. In 1980 he went to work for the Massachusetts Rate Setting Commission where he was in charge of policy development. While there, he staffed many of the negotiations with purchasers that came before the private health care coalition was established in 1982. In May 1972, Steven joined the Life Insurance Association, where he was influential in the implementation of Chapter 372. In 1990 he joined Blue Cross of Massachusetts, where he played a key role in the Chapter 495 negotiations.

25.   The reach of ERISA has been determined by the courts to be broad (Butler 1994; Chirba-Martin and Brennan 1994) and has complicated these states' efforts to regulate both health care financing and delivery. Several implementation strategies enacted by these states were identified as possibly raising an ERISA challenge. These strategies included efforts to require employers to provide basic benefit packages for their workers and dependents (Florida, Vermont, and Washington State); efforts to modify existing benefit packages (Hawaii); efforts to use uniform claims forms and to collect uniform data on health care use and expenditures for both providers and third-party payers (Minnesota and Vermont); efforts to finance reforms through a provider tax that would require employers either to insure their workers or dependents or to pay a tax to a public pool that would cover them the "pay-or-play" approach (Massachusetts, Minnesota, Oregon, Vermont, and Washington State); efforts to impose expenditure controls such as global budgets (Minnesota and Vermont); and efforts to regulate health plans and purchasing cooperatives (Florida and Washington State).

26.   Although congressional Republicans have historically favored state flexibility (and are vigorously pursuing it in other policy arenas), pursuing an ERISA exemption poses a different problem for them in that business—one of the Republicans' major constituencies—is adamantly opposed to approval of such an exemption. Thus, whether states can avoid the stifling effect ERISA may have on their major state efforts is an open question.

27.   By this, I mean vote them out of office. A politician's primary interest is most often in being reelected by his or her constituency. If an individual officeholder feels that casting an affirmative vote on a particular piece of legislation represents a significant threat to his or her reelection, the politician will most often not do so.

28.   For a discussion of these factors, see *Try, Try Again* (1994).

Part II

Key Contemporary Health Policy Issues

7 | The Political Economy Of Medicare

Bruce C. Vladeck

MY EPIPHANY, MY FLASH OF INSIGHT: An evening in August 1996, riding from the airport into Pittsburgh, prior to a seminar at the University of Pittsburgh the following morning. Few cities have so theatrical an entrance: If you're coming in from the airport, through the Fort Pitt tunnel, you emerge from the tunnel with all of downtown, across the river, laid out before you. At night especially, the taillights from the elevated expressway on the bluff above the river's north bank add motion to the more vertical tableau of the skyscrapers behind.

In the past, when the steel mills were operating, the view was even more spectacular. Lining both banks of the Monongahela, beginning just east of the Golden Triangle at the confluence with the Allegheny and extending miles upstream, stood the great industry that provided Pittsburgh its identity. During World War II, it is said, the mills on the Monongahela produced more steel than all of Germany's; Hitler and Tojo were defeated by western Pennsylvania. If you've never seen an operating open-hearth mill at night, it's difficult to imagine the orange-red brightness of the flames or the volume of smoke or the simple inhuman size of everything, with hard-hatted workers dwarfed by their tools.

By the mid-1980s the mills were all shut, made obsolete by mini-mills in Alabama and megamills in Korea and fuel-economy standards for cars. It must say something important about modern capitalist economies that the photographic images of closed factories rest more prominently in our memories than do the images of working mills.

But the scene as I emerged from the Fort Pitt tunnel that night more than two years ago was more dramatic still, for someone who remembered older times,

Reprinted from *Health Affairs*, 18, no. 1 (January/February 1999): 22–36. Copyright 1998. The People-to-People Health Foundation, Inc. All rights reserved. Used with permission.

because now the mills were gone altogether, torn down in the hope of urban regeneration from the brown fields cleared of rust and slag. My mind's eye played tricks, calling up the sight of enormous structures that were no longer there. In the Middle East, when one civilization succeeds another, it builds on top of the ruins of the old one. Here, we just leave the ghosts behind.

So we drove into town past the unmarked graves of the great steel plants, through the Medical Center, which was bustling on a summer night in the way that most American downtowns don't. Medical students carrying textbooks, stethoscopes proudly dangling from the pockets of their lab coats; housestaff and nurses grabbing a quick bite or just some fresh air, walking past brightly lit storefronts; cars double-parked on crowded streets. My hosts, two considerate health policy wonks, reminded me of what I already knew: that health care has replaced steel as Pittsburgh's largest industry, its major source of good jobs and economic growth.

Then I remembered something else. Western Pennsylvania has an especially high proportion of elderly citizens, second only to that of south Florida; as the mills dried up, young people left Homestead and Braddock and Carnegie and all of the other towns in the valley, while the old stayed. It's not just health care that is now the largest industry in Pittsburgh. The largest industry in Pittsburgh is Medicare.

For a Health Care Financing Administration (HCFA) administrator and life-long city boy and amateur urbanologist, that was a sobering and disconcerting thought; there is only so much responsibility one can take. It also clarified for me a whole gamut of perceptions and experiences from my four years on the job. It provided a framework and a perspective for much of what I had known and thought I had understood all along.

Every reader of *Health Affairs* knows that Medicare spends more than $200 billion a year. As they say, that's a lot of money, even by Washington standards, and although the political and ideological conflicts generated by that much money are familiar to most observers of the policy process, there are at least three other dimensions to that volume of expenditure that engender political processes of their own. To use some rather shopworn but still evocative termi-nology from political science, those dimensions are as follows: (1) Medicare as redistributive politics, in the sense of Medicare as a massive transfer program; (2) Medicare as special-interest politics, in the workings of what I call the "Medicare-industrial complex"; and (3) Medicare as distributive politics, in the allocation of financial benefits across regions and communities.

MEDICARE AS REDISTRIBUTIVE POLITICS

Medicare provides, through an insurance mechanism, a set of service benefits to many persons who otherwise would be unable to afford or obtain adequate access to health services. It has revolutionized access to health care for the elderly and disabled and thus has contributed to the demonstrable improvements in health status and life expectancy experienced by older Americans over the past thirty years. Not incidentally, Medicare also has been an extremely powerful weapon for reducing poverty for the elderly and disabled.

Medicare does so, however, at least in part by transferring income from working-age persons to retired or disabled former workers. On average, each working-age person contributes something over $1,250 a year to provide about $5,000 in benefits to each Medicare beneficiary. (The astute observer may interject at this point that Medicare funds are not in fact actually transferred to Medicare beneficiaries but rather to the providers that give them services— or, as the more cynically astute observers might argue, in the case of some managed care plans and some beneficiaries, providers that do not give them services. Certainly, unlike other Social Security programs, Medicare rarely puts cash into the hands of those who are described as its beneficiaries. But they benefit nonetheless. The politics of those who do cash the checks are the subject of the next section of this paper.) Although hardly anyone will say it out loud, the dynamics of this transfer—indeed, its very existence—lie not far below the surface of many of the most bitter and contentious political fights about Medicare that have erupted throughout its history, especially in the past five years.

Just under 60 percent of Medicare revenues—essentially all of the financing of Part A (hospital insurance)—comes from payroll taxes, which are mildly regressive since they apply uniformly to earned income at all levels and exclude all nonwage income. Since 1993, however, the payroll tax contribution to Medicare has been less regressive than Social Security's, since it now applies to all wage income, regardless of amount. Thirty percent of Medicare funds come from general federal revenues and are as progressive or regressive as those revenues are these days—which is to say, a lot less progressive than they used to be. The most regressive part of Medicare's income is the 10 percent derived from beneficiary premiums, but while the political debate has focused on the relatively small number of beneficiaries at the upper ends of the income distribution (fewer than 6 percent of beneficiaries live in households with incomes greater than $50,000 a year), the real regressivity in the flat premium structure arises from the millions with incomes just above the level of eligibility for additional subsidies through Medicaid who pay the same premiums that average beneficiaries pay.[1]

Medicare benefits, on the other hand, are distributed more progressively (as long as we continue, for purposes of this section, to attribute benefits to the recipients of the service, rather than to the recipients of the checks). Because lower-income beneficiaries tend to be sicker, just under three-quarters of all Medicare fee-for-service expenditures are on behalf of beneficiaries in the bottom two-thirds of the income distribution.[2] (The growth of Medicare managed care, by generating average expenditures for healthier-than-average beneficiaries, partially reverses this effect.) Over beneficiaries' lifetimes, however, this effect is greatly attenuated by the fact that more-affluent beneficiaries live longer.

As income-transfer programs go, in other words, Medicare isn't bad, in the sense that its revenue sources fall roughly in the middle of the total spectrum from progressivity to regressivity, and its benefits, in any given year, are highly progressive when viewed across society as a whole. It could be made much more progressive if a greater share of the financing were transferred from payroll taxes to general revenue (as was done to a small degree in the Balanced Budget Act, or BBA, of 1997) and a little more progressive if beneficiaries' premiums were related to income. Extending coverage to prescription drugs and long-term care would greatly increase the progressivity of benefit distribution.

But the very fact that Medicare is a mildly progressive income-transfer program underlies much of the contemporary political debate, even if that dimension is rarely acknowledged. Efforts to transform the program from one of defined benefits to defined contributions, to encourage medical savings accounts (MSAs), or to raise the share of program costs paid by beneficiaries are all part of the broader political and ideological attack on all policies that redistribute income or wealth from the more affluent to the less affluent (policies that redistribute income in the other direction remain much less controversial). Indeed, even much of the insistence that Medicare and Social Security face a "crisis" because of the aging of the baby boomers is rooted in visceral hostility to redistributive policy in all of its forms; the baby-boomer crisis simply goes away if one allows into the discussion the possibility of increased taxes on the more affluent.

There is no question, from an economic point of view, that this society could "afford" to support indefinitely a more generous Medicare program than the one we now have. The question is whether, politically, we want to do so. That question really comes down to the extent of our willingness to require the better-off to subsidize the less well off—a willingness that seems to be shrinking.

Nowhere is the redistributive dimension of Medicare politics more apparent than in the argument made by some proponents of radical change that it is imperative to do something soon, before a much larger share of the electorate is made up of Medicare beneficiaries or persons close to eligibility age, at which point the politics of the issue presumably would change. In fact, the views of Medicare beneficiaries, in responding to public opinion polls or in their voting behavior, do not differ substantially from those of forty- or fifty-year-olds regarding Medicare policies. This argument thus is less a reflection of reality and more of an anxiety that has persisted in American politics since the days of the Founding Fathers. The authors of *The Federalist,* after all, insisted that the separation of powers within a federal system was necessary to prevent the more numerous lower classes from abusing direct democracy to confiscate the wealth of the upper classes.[3]

The political behavior of lower-income Americans ever since has run largely counter to the Federalists' expectations: Most working Americans not only have identified themselves as "middle class" but generally have held "middle-class" views about taxation, inflation, and workers' solidarity, even when such views have run directly counter to their "objective" economic interests. That cultural reality has never sufficiently assuaged the paranoia of the more affluent, nor has it discouraged them from seeking to further tilt the political and economic systems in their own direction, as they continue to do in the Medicare debate. The image of hordes of voracious Medicare beneficiaries feasting on the hard-gotten gains of struggling, virtuous investment bankers has an almost Hogarthian tone to it, but such eighteenth-century imagery continues to dominate the conceptual map of much of the policy elite.

MEDICARE AS INTEREST-GROUP POLITICS: THE MEDICARE-INDUSTRIAL COMPLEX

Of course, James Madison's system works, most of the time, the way it was designed to, so American politics, most of the time, revolves not around the great redistributive issues but around narrower ones of primary concern to more focused interests. In that world of "normal" politics, Medicare's annual $200 billion is a major prize or, more precisely, an enormous aggregation of smaller prizes.

It is here that the fact that Medicare makes payments to providers of services, not directly to beneficiaries, becomes most relevant. Medicare is the largest single source of income for the nation's hospitals, physicians, home care agencies, clinical laboratories, durable medical equipment suppliers, and physical and occupational therapists, among others, and all of those groups work energetically to protect and advance their interests through the political process.[4]

The health care industry is so big, however, and Medicare is so complicated, that it is necessary to understand some of the subtleties of the process in order to understand the political dynamics of Medicare—and the ways in which those dynamics affect broader public policy concerns. A few examples help to illustrate that point.

Medicare accounts for as much as 40 percent of the income of the average U.S. hospital, but the hospital community is increasingly heterogeneous and internally fractious.[5] Medicare spends so much money on hospitals—more than half of its total outlays, if all hospital-delivered services are included—that at the highest levels of aggregation, hospital politics becomes indistinguishable from macrobudgetary politics, to the disadvantage of the hospital community. But most hospital politics around Medicare occurs at levels far lower than that of the hospital community as a whole. The BBA, for example, contains no fewer than half a dozen provisions targeted at individual hospitals or, at most, a mere handful; a large part of HCFA's administrative resources are devoted to evaluating claims on behalf of particular hospitals, or small groups of hospitals, advanced by individual members of Congress. With every passing year, the prospective payment system (PPS), which was touted by some of its initiators as a model of uniform, "scientific" national policy, looks less like a theoretical exercise in health economics and more like the Internal Revenue Code.

A little more broadly, PPS increasingly tilts toward particular classes of hospitals, especially teaching hospitals and those in rural communities. Teaching hospitals benefit from the American love of medical technology and the popular fascination with science, especially medical science. Rural hospitals play an important role in their communities and are especially dependent on Medicare as a share of their total revenues, but the basic Madisonian formula for representation in the U.S. Senate does them no harm, either.

Interest-group politics is not only a matter of narrowly focused interests seeking special consideration from the government. It is also a matter of organizational maintenance for interest-group representatives themselves. In Medicare politics this is reflected most clearly in the relationship with the American Medical Association (AMA). Although it occupies a central place in the literature on the politics of Medicare, largely because of its central role in delaying Medicare's enactment in the 1960s, the AMA, despite the size of its membership, the magnitude of its political contributions, and the number of lobbyists it employs, is much less influential on global issues of Medicare policy than is often believed. That is in part because of how closely the AMA has identified itself with the Republican party—a greater disadvantage, to be sure, when Democrats controlled the committees of jurisdiction, but a tactical disadvantage even today—and in part because, within the Republican party, the AMA continues to be outmuscled by the business and insurance interests with which it is so frequently in conflict.

The AMA's role in Medicare politics also must be understood as a manifestation of the dynamics of organizational maintenance. The AMA is implicated in Medicare's system of paying physicians because it helped to develop that system, but also because it holds the extremely lucrative copyright on the basic coding terminology, and because HCFA has largely delegated to it responsibility for maintaining many of the system's technical aspects. This requires the increasingly disputatious specialty societies to go through an AMA process to achieve some of their objectives. As HCFA administrator, I received hundreds of letters from the executive vice-president of the AMA, but the strongest and most urgent were always those that involved protection of the AMA's ministerial role.

In the U.S. political system, and especially in the current political climate, executive-branch agencies achieve what legitimacy they can by relying on private representatives for as many tasks as possible. The relationship between HCFA and the AMA is thus functional for both parties, although the extent to which it protects the interests of practicing physicians, even that fraction who belong to the AMA, is subject to increasing question.

Far more effective is the health maintenance organization (HMO) industry. Medicare beneficiaries still make up just a fraction of total HMO enrollment, but they represent the fastest-growing market and until recently accounted for a disproportionate share of all HMO profits, especially among the largest, publicly traded firms. Of all of the major types of Medicare providers, only HMOs incurred substantially smaller payment reductions in the BBA than were proposed by the Clinton administration, and they continue to enjoy a degree of support among the congressional leadership that is significantly at variance from the broader public perception.

Perhaps the most effective interest in the interest-group politics of Medicare is one that is rarely discussed or noticed—the *sine qua non* of effective interest-group politics—Medicare contractors. Contractors, of course, are the private insurance companies that perform the basic administrative tasks of the Medicare fee-for-service program: communicating with providers, reviewing claims, paying bills, and auditing cost reports. The Blue Cross/Blue Shield Association, its member plans, and the few commercial insurance companies still in the game operate under a set of contracting and procurement rules that differ in a number of critical respects from those that apply to almost all other government contractors. They have their own piece of statute, which is understood (let alone known about) by only a very small number of bureaucrats, congressional staff, and a few members of Congress, as well as the contractors themselves.

Public concern about health care fraud and abuse, the increasing eagerness of Medicare contractors to participate in the Medicare HMO program as part of their "private" businesses, and the fact that several contractors were caught in illegal activity, permitted a partial breach in this special arrangement in 1996 when, as part of the Health Insurance Portability and Accountability Act (HIPAA), HCFA was authorized to contract separately for audits, investigations, and other program integrity activities. However, the contractor community has continued to resist implementation of those provisions, as well as more far-reaching changes in the legal framework for contracting. If long-term reform of Medicare is to include modernization of the fee-for-service part of the program, as it almost certainly must, then modernization of the contractor process probably is a necessary precondition. For that precondition to be met, however, according to the general laws of interest-group politics, the issue of contractor reform probably will have to be redefined into part of a much larger issue.

Hospitals, doctors, HMOs, and Medicare contractors all have a major stake in Medicare policy and act as expected in the political system. Yet there are other service providers that essentially serve only Medicare customers. Literally thousands of home health agencies, durable medical equipment suppliers, and firms that contract for therapy services, as the most notable examples, have been formed to do business with Medicare. In most of these industries, individual entrepreneurs account for the large majority of suppliers, although large, national, publicly traded firms have become more important as a buoyant stock market has made equity capital easy to raise. These firms are really the foot soldiers in the Medicare-industrial complex.

Nothing is more frustrating to Medicare administrators, nor more puzzling to outside observers, than the fact that the payment methods—and even levels of payment—for so many things Medicare purchases are written into law, often at prices higher than a big buyer such as Medicare could obtain in the marketplace. Efforts to make Medicare a more "prudent purchaser" have been supported by administrations of both political parties for more than a decade. But Medicare suppliers occupy a political territory of classic dimensions in American political science: narrowly focused interest groups with an enormous specific stake in issues about which the rest of the body politic could really care less, seeking benefits of enormous importance to themselves, but almost invisible in the total aggregate of the federal budget. They thus have succeeded in resisting almost every effort to improve Medicare's purchasing by enlisting key members of Congress to defend their constituents from the depredations of the "big bad federal bureaucracy."

Medicare suppliers thus have built on the earlier successes of the more visible providers, such as hospitals and doctors, in turning the program from one that provides a legal entitlement to beneficiaries to one that provides a de facto political entitlement to providers. Part of that transformation dates to the attitudes of program administrators from the early days of Medicare, when officials were concerned (astonishingly enough, in retrospect) that not enough providers would be willing to participate in the program; part of it stems from some truly misguided decisions by the federal judiciary over the years. But the conversion of Medicare into an entitlement for thousands of smaller providers is also closely tied to the continued romancing of the small-business community by political leaders of both parties. Even though they exist for no purpose other than to sell services to a government program, and even though the government and its beneficiaries might be better off if there were fewer, larger, more efficient, and cheaper suppliers, these providers have acquired a kind of legitimacy in the political process that turns our conventional notions of the boundary between the public and private sectors upside down. Thus, we find the astonishing spectacle in which a presidential appointee in the Small Business Administration recently denounced, as inimical to small firms, the implementation of restrictions on home care agencies that had been announced as a presidential initiative barely a year earlier.[6]

The analogy to defense contractors is not totally far-fetched. There are plenty of $400 toilet seats in the Medicare program, because Medicare cannot deliver services to its beneficiaries without providers and because providers are major sources of employment, political activity, and campaign contributions in every congressional district in the nation. Although the average home care agency is very much smaller than the average military base, efforts to close either one produce the same kinds of congressional responses.

MEDICARE AS DISTRIBUTIVE POLITICS

The analogy between shutting down military bases and closing down Medicare providers also stands precisely at the boundary between Medicare as interest-group politics and Medicare as locality politics—the distributive dimension of Medicare's political economy. Medicare spends money in just about every city and town, and in every congressional district, in the United States. With the federal government reducing almost every other form of domestic spending, the geographic distribution of Medicare dollars has become a matter of increasing attention.

The very wide variation in health care spending from one community to another has long been accepted as a basic fact in health services research. Some of that variation is attributable to differences in demographic characteristics and health status across communities; some to differences in input prices and other price factors; and some—although an amount that is, in fact, hard to determine precisely and that may be less than often asserted—to differences in practice patterns among health professionals. Since Medicare buys health services from the existing system in every U.S. community, and since the prices it pays remain tied in some way to cost, even as the program moves to capitated or prospective payment, all of that variation is reflected in patterns of Medicare spending. Further, as noted above, the revenue that supports Medicare, as does federal revenue in general, varies with the differences in both total taxable income and payroll from one community to the next. As Sen. Daniel Patrick Moynihan (D-NY), among others, has noted repeatedly in recent years, the federal budget as a whole is significantly redistributive, spending money in poorer states and those with large military installations that is derived, net, from higher-income (but higher-cost-of-living) states in the Northeast and Midwest.

Examination of Medicare's "balance of payments" by state—comparing the state's share of Medicare expenditures to the state's share of Medicare revenues—produces no easy explanation for states' relative standing (Exhibit 7.1).[7] Michigan and Montana, for example, both pay a dollar in federal taxes for every ninety-two cents Medicare spends, but Michigan's per beneficiary expenditures are almost 40 percent higher. California, Kansas, and Georgia all have about the same Medicare balance of payments, but California spends a lot on each of its proportionately few beneficiaries; Kansas has more elderly people than Georgia, but Georgia has a higher proportion of Medicare disabled

EXHIBIT 7.1

Medicare Balance of Payments and Payments per Enrollee, by State, 1996 (Ranked in Descending Order by Balance-of-Payments Ratio)

State	Medicare Balance of Payments (Millions of Dollars)[a]	Medicare Balance-of-Payments Ratio[b]	Medicare Payments per Enrollee	
			Amount	Rank
DC	$ 638	2.12	$5,655	1
FL	6,822	1.74	5,027	6
LA	1,544	1.64	5,468	2
MS	588	1.41	4,189	21
WV	374	1.37	3,798	29
TN	1,139	1.34	4,441	14
OK	615	1.33	4,098	23
AL	803	1.32	4,454	12
PA	2,408	1.27	5,212	4
AR	352	1.25	3,719	32
MO	626	1.18	4,191	20
KY	347	1.15	3,862	27
ND	54	1.14	3,218	43
AZ	351	1.14	4,442	13
MA	611	1.12	5,147	5
RI	71	1.09	4,148	22
TX	831	1.07	4,703	10
SD	15	1.04	2,952	50
ME	20	1.03	3,464	36
OH	124	1.02	3,982	24
NC	−67	0.99	3,465	35
IN	−57	0.99	3,945	25
NY	−281	0.98	4,855	8
SC	−62	0.97	3,777	30
GA	−349	0.93	4,402	16
KS	−131	0.93	3,847	28
MT	−41	0.92	3,114	45
MI	−568	0.92	4,307	18
CA	−2,107	0.91	5,219	3
NV	−98	0.91	4,306	19
CT	−333	0.89	4,426	15
IA	−227	0.88	3,080	47
NE	−154	0.86	2,926	51

continued

EXHIBIT 7.1 *continued*

State	Medicare Balance of Payments (Millions of Dollars)[a]	Medicare Balance-of-Payments Ratio[b]	Medicare Payments per Enrolee Amount	Rank
DE	−81	0.85	4,712	9
IL	−1,508	0.84	4,324	17
WI	−569	0.84	3,246	42
NM	−159	0.83	3,110	46
OR	−385	0.82	3,285	41
NJ	−1,355	0.81	4,531	11
VT	−78	0.80	3,182	44
ID	−166	0.76	3,045	49
CO	−716	0.74	3,935	26
MN	−946	0.73	3,394	40
UT	−304	0.73	3,443	37
MD	−1,161	0.72	4,997	7
NH	−255	0.72	3,414	38
HI	−266	0.70	3,069	48
VA	−1,522	0.68	3,748	31
WA	−1,343	0.68	3,401	39
WY	−107	0.65	3,537	34
AK	−318	0.33	3,687	33

Sources: Health Care Financing Administration, "Estimated Benefit Payments for Fiscal Year 1996," unpublished data (Baltimore: HCFA, March 1998); Board of Trustees, Federal Hospital Insurance Trust Fund, 1997 *Annual Report of the Board of Trustees of the Federal Hospital Insurance Trust Fund* (Washington: U.S. Government Printing Office, April 1997), 30–31; Board of Trustees, Federal Supplementary Medical Insurance Trust Fund, *1997 Annual Report of the Board of Trustees of the Federal Supplementary Medical Insurance Trust Fund* (Washington: U.S. GPO, April 1997), 26; Tax Foundation, unpublished data (Washington: Tax Foundation, March 1998); J.H. Walder and H.B. Leonard, *The Federal Budget and the States: Fiscal Year 1996, 21st Edition* (Washington: U.S. Senate, September 1997), 85; and *Health Care Financing Review: Medicare and Medicaid Statistical Supplement, 1996* (1996): 211–213.
[a]The Medicare balance of payments for any state is calculated as follows: Medicare benefit payments in that state minus Medicare revenues contributed by state residents. Thus, a positive figure indicates that Medicare's spending in that state exceeded what its taxpayers paid in taxes toward Medicare. The contributions for the program were $188 billion.
[b]The Medicare balance-of-payments ratio is calculated as the ratio of Medicare benefit payments in the state to the tax contributions that the state's residents pay toward the Medicare program. Thus, a ratio of greater than one indicates that a state's residents receive more in benefits than the state's taxpayers paid in taxes toward Medicare.

beneficiaries. In general, western states have younger populations and relatively low per beneficiary costs, while the Southeast has lower per capita incomes and relatively higher health care spending, but there are exceptions all over the lot.

Whatever the actual results, however, issues of regional allocation increasingly affect Medicare policy. The most dramatic recent example is the treatment of payment rates for capitated plans in the BBA. Congress sought to respond to the complaints of rural representatives that the adjusted average per capita cost (AAPCC) formula, based as it was on actual Medicare costs in specific counties, penalized lower-cost (and therefore presumably more virtuous) rural counties, as well as such low-cost metropolitan areas as the Twin Cities and Portland, Oregon. At the same time, however, Congress responded to the concerns of teaching hospitals by carving out costs associated with Medicare's teaching hospital payments from capitated rates, to pay the money directly to the hospitals. Doing so by itself, however, would have produced significant rate reductions in major urban communities on both coasts, so Congress also established a hold-harmless provision in which each county was guaranteed a rate increase of at least 2 percent per year. The result was, in essence, a series of simultaneous equations that could not be solved. The BBA has produced the sought-after effect of substantial rate increases in rural counties, which has not yet been accompanied by any increase in the availability of capitated plans in most of those communities, and has produced modest rate increases in high-cost urban areas, but at the same time the Twin Cities and Portland have received almost no benefit.

There is no platonically "right" formula for allocating capitated payments across communities, especially since the dynamics of individual markets vary on a number of dimensions, only one of which is price. In fact, a strong case can be made that formula-driven administered prices are a fundamentally unsound way of setting capitated rates to begin with, a position that HCFA has long advanced in the face of considerable resistance from the HMO industry and Congress. But the health policy debate increasingly consists of high-sounding arguments cloaking relatively narrow, traditional regional and local issues.

THE POLITICAL ECONOMY OF PUBLIC ACTION

The three dimensions of Medicare's political economy—redistributive, interest-group, and distributive—come together in a particularly insidious set of arguments that are made with increasing frequency in the contemporary debate about the future of Medicare. The tendency of politicians and the interests to which they respond to behave as politicians and interest groups generally do is advanced as a rationale for moving responsibility for management of Medicare out of the public sector altogether, through some form of greater privatization such as a defined-contribution plan. The politics of Medicare, it is argued, makes more rational or more effective administration virtually impossible unless some mechanism is found to delink Medicare policy from the political process.

This argument, of course, is most frequently made by those parties who, the rest of the time, are most busily engaged in interest-group and distributive politics. As such, the argument is the moral equivalent of a junkie's seeking to be thrown in jail because it is the only way he or she knows to keep away from temptation. "Stop me before I sin again" might be the practical translation of this position. Apart from its dubious moral basis, this argument has two basic flaws.

First, the solution it proposes probably would not work. As the process of modifying capitation rates in the BBA demonstrates so well, when regional or local interests conflict with broader policy principles, the former often prevail, and those interests can be advanced or protected in a defined-contribution or voucher scheme almost as easily as in the current program. Those who think that it would be more difficult to promote interest-group or distributive politics under such an arrangement simply are not giving Congress enough credit; one has only to think for a moment about the Internal Revenue Code to realize that. Of course, Congress, executive-branch officials, and interest groups probably would have to think of new ways in which to bend a new system to their interests, and that might slow down the process for a year or two—but just think of the bonanza for new generations of consultants!

More basically, the argument that Medicare must somehow be insulated from the day-to-day workings of the political system is, at root, an argument that in some basic sense we have lost the capacity as a nation to govern ourselves. The flaws in our current political system are real and profound, and there is a long-standing tradition in American politics in which academic and social elites have sought to insulate one public function or another from "politics." That tradition has given us civil service; the Interstate Commerce Commission; and independent, ineffectual boards of public health. But that tradition is, at root, fundamentally antidemocratic.[8]

Inside the psychic Beltway occupied by the policy elites, there is broad consensus that "we" could run Medicare, or other parts of the health care system, much better if only the ugly exigencies of the political process could be pushed aside. But if we take that approach to Medicare—which affects almost every American family, reflects a profound and long-standing intergenerational compact, and often literally involves matters of life and death—then we are saying either that the American people cannot be trusted with something so large and so important or that we cannot trust our political processes to adequately protect the American people. Either conclusion would suggest that our problems are far worse than the pending insolvency of the Hospital Insurance trust fund or the economic impact of the retirement of the baby boomers.

Conversely, this means that the task of reforming Medicare in a way that serves all Americans, present and future, may be inseparable from the task of broader political reform. The corrosive influences of campaign contributions, media both bought and unbought, and widespread public disillusionment and apathy are generic political problems that are also specific to Medicare. Politics does matter.

As Medicare has gotten bigger, more expensive, and more important with each passing year, it has become more and more subject to the broader workings of the U.S. political system. That is something, I believe, that we cannot escape. More importantly, it is something, I also profoundly believe, that we should not try to escape. Doing so would break a bond far more basic than Medicare itself.

NOTES

The author thanks Danielle Holahan for her able and conscientious research support, and an anonymous reviewer for preventing some serious embarrassments. Preparation of this paper was supported by the Commonwealth Fund. The views presented here are those of the author and not necessarily those of the Commonwealth Fund or its directors, officers, or staff

1.   U.S. Department of Health and Human Services, Health Care Financing Administration, *A Profile of Medicare* (Washington: HCFA, May 1998), 16.

2.   Ibid., 18.

3.   Compare *The Federalist,* no. 10 (New York: Mentor Books, 1961), 77–83.

4.   K.R. Levit et al., "National Health Spending Trends in 1996," *Health Affairs* (January/February 1998): 35–51.

5.   Ibid.

6.   *BNA's Medicare* Report, 1 May 1998, 447.

7.   The data that make up these "balance-of-payments" tables are too extensive to be presented comprehensively in this paper. For more concisely prepared tables, contact the author at Institute for Medicare Practice, Mt. Sinai Medical Center, One Gustave Levy Place, Box 1077, New York, NY 10029, or via e-mail at Bruce_Vladeck@smtplink.mssm.edu.

8.   The historical ties between academe and the Progressive tradition pose what should be a worrisome parallel for this generation of health services researchers. Just as an earlier generation of social "scientists" provided much of the intellectual rationale through which dominant Protestant elites maintained sovereignty at the expense of newly emergent immigrant populations a century ago, so the increasing influence of health services research may serve, if health services researchers are not careful, to advance the interests of particular contemporary elites. In today's social sciences this danger is primarily the result of the simple fact that nothing ever works as well in practice as it does in theory, so no real program can ever compete with abstract microeconomic hypotheticals. The greater power that markets give to those with more wealth thus is reinforced in the political arena by analyses that confuse market models with reality.

8

A Framework for Considering Medicare Payment Policy Issues

Medicare Payment Advisory Commission (MedPAC)

Historically, Medicare has used a variety of methods to determine providers' payments, including retrospective reimbursement of allowable costs, allowed fees or charges, and prospective payment.[1] Today, payments for most services furnished by hospital outpatient facilities, home health agencies, inpatient rehabilitation facilities, long-term care hospitals, rural health clinics, and several other types of providers are still at least partially determined by the facility's incurred costs. Cost-based payment methods have long been criticized because they are complex, they result in unpredictable payments and spending for providers and Medicare, and they weaken providers' incentives for efficiency.

The Balanced Budget Act of 1997 (BBA) required the Health Care Financing Administration (HCFA) to replace cost-based methods with new prospective payment systems (PPSs) for many types of providers operating in the traditional fee-for-service program. New systems must be implemented for skilled nursing facilities (SNFs), hospital outpatient departments (OPDs), home health agencies, and inpatient rehabilitation facilities. Further, HCFA must submit a report to the Congress by October 1, 1999, on a PPS design for long-term care hospitals. The statute also modified the existing prospective payment systems for hospital inpatient care and physician services. In addition, HCFA has proposed revising its prospective payment system for ambulatory surgical centers (ASCs). Finally, the BBA changed the method for determining prospective capitation payments for health care organizations that enroll beneficiaries in the new Medicare+Choice program.

Reprinted from Medicare Payment Advisory Commission (MedPAC)'s *Report to the Congress: Medicare Payment Policy*, pp. 3–24 (Washington, D. C., March 1999).

Under the law, the Medicare Payment Advisory Commission (MedPAC) must review the design and implementation of these policies. In addition, we make annual payment update recommendations to the Congress for Medicare's payment systems (discussed in this report). To guide our analysis of payment issues in all of these settings, we have begun developing a payment policy framework. Our immediate goal is to lay out the issues that must be addressed in designing or updating prospective payment systems and a framework for thinking about them.[2] In the longer term, we intend to refine this framework and identify explicitly a set of consistent principles that policymakers should follow when they make payment policy decisions.

This chapter describes our policy framework by:

- outlining Medicare's payment objectives, the payment principles that flow from buying health care in local markets, and payment system design challenges for policymakers, and
- highlighting major design decisions, related payment system components, design options, and implementation issues.

The policy framework focuses on the issues policymakers confront in designing prospective payment systems. We illustrate key decisions and the factors that may influence choices among options by examining similar decisions that have been made in developing existing systems, such as those for hospital inpatient care and physicians' services. Because the same design issues must be resolved in setting payments for Medicare+Choice organizations, we also consider that payment system in this context. These illustrations suggest a set of common design questions that must be resolved in designing any prospective payment system. They also highlight some important design principles and show how their application may lead to different decisions across health care settings.

Common Design Questions

What is Medicare buying in a particular setting?
What factors account for predictable variation in the cost of producing these products?
How should we determine the level of payment?
How would we know if payment rates were too high or too low?
What factors should be considered in adjusting the payment rates over time?
Are similar services or products available in another setting?
Under what circumstances should Medicare pay more for a service in one setting than in another?

PAYMENT POLICY OBJECTIVES AND ENVIRONMENT

A framework for analyzing Medicare's payment systems must account for both payment policy objectives and the major features of the environment in which the payment systems will operate. Building a payment policy framework, therefore, raises several immediate questions:

- What are Medicare's payment policy objectives?
- What does buying health services from private providers in local markets imply for setting Medicare payment rates?
- What challenges must policymakers overcome in designing payment systems for multiple settings in a complex and dynamic health care delivery system?

MEDICARE'S PAYMENT POLICY OBJECTIVES

Medicare's primary goal is to ensure that its elderly and disabled beneficiaries have access to medically necessary acute care of high quality.[3] Federal spending to meet this goal is financed by a combination of payroll taxes, general revenues, and beneficiaries' premiums. To minimize the financial burden on taxpayers and beneficiaries, Medicare has an obligation to purchase appropriate care as efficiently as possible. Thus, Medicare's payment policies should promote efficient production and distribution of acute care products and services.

BUYING HEALTH CARE IN PRIVATE MARKETS

Medicare buys covered products and services from providers who compete for resources in private markets. Consequently, Medicare's payment systems should strive to establish payment rates that approximate the competitive prices that would prevail in the long run in local health care markets.

If the program's payment systems were successful in meeting this objective, then its payment rates would be:

- high enough to stimulate adequate numbers of providers to offer services to Medicare beneficiaries,
- sufficient to enable efficient providers to supply high quality services given the trade-offs between cost and quality that exist with current medical technology and local supply conditions for labor and capital inputs, and
- low enough to avoid imposing unnecessary burdens on taxpayers and beneficiaries through the taxes and the premiums they pay to finance the program.

Setting the Right Price

Approximating long-run market prices is not an easy task, partly because no one knows what they would be. Theoretically, long-run market prices in a competitive health care market would equal providers' long-run marginal costs per unit. This suggests that Medicare should pay rates that are equal to providers' long-run marginal costs, as long as those amounts also cover their long-run average costs (Pauly 1980).[4]

In the short-run, however, providers' costs may be above or below their long-run marginal costs. Moreover, substantial discrepancies between Medicare's prospective payment rates and providers' short-run costs may lead to serious problems for beneficiaries or taxpayers. When providers' marginal costs for individual patients may differ substantially from Medicare's payment rates, providers have incentives to engage in risk selection, seeking only the least costly patients and avoiding those who are likely to need unusually expensive care.[5] When payment rates fall short of the marginal costs of providing additional services, providers have incentives to stint on the services or inputs used to produce care. Thus, rates that are below marginal costs might cause access and quality problems for beneficiaries. Conversely, when rates are set above marginal costs, providers have incentives to furnish too many services, thereby exposing patients to unnecessary health risks and creating unwarranted financial burdens for beneficiaries and taxpayers.

These potential consequences suggest that Medicare's payment rates should be consistent with efficient providers' marginal costs. Providers' costs are difficult to determine, however, because the available measures are based on accounting costs, which may differ from true economic costs. Further, most health care providers produce multiple products and some operate across two or more settings—hospital inpatient and outpatient care, for instance—making it difficult to disentangle the costs associated with specific services. Nevertheless, markets for most products and services appear to accommodate a fairly substantial range of price and cost variation. Consequently, Medicare's payment rates need only to fall within that range.

Payment Rates, Incentives, and Unintended Consequences

In designing a PPS, it is crucial to keep in mind the potential for unintended consequences. Just like market-determined prices, Medicare's prospective payment rates create incentives for efficiency by placing providers at risk. Providers whose costs exceed the predetermined payment rate will take a loss; those whose costs remain below the payment rate keep the gain. Providers thus have an incentive to improve efficiency for the products and services included in the payment rate.

Providers can lower the risk of loss, however, by reducing their costs or increasing their revenues in ways that are inconsistent with Medicare's goals. As mentioned, these include risk selection, stinting, and increasing the volume of services provided. But others are possible as well even when the payment rates are neither too low nor too high: unbundling the product by shifting some component services to another setting; using the gray areas of diagnosis and procedure coding systems to overstate the complexity of care and receive higher payments; submitting false claims; or ceasing to participate in Medicare.

Each of these strategies has potential short-run and long-run costs for providers, such as loss of reputation, risk of malpractice claims, return of unwarranted payments, or loss of market share. These costs generally encourage providers to respond appropriately to payment incentives. But one or more of these responses may become attractive if Medicare's payment rates depart substantially from efficient providers' production costs. Consequently, payment system design decisions frequently involve carefully considering how the available options may raise or lower the likelihood of unintended responses.

CHALLENGES FOR POLICYMAKERS

Designing new payment systems and updating existing payment rates for a variety of health care settings raise several challenges for policymakers. First, circumstances differ among settings, so one challenge is to recognize differences among types of providers, the services they furnish, the beneficiaries they serve, and the tools and information available. As later discussion will show, payment system design is largely driven by policymakers' understanding of the clinical characteristics of the products Medicare is buying in each setting and the main features of providers' cost structures.

A second challenge arises because the delivery of health care is complex. In a single episode of care, for example, beneficiaries may receive physician visits, hospital outpatient diagnostic procedures, a surgical procedure during a hospital inpatient stay, physical therapy in an inpatient rehabilitation unit, post-acute care in a skilled nursing facility, and home health visits. At various points during the episode, the same or similar services could be furnished in two or more settings in which providers are paid under different payment systems with potentially different payment rates and financial incentives.

This complexity means that policymakers must recognize the potential for overlap among settings and avoid introducing inconsistencies among payment systems that might distort the behavior of providers or beneficiaries in determining the types and amounts of services consumed and the settings in which they are furnished. Other factors being equal, Medicare should pay the same amount for identical services regardless of the setting in which they are furnished. In applying this principle, however, policymakers need to be sure that services with the same description are in fact identical. This would not be true if the patients served in alternative settings present different clinical risks or needs for support services that may legitimately affect providers' costs. The challenge of appropriately addressing potential overlaps among settings has been growing with the introduction of new organizational arrangements for the delivery of care.

The dynamism of the health care system raises a final challenge. Continuing advances in medical science and technology and innovations in the organization and delivery of care alter the services available, where they can be produced, and providers' costs of production. Medicare's administered pricing systems (and those used by other health insurers), however, lack the full complement of competitive market feedback mechanisms.

Normal market feedback mechanisms generate prices that lead providers and consumers to adjust their behavior in response to changes in supply and demand conditions. Health care markets are unusual, however, because insured consumers face drastically reduced prices in purchasing services and because consumers and their physicians are both usually separate from the payer. One result is that consumers' decisions about service use are often distorted. Another is that shifts in demand among consumers in response to changes in product content or in service availability across settings do not automatically alter insurers' payment rates.

Consequently, Medicare must adjust its payment rates over time to reflect changes in prices that otherwise would occur automatically in a competitive market. This means that mechanisms for updating the payment rates and related factors must be designed and implemented in each setting to respond appropriately to changes in underlying supply and demand conditions. To support this effort, Medicare must devote substantial resources to monitoring and evaluating changes in the clinical technology and organization of care. In addition, the program must monitor beneficiaries' access to services, the quality of care they receive, and other indicators that suggest when payment rates diverge too far from providers' costs.

MAJOR DESIGN DECISIONS

All prospective payment systems must ultimately resolve the same set of issues:

- **Establishing the unit of payment.** Will providers be paid for an individual service or a bundle of services, such as an inpatient day, an inpatient stay, an episode of care or illness, or a month of care?
- **Establishing relative values.** How will payment rates based on the selected unit of payment be differentiated among distinct services, bundles of care, or beneficiary characteristics to recognize appropriate and predictable differences in providers' costs?
- **Defining local input price adjustments.** How will payment rates be adjusted to recognize differences in local prices for inputs such as labor and capital? Local input price differences, which reflect variations in supply

and demand conditions among market areas, may substantially raise or lower providers' costs. Payment rates must be adjusted accordingly to avoid creating arbitrary gains and losses for providers based solely on their location.

- **Defining other rate adjustments.** How will payment rates be adjusted to accommodate unusual circumstances of providers or special characteristics of services and beneficiaries that affect providers' costs but are not accounted for by the basic payment model? One example is how to adjust the payment rate when physicians perform surgery in an OPD or an ASC, thereby avoiding some costs that otherwise would be incurred in their offices. Another is how to adjust the payment rate when a patient's care turns out to be unusually costly.
- **Setting the initial level of payment.** How will the initial level of the payment rates be determined? Options include providers' historical costs or past Medicare spending for services in the particular setting.
- **Updating the payment rates over time.** How will payment rates and related factors be updated to reflect changes in technology, practice patterns, and market conditions? Update mechanisms must be designed to detect changes in these factors and make appropriate revisions to each of the main payment system components while maintaining the affordability of the program.

Policymakers' decisions on these issues define the components of a PPS. The essential character of any PPS primarily reflects choices on the unit of payment and the relative values. These two interrelated decisions define the products for which Medicare will pay. They also determine the scope of the payment system's incentives and its potential power to influence service use and program spending.

ESTABLISHING THE UNIT OF PAYMENT

Choosing a unit of payment depends on several issues:

- How well can the product be defined?
- Are effective product classification systems and related data available?
- How will policymakers balance trade-offs between the scope of the payment incentives and potentially undesirable provider responses?
- Is it desirable to bundle services furnished by complementary providers?
- What supporting rules are needed to define the boundaries of the payment unit?

How Well Can the Product Be Defined?

One of the most important factors influencing the unit of payment decision is how well the product or service can be defined. If the product cannot be defined

General Prospective Payment Formula

In a prospective payment system, the payment rate for a specific product in a particular market area is determined by the following general formula:

Payment rate for product A in market area B = Initial base payment amount × update factor × input-price adjustment factor for market area B × relative value for product A × other rate adjustment factors

The initial base payment amount is usually a national dollar amount for a specific year that reflects policymakers' decisions on the unit of payment and the appropriate initial level of payment for the average unit. The update factor adjusts the initial base amount for inflation and other factors to set the base level of payment for the rate year. The input-price adjustment factor then raises or lowers the national base amount to reflect the relative level of input prices in the particular market area compared with the national average. Next, the relative value adjusts the market-specific base amount to reflect the expected relative costliness of the particular product compared with that of the average unit. Finally, the local rate for the specific product may be modified by one or more additional rate adjustment factors designed to accommodate unusual characteristics of the provider, the service, or the specific patient.

well, setting payment rates that accurately reflect providers' expected costs will be difficult, and providers' gains and losses could be largely unrelated to their performance. It also would be difficult in this case to monitor providers' performance and ensure that they deliver what Medicare wants to buy. Moreover, a PPS based on a poorly defined product gives providers both incentives and opportunities to benefit financially without improving efficiency.

Ideally, the unit of payment should match the unit of service, which reflects the way providers think about the product and provides context for their decisions about care.[6] The unit of service for hospital inpatient care, for instance, is a hospital stay—a completed episode of acute inpatient care, beginning at admission and ending when the patient no longer needs the acute level of care hospitals offer. In contrast, the unit of service for physician care could be thought of as either an episode of care or as an individual instance of service.

Defining and measuring the product or service requires identifying the clinical factors that account for variation in the content and duration of care. In addition, reliable information on those factors must be readily available at the appropriate level (service, episode of care, or beneficiary). Lack of sufficient knowledge and information has often prevented policymakers from using a larger payment unit in some settings. For example, the recently implemented SNF payment system is based on a per diem payment unit rather than a complete stay because the clinical and other factors that account for differences in patients' lengths of stay are not well understood. Similarly, payment for home health care is based on visits rather than episodes of care because no one knows how to appropriately differentiate home care episodes.

Are Effective Product Classification Systems and Related Data Available?

Using a particular unit of payment requires a compatible and effective classification system that identifies distinct services, patient care products (types of days or cases), or beneficiaries that are expected to require different amounts of providers' resources. In the physician fee schedule, this function is performed by HCFA's Common Procedure Coding System (HCPCS). The hospital inpatient PPS is based on the diagnosis related groups (DRG). The Medicare+Choice program classifies beneficiaries based on their demographic characteristics and institutional status and soon will add health status. In each instance, the categories in the classification system define the products for which Medicare will pay.

The need for an effective classification system can be seen by considering how hospitals' financial incentives would change if Medicare paid a single fixed price for all inpatient stays. Although hospitals still would face strong incentives to reduce the cost of care for any patients they might serve, they also could realize large gains by engaging in risk selection, admitting only patients with relatively low-cost conditions. Conversely, they would experience large losses for patients with high-cost conditions, for example, those who required a bone marrow transplant or those with severe burns. Consequently, a per case PPS without an effective classification system like the DRGs would surely create access problems for beneficiaries with serious illnesses.

Effective classification systems generally meet two essential criteria. First, they account for a reasonably high proportion of the predictable variation in providers' costs. A successful system thus captures most of the systematic cost differences that result from clinical or other differences among services, patients, or beneficiaries. To the extent that this criterion is not met, providers have incentives for risk selection.[7] Equally important, providers that have established a reputation for expertise may attract patients who are more seriously ill and more costly than the average patient. When the classification system fails to capture such severity differences, these providers may be penalized because they cannot balance losses on high cost patients with gains from low cost ones.

Second, the classification variables, such as diagnoses or procedures, must be reasonably objective and easily monitored. If this criterion were not met, providers would have incentives to increase their revenues by manipulating the classification variables (called code creep) so that services or patients were assigned to higher paid categories.

The relevant information—procedures, patient diagnoses, or beneficiary characteristics—needed to assign services, patients, or beneficiaries to the appropriate classification categories also must be readily available. The lack of relevant data on beneficiary health status has retarded development of more effective classification systems and prevented payment system improvements in most post-acute care settings and in Medicare's managed care program for many years.

How Will Policymakers Balance Trade-offs Between the Scope of Incentives and Potentially Undesirable Provider Responses?

Other factors being equal, policymakers should choose a large unit of payment over a small one because it gives broader scope to providers' incentives for efficiency. This choice, however, also affects the potential undesirable actions providers might take. Whether this trade-off is important largely depends on the extent to which providers control product content and volume.

The scope of providers' incentives for efficiency depends on the size of the product or unit included in the price. Larger units include more services, thereby increasing the provider's opportunity to economize on the mix and quantity of services and related inputs used to produce the unit. Thus, a hospital inpatient stay or a month of care provides broad incentives for efficiency because many services are included in the product. In contrast, a narrow unit of payment—individual services, such as office visits or X-rays for instance—provides narrower incentives for efficiency. The provider's opportunities to reduce costs are limited to altering the mix and quantity of inputs used to produce each service.

Providers may respond to these incentives as intended, or some may respond in less desirable ways, such as stinting on services or inputs and increasing the number of units they furnish. The potential actions they might take, however, depend on the size of the payment unit, their control over the product, and the likelihood of oversight.[8]

When providers have direct control over product content and volume, a small payment unit—the service for instance—generally creates relatively little concern about stinting, but substantial concern about potential increases in the volume of units. Conversely, a large payment unit usually generates more concern about potential stinting but less about unintended changes in volume. Large payment units, such as hospital stays, generally include broad opportunities for stinting, but they often involve significant risks for patients and substantial costs and thus are more likely to attract oversight and review.

Providers' control over content and volume varies among care settings. In many facility settings, such as hospital inpatient units or ambulatory surgical centers, physicians' orders largely determine both the mix and quantity of services furnished and the number of patients served. In these settings, the potential for adverse responses to payment incentives by the facility provider may be limited to some degree by physician oversight. The strength of physician influence varies among settings, however, reflecting the extent to which they actively direct the care patients receive. Thus, the potential for both stinting on services and unintended volume growth might be of greater concern in a SNF payment system based on a per diem payment unit, for instance, than it would be in a hospital PPS with a per stay payment unit.[9]

Physicians' roles have been changing, however, raising some uncertainty about whether the traditional independence of their patient care decisions may be eroding. This uncertainty reflects physicians' growing interrelationships with other providers, especially hospitals and health care organizations, through contractual incentives that affect their compensation or through practice ownership.

Is It Desirable to Bundle Services Furnished by Complementary Providers?

Although a larger payment unit generally is preferred over a smaller one, the larger unit may be rejected because of concerns about the potential effects on patients. In the hospital inpatient PPS, for example, physician services related to a hospital inpatient stay could have been combined with the hospital facility services included in each DRG. This probably would have had little effect on the way in which diagnoses and procedures were grouped in defining the DRGs, but it certainly would have affected the relative values across DRGs and the initial level of payment.

Paying the combined rate to physicians would have potentially exposed them to high levels of financial risk. Although hospitals were better able to bear the financial risk, many physicians were concerned that giving hospitals control over the combined payment would compromise their independence in making patient care decisions. In the end, policymakers were persuaded that preserving physicians' independent patient advocacy role provided valuable protection for Medicare beneficiaries and outweighed potential efficiency gains that might have been obtained by using a broader payment unit.

What Supporting Rules Are Needed?

Payment policy cannot stand alone. Policymakers also must define the boundaries of the payment unit because providers facing a fixed payment rate have financial incentives to unbundle the product by billing separately for individual services that should be included in the payment unit or by shifting some of these services to another setting.

In the hospital inpatient PPS, for instance, hospitals have a strong incentive to shift diagnostic services to the outpatient department or a physicians' office. Hospitals also can reduce inpatient costs by discharging patients earlier to a long-term care hospital, rehabilitation facility, SNF, or home health care, all of which are paid under separate payment systems. SNFs have similar incentives to reduce per diem costs. Their ability to realize savings depends on how the boundary is defined between the bundle of services a SNF is expected to furnish and services that may be provided by an independent provider or in another setting— diagnostic imaging services furnished in a nearby hospital outpatient department, for instance.

To limit potential unbundling, HCFA has implemented a variety of rules. For example, hospital outpatient services furnished within 72 hours before a patient's admission for care are assumed to be part of the inpatient stay and may not be billed separately under the hospital outpatient payment system. To mitigate shifting of services at the end of a stay, hospitals' per discharge payments are reduced in 10 DRGs when a patient is discharged to a rehabilitation facility, long-term care hospital, SNF, or to related home health care after a stay that is two or more days shorter than the national average length of stay for the DRG.[10] The 10 DRGs include categories in which a high proportion of Medicare patients go on to use post-acute care.

ESTABLISHING RELATIVE VALUES

Relative values measure the expected costliness of a unit in each classification category compared with the overall average costliness of all units.[11] Relative values may be structured in different ways depending on policymakers' understanding of the clinical components of care and providers' cost structures. Thus, for each setting, policymakers must decide what components are combined to produce the product, how those components vary among product categories, and what factors are likely to affect efficient providers' component production costs. These decisions produce a model of provider cost structure, which identifies a set of factors that are expected to account for variation in the unit cost of services.

The model of hospital costs that is implicit in the hospital inpatient PPS, for example, is relatively simple. Hospitals' costs are assumed to be the sum of operating and capital costs. Each component is expected to vary in the same way across DRGs. Consequently, only one set of DRG relative values is needed to determine both the operating and capital components of a hospital's payment rates for all DRGs.[12]

The model of provider cost structure implicit in the physician fee schedule is more complicated. The value of each physician service is assumed to include three parts: physician work, practice expenses, and professional liability insurance costs. The value or cost of each component is expected to vary across the service categories of the HCPCS coding system, but the distribution is different in each instance. Consequently, three sets of relative values are needed to determine the payment rate for a service.[13]

In the Medicare+Choice payment system, the relative values are based on a risk adjustment model that estimates expected annual spending for all Medicare-covered services given a beneficiaries' demographic characteristics, eligibility for Medicaid benefits, and institutional status. HCFA has proposed using a new model that also takes into account beneficiaries' health status as indicated by the principal diagnosis for the most costly hospital stay (if any) they had during the previous year.

Constructing Relative Values

Relative values are often based on estimates of providers' costs. HCFA originally developed the DRG relative values for Medicare's hospital inpatient PPS, for example, using estimates of hospitals' average costs per case in each DRG. These estimates were derived from provider-specific billed charges and cost to charge ratios for each component type of service, adjusted to reflect national average input price levels.[14] Relative values for OPD services in HCFA's proposed outpatient PPS are determined similarly.

In the Medicare+Choice payment system, relative values are based on estimated average annual spending for Medicare-covered services for each beneficiary category. This method is appropriate because spending for covered services accounts for the overwhelming majority of a health plan's costs. These estimates are developed from HCFA's annual claims database, which includes all fee-for-service bills paid under the traditional program.

Sometimes, however, the data needed to estimate providers' costs at the product or component level are unavailable. In these instances, policymakers have used two alternative approaches. Occasionally, relative values have been based on a measure that reflects a major component of costs. Relative values for different categories of patient days in the recently implemented PPS for SNF services, for instance, were based on data from staff time studies. Although the mix and quantity of staff time accounts for much of the cost of a day of SNF care, this approach may result in payment errors if other components of costs follow a different pattern. Pending collection of data on actual cost differences among services, physicians' historical charges were used as a proxy for costs in developing relative values for the practice expense and professional liability insurance components of the physician fee schedule.

In other instances, relative values have been based on expert opinion. Service-specific data on resource use for the physician work component are almost unimaginable. To fill this void, panels of physicians assigned relative values to individual services by comparing them with a set of reference services usually performed by different physician specialists. These values were intended to measure the relative amount of work for each service based on several criteria, such as the amount of physician time, intensity of effort, skill and risk to the patient, compared with those for the reference services.

DEFINING LOCAL INPUT PRICE ADJUSTMENTS

Input-price differences among market areas may account for 50 percent or more of the observed nationwide variation in providers' costs for a given product. Consequently, an effective input-price adjustment is essential in setting appropriate payment rates for each market area.

Input-price adjustments are made using a price index, which compares prices in each market area with the national average. The index is applied to raise or lower all or a portion of the base payment amount to reflect each area's input-price level. The price index is based on two types of information: an input-price data set, which shows the average price in each market area for each type of resource; and a set of weights indicating the relative importance of each input in the production process, as indicated by its share of providers' costs.

Product Components that Are Affected by Input-Price Variation

Designing appropriate input-price adjustments requires decisions on three issues. First, policymakers must decide which product components—and corresponding portions of the base payment amount—should be adjusted for local price variation. This decision is based on knowledge of the production process, which identifies components whose inputs vary in price among local markets, and the proportion of component production costs that are affected. In the hospital inpatient PPS, for instance, HCFA has determined that 71 percent of hospital operating costs are affected by local variation in prices for labor. The other 29 percent is largely made up of supplies and minor equipment items, which are assumed to be purchased in national markets and thus need no adjustment.[15]

Defining Input Market Areas

In addition, policymakers must decide how market areas will be defined. This is critical both for measuring price differentials for specific inputs and for determining the adjustment that applies for any provider. HCFA generally has used metropolitan statistical areas and statewide rural areas to define market areas for most facility PPSs, such as those for hospitals, ASCs, and SNFs. In the physician fee schedule, market areas in some states are defined by administrative regions (called localities), and in others they are statewide. In the Medicare+Choice program, market areas are defined by collections of counties representing where each county's resident fee-for-service beneficiaries received care.

Measuring Input Prices

The third issue is how to measure input prices in each area. For each setting, policymakers must choose the specific inputs for which prices will be measured;

whether to use prices paid only by providers in a specific setting or prices for the same or similar inputs paid by a broader spectrum of providers; and how to account for differences among settings in the mix of inputs used. In recent years, HCFA has annually collected data on total wages and hours from most facilities, such as hospitals and SNFs. HCFA uses these data, without adjusting for differences in the mix of occupations employed, to calculate wage indexes for each type of facility in more than 300 market areas. The lack of an adjustment for occupational mix differences may cause the hospital and SNF wage indexes to overstate substantially the actual relative level of wages in some market areas and understate it in others.

For the physician fee schedule, HCFA calculates separate geographic practice cost indexes for physician work, practice expenses, and professional liability insurance expenses for 89 payment localities. To calculate these indexes, HCFA uses data from the decennial census, residential rent indexes, and other sources. Because each service is described by separate relative values that account for its particular mix of physician work, practice expenses, and professional liability expenses, the potential for systematic distortions across areas may be lower than that in the hospital and SNF wage indexes.

In the Medicare+Choice program, the most relevant inputs are the services that health plans purchase from physicians, hospitals, outpatient facilities, SNFs, and home health agencies. However, policymakers cannot easily obtain data on the prices health plans paid for a representative set of services, and many market areas have no health plans serving Medicare beneficiaries. Consequently, an input-price adjustment based on service prices is probably not a reasonable option in the near term.

Providers in virtually all health care settings employ workers in many of the same occupations, although the proportions probably vary substantially among settings. An alternative to the current approach thus might be to collect occupation-specific wage data from a representative set of providers operating in all health settings in each market area. These data then could be used with occupation cost shares for specific settings to obtain a set of indexes that could be applied in individual payment systems.

DEFINING OTHER RATE ADJUSTMENTS

Policymakers must decide whether and how to adjust the payment rate for a service or bundle of services to accommodate unusual characteristics of the patient or the services provided, the provider, or the market area in which the provider operates. Generally, rate adjustments should be applied for factors that would affect an efficient provider's costs and are beyond the provider's control. In some instances, policymakers also have added payment adjustments to provide explicit support for certain socially valued activities.

Special Characteristics of Patients or Services Provided

The product classification systems used in setting payment rates often fail to capture all of the patient characteristics that may affect providers' costs of delivering care. Some of these characteristics may be predictable. For example, extremely frail patients or those with severe cognitive impairment may require extra assistance for services as simple as a chest X-ray. In other instances, higher costs may be triggered by the occurrence of random events. Patients who suffer serious complications, such as a pulmonary embolism or a stroke during a hospital stay, can double or triple the hospital's costs compared with those for typical patients with the same underlying illness.

A payment system that fails to recognize predictable additional costs would give providers strong disincentives to treat patients who have high cost characteristics. Further, the extra costs associated with random catastrophic events could threaten providers' financial viability and thus beneficiaries' access to care.

In the hospital inpatient PPS, the latter problem is addressed by an outlier policy, which operates much like a mandatory reinsurance policy. Medicare makes additional payments to hospitals when costs for a patient exceed a DRG-specific loss threshold. The difference between the loss threshold and the usual DRG payment rate is a fixed loss amount, which acts like a deductible that must be exceeded before outlier payments begin. Payments above the deductible loss amount are subject to a 20 percent coinsurance (borne by the hospital) because Medicare pays only 80 percent of the additional amount. Outlier payments substantially reduce the losses hospitals otherwise would incur on unusually high cost patients, thereby limiting hospitals' incentives to avoid those who are seriously ill. These payments are financed by an equivalent aggregate reduction in all DRG payments, thus distributing the burden of unusually costly patients among all hospitals in proportion to their DRG revenue.

The physician fee schedule includes modifiers that a physician may apply to raise the physician work relative value when the services provided are greater than those usually required for a procedure. Other fee schedule modifiers may apply when a return trip to the operating room is required for a related or unrelated procedure during the postoperative period.

The opposite situation also may arise—when not all of the services included in the unit of payment are needed. This may occur, for instance, when a patient is transferred from one hospital to another after only a few days. To reflect the transferring hospital's lower costs, payment for these cases under the inpatient PPS is based on a DRG-specific per diem rate, which is equal to the hospital's full DRG payment rate divided by the national average length of stay for the DRG. This policy recognizes that the first day of care is usually much more costly than subsequent days of inpatient care. The transferring hospital thus receives twice the per diem rate for the first day and the per diem amount for each additional day, up to the full DRG rate.

Analogous adjustments are made in the physician fee schedule for situations in which the physician's service is less than that usually required. For example, modifiers are applied to reduce the relative value for the procedure if the physician acts as an assistant surgeon or if review of the medical record indicates that the usual services were not fully furnished. For many services, the practice expense component of the physician's payment is reduced by a site-of-service differential when the service is provided in a OPD or an ASC rather than the physician's office.

In the Medicare+Choice payment system, payments to an organization are reduced substantially when an enrolled beneficiary is employed and covered under the employer's health insurance plan. Under the law, the employer is primarily responsible for making payments to the plan and Medicare is considered the secondary payer. In this case, the organization's costs are unaffected, but it would be overpaid if Medicare made its usual payment.

Special Characteristics of Providers or Market Areas

Some providers offer specialized types of care that are not available from otherwise similar entities, thereby incurring unusual costs. Hospitals that provide organ transplant surgery, for example, bear highly variable costs for organ acquisition. Failing to recognize this extra burden would give hospitals strong incentives to cease offering transplant services. Consequently, these costs are excluded from the hospital inpatient PPS and paid separately based on the reasonable amount actually incurred. Other hospitals treat a disproportionate share of patients with end-stage renal disease (ESRD). To preserve access to care, the payment system accounts for the extra costs these facilities incur in providing dialysis services for ESRD patients when they are treated for unrelated conditions. The inpatient PPS thus makes extra payments based on the weekly cost of dialysis to hospitals in which more than 10 percent of Medicare patients have ESRD but are admitted for unrelated care.

Other providers serve sparsely populated or economically depressed market areas. One example is hospitals that are the sole providers in their communities. Another is physicians who practice in urban or rural health professional shortage areas. These providers may face higher costs or other disincentives to continue serving such markets. Both the hospital inpatient PPS and the physician fee schedule provide special treatment for providers in these circumstances.

Similarly, health care organizations participating in Medicare's managed care program (now the Medicare+Choice program) have been reluctant to serve counties with low payment rates. These counties may be unattractive because they have relatively small populations of beneficiaries or few hospitals and other providers with whom organizations might contract. To overcome these disadvantages and improve beneficiaries' access to health plans, the Congress established a floor payment rate, raising payment rates for some counties by 20 percent or more.

Explicit Subsidies for Socially Valued Activities

Developing a prospective payment system forces policymakers to make explicit decisions about whether to provide subsidies for certain socially valued activities. Before the hospital inpatient PPS was adopted, Medicare reimbursed hospitals for its share of the costs they incurred for certain activities, such as medical education and training programs. Unpaid costs incurred by hospitals that serve large numbers of poor patients generally were not reimbursed by Medicare unless they were related to the care furnished to Medicare patients. When the Congress adopted the inpatient PPS, it decided to make extra payments to hospitals to support both of these activities.

Extra payments for these activities generally have not been made in other settings. HCFA's proposed hospital outpatient PPS, for example, does not include payment adjustments for hospitals that operate teaching programs or those that serve a disproportionate share of poor patients (see Chapter 6). Moreover, policymakers generally have not been willing to adopt payment adjustments to support costs associated with other potentially valuable activities, such as hospitals' participation in trials of experimental therapies.

SETTING THE INITIAL LEVEL OF PAYMENT

Given the decisions they have made on the unit of payment, relative values, and payment adjustments, policymakers must establish the initial level of the base payment amount in each payment system. Combined with actual service use by type of service and location, the initial payment amount will determine the level of the payment rates, total program spending for the setting, and the level and distribution of beneficiaries' related copayments in the first payment year.

The base payment amount represents the amount Medicare pays for a standard service, product, or beneficiary in an area with national average input price levels. In the hospital inpatient PPS, for example, the base payment amount is Medicare's payment for an average case (a case in a DRG in which the relative value is 1.0) in a hospital located in an area with national average wage rates (the wage index equals 1.0), if no other adjustments are applicable.

Major Issues

The obvious issue is how to calculate an initial value for the base payment amount that is consistent with earlier payment design choices. The answer depends on three issues:

- whether pertinent information on providers' costs and payments, is available,
- whether, and how, to allow for regional differences in practice patterns, and
- whether the proposed payment system will be constrained to meet a specified aggregate spending target. A spending target may maintain aggregate spending at the level anticipated under the previous payment system (called budget neutrality) or achieve specified budget savings.

Availability of pertinent information. HCFA has used providers' reported costs and claims data to develop cost-based payment amounts when cost data have been available—for example, in payment systems for services provided in hospital inpatient and outpatient facilities, ASCs, SNFs, and home health agencies. When cost data have not been available, or relevant, HCFA has used data on claims payments and total spending instead, for instance in the physician fee schedule and in Medicare's managed care program.

Regional differences in practice patterns. Providers located in different regions may use varying amounts and mixtures of services and inputs to provide patient care.[16] As a result, providers' costs for a standard service unit or product may differ substantially among regions. In this case, policymakers face three options. One is to set payment rates based on a national base payment amount, thereby ignoring regional cost differences. With the same aggregate spending, this option would likely result in substantial redistribution of payments among providers based on their regional location. A key question in evaluating this option is whether any resulting changes in practice patterns would be harmful to beneficiaries. The answer depends on whether more costly practice patterns are associated with substantial improvements in patient outcomes.

A second option is to set payment rates based on separate regional base payment amounts, thereby fully recognizing regional differences in average cost. This approach would likely result in relatively little payment redistribution, and providers in all regions would face comparable incentives to alter their practice patterns to improve efficiency. On the one hand, this approach might seem attractive if higher cost practice patterns were associated with better outcomes. On the other hand, it would tend to freeze practice patterns for providers and beneficiaries in low cost regions, preventing them from realizing available quality improvements by adopting the practice patterns used in high cost regions.

The third option is a compromise, blending national and regional base payment amounts in specified proportions. This option may be used as a transition mechanism to blend national and regional amounts in varying proportions over time, thus allowing providers a reasonable period to make practice adjustments.

Moreover, the transition may end with a single national payment amount or with a specific permanent blend of national and regional amounts. Policymakers might choose a permanent blend if they were uncertain about the extent of the association between quality and cost.

Two examples illustrate how policymakers have addressed this issue. In the early 1980s, hospital inpatient operating costs per case exhibited substantial regional variation, partly because average lengths of stay were about twice as long in the Northeast and the Midwest as they were in the South and the West. After much debate, the Congress decided to include regional and national payment amounts in a transition mechanism that also included updated hospital-specific base year costs. The four-year transition ended with a PPS based on separate urban and rural base payment amounts which reflected a judgment that regional differences in practice patterns were not strongly associated with quality differences.

The second example concerns Medicare's original risk contracting program. Policymakers initially decided that managed care organizations should be able to provide all Medicare-covered services to beneficiaries in return for 95 percent of the estimated monthly per capita amount Medicare would expect to spend in the traditional fee-for-service program in each county. This decision recognized the full effects of differences in fee-for-service practice patterns on county per capita spending. For example, monthly per capita payment rates for managed care organizations in 1997 ranged from $221 to $767 among counties, with practice variation accounting for roughly 30 to 40 percent of the total variation (ProPAC 1997).[17]

The Congress revisited this issue in the BBA and decided to reduce substantially payment variation among counties by blending each county's updated base year payment rate with an input-price adjusted national average payment rate. At the end of the five-year transition period in 2002, the updated county and national rate components will each account for 50 percent of the county payment rate, thus recognizing one-half of the practice pattern variation in traditional Medicare spending among counties.

Constraining the payment amount to meet a spending target.   A budget neutrality requirement or other spending target shifts the policy focus from concerns about how the initial base payment amount should be developed to the assumptions that are made to ensure that actual spending reaches the target. This shift in focus occurs because a spending target, together with the other components of a payment system's design, fully determines the initial level of the base payment amount.

A spending target is sufficient to determine the initial base payment amount because of the way in which targets are implemented. First, HCFA develops a projection of the expected aggregate program payments that would be made under the current payment system during the initial year of the new system. This spending target is generally based on the most recent claims (and cost) data available and anticipated trends in factors that are expected to affect service use and costs in the projection year. HCFA then develops a similar projection of total program spending anticipated under the new payment system. This projection is based on the same data but takes into account the payment rates in the new system, and anticipated responses to those rates by providers and beneficiaries. Although aggregate spending under the new system cannot be estimated without plugging in an initial payment amount, this amount is not really needed. Because the spending target is known, HCFA can infer what the initial payment amount would have to be, given its data and assumptions, to produce projected spending equal to target spending.

To project spending under the new system, HCFA must decide how providers are likely to change their behavior in response to altered payment incentives. Among other responses, providers may unbundle services, improve the quality and completeness of diagnosis and procedure coding, or increase the volume of service units they furnish. All of these actions would increase spending within the particular setting, or in the case of unbundling, in other settings. HCFA often tries to capture the overall effect of such responses in a behavioral offset assumption. In implementing the physician fee schedule, for example, HCFA assumed a 50 percent behavioral offset; 50 percent of the savings that otherwise would accrue from the new system would be lost to the combination of these responses. This assumption played an important role in determining the initial level of the conversion factor and thus the level of physicians' fees.

SETTING THE INITIAL PAYMENT AMOUNT IN THE ABSENCE OF A SPENDING TARGET

Without a budget neutrality requirement or other spending target, policymakers must decide how to determine the initial level of the base payment amount using data on providers' costs, paid claims, and annual program spending. Three methods generally have been used. All three require prior development of the product classification system, relative values, and payment adjustment factors that will be applied in the proposed payment system.

The first method uses providers' historical cost information, Medicare claims data for the relevant services or products, and the proposed payment system components. HCFA combines these elements to build up a base payment amount for a standard product or service. Variations on this approach have been used to set base payment amounts for the hospital inpatient, outpatient, and SNF payment systems.

The second method uses claims data for all covered services, demographic characteristics for all fee-for-service beneficiaries living in each county, and relative values for demographic categories. HCFA uses these data to estimate per capita program spending for a standard beneficiary (one who has national average demographic characteristics) in a geographic area and in the nation. This approach has been used to establish a base payment amount per enrollee for each county in Medicare's managed care program.

The third method is based on claims data, estimated total spending for the relevant services (including both program spending and beneficiary copayments), and the proposed payment components. As in the budget neutrality calculation described earlier, HCFA combines these elements to infer the base payment amount that would generate the same expected total spending. This method has been used to establish conversion factors for the physician fee schedule.

BUILDING INITIAL PAYMENT AMOUNTS USING PROVIDERS' COSTS AND CLAIMS

The details of developing a base payment amount for the first payment year would vary somewhat according to the choice of method and the payment design decisions made earlier for a particular setting. HCFA has frequently used the first method based on cost and claims data because almost all types of facilities have been paid on the basis of incurred costs, making cost data for individual providers readily available. Using this method, however, raises three sets of issues:

- **Adjusting providers' base year costs.** Policymakers must decide how to adjust providers' reported base year costs to reflect earlier policy decisions about specific cost components and to improve comparability among providers. Cost elements that will be paid separately should be excluded from each provider's costs. Comparability may be improved by adjusting unaudited costs for the average effect of auditing and all providers' costs to reflect a common fiscal period rather than provider-specific reporting periods.
- **Standardizing for product mix, input prices, and other payment adjustments.** Policymakers also must decide how to adjust the revised provider-specific cost data to remove cost differences that reflect variations in service or product mix, local input-price levels, and other activities for which special payment adjustments will be made. These adjustments are necessary to make the base payment amount consistent with the various payment adjustments included in the payment system.
- **Computing and updating the base year amount.** The remaining decisions involve how to compute the base year amount per unit and update it to the first payment year. Policymakers could decide, for example, to compute the base year per unit amount using a simple average, a volume-

weighted average, or the median of providers' per unit standardized costs. Alternatively, policymakers could attempt to identify a subset of relatively efficient providers and use only their standardized costs to compute the base year amount per unit. Identifying efficient providers generally has proven to be difficult, however, partly because of the need to control for potential differences in product quality. The base year standardized amount per unit also must be updated to the first payment year.

UPDATING THE PAYMENT RATES AND RELATED FACTORS

Once a new payment system has been implemented, policymakers must decide how to update the payment rates and related factors to reflect changes in technology, practice patterns, and market conditions. Thus, policymakers must develop methods and data sources for updating three sets of payment components: the base payment amount, the classification system and relative values, and the various payment adjustments.

Policymakers also must decide how often each payment component should be updated. This depends on how rapidly market conditions, technology, and other factors change. In most payment systems, the base payment amount has been updated annually to reflect inflation in input prices and other factors that are expected to alter the level of providers' unit costs in the forthcoming year.

The timing of updates may differ for other payment components. For example, although input prices may rise annually with inflation, the relative structure of prices across market areas may change less rapidly. Consequently, input-price indexes may not need revision more often than every three or four years. Similarly, the relative costliness of different products may be affected by changes in technology and practice patterns, but this is usually a slow process. The classification system and relative values in many settings may thus need only minor revisions each year, with major revisions at longer intervals. Some of the other payment adjustments, such as outlier loss amounts for instance, may require annual updates, while others may be revised rarely, if at all.

Updating the Base Payment Amount

Among these update issues, the lion's share of policymakers' attention has been focused on how to determine annual updates to the base payment amount in each payment system. This focus reflects the powerful role the base amount plays in determining the level of the payment rates and its strong influence on total program spending.

It is important to note that the update affects all payment rates equally. Although it influences the total amount of spending for a class of services or products, the update does not affect the distribution of spending among providers or regions. Consequently, the update has nothing to do with the question of whether Medicare's payment rates are at the right level for any specific service or in any particular market. Rather, the focus is on two questions:

- Is the overall national structure of the payment rates at the right level?
- What factors should be taken into account in deciding how much to change that level over time?

Payment updates often are used to address both questions at the same time. It is important to keep these questions distinct, however, because each requires different types of information and different judgments. The first question asks policymakers to consider what has been happening in the recent past that might signal a substantial divergence between the base payment amount and providers' current costs. The answer is important because payment rates that are too low may lead to a reduction in beneficiaries' access to care or the quality of care they receive, while rates that are too high may encourage overproduction of services, which would burden beneficiaries and taxpayers.

If the analysis suggests that the base payment amount has strayed too far from providers' costs, then policymakers should make a corresponding adjustment. This is sometimes called rebasing because a similar adjustment would result if providers' most recent cost data were used to recalculate the base payment amount. Adjusting the base rate in this way does not recoup past over- or underpayments to providers. Rather, it simply makes the base payment rate more consistent with providers' costs in the future.

The second question asks policymakers to consider what objectives they want update policy to achieve. Update objectives may be limited to keeping the payment rates consistent with providers' costs, thereby focusing attention on factors that should legitimately affect those costs in the forthcoming year. Alternatively, policymakers also may seek to control growth in program spending for a particular set of services. This involves considering whether recent spending growth has been above or below the desired level and adjusting the update appropriately to rectify any discrepancy. In this case, policymakers use payment updates deliberately to signal providers that they have been producing too many or too few services.

These decisions about update objectives suggest the kinds of factors that should be considered in determining how much to raise payment rates for the forthcoming year. Assuming that the base payment amount is at the right level today, policymakers can use their knowledge of the recent past and their expectations about the future to develop a quantitative projection for each factor. These projections can then be combined to determine a specific update percentage. Finally, the resulting update percentage may be added to any rebasing adjustment determined earlier to produce a consolidated update for the coming year.

Evaluating the current level of payment. Policymakers may examine a broad array of information to evaluate whether the current base payment level is consistent with providers' costs. The direct relevance, availability, cost, and quality of each type of information will vary by industry and setting:

- **Market prices and costs.** Policymakers could compare Medicare's payment rates directly with market prices and costs for services and products in each setting. Observing market prices and costs often is not feasible, however, because providers' posted fees or charges generally differ from the payments they actually receive from public and private payers. Moreover, measuring actual prices is difficult and extremely costly, partly because they often are determined in private negotiations between individual providers and payers, and neither party wants competitors to know the agreed amounts.
- **Access and quality of care.** Evidence of widespread access or quality problems for beneficiaries might suggest that Medicare's payment rates are too low. In the absence of such evidence, Medicare's rates could be either about right or too high.[18]
- **Entry and exit.** Rapid growth in the number of providers participating in Medicare across many market areas could indicate that Medicare's payment rates are too high. Conversely, widespread provider withdrawals from Medicare could suggest that the rates are too low.
- **Volume growth.** Rapid growth in the volume of services could suggest that Medicare's rates are too high. Declines in volume could indicate the opposite. Either trend, however, also could be explained by changes in technology, beneficiaries' preferences, or practice patterns.
- **Providers' costs, revenues, and margins.** Information on providers' costs and revenues sometimes can be obtained from HCFA's administrative files or from industry surveys. This information often is incomplete because it lacks accurate measures of each provider's overall product mix, and it is available only for some types of providers. As noted earlier, accounting costs may differ from providers' true economic costs. Such cost and revenue data are valuable, however, because they provide a good picture of providers' overall financial condition and financial performance on their Medicare business. Often, these data provide fairly strong evidence about the overall relationship between Medicare's payment rates and providers' Medicare costs for broad sets of services, such as hospital inpatient and outpatient care. They also allow policymakers to track trends in providers' average costs.
- **Changes in the product.** Medicare administrative data and industry surveys also enable policymakers to examine broad trends in the nature of the providers' product. For example, recent declines in hospitals' inpatient

costs per discharge partly reflect substantial declines in lengths of stay. Some part of both trends certainly results from ongoing changes in technology (new drugs and improvements in surgical techniques and anesthesia, for instance), but another part reflects a substantial shift in the site of care. More beneficiaries are using post-acute services in rehabilitation facilities, long-term care hospitals, SNFs, or home health care, and they are being discharged to these settings earlier than in the past. The shift in site of care has helped to reduce hospitals' costs per case, but it has not reduced Medicare's per case payment rates. These trends suggest that Medicare's current base payment amount for hospital inpatient care may be too high (see Chapter 3).

In isolation, none of these indicators provides direct evidence about the appropriateness of Medicare's current base payment amounts in any of its payment systems. Collectively, however, they often provide enough evidence for policymakers to make reasonable judgments for at least some settings, such as hospital inpatient care.

Policy objectives and update methods. Once policymakers have decided whether to change the current base payment, they also must decide what factors should be considered in determining the update for the forthcoming year. This decision is driven by their update policy objectives. The objective of maintaining consistency with providers' costs in the next year is common to all update methods. But policymakers also may want to control total program spending.

Historically, differences in update objectives have led policymakers to determine updates using three approaches. One builds the percentage update by examining historical trends and future projections for factors that are expected to affect providers' costs in the forthcoming year. Although some factors may be quantified with reasonable precision, others require substantial judgment. This approach has been used by MedPAC and HCFA in developing update recommendations for most facility-based services, such as hospital inpatient care, SNF services and home health care (see Chapters 3 and 5).

The second approach takes some of the same kinds of factors into account but also considers whether cumulative changes in program spending are likely to be sustainable in light of projected changes in overall economic conditions. This approach, called the sustainable growth rate (SGR) system was adopted in the BBA to set updates for the conversion factor in the physician fee schedule. HCFA annually makes estimates of the update components specified in the law and applies the resulting update to the conversion factor. Technical judgment is required in making these estimates, but there is little room for policymakers' judgment. In this report, the Commission recommends that the Congress consider adopting a somewhat modified form of this approach to set coordinated updates for all ambulatory care payment systems, including those for physician services, hospital outpatient care, ASC services, and various primary care clinics (see Chapter 6).

In the third approach, the update is based only on the projected growth in spending under the traditional fee-for-service program. This projection is used without considering changes in factors that might appropriately affect providers' costs or the affordability of any changes in program spending that might result. HCFA has used this approach in updating county payment rates for Medicare+Choice organizations (see Chapter 2).

Updates based on factors that affect costs. MedPAC and HCFA both use similar conceptual frameworks to arrive at recommendations for updating base payment amounts and cost limits for various facility services. Both frameworks explicitly consider five factors that are expected to affect efficient providers' costs:

- **Projected inflation in input prices.** Input-price inflation generally raises providers' costs, though probably not to the full extent of the rise in prices. Anticipated input-price inflation is indicated by the forecasted increase in an industry-specific (hospitals, for example) national input-price index called a market basket index. A market basket index tracks national average price levels for labor and other inputs, weighted to reflect the relative importance of each input category in the specific industry.
- **Anticipated scientific and technological advances.** This factor is intended to raise Medicare's payment rates to accommodate the expected effects of new technologies that improve quality of care but also increase costs. The idea is to ensure that the payment rates are high enough to allow providers to adopt significant cost-increasing innovations. The size of this factor is a judgment based on literature review and other surveillance methods designed to identify major innovations as they appear.
- **Expected productivity improvements.** This factor reflects the expectation that, in the aggregate providers should be able to reduce the quantity of inputs required to produce a unit of service while maintaining service quality. Further, the Medicare program should benefit from some portion of this productivity improvement through lower payment rates, just as consumers in private markets do. The size of this downward adjustment is also a judgment. It is often based on analysis of past trends in the specific industry but also considers that the available productivity measures may be inaccurate because they lack adjustments for changes in the quality of care.
- **Site substitution.** This factor is intended to adjust the base payment amount to account for past changes in the product that have altered

providers' costs without corresponding changes in Medicare's payment rates. The site substitution factor is a specific instance of the more general rebasing adjustment discussed earlier. Policymakers would apply this adjustment only if they believed that current Medicare payment rates had strayed too far from providers' costs. An adjustment for site substitution has been applied only in developing a consolidated update for hospital inpatient payments. In principle, the adjustment could either lower or raise the base amount. Substitution of post-acute care for hospital inpatient care, for example, may lead policymakers to conclude that the base amount for hospital inpatient payments should be reduced. The same shift, however, might result in an increase in the average severity of SNF patients, which would require more nursing care per day than in the past. Thus, it might be appropriate to raise the base payment amount for SNF services.

- **Case-mix change.** This factor is intended to adjust Medicare's payment rates to reflect the real net change in resource requirements that results from measured and unmeasured changes in the mix of services or products. When the reported (billed) mix of services or cases shifts, the associated relative values ensure that providers' payments rise or fall appropriately. But changes in providers' coding practices could raise relative values and payments with no change in resource use. Conversely, payments would not increase appropriately if patients' average severity levels rose within each product category. This might happen if improvements in technology were to allow healthier patients to receive their care in other settings. The adjustment for case-mix change is intended to raise or lower the payment rates in the forthcoming year to reflect the net effect of this year's changes in coding and within-category severity levels.

Except for input-price inflation, the factors in this framework cannot be estimated with precision. Consequently, the Commission usually identifies a range of potential adjustments for each of the other four factors. The overall update recommendation that results from the framework, thus, is usually stated as a range of reasonable changes in the base payment amount that would keep Medicare's payment rates consistent with providers' costs in the forthcoming year.

This update framework is applied annually, but because judgments are based on both past trends and future projections, update recommendations generally are closely related from year to year. Nevertheless, this approach does not explicitly consider trends in total program spending for each type of service or whether recent spending trends are consistent with anticipated changes in overall economic activity. Consequently, updates based on this framework are not designed to recoup past discrepancies between desired and actual program spending. Instead, these updates are intended to ensure that the payment rates are at the appropriate level in the future.

The sustainable growth rate system.   Like the cost-based update approach, the SGR begins with the projected increase in providers' input prices as the base for the annual update. It then adds an update adjustment factor that explicitly considers whether cumulative actual Medicare spending for the specified services is above or below the cumulative level that policymakers believe would be sustainable. If cumulative actual spending exceeds the allowed level, the update is reduced to reestablish projected equality during the forthcoming year. Conversely, if cumulative actual spending is less than the allowed level, the update is increased enough to achieve projected equality. Consequently, updates based on this approach are designed to fully offset past discrepancies in program spending in a single year, if possible.[19] The SGR approach is currently applied only in determining annual updates to the conversion factor in the physician fee schedule, but it could be extended to payments for other services.

To use this method, policymakers must decide how to measure anticipated changes in providers' input prices and what factors to consider in estimating the cumulative level of allowed spending. Anticipated increases in physicians' input prices are measured by a projection of the Medicare economic index (MEI), which tracks changes in physician's earnings, staff salaries, and prices for supplies, equipment, and professional liability insurance.

To determine allowed spending growth, policymakers must identify factors that are likely to cause legitimate changes in Medicare fee-for-service spending for physicians' services and are beyond physicians' control. In addition, they must choose a measure of the nation's capacity to afford increases in spending. Currently, annual allowed spending growth is based on four factors:

- **The percentage change in physicians' input prices.** If the mix and volume of physicians' services remain unchanged, allowed program spending should increase enough to accommodate inflation in input prices for the goods and services physicians purchase to produce care. This factor is measured by the MEI.
- **The percentage change in Medicare Part B enrollment.** Allowed spending should reflect changes in the number of beneficiaries eligible to receive Medicare-covered physicians' services under the traditional fee-for-service program.
- **The percentage change in spending that results from changes in law or regulation.** Allowed spending should include the full effects of policy changes enacted in law and implemented in regulations.
- **The percentage change in real gross domestic product (GDP) per capita.** This factor is intended to measure the nation's capacity to afford additional increases in spending that are to some extent within physicians' control. It thus establishes a limit on increases in spending that result from growth in the volume and intensity of services. As long as per capita GDP is growing, however, it allows some increases in spending to

accommodate advances in medical science and technology that enhance medical capabilities.

HCFA combines estimates for these four factors to determine a SGR for each year. Allowed spending is estimated by multiplying actual spending in 1997 by the SGRs for the years between then and the current year. Cumulative allowed spending (the sum of allowed spending from 1997 to the current year) is then compared with estimated cumulative actual spending to determine the update adjustment factor that will be applied for the forthcoming year. Finally, the actual update is calculated as the product of the projected change in the MEl and the update adjustment factor.

This approach to update policy is attractive for two reasons. First, it sets some limits on the growth in program spending. Second, by restraining payment rates for services, it may create financial incentives for providers to consider the marginal benefits and costs of providing additional services.

This policy also poses some potential risks. If the update adjustment factors consistently lead to large increases or decreases in the base payment updates over a period of several years, Medicare's payment rates could diverge significantly from providers' costs. This risk is difficult to evaluate because changes in providers' costs are likely to be driven by a range of factors that are unrelated to Medicare's policies. At the same time, however, the potential for divergence under this policy may not be any greater than it would be under the alternative cost-based update approach. Thus, careful monitoring probably should be given a high priority under either update method.

ENSURING PAYMENT CONSISTENCY ACROSS SETTINGS

In designing a new payment system for specific services or products, policymakers tend to focus their attention narrowly on developing system components that appear to provide the best fit given the nature of the services, patients, and providers in the particular setting. Making these decisions in isolation for each setting, however, may lead to unintended inconsistencies in payment rates across payment systems. These inconsistencies could create inappropriate financial incentives to select one site of care over another in situations where comparable products or services are paid at different rates in two or more settings. Similarly, where either the payment rate or the basis for calculating beneficiary coinsurance differs, beneficiaries could have strong incentives to favor one setting over another.[20]

Policymakers' concerns about the potential for inappropriate site selection have increased substantially in recent years. In the past, most facilities were paid on the basis of incurred costs, which obscured payment differentials across settings for individual services and products. But the adoption of prospective payment systems has been making payment differentials increasingly explicit and visible. In addition, as discussed earlier, physicians, hospitals, other facilities, and health plans now are much more likely to be financially interdependent than they were only a decade ago. These financial interrelationships may have increased the likelihood that payment inconsistencies across settings would sometimes lead to inappropriate shifts in the site of care.

Policymakers should be concerned about this problem for two reasons. First, decisions about the site of care should be driven by the patient's clinical needs rather than opportunities for financial gain. Second, when those clinical needs can be met equally in different settings, however. Medicare should not pay more for a service in one setting simply because the providers' costs historically have been higher.

Other factors being equal, Medicare thus should pay the same price for the same service regardless of the setting in which it is furnished. This principle has some implications for payment systems design in settings where providers produce common sets of services. But it also begs the question of when services that look the same might still be paid appropriately at different rates, such as when a service is delivered to patients with substantial differences in health status.

Ambulatory Care Services

Most ambulatory care services can be provided in a number of settings, such as a physician's office, OPD, or ASC. The Commission's analysis, however, suggests that most types of ambulatory services are provided almost entirely in one setting. In part, this reflects Medicare coverage rules that limit the procedures that may be performed in an ASC. But it also may reflect clinical and economic factors that influence physicians' decisions about the appropriate site of care. Clinical factors may include patient frailty or comorbidities and other risk factors that raise the likelihood that backup services will be needed. Alternatively, many physicians' practices may lack sufficient volume to support ownership of needed equipment or employment of the specialized staff required to perform many imaging or invasive services in the office.

HCFA has not yet implemented its proposed PPS for hospital outpatient services or its revised payment system for ASC services. When these systems are implemented, the payment rates for many services in these settings likely will be higher than the analogous practice expense payments physicians would receive if they performed the same services in the office. These payment differentials might lead to inappropriate shifts in the site of care, away from physicians' offices and toward OPDs and ASCs. The physician's fee schedule payment, however, is largely the same regardless of where a service is provided.[21] Consequently, physicians do not appear to have strong direct financial incentives to shift services among alternative sites of care.

Nevertheless, the potential for inappropriate shifts should not be ignored in designing the OPD and ASC payment systems. Policymakers should build in the capability to compare like services and monitor changes in care settings. This means, at minimum, that like services should be defined in the same way across ambulatory care settings.

Even if services do not shift among ambulatory settings when these payment systems are adopted, it may be appropriate to begin moving toward paying similar rates for the same services across these settings. Moving in this direction raises the question of the circumstances in which services that have the same identifier might appropriately be paid at different rates. One likely possibility is that the same service may have different costs because of differences in patient condition. To explore this possibility, patient characteristics, such as health status differences, should be analyzed for patients who receive the same service within and across these settings. If providers' costs vary in response to differences in patient condition, then specific payment adjustments should be developed to account for such differences. These adjustments should be applied, if possible, at the patient level, rather than the facility level, so that providers are automatically paid appropriately for the mix of patients they actually treat. However, in the absence of the data necessary to identify patients with special needs, a facility-level adjustment may be necessary if such patients are concentrated in certain types of facilities.

Low volume providers in isolated rural communities also may have higher costs for comparable services. If these providers faced the same payment rates that would be appropriate for high volume providers, they might cease providing services, thereby forcing Medicare beneficiaries to travel elsewhere to obtain access to care. This possibility suggests the need to examine cost differences in OPDs and ASCs to see if those located in isolated areas exhibit higher costs. If they do, then it might be appropriate to develop a special payment adjustment, like that for sole community hospitals, which would protect beneficiaries' access to care.

Skilled Nursing Facilities and Rehabilitation Hospitals

The principle of payment consistency raises somewhat different issues in the development of a payment system for rehabilitation facilities. Both rehabilitation hospitals (and rehabilitation units of general hospitals) and some SNFs treat patients who need high intensity rehabilitation therapy. Most of these patients, who must be able to tolerate three hours of intensive therapy per day, are treated in hospital facilities. Some SNFs, however, have developed specialized rehabilitation units to which they admit such patients. Often, these units have been developed because local hospitals do not provide sufficient rehabilitation capacity.

Under the recently implemented SNF prospective payment system, SNFs treating these patients are paid a per diem rate for each day of care. HCFA argues that rehabilitation hospitals also should be paid per diem rates as the first step toward paying the same rate for the same rehabilitation services. Rehabilitation hospitals, however, have been paid under per discharge cost limits for more than 15 years. Moreover, intensive rehabilitation treatment protocols are well defined, and a suitable classification system has been developed for rehabilitation stays.

In choosing the unit of payment for rehabilitation hospitals, policymakers face unattractive trade-offs. The preconditions for payment consistency could be achieved by selecting a per diem unit of payment, matching the SNF payment unit. In a second option, HCFA could adopt the more appropriate per case payment unit. But selecting this option without also changing the recently implemented SNF payment system would sacrifice the potential for payment consistency. In a third option, HCFA could change the recently implemented SNF payment system to adopt the per case payment unit only for intensive rehabilitation patients. HCFA would have to continue using a per diem payment unit for other SNF patients because an effective per stay classification system for all SNF patients does not exist. Elsewhere in this report, the Commission is recommending that HCFA pursue the third option (see Chapter 5).

CONSIDERING IMPLEMENTATION ISSUES

Implementing new payment systems raises two additional issues that policymakers need to consider. One is that applying a new system will frequently cause a substantial redistribution of payments among providers. To avoid potentially serious disruptions in access to care or quality of care, transition mechanisms often must be developed. These mechanisms are designed to cushion the immediate effects of the new system and allow providers time to adjust to the change in their circumstances.

The second issue concerns the administrative systems and other supporting mechanisms that are needed to operate and maintain a new system over time. The earlier discussion of design issues frequently identifies specific tools and information that are needed to establish the various payment system components. It also describes some of the companion rules and procedures necessary to operate a payment system once it is implemented. Finally, the discussion also highlights the crucial role for monitoring payment system performance, especially beneficiary access to care and the quality of care.

Transition Mechanisms

In implementing a new payment system, policymakers must decide whether, and how, to manage the transition from the old payment method to the new one. A transition is more likely to be needed when the potential effects on individual providers' payments may be large, or when policymakers are highly uncertain about providers' responses to the new system. At the same time, program savings anticipated from the new payment system generally would be reduced by any transition method, although the loss of savings may be greater with some methods than it would be with others. Likewise, any improvement in providers' incentives generally would be weakened by any transition method.

Choices among transition methods often involve trade-offs between establishing absolute limits on the percentage change in any provider's payments and the administrative burden for HCFA and providers. Alternative methods also may affect providers' payment incentives in somewhat different ways.

Several transition methods have been used in implementing new payment systems:

- hold-harmless and minimum increase methods, which ensure that each provider's payments under the new system would be at least equal to its base year payments or a specified percentage above those payments,
- corridor limits on the percentage change in payments, which ensure that a provider's payments would neither decrease nor increase by more than the specified percentage each year, and
- a blend approach, which mixes payment amounts under the old system with those under the new one in specified proportions that change each year.

Supporting Administrative Systems

All payment systems require a substantial supporting infrastructure. This administrative infrastructure performs a variety of functions, such as defining covered services, identifying which providers may furnish specific types of services, and ensuring the availability of data needed to establish and maintain the payment rates and related factors.

Coverage policies may play an especially important role in settings where the product is not well defined, consensus about the medical necessity of services is weak, physician oversight or involvement is limited, or there is a large potential for shifts in the site of care. One reason that home care episodes are difficult to define, for example, is that the related coverage policies are vague or ill-defined. Coverage policies limiting the procedures that may be performed in an ASC, however, may have prevented some appropriate as well as inappropriate shifts in services from OPDs to ASCs.

Smoothly functioning data systems are essential because most components of a payment system are data driven. The payment amounts, relative values, and other payment adjustments often can be updated based on analyses of provider cost, claims, and spending data drawn from standard administrative files. But special studies based on other data sources also are needed periodically to provide information about specific payment or update components for some settings or services. For instance, information about staff time use for the relative values in the SNF payment system must be collected in special surveys.

As a tool for achieving Medicare's overall goals, payment policy has limits. Payment policy alone cannot simultaneously ensure that the production and distribution of health care services is efficient and that beneficiaries have appropriate access to high quality care. Other administrative systems are needed to help reach these goals, such as access and quality monitoring systems. Although data and monitoring systems are reasonably well developed for hospital inpatient care, similar systems are much less fully developed for ambulatory and post-acute care services, where they are arguably more essential.

The need for this supporting infrastructure inevitably raises issues about the appropriate level of funding for the many administrative activities carried out by HCFA and its private contractors. In addition, the number and complexity of decisions required to maintain and coordinate many payment systems in a rapidly changing environment suggests that HCFA needs a substantial amount of flexibility to fashion appropriate and timely changes in policy and meet its obligations to beneficiaries and taxpayers. MedPAC endorses the views recently expressed on these topics in an open letter published in the journal *Health Affairs*.

Open Letter to Congress and the Executive

Crisis Facing HCFA and Millions of Americans. The signatories to this statement believe that many of the difficulties that threaten to cripple the Health Care Financing Administration (HCFA) stem from an unwillingness of both Congress and the Clinton administration to provide the agency the resources and administrative flexibility necessary to carry out its mammoth assignment. This is not a partisan issue, because both Democrats and Republicans are culpable for the failure to equip HCFA with the human and financial resources it needs to address what threatens to become a management crisis for the agency and thus for millions of Americans who rely on it. This is also not an endorsement of the present or past administrative activities of the agency. Congress and the administration should insist on an agency that operates efficiently and in the public interest.

Over the past decade Congress has directed the agency to implement, administer, and regulate an increasing number of programs that derive from highly complex legislation. While vast new responsibilities have been added to its heavy workload, some of its most capable administrative talent has departed or retired; other employees have been reassigned as a consequence of reductions in force. At the same time, neither Democratic nor Republican administrations have requested administrative budgets of a size that were in any way commensurate with HCFA's growing challenge.

The latest report of the Medicare trustees points out that HCFA's administrative expenses represented only 1 percent of the outlays of the Hospital Insurance trust fund and less than 2 percent of the Supplementary Medical Insurance trust fund. In part, these low percentages reflect the rapid growth of the denominator—Medicare expenditures. But, even accounting for Medicare's growth, no private health insurer, after subtracting its marketing costs and profit, would ever attempt to manage such large and complex insurance programs with so small an administrative budget. Without prompt attention to these issues, HCFA will fall further behind in its implementation of the many significant reforms mandated by the Balanced Budget Act (BBA) of 1997. In the future the agency also has to cope with a demographic revolution that it is ill equipped to accommodate and with changes in medical technology that will increase fiscal pressures on the programs it administers.

As the Bipartisan Commission on the Future of Medicare grapples with the problem of reshaping the Medicare program for the next millennium, it would do well to consider two important reforms concerning HCFA's administration. First, the commission should recommend that Congress and the Clinton administration endow the agency with an administrative capacity that is similar to that found in the private sector. Second, the commission should consider ways in which the micromanagement of the agency by Congress and the Office of Management and Budget could be reduced. Congress and the public would be better served by measuring the agency's efficiency in terms of its administrative outcomes (such as accuracy and speed of reimbursement of various providers), rather than by tightly controlling its administrative processes. Only if HCFA has more administrative resources and greater management flexibility will it be able to cope with the challenges that lie ahead.

The mismatch between the agency's administrative capacity and its political mandate has grown enormously over the 1990s. As the number of beneficiaries, claims, and participating provider organizations; quality and utilization review; and oversight responsibilities have increased geometrically, HCFA has been downsized. When HCFA was created in 1977, Medicare spending totaled $21.5 billion, the number of beneficiaries served was twenty-six million, and the agency had a staff of about 4,000 full-time-equivalent workers. By 1997 Medicare spending had increased almost tenfold to $207 billion, the number of beneficiaries served had grown to thirty-nine million, but the agency's workforce was actually smaller than it had been two decades earlier. The sheer technical complexity of its new policy directives is mind-boggling and requires a new generation of employees with the requisite skills.

HCFA's ability to provide assistance to beneficiaries, monitor the quality of provider services, and protect against fraud and abuse has been increasingly compromised by the failure to provide the agency with adequate administrative resources. Even with the addition of $154 million to its administrative budget that Congress included in its latest budget bill, the likelihood that HCFA can effectively implement all of its varied assignments is remote. The Health Insurance Portability and Accountability Act of 1996 assigns many new regulatory responsibilities to HCFA, but a far larger task is implementing the BBA of 1997. The BBA has more than 300 provisions affecting HCFA programs, including the Medicare+Choice option, which will require complex institutional changes and ambitious efforts to educate beneficiaries.

Medicare spending accounts for more than 11 percent of the U.S. budget. Workable, effective administration has to be a primary consideration in any restructuring proposal. Whether Medicare reform centers on improving the current system, designing a system that relies on market forces to promote efficiency through competition, or moving toward an even more individualized approach to paying for health insurance, Congress and the administration must reexamine the organization, funding, management, and oversight of the Medicare program. Doing anything less is short-changing the public and leaving HCFA in a state of disrepair.

Stuart M. Butler, Heritage Foundation
Patricia M. Danzon, University of Pennsylvania
Bill Gradison, Health Insurance Association of America
Robert Helms, American Enterprise Institute
Marilyn Moon, Urban Institute
Joseph P. Newhouse, Harvard University
Mark V. Pauly, University of Pennsylvania
Martha Phillips, Concord Coalition
Uwe E. Reinhardt, Princeton University
Robert D. Reischauer, Brookings Institution
William L. Roper, University of North Carolina at Chapel Hill
John Rother, AARP
Leonard D. Schaeffer, WellPoint Health Networks. Inc.
Gail R. Wilensky, Project HOPE

Source: *Health Affairs* January/February 1999, Vol. 18 No 1, p. 8–10.
Note: Reprinted with permission.

CONCLUSIONS

The primary goal of Medicare's payment policies should be to help beneficiaries obtain medically necessary acute care of reasonable quality in the most appropriate clinical setting. At some level, this goal is the ultimate touchstone for all program policies. It is especially important for payment policies, however, because of their power to affect providers' willingness and ability to furnish good care. Therefore, when policymakers are designing or evaluating a payment system, they should repeatedly ask how it will work for all beneficiaries and especially for those who are vulnerable because of their circumstances.

To avoid serious problems for beneficiaries or taxpayers and promote efficient production and distribution of acute care services, Medicare's payment rates must be consistent with providers' costs. But Medicare buys a wide range of health care products furnished in a variety of settings by different types of providers who must compete for scarce resources in local private markets. Consequently, Medicare's payment systems must appropriately account for:

- the types of products Medicare is buying,
- the clinical and economic factors, including differences among patients, that account for legitimate variation in costs among products, types of providers or settings for care, and local markets, and
- the factors that are likely to cause appropriate changes in costs over time.

Successfully setting and maintaining payment rates consistent with providers' costs in many provider-specific payment systems thus raises a host of practical and policy questions that must be answered to make decisions about units of payment, product definitions and relative values, and other payment system components.

What Is Medicare Buying in a Particular Setting?

- What are the clinical components of the care provided?
- What are the clinical factors that distinguish among types of services, patients, or beneficiaries?
- What services are included in each type of product?

What Factors Account for Predictable Variation in the Cost of Producing these Products?

- What does the provider's production process look like?
- What are the components of costs?
- What factors account for predictable cost variation among types of services, patients, or beneficiaries?
- What factors account for regional or local cost variation?
- What special circumstances should be taken into account to protect access to care?

How Should We Determine the Level of Payment?

- Providers' historical costs?
- Anticipated program spending?

How Would We Know if Payment Rates Were Too High or Too Low?

- Provider entry or exit?
- Rapid changes in volume?
- Widespread access or quality problems?
- Providers' financial condition?

What Factors Should Be Considered in Adjusting the Payment Rates Over Time?

- Anticipated changes in factors that affect providers' unit costs?
- Growth in program spending compared with that of the overall economy?

Are Similar Services or Products Available in Another Setting?

- What is the extent of the overlap?
- Who chooses the site of care and what incentives do they face?

Under What Circumstances Should Medicare Pay More for a Service in One Setting Than in Another?

- Differences in patient condition?
- Unusual market conditions?

Empirical analysis can illuminate many of these questions, depending on available data. All of the policy questions, however, inevitably involve making trade-offs between potentially desirable and undesirable outcomes. Moreover, balancing these trade-offs is often complicated by two factors. One is uncertainty about the extent of providers' opportunity and inclination to respond to payment incentives in undesirable ways. The other is the lack of tools and information needed to develop payment adjustments that would focus payment more appropriately on the patient and the service rather than the provider or setting in which it is furnished.

Nevertheless, trade-offs must be evaluated and design choices must be made in the short term. In this regard, the Commission's policy framework may prove especially useful in explicitly highlighting the gains and sacrifices associated with specific choices as well as alternatives that should be pursued in the future.

REFERENCES

Pauly MV. *Doctors and Their Workshops: Economic Models of Physician Behavior.* Chicago, The University of Chicago Press. 1980.

Prospective Payment Assessment Commission. Report to the Congress: Medicare and the American Health Care System. Washington (DC), ProPAC. June 1997.

NOTES

1.   Under prospective payment, a provider's payment is based on predetermined rates and is unaffected by its incurred costs or posted charges. Examples of prospective payment systems include the one Medicare uses to pay hospitals for inpatient care and the physician fee schedule.

2.   Payments also could be based on negotiated rates or on amounts set by competitive bidding. This chapter focuses on prospective payment systems because Medicare is required by law to use that approach for most services.

3.   Medicare also provides limited coverage of long-term care furnished in a skilled nursing facility or through home health visits; it does not cover custodial care.

4.   Some local markets—for example, those that have only one hospital or one specialist physician—may not be competitive now or in the future. In these and some

other situations, providers' long-run average costs may be higher than their long-run marginal costs. Because technology changes and capital assets deteriorate, however, Medicare's payment rates ultimately must cover providers' long-run average costs. Thus, in some instances, Medicare may have to set payment rates that are higher than the prices that might have prevailed in a hypothetical competitive market.

5.   To act on this incentive, providers would have to be able to identify patient characteristics that predictably lead to relatively high or low marginal costs

6.   The unit of payment may be changed intentionally to alter the mindset of providers. In the early 1980s, HCFA replaced per diem limits on hospitals' allowable costs for routine inpatient care (room, board, and nursing care) with per case payments, partly to stimulate changes in hospitals' and physicians' thinking about the production of inpatient care.

7.   Medicare generally does not pay for physicians' services based on episodes of care because it lacks an effective episode-based classification system. One exception is surgical episodes in which pre- and post-operative office visits are bundled together with the surgical procedure and paid under a global surgical fee. Another is end-stage renal disease; Medicare pays for physician management of dialysis services on a monthly capitation basis.

8.   The likelihood that providers would take undesirable actions also may be affected by other factors, such as related potential costs (loss of reputation, for example), how well the product is defined, and the degree of consensus about its medical necessity. Personal and professional ethics and values also play a significant role.

9.   The potential for unintended volume growth has been a major concern in the physician fee schedule and in other ambulatory care settings where the payment unit is the individual service.

10.   Such early discharges are considered transfers, and the hospital is paid based on a per diem rate up to a maximum of the full per discharge payment rate for the DRG.

11.   Relative values also may be thought of as measuring the relative worth of each product or service compared with that of all services in the particular setting. Conceptual distinctions between cost, worth, and value, however, generally have little practical significance.

12.   Other factors differ between the operating payment rates and those for capital—geographic input-price adjustments for example—but the DRG relative values are the same. Although it is highly likely that the distribution of capital costs among DRGs differs from that for operating costs, it would be difficult to measure accurately capital costs by DRG. Moreover, policymakers anticipated that the capital and operating payment rates eventually would be combined in a single rate for each DRG. Consequently, they chose to use the same relative values for both components.

13.   Anesthesia services are priced separately using a single set of relative values based on the sum of a fixed component and a time-based component, which varies by procedure.

14.   Later analysis showed that adjusted costs per case were highly correlated with adjusted charges among DRGs. Consequently, DRG relative values have been based on billed charges for more than a decade.

15.   A cost of living adjustment is applied to adjust the nonlabor component for hospitals in Alaska and Hawaii.

16.   This variation may have developed in response to differences among market areas in the supply of specific resources or as a result of historical factors, such as state policies, that influenced the organization of care. Long-term care hospitals and ASCs, for example, tend to be highly concentrated in certain regions.

17.   The Prospective Payment Assessment Commission (ProPAC) estimated that adjusting the county payment rates for variation in input prices would reduce the range by roughly one-half. The remaining variation comprises some combination of unmeasured differences in average risk (expected costliness) for the beneficiaries in each county and differences in the mix and quantities of services used (practice variation). If the former represents roughly 10 to 20 percent of the total variation, the latter must account for 30 to 40 percent.

18.   Issues regarding beneficiaries' access to care and the quality of care will be addressed in the Commissions June report to the Congress.

19.   To prevent excessive annual volatility in the payment rates, the update adjustment factor for any year may not be greater than three percentage points or less than minus seven percentage points.

20.   Note that this problem differs from the unbundling problem discussed earlier. Even if payment rates for similar services were the same across settings, providers facing a large payment unit would still have incentives to shift some component services to other sites and thereby reduce their costs.

21.   The practice expense component is reduced for certain services when they are performed in a hospital or on ASC.

9 | **The Dilemmas of
Incrementalism:
Logical and
Political
Constraints in the
Design of Health
Insurance Reforms**

Thomas R. Oliver

INTRODUCTION

In the first half of the 1990s, concerns about the nation's health care system moved into the mainstream of political consciousness and debate. The early movement occurred in the states, where recognition of urgent problems generated widespread study and a variety of legislative responses. Then came the battle royal in Washington. In the wake of the 1992 election that, to many, promised to end a deadlock on domestic policies, President Bill Clinton sought to erase a century of failure by giving Americans "health care that can never be taken away."

That attempt to establish universal health insurance coverage suffered the same fate as several earlier attempts, as defenders of the current patchwork system of public and private insurance emerged victorious [e.g., Starr, 1982; Rothman, 1993]. The president retreated in the fall of 1994, lost Democratic

Reprinted with permission from *Journal of Policy Analysis and Management,* 18, no. 4 (Fall 1999): 652–83.

The study was supported in part by an Investigator Award in Health Policy Research from the Robert Wood Johnson Foundation.

majorities in both houses of Congress, and thereafter pursued a strategy of supporting incremental, bipartisan reforms championed by legislators instead of the administration.

The ambivalence of public opinion, strategic errors, opposition tactics, and the sheer scale of the proposed reforms undermined the considerable effort and commitment of the president and his allies [Skocpol 1996; Johnson and Broder, 1996]. Other observers noted that whatever the merits or flaws of the Clinton proposals, the most formidable barriers to action have little to do with health care per se, but rather are endemic features of American political institutions [Steinmo and Watts 1995]. Hugh Heclo [1995] endorsed this analysis, concluding:

> Social policy reformers must struggle in an institutional system that tilts the survival odds in favor of incremental action or inaction and against big new expressions of public authority. More recent developments in our informal, unwritten constitution—declining attachments to political parties, reforms in Congress, proliferating interest groups, widening access to policy litigation in the courts, and so on—have only added to the formal constitutional fragmentation of power. The result, spread across the historical record, is that major social reform efforts rarely succeed. It is the weasely, piecemeal adjustments to social policy that make up the bulk of successful reform efforts (p. 87).

In the wake of the Clinton plan's demise, the conventional wisdom has been that a variety of piecemeal adjustments are not only politically feasible but also reasonably effective ways to improve how substantial segments of the American population are served by the health care system.

This article focuses on one class of reforms, those that aim to make private health insurance more accessible and more affordable, especially to individuals and workers in small firms. The policy changes considered here are at best incremental, since they do very little to expand insurance coverage for more than 40 million uninsured Americans and do not reach far enough to provoke systemwide cost containment [McLaughlin and Zellers, 1992; Cantor, Long, and Marquis, 1995].[1]

Nonetheless, insurance reforms that only marginally impact the system could significantly affect the income and security of many individuals. A built-in feature of our patchwork insurance system is a "revolving door" through which a substantial proportion of the population regularly changes coverage because individuals switch or lose jobs, enter adulthood, have a child, leave a marriage, or suffer an illness. In 1993, more than 51 million Americans had no health insurance at some time during the year [Rowland et al., 1994]. It follows that individuals (and their families or firms) who pose a financial risk to an insurer because of an existing or new medical condition may find it difficult to return through the revolving door and obtain coverage—because they either face large premium increases or are denied any coverage at all.

Insurance regulations such as guaranteed access and renewal, community rating, and limits on pre-existing condition clauses could serve as small but important steps, therefore, toward a health insurance system based on social solidarity rather than actuarial risk. If, as Deborah Stone [1993] argues, the basic question for our society is whether medical care will be distributed as a right of citizenship or as a market commodity, these reforms represent attempts to reverse the trend toward commodification of health insurance. In an important way, they promote a vision of distributive justice and community different from the vision intrinsic to the unregulated marketplace.

Insurance reforms may also promote efficiency in the administration of insurance and delivery of health services. Some provisions aim to reduce competition among insurers based on avoiding sick or potentially sick patients, and to increase competition based on efficiently delivering needed services to patients regardless of their health status and actuarial risk. Other provisions, such as purchasing cooperatives, offer greater economies of scale to employers and insurers in the small-group market. In addition, they might enhance the information, choices, and bargaining power of consumers vis-à-vis insurers in the marketplace [Enthoven and Singer, 1995; Ellwood and Enthoven, 1995].

The supposed capstone reform in this area is the Health Insurance Portability and Accountability Act of 1996 (HIPAA). Brian Atchinson and Daniel Fox [1997, p. 146] suggested that HIPAA "could be the most significant federal health care reform in a generation . . . affecting all working Americans and their employers, three federal agencies, and the governments of all fifty states." The legislation set standards for access to insurance, as well as portability and renewability of coverage for both groups and individuals.

A recent study casts doubt on the effectiveness of this class of reforms, however. A year and a half after enactment of HIPAA, the U.S. General Accounting Office (GAO) reported that "many consumers who had lost group coverage experienced difficulty obtaining individual market coverage . . . or paid significantly higher rates for such coverage. Some carriers have discouraged individuals from applying for the coverage or charged them rates 140 to 600 percent of the standard premium" [U.S. Congress, 1998, p. 2]. In some states, insurance carriers advised agents against referring HIPAA-eligible applicants, or they reduced or eliminated commissions for agents who sold those policies. James Jeffords (R-VT), chairman of the Senate Labor and Human Resources Committee, summarized the main issue in an oversight hearing: "Health insurance policies that are clearly intended to be unaffordable violate the spirit of the law and will prevent many individuals from taking advantage of HIPAA's expanded access provisions. From the report, it is clear that some insurance companies are using marketing practices to avoid enrolling those who need health care the most" [Jeffords, 1998]. The *Washington Post* [1998] echoed that criticism:

The president said when he signed the bill two years ago that it "seals the cracks that swallow as many as 25 million Americans who can't get insurance or fear they'll lose it. Now they're going to be protected." Just about everyone at the signing ceremony understood the bill would do much less than that even if enforced. . . . If they're going to pass incremental legislation, at least let the increments be real. (p. A22)

One response of the health insurance industry to the criticism was to defend its members' actions, noting that insurers warned policymakers that HIPAA requirements could result in "unacceptable premium increases." The principal response of the industry, however, was that insurers need more time to implement the new regulations; and that federal agencies need more resources to meet the current "regulatory overload" created by HIPAA and subsequent provisions for children's health insurance, Medicare, and Medicaid in the Balanced Budget Act of 1997 [Gradison, 1998].

The industry's behavior and arguments would be more credible if HIPAA were broaching an entirely new area of public policy. In fact, reforms in this area have been under way since the beginning of the decade. While national policymakers contemplated insurance market reforms beginning in the Bush administration [Advisory Council, 1991], the states instituted many changes on their own. Indeed, HIPAA is only a modest addition to reforms adopted by a vast majority of states in the early 1990s. *Thus, it is likely that the problems documented by the GAO are not short-term problems with policy implementation, but rather long-term problems with policy design.*

The purpose of this article is to describe and analyze the design of insurance market reforms adopted by states and the federal government in the past several years. It is based on the proposition that policy design is substantially a political, not technical, process [e.g., Stone, 1988; Palumbo and Calista, 1990; Bosso, 1994]. Judith Feder and Larry Levitt [1995] asserted that even though insurance reforms were regarded as the "motherhood and apple pie" issues of health care reform, the perception that everyone agreed on what to do reflected limited debate (at the national level) instead of genuine consensus. Some of the specific provisions turned out to be highly controversial, with substantial disagreements on what insurance practices to regulate and what populations they should apply to. In addition, there was little empirical evidence with which to estimate the effects of incremental insurance reforms—the same problem confronting the major reform proposals offered in the Clinton plan [Thorpe, 1995].

The article begins by setting forth the ideas for reforming the private health insurance system—the assumptions about current problems in the system and specific alternatives to improve its performance. This analysis demonstrates that even though increasing access is a worthy and widely supported goal, it is difficult to accomplish in a system where insurance coverage is largely voluntary and the purchase of insurance (and sharing of risk) is so fragmented.

The reality is that mending one part of the system simply means another part becomes relatively weakened and threatens to unravel—greater access for some can easily create less access for others. To account for all of the potential problems requires a set of new institutions and rules that, while far short of those envisioned in the Clinton plan, are still broad in scope and largely untested at either the state or federal level. Ultimately, there are difficult tradeoffs for every element of a small-group insurance reform package, and uncertainty prevents experts from agreeing upon a package of policy recommendations.[2]

The article then examines several key provisions adopted in state reforms between 1990–1995 and in the federal legislation in 1996. It demonstrates that, despite political consensus that pushed this issue to the top of the governmental agenda, there was little policy consensus, and relatively few design features were universally accepted. There is substantial variation in the policies adopted across the states, and HIPAA ended up requiring a minimal degree of regulation rather than a broad reform of insurance practices.

Finally, the article discusses the implications of this pattern of state and federal action for policy performance. It concludes that few of the reforms present a serious challenge to existing practices and interests of the insurance industry. The reforms represent some progress on nominal access to insurance but little progress on the affordability of insurance for individuals and small groups. Even amid a historic political opportunity where incremental insurance reforms were viewed as barely minimum achievements, the policy choices made in Washington and most states were more a product of "muddling through" [Lindblom, 1959] than progressive steps toward a stronger system of social insurance.

ASSUMPTIONS, CHOICES, AND TRADE-OFFS IN THE DESIGN OF HEALTH INSURANCE MARKET REFORMS

Why and how should government regulate private health insurance—what are the main options for intervention? This section outlines the key arguments made by expert analysts to justify reforms in the health insurance system and the options and tradeoffs that must be considered in their design.

The reforms examined below are primarily aimed at what is referred to as the small-group health insurance market. This typically includes business firms or associations covering 2 to 50 persons, although some reforms apply to individuals and other reforms extend to groups of up to 100. These actions reflect the fact that the greatest barriers to insurance coverage originate in that market. It surprises many casual observers of the health care reform debate to learn that over three-quarters of Americans without insurance are gainfully employed or are dependents of employees. Two-thirds of these "working uninsured" are associated with firms with 100 or fewer employees, and one-half are in firms with 25 or fewer employees [Thorpe, 1992a; Helms, Gauthier, and Campion, 1992].

The prevalence of small-group market reforms also reflects the fact that states have been barred by the federal Employment Retirement Income Security Act (ERISA) of 1974 from regulating the health plans of employers who elect to self-insure. Nationally, ERISA exempts between one-third and one-half of the private insurance market from state regulation, making effective marketwide reform at the state level difficult, if not impossible [U.S. Congress, 1991, 1992; Helms, Gauthier, and Campion, 1992]. So states have chosen a path of less resistance, regulating a part of the health care system that is clearly within their jurisdiction.

HIPAA is potentially important because it represents the first time the federal government has enacted direct regulation of private health insurance. It supplements state regulation because it covers individual subscribers as well as groups, and it supercedes ERISA and applies to all health plans, whether the sponsor is self-insured or not.

The broad goals of these reforms are: (1) to create greater access to health insurance for higher risk groups; (2) to restrict the ability of insurers to compete based on subscriber risks; (3) to restructure the marketplace to encourage price and quality competition among insurers; and (4) to reduce the administrative costs of providing health insurance to these populations.

Policymakers have attempted to achieve these goals by regulating insurance underwriting and marketing practices, by controlling variation in premiums, and by establishing or enabling the formation of health plan purchasing cooperatives (also referred to as purchasing pools or alliances). The following section describes the main elements of small-group insurance reforms and some of the choices facing policymakers. Table 9.1 summarizes the key policy goals, available instruments, and trade-offs involved in policy design.

ENHANCING ACCESS TO HEALTH INSURANCE

Under traditional regulations, an insurer may decline to offer coverage to groups or individuals that it deems too risky. For example, it is not unusual for insurers to "redline" certain employers such as construction firms or ski resorts [Glazner et al., 1995, p. 225]. Similarly, if an insurer has an unprofitable experience with a group, it may refuse to renew that group's coverage.

Guaranteed Issue and Renewal of Health Plans

A mandate requiring insurers to guarantee the issue and renewal of health insurance policies improves access for these higher-risk populations. At the same time, it is likely to increase the costs for insurers if these populations do in fact use more medical services. Consequently, insurers faced with such

TABLE 9.1

Policy Goals, Instruments, and Key Trade-offs

Policy Goals and Instruments	Intended Policy Results	Policy Trade-offs
Improved access		
Guaranteed renewal	Prevents insurers from cancelling insurance due to poor health or high medical expenses.	Higher premiums as poorer risks are retained in group's risk pool. Increased difficulty in obtaining initial insurance coverage.
Guaranteed issue	Guarantees that health insurance is available regardless of health status or past medical expenses.	Higher premiums as poorer risks are retained in group's risk pool. Higher premiums may drive the "better" health risks from insurance market.
Limits on preexisting condition exclusion clauses	Enhances portability of insurance, since coverage of a condition cannot be denied if previously insured and reduces waiting period for coverage if previously uninsured.	Creates a disincentive to purchase health insurance before it is needed.
Social solidarity in rating & underwriting		
Limits on variation in premium	Narrows the variation in premium between and within groups due to real or perceived health risks (reducing premiums for poorer risks) and broadens the pool across which such risk is spread.	Higher premiums for better risks, perhaps driving them from the insurance market. Potentially reduces incentives for healthier lifestyles.

continued

TABLE 9.1 *continued*

Policy Goals and Instruments	Intended Policy Results	Policy Trade-offs
Limits on use of group characteristics in rating and underwriting	Reduces the ability of insurers to use selected groups' characteristics as a basis for issuing and pricing insurance.	Higher premiums for better risks, perhaps driving them from the insurance market.
Community and modified community rating	Broadens the pool across which risk is spread and restricts characteristics for rating purposes. Improves access and reduces cost for the highest risk groups.	Higher premiums for better risks, perhaps driving them from the insurance market.
Fair and efficient market competition		
Standardized benefit plans	Increased competition from product comparison on cost. Expected to create downward pressure on premiums.	No ability to design plans to meet specific needs of group. Potential for adverse selection when not mandated for entire market.
Fair marketing rules	Eliminates the most egregious strategies for risk selection and discloses insurer rating practices.	Inserts government into operation of market.
Limits on premium increases	Maintains affordability and increases retention of insurance coverage.	Impedes the free operation of market forces.
Health plan purchasing cooperative (HPPC)	Can reduce administrative and commission costs, especially for smallest groups.	Potential for adverse selection when market rules are not uniform inside and outside the HPPC.

a mandate can be expected to increase their premiums. In addition, where insurance coverage is voluntary, guaranteed issue may encourage individuals and groups not to purchase insurance until it is actually needed. This form of adverse selection may reduce the overall rate of insurance coverage in the market and raise the average premiums for those who do purchase coverage [Hall, 1992, p. 120].[3]

Where insurers are mandated to guarantee the issue and renewal of government-certified "standard" plans but not all plans, there is also a risk of adverse selection because those plans are likely to attract groups that would otherwise be denied coverage. This creates an incentive for insurers to avoid offering the standard plans unless they are required to do so—and even then they can limit marketing efforts for those plans.

Provisions for guaranteed issue and renewal help ensure access to health insurance, but they clearly create concerns about adverse selection and cost containment that must be addressed through other elements of reform proposals.

Preexisting Condition Causes

Under a preexisting condition clause, an employee's medical condition that manifested itself prior to the effective date of the policy will not be covered by the insurer for a specified period of time. This saves the insurer from paying for treatment that individuals have postponed and sought only after obtaining insurance coverage. But such clauses are particularly onerous for millions of individuals for whom a change in employment means a change in insurance. Reforms to limit preexisting condition clauses help increase the "portability" of insurance and reduce "job lock," so individuals can accept a preferred job or start a new business without jeopardizing insurance coverage for themselves or family members with a chronic health condition.

In the absence of universal, compulsory health insurance, preexisting condition clauses discourage currently healthy individuals from going uninsured and reduce the amount of adverse selection that might otherwise occur [Enthoven and Singer, 1995, p. 117]. Establishing rules for such clauses requires policymakers to balance the need for access and fairness to individuals with chronic conditions against the costs of adverse selection and free-riding.[4] A logical way to maintain incentives to carry insurance coverage and also enhance fairness is to prohibit insurers from applying preexisting clauses to individuals who are merely switching from one source of insurance coverage to another.

Community Rating of Insurance Premiums

Most insurers use rating categories based on such factors as age, gender, geographic location, business or industry, occupation, claims experience, and health status to predict risk and set premiums in the small-group market. The resulting variation in premiums—if these factors accurately predict beneficiaries' use of services and expenses—conforms to the principle of actuarial fairness under which individuals with the highest health risks pay the highest premiums. This is consistent with industry practices in life, auto, and property insurance [Stone, 1993].

There are several objections to these practices in health insurance, however. First, the actuarial methods used by insurers to predict risk are often not particularly accurate. Prospective medical screening, for example, does not do a good job of predicting use of services in the small-group market [Glazner et al., 1995].[5] Even experience-rating techniques are able to predict only about 10 percent of the observed variation in the individual use of services [Aaron and Bosworth, 1994]. Second, many methods of risk classification reflect cultural biases rather than firmly established financial experience [Stone, 1993]. Thus, certain kinds of groups—for example, those having members with chronic illness or disability—may be charged higher premiums than their actual use of services warrants.[6] Third, since a perfectly fair market requires *individual* premiums, no classification scheme results in actuarially fair premiums as long as insurance is provided through employers or other social groups. Within an arbitrary group (the firm), there will always be individuals with substantially higher risks than others, yet all members pay the same rate for coverage. In small firms, an illness that strikes one or more employees may cause a large increase in premiums for their colleagues. So workers with identical risks in two different firms may pay substantially different insurance premiums—a violation of the principle of horizontal equity in social policy.[7]

In an actuarial sense, horizontal equity is possible only if companies abandon health plans altogether and force their employees to obtain insurance in the individual market. What the current insurance system really does is substitute certain bases of social solidarity and cross-subsidy (membership in a company and other risk categories) for other bases of social solidarity used in the past or in other places (membership in a community or nation).

The rationale for limiting variation in insurance premiums extends well beyond these criticisms. The key argument is that medical care is not a commodity but an object of mutual aid. It should be distributed, therefore, on the basis of one's medical need, not one's ability to pay. Indeed, the onset of sickness and disability often means that those in greatest need are least able to pay for medical services. So the main issue for policymakers to resolve is defining what conditions are deserving of mutual aid—and implicitly, what cross-subsidies are acceptable to members of society.[8]

Under pure community rating, everyone in a specified geographic area would pay the same premium for health insurance, regardless of their current age, employment, or health status. This policy would result in lower-risk individuals subsidizing the cost of health insurance for higher-risk individuals. Even if this is politically feasible, there are potential trade-offs to consider.

One concern is that community rating will cause further erosion of insurance coverage and undermine the goals of greater risk pooling and mutual aid. Where insurance coverage is not compulsory, community rating will increase premiums for lower-risk groups and cause them to seek self-insurance or withdraw from the insurance market entirely [Hall, 1992, p. 120; Stone, 1993, p. 292; Enthoven and Singer, 1995, p. 106]. New York's adoption of community rating in 1993 is alleged to have produced this undesirable side effect, at least in the short term, as the overall insured population dropped by an estimated 25,000 during the first year following the reforms [Alpha Center, 1994].

Another concern is that pure community rating might reduce price competition in the market by eliminating the opportunity for employers to negotiate lower premiums and for insured individuals to benefit from health-promoting behaviors [Aaron and Bosworth, 1994, p. 270; Enthoven and Singer, 1995, p. 108]. The latter argument assumes that current rating practices are accurate risk predictors and that individuals are substantially rewarded or penalized for their health-related behaviors under the current system. Aaron and Bosworth [1994, p. 271] argue that neither of these assumptions is true, so the potential effect of rating regulations on individual incentives should be a minor concern.

These concerns may lead policymakers to reject pure community rating and instead accept "rate bands," which allow a range of premiums for a given health plan based on a limited set of rating categories. Under a rate band, premiums offered to groups or individuals are permitted to vary by a certain percentage compared to the average premium in that class of subscribers.

ENHANCING MARKET COMPETITION AND EFFICIENCY

Most of the insurance reforms discussed above attempt to modify market practices to increase social equity and reduce the economic penalties for becoming sick. In contrast, other reforms attempt to improve the efficiency of the health care system by strengthening the market tendency to force those who use more health services to pay higher costs. Here, the assumption is not that the market works too well, but that it does not work well enough.

Employee Choice of Health Plans

Part of the reason for high costs in the small-group insurance market is that price competition among health plans is often quite limited. Some analysts, therefore, advocate increasing price elasticity by requiring employers to offer a number of competing health plans and allowing individual employees to choose their individual plan. In addition, employees must pay some of the cost of a health plan as an incentive to limit their demand for services [Enthoven and Singer, 1995, p. 111]. These provisions, it is argued, will lead to more prudent purchasing of insurance and result in plans better tailored to what consumers really need.

If policymakers decide to expand the choice of health plans, they must also decide whether and how to limit the number of choices. The main concern is that choices must be numerous enough and diverse enough to satisfy consumers, but not so large as to make a meaningful comparison of plans impossible.

Standard Benefit Plans

One way to enhance consumer choice of health plans is to make side-by-side comparisons easier. This can be done by requiring or encouraging insurers to offer one or more plans with standard benefits. In theory, simplifying and standardizing contractual benefits forces insurers to compete on overall price and quality instead of using selective benefits to lure the best risks. Without this kind of market regulation, health plans can be designed to attract or discourage certain kinds of subscribers. The range of physician choice, the level of cost-sharing, and particular benefits affect the potential number and actuarial risk of subscribers. Any attempt to reduce risk-based competition, therefore, requires some controls over plan design and benefit packages [Chollet and Paul, 1994; Enthoven and Singer, 1995].

Authorizing standard benefit plans is a way to broaden access as well as equalize competition among insurers. A fairly broad benefit package can help guarantee the availability of services that consumers might have difficulty obtaining in an unregulated market (e.g., AIDS therapy, mental health, physical rehabilitation).

An obvious problem for policymakers is that creating a standard benefit package becomes a political and ethical exercise as provider and patient advocates lobby for particular services. Clearly, any package will exclude benefits that would be of considerable value to some individuals. In addition, it creates an economic dilemma in that each added benefit can make the package less affordable to the small businesses and individuals that policymakers are trying to extend insurance to in the first place [Thorpe, 1992a].

The choice to adopt standard benefit plans is also complicated by the need to decide whether insurers will be allowed to offer nonstandard plans. If there are parallel systems, then adverse selection may follow as the standard plans become "dumping grounds" for the bad risks. This could cause access to the guaranteed benefit package to decline as the premiums become less affordable and as insurers restrict marketing efforts for the unprofitable standard plans.

Information on the Quality of Health Plans

Making consumers more cost-conscious in their choice of health plans requires better information about the quality of services as well as premiums. The concept of "accountable health partnerships" advanced by the Jackson Hole Group suggests that market competition can be facilitated by indicators of patient satisfaction, clinical status, function, well-being, and other aspects of quality [Ellwood, Enthoven, and Etheredge, 1992].

While this kind of information is being developed in both public and private settings, the state of the art in clinical information systems and outcomes management is far away from providing uniform and valid measures of quality for insurers, providers, and purchasers of health plans [Alpha Center, 1994, p. 12; Jewett and Hibbard, 1996]. Thus, policymakers interested in fostering a more efficient insurance market need to recognize that quality standards and data are a critical public good, and must work with all stakeholders to create an information infrastructure that will encourage greater health plan performance and consumer satisfaction.

Risk Adjustment Mechanisms

The stakes for insurers in accurately predicting or avoiding high-risk individuals are sizable, as about 5 percent of the population accounts for half of all annual health care spending, and 10 percent of the population accounts for 70 percent of expenditures.[9] Even if risk-based competition were totally eliminated, however, high-risk individuals are unlikely to be evenly distributed among insurers. The chance of drawing a significant number of high-risk subscribers causes all insurers to raise their costs to protect against such an eventuality. It is also likely that reforms would not eliminate all ability to engage in risk selection strategies, in which case some insurers would be favorably advantaged in comparison to others.

One solution is to adopt a risk adjustment mechanism to transfer revenues from health plans with below-average risks to plans with above-average risks. Such a policy would act as a disincentive to risk-based competition by eliminating the fruits of such a strategy, and prevent some insurers being forced out of the market because they have ended up, by chance, serving a riskier population [Enthoven and Singer, 1995, pp. 108, 112]. A risk adjustment mechanism is also desirable to encourage health plans to develop specialty services for populations with demonstrably higher risks and costs. It is an important step, therefore, toward competition that rewards overall quality and efficiency instead of the lowest, unadjusted price.

The challenge, however, is that an accepted method of risk adjustment is another missing link on the path to fair market competition [Newhouse, 1994; Shewry et al., 1996]. To work properly, a method must be constructed to adjust only for differences in risk as nearly as possible. It must not become a means to subsidize inefficient health plans and thereby reduce incentives to improve the value of services for a given premium.

Health Plan Purchasing Cooperatives

A relatively new way to reshape the small-group insurance market is to create health plan purchasing cooperatives.[10] Allowing small employers (and possibly individuals) to purchase insurance through a public or private cooperative reduces an insurer's risk for any given employer by increasing the size of the risk pool. In addition, purchasing cooperatives reduce the high administrative expenses that insurers incur in the small-group market for marketing, enrollment, collection of premiums, claims administration, and so forth.[11]

These reductions in risk and administrative overhead should permit insurers to offer lower and more uniform premiums through a purchasing cooperative than if they deal with individual employers [Thorpe, 1992b; Wicks, Curtis, and Haugh, 1993; Enthoven and Singer, 1995; Cantor, Long, and Marquis, 1995]. The pooling of risk reduces the need for medical screening, making more firms and individual employees eligible for coverage. The lower premiums should also expand access to insurance.

There are a number of key choices in the design of purchasing cooperatives. The first choice is sponsorship. Since most if not all the functions of a purchasing cooperative can be performed by either a public or private entity, a judgment must be made as to which offers the proper mix of flexibility and accountability. This choice is partly a matter of ideology as well: Alain Enthoven and Sara Singer [1995, p. 106] promote private cooperatives based on a rhetorical assertion that public agencies are "often associated with waste, complexity rigidity, and coercion."

The second choice is whether to authorize a single purchasing cooperative in a state, a network of regional cooperatives, or multiple cooperatives in any jurisdiction. This choice depends on whether competing cooperatives will have sufficient size to effectively pool risks, achieve economies of scale and, if authorized to do so, negotiate premiums. In addition, a judgment is necessary as to whether the insurance system will perform better if dissatisfied employers can join other cooperatives or can only return to the conventional small-group market. Finally, the choice depends on whether there is sufficient administrative expertise to organize and operate several cooperatives. This is a perennial problem for public agencies [Sapolsky, Aisenberg, and Morone, 1987] and presumably would limit the number of effective private cooperatives as well. Overall, policymakers need to consider whether the presumed advantages of choice and redundancy [Hirschman, 1970; Landau, 1987; Bendor, 1985] can be realized without compromising the effectiveness of all purchasing cooperatives.

A third design choice is whether to allow purchasing cooperatives to select participating insurers and negotiate premiums. The recent experience of major health care purchasers such as state employee programs, Medicaid programs, and private large-employer purchasing cooperatives demonstrates that selective contracting or price negotiation results in lower premium increases than in the market as a whole [U.S. Congress, 1994; Borger, 1995; Ramey, 1995]. Overall, the history of health policy suggests that governmental agencies with central bargaining power are the common ingredient in effective cost containment [Thorpe, 1993; Hackey, 1993; Sparer, 1993; Brown 1992].

A fourth choice is whether purchasing cooperatives should market plans through insurance agents and brokers. Since employers can obtain insurance directly from the cooperative, agents and brokers are theoretically superfluous to insurance administration and their fees represent excess costs to subscribers. Substantial savings are possible—perhaps 10 to 12 percent of total premiums— if agents and brokers are cut out of the system [Ramey, 1995]. On the other hand, agents and brokers may provide small business owners and employees with valuable advice about the quality of health plans and additional concerns; in addition, the economic incentives of agents and brokers to sell insurance may translate into broader coverage among small groups than if health insurance was not marketed in the context of the company's other insurance needs. Ultimately, the judgment policymakers face is whether small employers will find their way to purchasing cooperatives without the guidance of agents and brokers. This judgment enters into the decision of how much to provide in compensation: the purchasing cooperative can pay agents and brokers who bring in business a percentage commission or it can pay them a flat fee or it can pay them nothing. The cooperative must also decide whether to include the fees in the premium, leaving the amount unstated to employers, or publish the fees showing the added cost to the employer. California, for example, has chosen to make the use of agents and brokers voluntary and allow the employer to decide whether to pay a fee on top of the premium. Given that employers are not mandated to use the purchasing cooperative, policymakers must consider whether agents and brokers might boycott the cooperative and the participating insurers if they can receive substantially greater compensation doing business with plans outside the pool.

STATE ACTIONS TAKEN TO REFORM HEALTH INSURANCE MARKETS

The preceding section outlined the possible actions that policymakers might take to reform the small-group insurance market, the rationale for those actions, and the possible consequences of various policy choices. This section examines how states actually designed their reforms. It is based on a review of statutes in

FIGURE 9.1

Timing of Access Reforms, 1990–1995

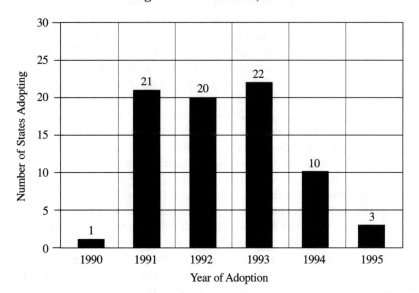

Source: Adapted from Oliver and Fiedler [1997].

45 states that adopted small-group health insurance reforms between 1990 and 1995, available reports on those reforms, and interviews with state officials and executives of public and private health plan purchasing cooperatives.[12]

The analysis begins by identifying notable patterns across the states in this area of legislation. What does the timing of these reforms suggest about the relationship of these incremental reforms to the push for national health care reform? On what elements of policy design was there nearly universal acceptance and on what elements was there substantial variation? Then it discusses the implications of the observed patterns in policy design.

TIMING OF SMALL-GROUP INSURANCE REFORMS

The first notable pattern is the timing of the small-group reforms. The data in Figure 9.1 indicate that 22 states debated and enacted their initial small-group market reform measures prior to 1992, when health care reform became an important issue in the U.S. presidential campaign. An additional 12 states enacted an initial reform package in 1992.

A total of 34 states acted before President Clinton formed his task force in 1993, while only 11 states initiated small-group reforms once the design of

FIGURE 9.2

Size of Groups Covered by State Insurance Reforms, 1990–1995

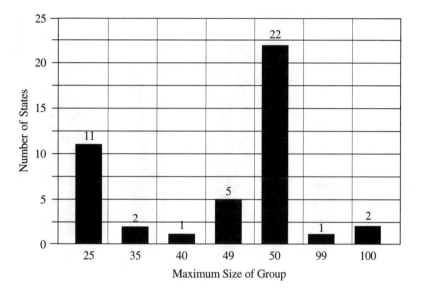

Source: Adapted from Oliver and Fiedler [1997].

the Clinton plan and the national debate were under way. (The yearly totals in Figure 1 include both states that enacted initial legislation and states that adopted followup legislation to earlier reforms.) This timing strongly suggests that the states were leaders in this area of reform, at once sensing the importance of the health insurance issue and responding to inaction at the national level.

RESTRICTING INSURANCE UNDERWRITING PRACTICES

The data in Figure 9.2 compare the size of groups targeted by the various state small-group insurance reforms. The vast majority of the state reforms covered groups of 50 or fewer individuals. Eleven states applied their reforms to groups of up to 25 members, while 30 states set the maximum size of groups between 25 and 50 members. Only Kentucky, New Hampshire, and Virginia included groups of up to 100. Some states extended the upper and lower bounds of the small-group market. Approximately half of the states folded self-employed individuals into the reforms. Other states applied some of the reform measures beyond the confines of small groups. Washington and Minnesota, for example, mandated that insurers guarantee the issue and renewal of at least some health benefit plans regardless of group size, including individuals.

FIGURE 9.3

Adoption of Access Reforms

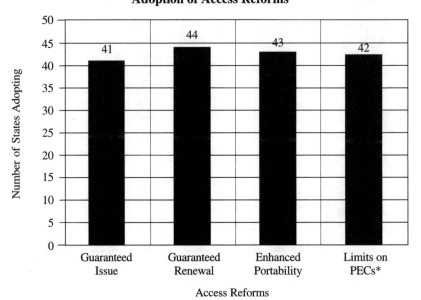

Source: Adapted from Oliver and Fiedler [1997].
*Preexisting condition exclusion.

The data in Figure 9.3 show the pattern of state reforms intended to improve access to health insurance. Nearly every state introduced new rules in this area. Each of the 45 states that adopted reforms of some kind required insurers to guarantee the issue or renewal of at least some health benefit plans in the small-group market. These requirements often applied only to "basic" or "standard" health benefit plans established by the state insurance department or some other designated body. Other states went further, requiring guaranteed issue and renewal for all health benefit plans offered in the small-group market.

Every state continued to permit some exclusions from coverage due to preexisting conditions. A total of 42 states introduced new limits, however. The reforms defined what will constitute a preexisting condition (although these definitions are not narrowly drawn) and restricted the period of exclusion from coverage, usually to a maximum of six to twelve months.

To encourage a greater sense of personal security, virtually all states adopted provisions that enhance the portability or continuity of health insurance coverage by prohibiting preexisting condition exclusions for individuals who join a new plan within one or two months after their previous coverage ends. A few states adopted special rules for persons whose involuntary unemployment interrupts their health benefit plan coverage.

CONTROLLING VARIATION IN PREMIUMS

The data in Figure 9.4 show that a large majority of states introduced policy instruments that can be used to restrict the characteristics used to assess group risk and set premiums, as well as to constrain the variation in premiums among groups and overall premium increases. The strength of those market restrictions was quite modest, however, in all but a few states.

Historically, insurers have used a wide variety of factors as a basis for setting the premiums charged to a group. Some factors are discrete (age, gender, family size and composition) and others tend to be more ambiguous or subjective (occupation, perceived health status). Age and health status together have been found to account for a 500 percent or more variance in health insurance premiums [Institute for Health Policy Solutions, 1995]. Most states continued to allow the use of certain discrete factors for establishing comparable groups. A few states specifically prohibited gender as a rating factor. The factors that states most frequently prohibited insurers from using to establish rates are claims experience, health status, and duration of insurance coverage.

In groups classified according to discrete factors, many states restricted the variance between the highest and lowest premium based on additional, more subjective factors. Most importantly, however, no state restricted the variation in premiums between the highest and lowest risk groups in the entire small-group market.

Pure community rating, according to the American Academy of Actuaries [1994], allows premiums to vary only according to family composition, geographic location, and the design of the health benefit plan. Only the New York reforms meet those criteria. Thirteen other states adopted legislation requiring a modified form of community rating (sometimes heavily modified). Of those states, only Connecticut and Vermont expressly excluded age as a basis of risk classification. Gender was excluded as a risk characteristic in Connecticut, Montana, New Hampshire, and Vermont. None of the states with modified community rating permitted risk classification on the basis of health status, claims experience, or duration of coverage. Only two of the thirteen permitted risk classification on the basis of industry or occupation.

The majority of states did not adopt even modified community rating as a part of their small-group reform initiatives. Actuarial rating in these markets is extraordinarily complicated. To begin with, insurers create many "classes" of business that involve distinct marketing strategies or administrative costs. Each small group within a business class is then rated by "case characteristics" such as age, gender, industry, and so forth.

FIGURE 9.4

Regulation of Rating Practices and Premiums

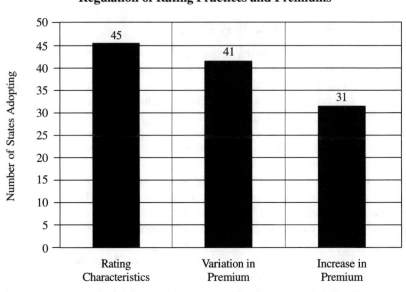

Source: Adapted from Oliver and Fiedler [1997].

In addition to this two-part risk classification, almost all states still allowed rate variation within the permitted risk classes, often including consideration of the claims experience and health status of a group. However, many rating reforms did restrict the variation in premiums so that an individual insurer could not charge one group more than a set percentage (e.g., 200 percent) of the lowest premium that is charged to another group in the same risk class, regardless of the group's claims experience or health status.

Closer approximations to community rating were incorporated into some of the state purchasing cooperatives. California, for example, established fairly tight rate bands within its health plan purchasing cooperative (HPPC): as of 1996, insurers had to offer potential subscriber premiums within 10 percent of the insurer's average premium for a given plan, with additional variation permitted only for specified age categories, geographic location, and family composition.

REGULATING INSURANCE MARKETING PRACTICES AND PRODUCTS

The data in Figure 9.5 illustrate the policy instruments that states adopted to regulate marketing and the scope of insurance benefits. Twenty-eight states

FIGURE 9.5

Standardized Plans and Fair Marketing Rules

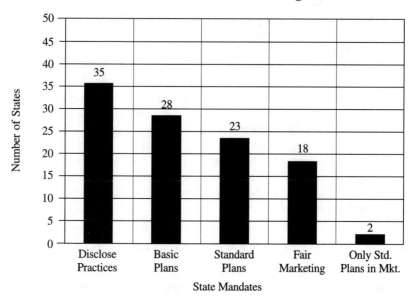

Source: Adapted from Oliver and Fiedler [1997].

authorized the creation of one or more benefit packages for the small-group market. The design of such plans was delegated to regulatory bodies or independent commissions and varies between states. The "standard" plans were generally comparable to the health benefit plans of public and private employers in the market as a whole. The "basic" plans provided less comprehensive benefits, reflecting an effort to reduce premium costs and attract employers that do not presently offer a health plan for their workers.

Only Kentucky and Maryland required insurers to offer only state-authorized benefit packages. The half-way regulation in the rest of the states will continue to make it difficult for small-group sponsors and members to easily compare all available insurance plans, and makes it likely that insurers will continue to engage in risk-selection strategies by promoting insurer-designed plans through insurance agents and brokers.

Eighteen of the states with standard or basic plans adopted new rules of disclosure and fair marketing, which suggests that legislators recognized that where the state-authorized plans must compete with traditional insurer-designed plans, efforts must be made to prevent insurers from seeking out low-risk groups through their marketing practices.

Another policy to reduce risk-based competition is to mandate risk adjustment among health plans. The extent to which this policy was adopted is unclear, because most of the data for this study were drawn from statutory provisions, and risk adjustment mechanisms may have been adopted by state officials in subsequent implementing regulations.

In many states that promoted purchasing cooperatives, however, policymakers chose to include risk adjustment with other provisions for market restructuring. Of the nine states with HPPC enabling legislation, Kentucky, Maine, and North Carolina mandated the use of risk adjustment in their legislation. The remaining six states left it to the discretion of the purchasing cooperative or a regulatory body, or else failed to address the issue explicitly. The purchasing cooperatives in California, Kentucky, and Utah each reported that risk adjustment mechanisms were adopted and implemented. The Minnesota Employer's Insurance Program also reported using risk adjustment, though there was no enabling HPPC legislation. The remainder of the states had not developed their mechanisms or had no plans to do so.

PROMOTING HEALTH PLAN PURCHASING COOPERATIVES

As of 1996, nine states had enacted legislation to create small-group health plan purchasing cooperatives or to specifically enable their creation. The insurance reforms in some other states may permit the creation of HPPCs, but the legislation did not make explicit policy decisions regarding their structure and operations.

States chose three basic approaches for purchasing cooperatives: (1) a HPPC operated and controlled by a public agency, (2) a HPPC operated privately but controlled by a publicly appointed board, or (3) a HPPC operated and controlled by private organizations.

The data in Table 9.2 compare the operational design of individual HPPCs controlled by public agencies or public boards, based on legislation and implementing regulations. Five of the nine states that adopted HPPC legislation authorized operation by a public agency or public appointment of the HPPC boards. California and Kentucky HPPCs were operated by public agencies, while Florida, North Carolina, and Texas HPPCs were private not-for-profit organizations whose boards were appointed by public officials. In addition to these five states with HPPCs devoted specifically to the small-group market, Minnesota and Washington provided small groups access to health insurance through state agencies that offer health plans to public employees. Thus, a total of seven states opted for public sector control of HPPCs while four (Colorado, Maine, South Carolina, and Utah) opted for wholly private control.[13]

As of 1996, the publicly sponsored or publicly enabled cooperatives were statewide except for the regional organizations in Florida and South Carolina.

TABLE 9.2

**Design Elements of Seven Health Plan Purchasing
Cooperatives with Publicly Appointed Boards**

Design Choices	*Number of States Using Specific Design Elements*	
Operating entity (public or not-for-profit)	4	Public agency, board, or commission
	3	Private not-for-profit entities
Employer contribution (mandated or voluntary)	5	Mandate an employer contribution to premium
	2	Voluntary
Carrier participation (open to qualified carriers or selective contracting)	2	By statute, all qualified carriers must be permitted to participate
	4	Participation open to most carriers
	1	Selective contracting arrangement
Number of carriers participating by participation type (open or selective)	6	Between 10 and 32 carriers in the HPPCs "open" to carriers
	1	Only 3 carriers in the HPPC with selective contracting
Employee choice of carriers (employee or employer selection of carrier)	6	Employee choice from available carriers
	1	Choice limited if employer contributes 70% or more of premium
Number of available health benefit plans	6	Between 2 and 4 standardized plans are available
	1	Only a single standardized plan is available
Health benefit plan pricing (negotiation, requests for proposal, combination)	6	Requests for proposal (RFP)
	1	Negotiation (only)
	4	Combination of RFP and negotiation
Insurance agent/broker fees (commissions and use limited or open)	4	Some limits on commissions
	3	No limits on commissions
	3	Mandate use of insurance agents or brokers
	4	Use of insurance agents or brokers is permitted
Risk adjustment mechanisms	2	In use and unique to HPPC
	1	Under development
	1	Pools all claims of $50,000 or more
	3	No risk adjustment mechanism
Use of comparative cost and quality data	7	Use and distribute comparative cost data
	0	Use and distribute comparative quality data (under development)
Development of marketing materials (by HPPC, carrier, or combination)	2	Materials developed by HPPC or its third-party administrator
	1	Materials by HPPC and adds selected materials from carriers
	4	Materials developed by the HPPC and the carriers

In contrast, only two private purchasing cooperatives operated on a statewide basis (in Connecticut and Utah), while all the others were regional entities.

Requirements for employer participation were generally not established by state legislatures. Most public and private HPPCs established their own participation rules to protect against adverse selection, however. A minimum percentage of employees, most commonly 70 percent, must purchase coverage for the group to participate in the HPPC. The public HPPCs generally required employers to make a contribution of 50 percent of the lowest cost plan available through the HPPC while the private HPPCs generally did not impose such a requirement.

No legislature mandated that insurers participate in HPPCs in order to do business in the state. On the other hand, insurers were typically not guaranteed participation, either. Almost all of the purchasing cooperatives were able to select participating insurers. Only Florida and North Carolina required the cooperatives to accept all certified plans. The public cooperatives were not typically very restrictive in the number of insurers and plans they offered, however. Several state programs offered plans from about 20 different insurers, and Minnesota was the only cooperative with fewer than 10 participating insurers. In contrast, only one of the private cooperatives had more than four participating insurers.

Almost all HPPCs, both public and private, negotiated premiums with insurers in some fashion. Again, only Florida and North Carolina prohibited selective contracting. Because participation by insurers in the cooperatives is voluntary, however, price negotiation was not necessarily coercive. In California, for example, "negotiation" consisted of providing insurers general feedback on where their proposed premiums fit in relation to those of all plans, and allowing them a week to adjust their price if they desired to do so. Insurers were not given any information about specific competitors, nor were they told the exact rankings of the proposed premiums (according to Sandra Shewry, Deputy Director of the California Managed Risk Medical Insurance Board, in a personal communication, July 1995).

The publicly sponsored or publicly enabled cooperatives provided distinctly greater choice for employees than do the private cooperatives. Florida mandated that employees be able to choose from between a minimum of two insurers. California, Kentucky, and Washington provided for full employee choice of benefit plan (basic or standard) and insurer. While Minnesota and Texas permitted the employer to select the benefit plan, employees were free to select their preferred insurer. And North Carolina required free employee choice unless the employer contributed 70 percent or more of the premium. In contrast, private HPPCs had varying degrees of employee choice, with some reserving all choice to employers and others providing employees full choice unless the participating employer objected.

With the exception of Kentucky, it appears that states were willing to risk adverse selection by permitting insurers to market their own small-group plans outside the HPPC in direct competition with the state-designed benefit plans within the HPPC.[14] When insurer-designed plans are marketed outside of a HPPC, they may attract better risks and leave the HPPC and its standardized products as "dumping grounds" for the relatively poorer risks. Members of the program staff of the Independent Health Alliance of Iowa (telephone interviews, July 1996), now out of business as a HPPC, identified this form of risk selection and differences in rating methodologies as key factors in its failure.

The desire to increase competition between insurers on the basis of cost and quality rather than risk was one of the driving forces behind the small-group reforms. The prevalence of employee choice and the use of state-designed benefit plans have aided progress toward this goal within the state HPPCs. The availability of another means to fair and efficient competition—comparative information on health plan quality—has yet to be realized. Although every state with a publicly sponsored or publicly enabled HPPC had committed itself to developing quality measures and consumer information on plan performance in the future, the systems to accomplish that were still being developed. Private HPPCs that offered subscribers a choice among competing insurers were even further behind in this crucial area of market regulation.

No purchasing cooperative in either the public or private sector had eliminated the use of agents and brokers for enrolling subscribers. Officials in various HPPCs acknowledged the importance of agents, arguing that health insurance is a product that must be *sold* in the small-group market because it is not actively *bought*. While every cooperative either mandated or permitted the use of agents and brokers, however, most public sector cooperatives offered lower commissions or fees. This is consistent with the fact that much of the market information normally available only through agents is provided by the cooperatives themselves, thereby reducing the value of the service that agents can provide. The early evidence showed that cooperatives relied on agents and brokers for a majority of their enrollment, even where their use was not mandatory. In California, nearly 80 percent of subscribers used agents and brokers when the state purchasing cooperative first started up in 1993. Two years later, direct enrollment was slowly increasing but 65 percent of subscribers were still referred by agents and brokers.

As of 1996, the enrollment in small-group HPPCs ranged from a few hundred to over 100,000 subscribers in California. It is clear that the public HPPCs had achieved a greater penetration of the small-group market than their private sector counterparts. It is not clear, however, whether the early differences in enrollment were due to initial resources for staffing and marketing, perceptions of need for HPPC services across the states, leadership skills of HPPC staff, or other factors.

NATIONAL ACTION TO REFORM HEALTH INSURANCE MARKETS: THE HEALTH INSURANCE PORTABILITY AND ACCOUNTABILITY ACT OF 1996

Since 45 of the 50 states adopted small-group health insurance reforms during the first half of the 1990s, one might expect federal legislation to build upon those state initiatives and establish stronger regulation of the insurance industry. The main function, however, was to set a floor of minimum expectations rather than a national commitment to structural reform of insurance practices.

The bipartisan bill drafted in 1995 by Senator Nancy Kassebaum (R-Kansas) and Senator Edward Kennedy (D-Massachusetts) began as the Health Insurance Reform Act, with its sights set on establishing a new regulatory infrastructure that could deliver long-term improvements in insurance accessibility and affordability, if not immediate results. Their initiative ended up merely as the Health Insurance Portability and Accountability Act of 1996, and, true to its title, it enhanced portability of health insurance coverage while doing little else.[15] The primary distinction is that the federal act, unlike the state reforms, reached beyond the small-group market and applied its standards to individuals and all groups, large and small, who have conventional insurance plans or are self-insured.[16]

HIPAA prohibited health plans from excluding for more than 12 months coverage of any medical condition for which medical advice, diagnosis, care, or treatment was recommended or received within six months of the effective date of coverage. The 12-month exclusion was reduced or eliminated altogether for individuals who have been insured prior to obtaining the new coverage. This standard was consistent with many existing state small-group market reforms in the use of preexisting condition exclusionary clauses. Tougher state requirements were expressly permitted by the federal law.

Complementing the restrictions on the use of preexisting condition clauses were provisions that preclude health plans from charging individuals within a group different premiums on the basis of health status, medical condition, claims experience, receipt of health care, medical history, genetic information, evidence of insurability, or disability. These rating restrictions were meant to enhance equity within insured groups and ensure that the costs of insurance would be borne by the group as a whole rather than the individual.

Congress, unlike the majority of the states, was unable to adopt insurance rating reforms designed to reduce risk selection and risk competition by health insurers or to broaden the insurance pool. With little agreement among the states as to the specific formula for such reforms, it is perhaps unsurprising that insurance rating reform, traditionally an area exclusively regulated by the states, was left alone.

Ultimately, Congress also hesitated to advance regulation of insurance purchasing and marketing. The earlier Kassebaum-Kennedy bill included several provisions for the formation of private health plan purchasing cooperatives and marketing information provided by insurers to HPPC enrollees. It would have required each state to adopt a certification program for HPPCs, and, if a state failed to do so, it would possibly be subject to a federal certification program. The HPPCs were to be controlled by a board composed of both employers and enrollees, and were to provide an ombudsman for enrollees. In addition, the Kassebaum-Kennedy proposal would have required HPPCs to provide comparative cost and quality information on health plans and leave the choice of plans to individuals, not their employers. This was a notable shift from existing private purchasing cooperatives or other group purchasing arrangements that primarily served the interests of the employers that sponsor them.

The final legislation, however, eliminated provisions for insurance purchasing reforms. With its already timid approach to rating reforms, HIPAA amounted to this: It ratified a single, widely adopted, and relatively uncontroversial component of state initiatives—portability of coverage—and provided it for residents of every state and every source of insurance. In all other respects, it failed to encompass even the modest achievements of the majority of recent state reforms. Most importantly, as the GAO report makes clear, it failed to ensure that individuals forced to change insurance plans could afford their new coverage—inaction that threatened to make portability a hollow promise [U.S. Congress, 1998; National Journal, 1998].

THE CONSTRAINTS ON POLICY DESIGN AND PERFORMANCE

What lessons can be drawn from this pattern of state and federal health insurance reforms? These reforms may be designed mostly by analysts and advocates steeped in the mechanics of finance and the health care system, but even the most incremental actions are a result of "how people fight over visions of the public interest or the nature of the community—the truly significant policy questions" [Stone, 1988, p. 7]. The policies that emerge reflect the intellectual, political, and institutional contexts in which debates arise and are resolved.

It is clear that the main idea underpinning insurance reforms is how to modify market structures and transactions to achieve a "fairer" distribution of medical care and medical care costs. People who happen to work for small businesses should not have to pay more for health insurance, nor should insurance be unavailable to the very people who need it most. In the typology of social groups proposed by Anne Schneider and Helen Ingram [1993], this "dependent" population, unable to organize itself in the health care market, would be regarded as deserving of intervention by policymakers. There seems to be genuine concern that health insurance maintain at least some degree of risk sharing and not degenerate further toward a pure market commodity. This accounts for why guaranteed issue and renewal of policies, restrictions on exclusions for preexisting conditions, and at least weak limits on how much premiums can vary are nearly universal elements of these reforms.

On the other hand, the relatively light controls on pricing and marketing in most states and the lack of such regulation in HIPAA reflect the logical and political constraints of incrementalism. In a system where insurance coverage is voluntary, changes to increase access for one group (individuals with costly medical conditions or other high-risk characteristics) tend to increase costs and thereby decrease access for another segment of the population (low-wage workers). Only in a compulsory insurance system can these forms of regulation be instituted without serious economic and political trade-offs. In addition, because these incremental reforms will not attract sustained attention and support from the general public, it is politically difficult to alter existing practices and impose substantial new regulation on a powerful industry. Thus, the pattern of policy design is consistent with Schneider and Ingram's theory: even groups that are perceived as especially needy or deserving do not necessarily receive substantial assistance if the costs will fall on politically powerful groups. On health insurance issues, "dependent" interests (deserving but not powerful) are matched against "contending" interests (undeserving but powerful). This alignment is likely to result in primarily symbolic burdens on the contending interests of the insurance industry.[17]

In fact, the prevalence and forms of the policy instruments shown in Figure 9.6 are not a severe threat to the insurance industry—indeed, the industry worked closely with the National Association of Insurance Commissioners (NAIC) to promulgate model legislation for the small-group market. A few states went beyond the minimalist NAIC recommendations and mounted a direct challenge to current insurance practices. Only nine states adopted legislation with a relatively full scope of regulations on access to coverage, rating of premiums, and marketing and purchasing of plans. And within each area of regulation, few states opted for the strongest possible provisions.

Throughout this decade, the media and consumer interest groups have continually publicized the tragedies that befall individuals and families denied insurance coverage. Yet only a handful of states adopted policies approaching community rating of insurance and only one state required pure community rating. Because the current voluntary system falls well short of universal coverage, no state is in a position to eliminate exclusions on the coverage of preexisting conditions without risking massive disenrollment in the small-group market.

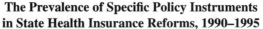

The Prevalence of Specific Policy Instruments
in State Health Insurance Reforms, 1990–1995

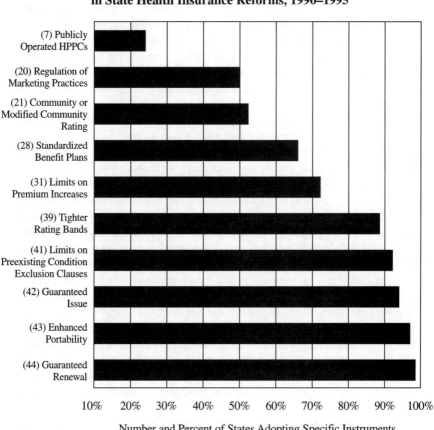

Number and Percent of States Adopting Specific Instruments
(Among States Enacting Small-Group Market Reforms)

Source: Adapted from Oliver and Fiedler [1997].

To date, the effort to reduce industry incentives for selective marketing and avoiding subscribers with potentially high-cost conditions has been minimal. Federal regulations for HIPAA implementation allow states to meet the porta-bility requirements by routing individuals whose coverage runs out into high-risk pools, which encourages screening and "dumping" into the common pool (with risks divided up among insurers) and raises the cost of coverage for those assigned to the pool. The recent development of risk adjustment in the California purchasing cooperative serves as a reminder that regulating marketing practices is a highly political process: policymakers must gain the cooperation of insurers to create a risk adjustment mechanism at all, and even then the adjustment and resulting transfer of revenues between plans is limited to boundaries of risk that the plans themselves are willing to negotiate [Shewry et al., 1996]. Finally, no state has gone so far as to make purchasing cooperatives the main field of competition for the small-group market by preventing insurers from offering nonstandard benefit plans outside of the cooperative for groups with the most attractive risks.

Other than pure community rating, it appears that the most difficult change in policy design is to establish a purchasing cooperative. In the early stages of HPPC development, the public sector approach was more successful than strictly voluntary organization, as reflected in both the number and size of each kind. The pattern suggests that establishing purchasing pools for small groups and individuals is a collective action problem that often requires governmental support, because the stakes for a given participant are not great enough to justify the costs of organizing a cooperative in the private sector. Until a "learning curve" in HPPC development has been established, private sector cooperatives will appear only in the presence of skillful entrepreneurs [Salisbury, 1969] or in places like the Twin Cities, where a small-group cooperative can form as a "little brother" to an established purchasing group like the Buyers Health Care Action Group for the region's large employers. The comparatively large enrollment in the California and Florida cooperatives suggests that governmental sponsorship also speeds up the implementation process, either because it provides greater material resources or more likely because public endorsement signals insurers that the cooperative will provide them a substantial pool of potential customers, making it more immediately rewarding to do business there.

It can be argued that these initiatives, however well publicized, have little impact on the insurance market. While it is too soon to tell what the ultimate numbers will look like, in a market of tens of millions of individuals, there were tiny enrollments in most of the state purchasing cooperatives. Except in California (106,000) and Florida (77,000), there were no more than 30,000 subscribers participating in any cooperative as of late 1996; and in California fewer than one-quarter of the new subscribers were previously uninsured. The numbers could increase if purchasing cooperatives demonstrate they are capable of delivering substantial savings to employers; it will be many years, however, before these new institutions can become an integral part of the insurance system.[18]

So the most important question to be asked about insurance reforms is: If states or the federal government build them in a voluntary system, will anybody come? Many of the access and pricing regulations help only if the intended beneficiaries have some purchasing power in the first place. One survey of small employers showed that for those not currently offering health benefits, 60 percent were simply not willing to contribute anything toward employee health benefits, regardless of accessibility and cost [Cantor, Long, and Marquis, 1995]. Other studies noted that despite a slight increase between 1989 and 1996 in the proportion of small employers offering health insurance, fewer employees actually enrolled because of increases in the financial contributions required by employers [Cooper and Schone, 1997; Ginsburg, Gabel, and Hunt, 1998]. Thus, the impact of these reforms will likely be modest, if only because they fail to address the heart of the insurance access problem—paying for those who cannot afford coverage on their own [National Journal, 1998].

Perhaps the most compelling evidence of the political constraints on this class of reforms is this: Under HIPAA, states are allowed to set up their own regulatory apparatus or they may opt to have the federal Department of Health and Human Services (HHS) enforcement provisions that are not included in state reforms. Even though most states already enacted similar or even stronger insurance market reforms overall, many did not include certain provisions such as guaranteed access to insurance if a person moves from group to individual coverage. In the current climate, many states are unwilling to make additional changes and have chosen to allow the federal government to enforce HIPAA rather than do it themselves. As of early 1998, these states included California, Massachusetts, Michigan, Missouri, and Rhode Island and many more were in a position to require federal enforcement. The GAO [U.S. Congress, 1998, p. 18] noted this surprising development: "According to HHS officials, the agency as well as the Congress and others assumed HHS would generally not have to perform this role, believing instead that states would not relinquish regulatory authority to the federal government. However, several states reported that they did not pass legislation implementing key provisions of HIPAA, thus requiring HHS to actively regulate insurance plans in these states." This demonstrates how difficult a job it is to monitor the insurance industry and how little political reward there is at this time for doing so. In an era when devolution of many other policies is desired (welfare, Medicaid, children's health insurance), it is telling that states would ask federal regulators to enter into an arena that has been almost entirely a state responsibility until now.

CONCLUSION

The bottom line is that government is willing to modify the market on behalf of deserving interests, but there are severe constraints on how far it can go. Those constraints include the potential side effects of these incremental reforms, entrenched practices in the insurance market, and political interests that can mobilize vast resources to defeat or reduce initiatives in scope, scale, and duration. For observers of public policymaking, the wide variation in state actions and limited interventions of the federal government during the past few years should confirm that, in health care, even minor reforms are complex and there is little likelihood of experts developing a "model" reform package that can diffuse with little modification across jurisdictions.[19]

For supporters of a more equitable and efficient health care system, the most obvious lesson from the recent era of reform is that broad agreement on fundamental problems and goals is not sufficient to guarantee effective governmental action. It took a historic amount of political capital to achieve even these incremental changes, and perhaps only a continuing threat of large-scale reform will ensure that they become real accomplishments instead of "ridiculous overpromises" [Broder, 1998]. In the absence of this threat, it will require remarkable skill and leadership to turn these new institutions into building blocks for a system that can meet much higher aspirations.

REFERENCES

Aaron, H.J., & Bosworth, B.P. (1994). Economic issues in reform of health care financing. In M.N. Baily, P.C. Reiss, & C. Winston (Eds.), Brookings papers on economic activity: Microeconomics 1994. Washington, DC: Brookings Institution.

Advisory Council on Social Security (1991). *Commitment to change: Foundations for reform*. Washington, DC: Government Printing Office.

Alpha Center (1994, July/August). State initiatives in health care reform, 7, 1.

American Academy of Actuaries (1994). An analysis of mandated community rating. Washington, DC: American Academy of Actuaries.

Atchinson, B.K., & Fox, D.M. (1997, May/June). Politics of the health insurance portability and accountability act. *Health Affairs*, 16, 146–150.

Bendor, J.B. (1985). Parallel systems: *Redundancy in government*. Berkeley: University of California Press.

Blumberg, L.J., & Nichols, L.M. (1996, Fall). First, do no harm: Developing health insurance market reform packages. *Health Affairs*, 15, 35–53.

Borger, J.Y. (1995, 30 July). *Employers take aim at health plans*. St. Paul: Pioneer Press, p. 1A.

Bosso, C.J. (1994). The practice and study of policy formation. In S.S. Nagel (Ed.), *Encyclopedia of policy studies* (2nd ed.). New York: Marcel Dekker.

Broder, D.S. (1998, 29 July). Patients' rights: No pain, no gain . . . *Washington Post*, p. A21.

Brown, L.D. (1992, Winter). Political evolution of federal health care regulation. *Health Affairs*, 11, 17–37.

California Legislature, Assembly (1992, 26 August). Analysis of the conference committee report on A.B. 1672.

Cantor, J.C., Long, S.H., & Marquis, M.S. (1995, Summer). Private employment-based health insurance in ten states. *Health Affairs*, 14, 199–211.

Chollet, D.J., & Paul, R.R. (1994). *Community rating: Issues and experience*. Washington, DC: Alpha Center.

Cooper, P.F., & Schone, B.S. (1997, November/December). More offers, fewer takers for employment-based health insurance: 1987 and 1996. *Health Affairs*, 16, 142–149.

Ellwood, P.M., Enthoven, A.C., & Etheredge, L. (1992). The Jackson Hole initiatives for a twenty-first century American health care system. *Health Economics*, 1, 149–168.

Ellwood, P.M., & Enthoven, A.C. (1995, Summer). Responsible choices: The Jackson Hole group plan for health reform. *Health Affairs*, 14, 24–39.

Enthoven, A.C. (1980). *Health plan*. Reading, MA: Addison-Wesley.

Enthoven, A.C. (1988). *Theory and practice of managed competition in health care finance*. New York: Elsevier Science Publishers.

Enthoven, A.C., & Singer, S.J. (1995, Spring). Market-based reform: What to regulate and by whom. *Health Affairs*, 14, 105–119.

Feder, J., & Levitt, L. (1995, Spring). Steps toward universal coverage. *Health Affairs*, 14, 140–149.

Ginsburg, P.B., Gabel, J.R., & Hunt, K.A. (1998, January/February). Tracking small-firm coverage, 1989–1996. *Health Affairs*, 17, 167–171.

Glazner, J., Braithwaite, W.R., Hull, S., & Lezotte, D.C. (1995, Summer). The questionable value of medical screening in the small-group health insurance market. *Health Affairs*, 14, 224–234.

Gradison, B. (1998). Written testimony before the U. S. Senate Labor and Human Resources Committee, 18 March 1998. Washington, DC: Federal Information Systems Corporation.

Hackey, R. (1993, Summer). Regulatory regimes and state cost containment programs. *Journal of Health Politics, Policy and Law*, 18, 491–502.

Hall, M.A. (1992, Summer). The political economics of health insurance market reform. *Health Affairs*, 11, 108–124.

Heclo, H. (1995, Spring). The Clinton health plan: Historical perspective. *Health Affairs*, 14, 87–98.

Helms, W.D., Gauthier, A.K., & Campion, D.M. (1992, Summer). Mending the flaws in the small-group market. *Health Affairs*, 11, 7–27.

Hirschman, A.O. (1970). *Exit, voice, and loyalty*. Cambridge, MA: Harvard University Press.

Institute for Health Policy Solutions (1995). State experience with community rating and related reforms. Washington, DC: Kaiser Family Foundation.

Jeffords, J.M. (1998). The Health Insurance Portability and Accountability Act of 1996: First Year Implementation Concerns. Floor statement to the U.S. Senate Labor and Human Resources Committee, 18 March 1998. Washington, DC: Federal Information Systems Corporation.

Jewett, J.J., & Hibbard, J.H. (1996, Fall). Comprehension of quality care indicators:

Differences among privately insured, publicly insured, and uninsured. *Health Care Financing Review*, 18, 75–94.

Johnson, H., & Broder, D.S. (1996). *The system: The American way of politics at the breaking point*. Boston, MA: Little, Brown.

Landau, M. (1987). Redundancy, rationality, and the problem of duplication and overlap. In D.L. Yarwood (Ed.), *Public administration: Politics and the people*. New York: Longman.

Lindblom, C.E. (1959, Spring). The science of "muddling" through. *Public Administration Review*, 19, 79–88.

MacRae, D., Jr., & Wilde, J.A. (1979). *Policy analysis for public decisions*. North Scituate, MA: Duxbury Press, 65–67.

McLaughlin, C.G., & Zellers, W.K. (1992, Summer). The shortcomings of voluntarism in the small-group insurance market. *Health Affairs*, 11, 28–40.

National Journal (1998, 12 March). Study: Insurers hiking rates under portability law. CongressDaily. Washington, DC: author. Available online: *http:nationaljournal.com*.

Newhouse, J.P. (1994, Spring I). Patients at risk: Health reform and risk adjustment. *Health Affairs*, 14, 132–146.

Oliver, T.R., & Dowell, E.B. (1994, Spring II). Interest groups and the political struggle over expanding health insurance in California. *Health Affairs*, 13, 123–141.

Oliver, T.R., & Fiedler, R.M. (1997). State government and health insurance market reform. In H.M. Leichter (Ed.), *Health policy in America: Innovations from the states* (2nd ed., pp. 47–100). Armonk, NY: M.E. Sharpe.

Palumbo, D.J., & Calista, D.J. (1990). Opening up the black box: Implementation and the policy process. In D.J. Palumbo & D.J. Calista (Eds.), *Implementation and the policy process: Opening up the black box* (pp. 3–17). Westport, CT: Greenwood Press.

Rothman, D. (1993, Summer). A century of failure: Health care reform in America. *Journal of Health Politics, Policy and Law*, 18, 271–286.

Rowland, D., Lyons, B., Salganicoff, A., & Long. P. (1994, Spring II). A profile of the uninsured in America. *Health Affairs*, 13, 283–287.

Salisbury, R.H. (1969, February). An exchange theory of interest groups. *Midwest Journal of Political Science*, 13, 1–32.

Sapolskv, H., Aisenberg, J., & Morone, J.A. (1987, March/April). The call to Rome and other obstacles to state-level innovation. *Public Administration Review*, 47, 135–142.

Schneider, A., & Ingram, H. (1993, June). Social construction of target populations: Implications for politics and policy. *American Political Science Review*, 87, 334–347.

Shewry, S., Hunt, S., Ramey, J., & Bertko, J. (1996, Spring). Risk adjustment: The missing piece of market competition. *Health Affairs*, 15, 171–181.

Skocpol, T. (1996). *Boomerang: Clinton's health security effort and the turn against government in U.S. politics*. New York: W.W. Norton.

Sparer, M. (1993, Summer). States and the health care crisis. *Journal of Health Politics, Policy and Law*, 18, 503–513.

Starr, P. (1982). *The social transformation of American medicine.* New York: Basic Books.

Steinmo, S., & Watts, J. (1995, Summer). It's the institutions, stupid! Why comprehensive national health insurance always fails in America. *Journal of Health Politics, Policy and Law,* 20, 329–372.

Stone, D.A. (1988). *Policy paradox and political reason.* New York: Harper Collins.

Stone, D.A. (1993, Summer). The struggle for the soul of health insurance. *Journal of Health Politics, Policy and Law,* 18, 287–317.

Thorpe, K.E. (1992a, Summer). Expanding employment-based health insurance: Is small group reform the answer? *Inquiry,* 29, 128–136.

Thorpe, K.E. (1992b, Summer). Inside the black box of administrative costs. *Health Affairs,* 11,41–55.

Thorpe, K.E. (1993, Summer). The American states and Canada: A comparative analysis of health care spending. *Journal of Health Politics, Policy and Law,* 18, 477–489.

Thorpe, K.E. (1995, Spring). A call for health services researchers. *Health Affairs,* 14, 63–65.

U.S. Congress, General Accounting Office (GAO) (1991). Private health insurance: Problems caused by a segmented market (Doc. No. GAO/HRD-91-114). Washington, DC: GAO.

U.S. Congress, General Accounting Office (GAO) (1992). Access to health care: States respond to growing crisis (Doc. No. GAO/HRD-92-70). Washington, DC: GAO.

U.S. Congress, General Accounting Office (GAO) (1994). Health reform: Purchasing cooperatives have an increasing role in providing access to insurance (GAO/T-HEHS-94-196). Washington, DC: GAO.

U.S. Congress, General Accounting Office (GAO) (1998). Health insurance standards: New federal law creates challenges for consumers, insurers, regulators (GAO/HEHS-98-67). Washington, DC: GAO.

Washington Post (1998, 13 April). Pulling back on health care.

Wicks, E.L., Curtis, R.E., & Haugh, K. (1993, March/April). The ABCs of HIPCs. *Journal of American Health Policy,* 29–34.

NOTES

The author would like to thank Robert Fiedler for his research assistance, and Marvin Mandell and two anonymous reviewers for their comments and suggestions on earlier versions of this article.

1. For example, official estimates accompanying the 1992 California legislation predicted that only about 100,000 additional individuals would receive employer-based insurance coverage, less than 2 percent of the estimated six million state residents then uninsured [California Legislature, 1992].

2. Throughout, this article employs arguments and evidence from a study of insurance reforms adopted by the state of California. The creation and early operation of a state-sponsored health plan purchasing cooperative for small employers is one case

in a larger study of "Public Entrepreneurship and Health Policy Innovation" supported by an Investigator Award in Health Policy Research from the Robert Wood Johnson Foundation.

3.   The rise in premiums due to adverse selection—where people who need more services are the ones most likely to purchase insurance—is exacerbated by the "moral hazard" introduced by insurance coverage: once people have insurance coverage, they are more likely to use covered services than if they pay out of pocket for each service.

4.   Free-riding refers to the fact that many uninsured persons still receive medical treatment if they are injured or become ill. The costs of treating the uninsured are covered by providers, by public or philanthropic funds, or by raising premiums for insured individuals.

5.   This study reviewed the claims experience of employees in firms that were subject to medical screening compared to those that were not screened and found no significant difference in the average claims per employee over a six-year period. If insurance agents and brokers informally screen firms under the assumption that some applications will be rejected, however, then formal medical screening by insurers may discourage firms with the worst risks from applying for coverage in the first place.

6.   The chairman of the California Managed Risk Medical Insurance Board, Clifford Allenby (personal communication, September 1994), says that the experience with the state's high-risk insurance pool (which provides subsidized coverage for individuals who have been rejected by private insurers) demonstrates that traditional medical underwriting is likely to overestimate medical care use by individuals with preexisting conditions. The state program has been able to cover nearly twice as many individuals as anticipated in the original actuarial projections.

7.   On the application of horizontal equity as a criterion for public policy, see MacRae and Wilde [1979, pp. 65–7].

8.   The current private insurance system explicitly subsidizes coverage for spouses and large families, for example. Single individuals pay substantially higher per person insurance premiums than individuals with dependents, and beyond a certain number of children there are no increases in premiums at all.

9.   These are the figures cited by officials in the Maryland Department of Health and Mental Hygiene; similar figures are cited in Enthoven and Singer [1995].

10.   The purchasing cooperative can be viewed as a variation on the Federal Employees Health Benefits Plan, which began operation in the early 1960s (according to Scott Fleming, former vice-president of the Kaiser Foundation Health Plans, in a personal communication, July, 1995). It served as the original model for a series of proposals to extend market competition throughout the insurance market [Enthoven, 1980; Enthoven, 1988; Ellwood, Enthoven, and Etheredge, 1992; Ellwood and Enthoven, 1995].

11.   The cost of acquiring a new subscriber is somewhere between $1,000 and $3,000 in the conventional small-group market, well above the costs of acquiring new business through a purchasing cooperative (according to John Ramey, Director of the California Managed Risk Medical Insurance Board in a personal communication, July, 1995).

12.   The specific provisions in individual states are presented in Oliver and Fiedler [1997].

13.   Data on the design of privately operated HPPCs as of July 1996 are available from the author.

14.   Maryland, which has no HPPC legislation, has mandated that insurers can offer only standardized health benefit plans in the small-group market.

15.   Senator Kassebaum introduced her original bill, S. 1028, on 13 July 1995. A substitute version of the bill, HR. 3103, was unanimously approved 100–0 by the Senate on 23 April 1996. Reconciliation with the legislation passed in the House of Representatives was approved by both houses of Congress on 2 August 1996. H.R. 3103, the Health Insurance Portability and Accountability Act of 1996, was signed by President Clinton on 21 August 1996.

16.   HIPAA did include several provisions outside of the kind of insurance regulation discussed in this article. It strengthened tax incentives for self-employed individuals to purchase insurance and for long-term care insurance, permitted seriously ill individuals to receive life insurance benefits to cover the cost of health care, authorized further development of electronic medical records, increased oversight of health care fraud and abuse, and endorsed an experiment to test the viability of personal medical savings accounts.

17.   It can be argued that the social construction of small-business interests would be "advantaged" (deserving and powerful), but until the debate over the Clinton health plan, small business was not very engaged on health insurance issues and was a fringe interest as a result [Oliver and Dowell, 1994]. During and after the national debate, small-business organizations have appeared more interested in avoiding obligations to employees than in seeking benefits for them. Individual small-business owners may be less ideologically opposed to providing health benefits, but must nonetheless pass on the costs to employees to remain in business. Although more small employers in fact offer health insurance than in the past, they require higher employee contributions as well [Ginsburg, Gabel, and Hunt, 1998].

18.   As of May 1998, enrollment in the Health Insurance Plan of California was 136,434 and enrollment in the Florida Community Health Purchasing Alliances was 92,571.

19.   Blumberg and Nichols [1996] outlined one such set of model health insurance reforms for states. The patterns of actual state reforms described in this article differ considerably from their proposed models, however, revealing how policymakers apply different criteria and make different trade-offs in policy design than detached analysts.

10 | Setting Performance Standards and Expectations for Patient Safety

Janet Corrigan,
Linda Kohn, and
Molla Donaldson, Editors;
Committee on Quality of
Health Care in America,
Institute of Medicine

The development and availability of standards for patient safety can serve several purposes. They can either establish minimum levels of performance or can establish consistency or uniformity across multiple individuals and organizations. Another purpose for standards is that they set expectations. The process of developing standards can set expectations for the organizations and health professionals affected by the standards. The publication and dissemination of standards additionally helps to set expectations for consumers and purchasers.

Standards can be developed and used in public regulatory processes, such as licensure for health professionals and licensure for health care organizations, such as hospitals or health plans. Standards can also be developed through private voluntary processes, such as professional certification or organizational accreditation.

Although there are many kinds of standards in health care, especially those promulgated by licensing agencies and accrediting organizations, few standards

Reprinted with permission from Corrigan, Kohn, and Donaldson (eds.), *To Err Is Human: Building a Safer Health System*, pp. 114–33 (Washington, D.C. 1999). Copyright 1999 by the National Academy of Sciences. Courtesy of the National Academy Press, Washington, D.C.

focus explicitly on issues of patient safety. Furthermore, the current lack of safety standards does not allow consumers and purchasers to reinforce the need for safe systems from the providers and organizations with whom they have contact. All existing regulatory and voluntary standard-setting organizations can increase their attention to patient safety and should consistently reinforce its importance.

Expectations for the performance of health professionals and organizations are also shaped by professional groups, purchasers and consumers, and society in general. Professional groups and leaders play a particularly important role in establishing norms and facilitating improvements in performance through educational, convening and advocacy activities. Large public and private group purchasers and purchasing coalitions also have the opportunity to shape expectations through marketplace decisions.

This chapter describes how performance standards and expectations can foster improvements in patient safety. Although this report has described the importance of a systems approach for reducing errors in health care, licensing and accreditation of individual practitioners and organizations can also play a role in reinforcing the importance of patient safety. The primary focus is on how existing models of oversight can be strengthened to include a focus on patient safety. In this report, the committee did not undertake an evaluation of the effectiveness of public and private oversight systems to affect quality of care. The committee recognizes, however, that as the organizational arrangements through which health care is delivered change, an evaluation may be appropriate since the existing models of oversight may no longer be adequate.

RECOMMENDATIONS

In the health care industry, standards and expectations about performance are applicable to health care organizations, health professionals, and drugs and devices. The committee believes there are numerous opportunities to strengthen the focus of the existing processes on patient safety issues.

RECOMMENDATION 1—Performance standards and expectations for health care organizations should focus greater attention on patient safety.

- **Regulators and accreditors should require health care organizations to implement meaningful patient safety programs with defined executive responsibility.**
- **Public and private purchasers should provide incentives to health care organizations to demonstrate continuous improvement in patient safety.**

Changes within health care organizations will have the most direct impact on making care delivery processes safer for patients. Regulators and accreditors have a role in encouraging and supporting actions within health care organizations by holding them accountable for ensuring a safe environment for patients.

Health care organizations ought to be developing patient safety programs within their own organizations. After a reasonable period of time for health care organizations to set up such programs, regulators and accreditors should require patient safety programs as a minimum standard.

The marketplace, through purchaser and consumer demands, also exerts influence on health care organizations. Public and private purchasers have three tools that can be employed today to demand better attention to safety by health care organizations. First, purchasers can consider safety issues in their contracting decisions. Second, purchasers can reinforce the importance of patient safety by providing relevant information to their employees or beneficiaries. There is increasing attention in providing information to aid in the selection of health coverage. Information about safety can be part of that process. Finally, purchasers can communicate concerns about patient safety to accrediting bodies to support stronger oversight for patient safety.

RECOMMENDATION 2—Performance standards and expectations for health professionals should focus greater attention on patient safety.

- **Health professional licensing bodies should**

  (1) implement periodic reexaminations and relicensing of doctors, nurses, and other key providers, based on both competence and knowledge of safety practices; and
  (2) work with certifying and credentialing organizations to develop more effective methods to identify unsafe providers and take action.

- **Professional societies should make a visible commitment to patient safety by establishing a permanent committee dedicated to safety improvement. This committee should**

  (1) develop a curriculum on patient safety and encourage its adoption into training and certification requirements;
  (2) disseminate information on patient safety to members at special sessions at annual conferences, journal articles and editorials, newsletters, publications and websites on a regular basis;
  (3) recognize patient safety considerations in practice guidelines and in standards related to the introduction and diffusion of new technologies, therapies, and drugs;
  (4) work with the Center for Patient Safety to develop community-based, collaborative initiatives for error reporting and analysis and implementation of patient safety improvements; and
  (5) collaborate with other professional societies and disciplines in a national summit on the professional's role in patient safety.

For most health professionals, current methods of licensing and credentialing assess knowledge, but do not assess performance skills after initial licensure. Although the state grants initial licensure, responsibility for documenting continued competence is dispersed. Competence may be considered when a licensing board reacts to a complaint. It may be evaluated when an individual applies to a health care organization for privileges or network contracting or employment. Professional certification is the current process for evaluating clinical knowledge after licensure and some programs are now starting to consider assessment of clinical skills in addition to clinical knowledge. Given the rapid pace of change in health care and the constant development of new technologies and information, existing licensing and accreditation processes should be strengthened to ensure that all health care professionals are assessed periodically on both skills and knowledge for practice.

More effective methods for identifying unsafe providers and better coordination between the organizations involved are also needed. The time between discovery of a problem, investigation, and action can currently last several years, depending on the issue and procedures for appeal or other processes. Efforts should be made to make this time as short as possible, while ensuring that practitioners have available the due process procedures to which they are entitled. States should also be more active in notifying other states when a practitioner's license is rescinded. Although unsafe practitioners are believed to be few in number and efforts to identify such individuals are not likely to improve overall quality or safety problems throughout the industry, such efforts are important to a comprehensive safety program.

Finally, professional societies and groups should become active leaders in encouraging and demanding improvements in patient safety. Setting standards, convening and communicating with members about safety, incorporating attention to patient safety into training programs, and collaborating across disciplines are all mechanisms that will contribute to creating a culture of safety. As patient advocates, health care professionals owe their patients nothing less.

RECOMMENDATION 3—The Food and Drug Administration (FDA) should increase attention to the safe use of drugs in both pre- and post-marketing processes through the following actions:

- **develop and enforce standards for the design of drug packaging and labeling that will maximize safety in use;**
- **require pharmaceutical companies to test (using FDA-approved methods) proposed drug names to identify and remedy potential sound-alike and look-alike confusion with existing drug names; and**
- **work with physicians, pharmacists, consumers and others to establish appropriate responses to problems identified through postmarketing surveillance, especially for concerns that are perceived to require immediate response to protect the safety of patients.**

FDA's role is to regulate manufacturers for the safety of their drugs and devices; however, even approved drugs can present safety problems when used in practice. Drugs may be prone to error in use due to sound-alike or look-alike names, unclear labeling, or poorly designed packaging. FDA standards for packaging and labeling of drugs should consider the safety of the products in actual use. Manufacturers should also be required to use proven methods for detecting drug names that sound or look similar. If necessary, Congress should take appropriate action to provide additional enabling authority or clarification of existing authority for FDA to implement this action. Since not all safety problems can be predicted or avoided before a drug is marketed, FDA should also conduct intensive and extensive monitoring to identify problems early and respond quickly when serious threats are discovered in the actual use of approved drugs.

CURRENT APPROACHES FOR SETTING STANDARDS IN HEALTH CARE

Generically, standards can be used to define a process or outcome of care. The Institute of Medicine defines a quality standard as a minimum level of acceptable performance or results *or* excellent levels of performance or results *or* the range of acceptable performance or results.[1] Other definitions for standards have been enacted through legislation, such as the Occupational Safety and Health Act of 1970, which defines a safety and health standard as one that requires conditions, or the adoption or use of one or more practices, means, methods, operations or processes, reasonably necessary or appropriate to provide safe or healthful employment and places of employment.[2] A variety of standards have also been defined through private organizations, such as the American Society for Testing and Materials. The committee does not recommend one definition or type of standard over another, but recognizes that standards can be quite varied and that as standards specific to safety are developed, they could take multiple forms and focus.

In health care, standards are set through both public, regulatory initiatives and private, voluntary initiatives. Standards can apply to health care organizations, health professionals, and drugs and medical devices. For health care organizations (e.g., health plans. hospitals, ambulatory care facilities), standards are set through licensure and accreditation and, to some extent, requirements imposed by large purchasers, such as Medicare and Fortune 500 companies. For health care professionals, standards are set through state licensure, board certification, and accrediting and credentialing programs. For drugs and devices, the FDA plays a critical role in standard setting.

In general, current standards in healthcare do not provide adequate focus on patient safety. Organizational licensure and accreditation focus on the review of core processes such as credentialing, quality improvement, and risk management, but lack a specific focus on patient safety issues. Professional licensure concentrates on qualifications at initial licensure, with no requirements to demonstrate safe and competent clinical skills during one's career. Standards for drugs and medical devices concentrate on safe design and production, with less attention to their safe use. Current standards in health care leave serious gaps in ensuring patient safety.

PERFORMANCE STANDARDS AND EXPECTATIONS FOR HEALTH CARE ORGANIZATIONS

Standards and expectations for health care organizations may be established through oversight processes, primarily licensing and accreditation requirements. Additionally, large public and private purchasers may also impose demands on health care organizations. Each is discussed in this section.

LICENSING AND ACCREDITATION

There is a great deal of variation in state licensure requirements for health care organizations. Responsibility for licensure rests at the state level, with each state setting its own standards, measurement, and enforcement. Although standards and measurement can be made more similar, enforcement is always likely to vary to some extent depending on the level of resources devoted by a state to this activity.

In many states, licensure and accreditation are intertwined. For hospital licensure, 44 states accept the Joint Commission on Accreditation of Healthcare Organization's evaluation, in whole or in part, as a condition for licensure (Personal communication, Margaret VanAmringe, JCAHO, February 23, 1999). Some states may additionally require compliance with other standards related to building safety or medical care issues that are tracked in that particular state. The remaining states do not link hospital licensure and accreditation. Although the overwhelming tendency to use JCAHO increases the consistency of standards nationally, differences in application also contribute to the variation in ensuring patient safety. For licensure of health maintenance organizations (HMOs), some states rely on private accrediting bodies, primarily the National Committee for Quality Assurance (NCQA), to conduct reviews of health plans. It should also be noted that other health facilities, such as some ambulatory care centers or physicians offices, may not be licensed at all and are generally not subject to traditional methods of oversight. One of the few mechanisms in place today that more broadly examines care in the ambulatory setting is managed care organizations.

Three private-sector agencies play a role in organizational accreditation: JCAHO, NCQA, and the American Accreditation Healthcare Commission/

URAC. Each effort, to some degree, encompasses aspects of standard setting and performance measurement.

JCAHO accredits more than 18,000 health care organizations, including hospitals, health plans, home care agencies, and others.[3] Its longest-standing accreditation program applies to hospitals. JCAHO accredits hospitals for three-year periods based on compliance with its standards in the areas of patient rights and patient care: organizational performance; leadership; information management; and nursing and medical staff structures. Approximately 85 percent of hospitals are accredited by JCAHO. Both Joint Commission–accredited hospitals and those accredited by the American Osteopathic Association are deemed to meet Medicare conditions of participation. JCAHO is incorporating performance information into the accreditation process through its Oryx system, in which hospitals will collect clinical data on six measures and submit performance data on these measures. This system was introduced in 1997 and is required by the Joint Commission for a hospital to be accredited. Eventually hospitals will have to demonstrate specific Oryx performance to maintain their accreditation status.

NCQA accredits health plans for periods of one, two, or three years. The accreditation process covers areas related to quality improvement, credentialing, members' rights and responsibilities, preventive health services, utilization management, and medical records. Approximately 14 states incorporate accreditation into their licensure requirement for health plans; another six states require that health plans have external reviews, most of which are done by NCQA (Steve Lamb, NCQA, personal communication, March 2, 1999). A number of states also require that health plans serving public employees and/or Medicaid enrollees be accredited. NCQA's performance dataset, the Health Plan Employer Data and Information Set (HEDIS), looks at indicators of effectiveness of care, access or availability, satisfaction, health plan stability, use of services, and costs. Beginning in July 1999, accreditation criteria began to incorporate HEDIS measures, initially being used only if they increase a health plan's overall score.[4] Accreditation status will also change with the top 20 percent of health plans earning the status of "excellent."

URAC was established in 1990 and offers nine different accreditation programs for managed care organizations, such as health plan accreditation, health network accreditation, health utilization management accreditation, and network practitioner credentialing.[5] Individual managed care organizations can seek accreditation under different sets of programs depending on the range of services they offer. URAC accreditation focuses on preferred provider organization (PPO) and point-of-service (POS) plans. Approximately 22 states have incorporated Commission/URAC accreditation into their regulatory structures.

PURCHASER REQUIREMENTS AND DEMANDS

Both private and public purchasers have the ability to encourage health care organizations and providers to pursue continuous improvements in patient safety. Large group purchasers, such as Fortune 500 companies or the Health Care Financing Administration, and purchasing coalitions that provide insurance to large numbers of people are well positioned to exert considerable leverage in the marketplace.

PRIVATE GROUP PURCHASERS

There are numerous examples of large private employers that incorporate quality issues into their decision-making process when selecting health plans and providers to offer to employees.[6] Xerox Corporation ranks health plans according to various quality indicators, including accreditation status, satisfaction ratings, and quality indicators. ARCO evaluates health plans based on 50 different quality and access criteria, and ties the employer contribution to the premium level of the highest-ranking plan. In a survey of 33 large purchasers in four states, 45 percent reported using HEDIS data (i.e., NCQA's Healthplan Employer Data and Information Set quality indicators), 55 percent reported using accreditation data, and 53 percent reported using consumer satisfaction survey data to choose a health plan.[7]

Although some large employers have incorporated quality considerations into their purchasing decisions, this is not the norm. A 1997 survey of 325 U.S. companies found that most employers consider provider network characteristics, but only a fraction consider quantifiable measures of access, quality or outcomes.[8] Another survey found that nearly two-thirds of midsize and large employers are unfamiliar with NCQA accreditation, the most widely used accreditation program for health plans.[9]

Clearly, there is much opportunity to for large employers to place greater emphasis on quality, and specifically patient safety, issues when making decisions to contract with a specific health plan and in the design of payment and financial incentive systems to reward demonstrated quality and safety improvements.

HEALTH CARE FINANCING ADMINISTRATION

As a major national purchaser of health care services, HCFA sets standards through payment policies and conditions of participation for the organizations with which it contracts. HCFA provides health insurance for 74 million people through Medicare, and in partnership with the states, Medicaid, and Child Health Insurance programs.[10] It also performs a number of quality-focused activities, including regulation of laboratory testing, surveys and certification, development of coverage policies, and quality improvement initiatives.

The peer review organizations (PROs) monitor the utilization and quality of care of Medicare beneficiaries through a state-based network.[11] They have three functions. First, they conduct cooperative quality improvement projects in partnership with other quality-focused organizations. Among the current projects are programs on diabetes, end-stage renal disease, influenza campaign, and quality improvement systems for managed care. Second, PROs conduct mandatory case review in response to beneficiary complaints, as well as educational and outreach activities. Third, they oversee program integrity by ensuring that Medicare pays only for medically necessary services. Patient safety has not been identified as a priority to date, however, HCFA is giving serious consideration to making patient safety a higher priority.[12]

Medicare and Medicaid survey and certification activities are aimed at ensuring that providers and suppliers for these programs meet health, safety, and program standards.[13] They deal with issues related to the effective and efficient delivery of care to beneficiaries, ensuring their safety while in health care facilities and improving their quality of care. HCFA relies on state health agencies as the principal agents to perform certification activities through their licensure activities. As already noted, state health departments, in turn, often rely on JCAHO as part of licensing a hospital.

STANDARDS FOR HEALTH PROFESSIONALS

Performance standards and expectations for health professionals may be defined through regulatory and other oversight processes, such as licensing, accreditation, and certification. Standards and expectations may also be shaped by professional societies and other groups that voluntarily promulgate guidelines or protocols and sponsor educational and convening activities.

LICENSING, CERTIFICATION AND ACCREDITATION

Compared to facility licensure (as discussed in the previous section) there is even greater variation found in professional licensure. There are several reasons for this. First, professional licensure is structured through individual licensing boards for each regulated profession in the state.[14] The result is variation both within states and across states. Within states, there is little coordination of management or dissemination of information among different boards.[15] Across states, there is variation in what is considered a complaint and in the rate at which disciplinary action is taken. Variation in what is considered a "complaint" influences what is investigated and what can be shared and when. A call to the licensing board may be considered a complaint, or a complaint may be recognized only when there is a formal charge. It is not clear, therefore, when information can be shared: when something is filed (which may or may not

lead to a charge), while it is being investigated, after there is a charge, or
only if disciplinary action is taken. Inconsistencies permit unsafe practitioners
to move to different jurisdictions before a complaint can be investigated and
handled.[16]

Although not a comprehensive measure of effectiveness, there is wide
variation in the rate at which state licensing boards take serious disciplinary
actions against physicians, ranging from 0.85 per 1,000 physicians in Louisiana
to 15.40 per 1,000 physicians in Alaska, based on data from the Federation
of State Medical Boards.[17] Across the country, the rate was 3.76 actions per
1,000 physicians in 1998. States that appeared to be doing a better job (more
disciplinary actions) tended to have better funding, and more staff, conducted
proactive investigations (as opposed to waiting for complaints), used other
available data (e.g., Medicare or Medicaid data), had good leadership, were
independent from state medical societies and other parts of state government,
and had a reasonable statutory framework for conducting their work. Board
action can also be quite slow. For example, the Virginia Board of Medicine
takes an average of more than two and a half years to resolve a case.[18]

The National Council of State Boards of Nursing has endorsed a mutual
recognition model for interstate nursing practice to encourage reciprocal arrangements between states for licensing and disciplinary action (Carolyn Hutch-
erson, National Council of State Boards of Nursing, personal communication,
June 1, 1999).[19] The goal would be to make licensure more like the rules used
for a driver's license. That is, licensure is recognized across state lines, but the
nurse would still be subject to the rules of a state while in that state (e.g., even
if a driver's residence is in Maryland, the driver can still get a speeding ticket
in Texas).

Another issue related to professional licensure is that there is no continuing
assessment or required demonstration of performance after initial licensure is
granted, except for physician assistants and emergency medical technicians.[20]
In general, the state is involved in initial licensure or follow-up of complaints;
processes for documenting continued competence are voluntary.

For example, physicians may voluntarily seek board certification through
one of 24 specialty medical boards that have been approved by the American
Board of Medical Specialties (ABMS).[21] The specialty boards set professional
and educational standards for the evaluation and certification of physician
specialists. Initial certification is granted by passing written and oral examinations. Recertification occurs at seven- to ten-year intervals, although not
all boards require recertification. Recertification is granted based on self-
assessment, examinations, and credentialing (e.g., unrestricted license, good
standing in practice, hospital privileges; Linda Blank, American Board of Internal Medicine, personal communication, May 18, 1999). A minimum number
of continuing education credits may also be required. At the present time,

there is no assessment of practice skills, although some specialty boards have committed a broader and more timely assessment of competence.[22]

Another voluntary approach is the American Medical Accreditation Program (AMAP), which is being developed by the American Medical Association. AMAP is a voluntary process, begun in 1998, for the accreditation of individual physicians that is designed to measure and evaluate individual physicians against national standards and peer performance.[23] The program will evaluate physicians in five areas: (1) credentials; (2) personal qualifications (including ethical behavior and participation in continuing medical education, peer reviews, and self-assessment of performance); (3) environment of care (including a site review of office operations and medical records); (4) clinical processes (including standardized measures of key patient care processes and comparative feedback to the physician); and (5) patient outcomes (including standardized measures of patient outcomes, perceptions of care, and health status). Although this is a national program, it is being implemented on a state-by-state basis.

A comparable process is found in nursing, which recognizes specialty practice through board certification. One such specialty certifying body is the American Nurses Credentialing Center (ANCC), a subsidiary of the American Nurses Association. Specialty certifying boards set professional and educational standards for the defined specialty and determine a mechanism for establishing continued competency through the recertification process, which occurs every three to five years, depending on the specialty. Although safety is not an explicit focus of certification exams, areas covered may relate to safety, for example, medication errors. Nurses may pursue certification voluntarily, although some states require it for licensure at advanced levels such as nurse practitioner (Ann Carey, R.N., American Nurses Credentialing Center, personal communication, July 20, 1999). Certifying organizations are exploring alternative ways to validate continued competency in addition to continuing education.

Health care organizations are also involved in assessing the continued performance of professionals when hiring nurses or credentialing physicians for hospital privileges, network membership, or employment. Again, there is little consistency in the standards used and little opportunity for communication across organizations. For example, an unsafe provider may be dismissed from one hospital, with no notification to the licensing board and limited ability for the next hospital to find out the reasons for the dismissal.

The Pew Health Professions Commission conducted an extensive investigation of licensure and continued competency issues. Its report identifies four places in which assessment of competency can occur: upon entry into practice, for continuing authorization to practice, reentry to practice, and after disciplinary action.[24] The report recommended increased state regulation to require health care practitioners to "demonstrate their competence in the knowledge, judgment, technical skills and interpersonal skills relevant to their jobs throughout their career." They note that considerations of competence should include not only the basic and specialized knowledge and skills, but also other skills such as "capacity to admit errors." In their view, the current system that relies on continuing education and disciplinary action after a problem has occurred is insufficient. The trend toward computer-based testing should facilitate greater attention to skill assessment in the future. Physician licensure tests and physician recertification are moving toward interactive, computer-based testing, and nursing is also testing a computerized system for initial licensure.[25]

THE ROLE OF HEALTH PROFESSIONAL SOCIETIES AND GROUPS

Professional societies, groups, and associations can play an important role in improving patient safety by contributing to the creation of a culture that encourages the identification and prevention of errors. Few professional societies or groups have demonstrated a visible commitment to reducing errors in health care and improving patient safety. Although it is believed that the commitment exists among their members, there has been little collective action. The exception most often cited is the work that has been done by anesthesiologists to improve safety and outcomes for patients.

Anesthesiology has successfully reduced anesthesia mortality rates from two deaths per 10,000 anesthetics administered to one death per 200,000–300,000 anesthetics administered. This success was accomplished through a combination of:

- technological changes (new monitoring equipment, standardization of existing equipment);
- information-based strategies, including the development and adoption of guidelines and standards;
- application of human factors to improve performance, such as the use of simulators for training;
- formation of the Anesthesia Patient Safety Foundation to bring together stakeholders from different disciplines (physicians, nurses, manufacturers) to create a focus for action; and
- having a leader who could serve as a champion for the cause.[26]

To explore the ways that professional societies could improve patient safety, the Institute of Medicine (IOM) convened a one-day workshop on September 9, 1999 with 14 health professionals representing medicine, nursing, and pharmacy (workshop participants are included in the acknowledgments). These leaders are interested and involved in issues related to patient safety and are active in professional societies, although they did not participate in the workshop as representatives of these societies. Four broad roles were identified that could be employed, individually or in combination, to create a culture of safety. These roles are: (1) defining standards of practice; (2) convening and collaborating among society members and with other groups; (3) encouraging research, training and education opportunities; and (4) advocating for change.

One way that professional societies contribute to standards of practice is through the promulgation and promotion of practice guidelines. A number of professional groups have produced practice guidelines and defined best practices in select areas. Guidelines produced by the American College of Cardiology (ACC) and the American Heart Association Task Force of Practice Guidelines are consistently cited models. They have produced sixteen guidelines ranging from coronary artery bypass graft (CABG) to management of chronic angina.[27]

Pharmacy has also devoted significant attention to patient safety. The American Society of Health-System Pharmacists (ASHP) has published extensively on safe medication practices. Reduction of medication errors has been an identified priority for a decade and is reflected through publications in professional and scientific journals, educational programming, and advocacy. Included among the standards and guidelines is a widely disseminated list of the top priority actions for preventing adverse drug events in hospitals.

Practice guidelines can also be written through a more interdisciplinary approach, such as the perinatal guidelines published jointly by the American College of Obstetricians and Gynecologists (ACOG) and the American Academy of Pediatrics. There is now a fourth edition of these guidelines. As recognition has grown that errors are caused by failures in systems, interdisciplinary collaboration may become increasingly necessary for redesigning complex systems of care. Participants at the workshop suggested that professional societies develop guidelines devoted specifically to patient safety and the incorporation of patient safety considerations into other guidelines.

One of the most visible activities of professional groups is their convening function. Through annual conferences and specialty meetings, professional groups can develop and communicate standards, values, and policy statements to membership and key opinion leaders. Meeting conclusions may also be disseminated through their own and other journal publications. There are few examples of specialty meetings or conferences where patient safety has been explicitly included on the agenda. Additionally, there are few interdisciplinary conferences devoted to issues of patient safety. Participants at the workshop proposed a national conference that would bring together all health professions and professionals from other disciplines (e.g., industrial engineering, human factors analysis) and other industries (e.g., airline pilots).

Clinical training and education is a key mechanism for cultural change. Colleges of medicine, nursing, pharmacy, health care administration, and their related associations should build more instruction into their curriculum on patient safety and its relationship to quality improvement. One of the challenges in accomplishing this is the pressure on clinical education programs to incorporate a broadening array of topics. Many believe that initial exposure to patient safety should occur early in undergraduate and graduate training programs, as well as through continuing education. Clinical training programs also need to ensure that teaching opportunities are safe for patients. One workshop participant told of a monitoring device used to alert staff to possible problems with the patient that was turned off because it was seen as interfering with the teaching experience.

The need for more opportunities for interdisciplinary training was also identified. Most care delivered today is done by teams of people, yet training often remains focused on individual responsibilities, leaving practitioners inadequately prepared to enter complex settings. Improving patient safety also requires some understanding of systems theory in order to effectively analyze the many contributing factors that influence errors. Again, the "silos" created through training and organization of care impede safety improvements. Instruction in safety improvement requires knowledge about working in teams, using information and information technology, quality measurement, and communicating with patients about errors. A background in other disciplines is also relevant, such as cognitive psychology, systems theory, and statistics.[28] Principles of crew resource management used to train personnel who work together in airline cockpits might also be applicable to health care. Training should also emphasize better communications across disciplines. This is important when the members of a care team are in one physical location, such as a hospital or office setting, but becomes even more important when the care team may not be in one place, such as a team providing home care.

Few professional groups have sufficient resources to devote to research support, although many have established research and education foundations. The need for greater collaboration in developing regional databases was noted. A key advantage of establishing these at the regional level is the ability to obtain a sufficient number of cases for meaningful analysis. The number of cases of any particular event in a single hospital or clinical setting is usually too small to be able to generalize across cases and identify a way to make system improvements. Regional data systems can increase numbers to improve analytic power and can facilitate collaboration to understand the extent and nature of errors in health care. Professional societies and groups could participate in efforts to coordinate a research agenda and the development of databases to provide information on the extent and nature of errors in health care.

Professional groups can also serve as advocates for change. Professional groups have been able to call attention to a health risk and create awareness. For example, pediatricians have been active in promoting increased immunization rates, the American Heart Association has promoted diet and exercise to prevent heart disease, and the American Medical Association (AMA) has been an outspoken opponent against smoking. Professional groups have not been as visible in advocating for patient safety and communicating such concerns to the general public and policy makers. A notable exception has been the formation of the National Patient Safety Foundation (NPSF) by the AMA in 1997. The NSPF has taken a visible role in advocating for improvements in patient safety and communicating with a broad array of audiences. Professional societies can play a role not only in informing their members about patient safety, but also in calling attention to the issue among the general public.

Implementation of activities to increase the role of health professionals in patient safety must occur at multiple levels. Although some professional groups influence and communicate with just their own members, other groups have the potential to influence many audiences. For example, the American Board of Medical Specialties has the potential to influence 24 professional medical societies. The Accreditation Council for Graduate Medical Education and the American Association of Colleges of Nursing have the potential to influence numerous training programs. The Association of American Medical Colleges can influence multiple medical schools and academic medical centers. There are many other similar groups that coordinate across multiple organizations. These "high leverage" groups are critical players in encouraging action among their constituent organizations. They should use their influence to promote greater awareness of patient safety and to consistently reinforce its importance.

STANDARDS FOR DRUGS AND DEVICES

The Food and Drug Administration is a major force in setting standards for medical products and monitoring their safety. FDA regulates prescription and over-the-counter drugs, medical and radiation-emitting devices, and biologics, among other things. This discussion focuses on its activities related to drugs and devices. It should be noted, however, that the FDA regulates manufacturers, not health care organizations or professionals. There are two opportunities for FDA to ensure and enhance patient safety: during its approval process for drugs and devices, and through postmarketing surveillance.

FDA has regulatory authority over the naming, labeling, and packaging of drugs and medical devices. FDA approves a product when it judges that the benefits of using the product outweigh the risks for the intended population and use.[29] For drugs, the approval process examines evidence of the effectiveness of the drug and the safety of the drug when used as intended. For devices, FDA looks at the safety and effectiveness of the device compared to devices already on the market or else looks for reasonable assurance of safety and effectiveness.

A major component of postmarketing surveillance is conducted through adverse event reporting.[30] Reports may be submitted directly to the FDA or through MedWatch, FDA's reporting program. For medical devices, manufacturers are required to report deaths, serious injures, and malfunctions to FDA. User facilities (hospitals, nursing homes) are required to report deaths to both the manufacturer and FDA, and to report serious injuries to the manufacturer. For suspected adverse events associated with drugs, reporting is mandatory for manufacturers and voluntary for physicians, consumers, and others. All reports are entered into the Adverse Event Reporting System (AERS) or another database, which is used to identify problem areas or increased incidence of an event.

FDA receives approximately 235,000 reports annually for adverse drug events and approximately 80,000–85,000 reports on device problems. Despite the extensive testing that FDA requires before drugs and devices are approved, side effects or other problems invariably show up after they have been released and used widely. Not all risks are identified premarketing because study populations in premarketing trials are often too small to detect rare events, studies may not last long enough to detect some events, and study populations may be dissimilar from the general population.[31] Some of these initially unknown risks can be serious or even fatal. The problem is likely to continue and possibly worsen in the future because of the number of new drugs being introduced. In 1998 alone, FDA approved 90 new drugs, 30 new molecular entities (drugs that have never been marketed in this country before), 124 new or expanded uses of already approved drugs, 344 generic drugs, 8 over-the-counter drugs, and 9 orphan drugs, or almost two actions every day of the year.[32] Approximately 48 percent of the prescription drugs on the market today have become available only since 1990.[33] Medications are also the most frequent medical intervention, with an average of 11 prescriptions per person in the United States.[34]

FDA has three general strategies it pursues for corrective action. The first (and most commonly pursued) is negotiation with the manufacturer to make the desired changes. The extent of cooperation from the manufacturers can vary. In terms of drugs, names are the most difficult to change, particularly once a name has been trademarked by the company (OPDRA, personal communication, May 4, 1999). Second, FDA may take regulatory action against manufacturers to require changes. This could include name changes or withdrawal of a product from the market. The final type of action that FDA can take is communication about risks, including letters to physicians, pharmacists, and other health professionals, postings on the Internet, and publication of clinical and consumer journals. FDA decisions about corrective action are made on a case-by-case basis, by considering the unexpectedness and seriousness of the event, the vulnerability of the population affected, and the preventability of the event.[35]

Some concerns have been expressed over the responsiveness of FDA to reported problems. Concerns have related to the timeliness and effectiveness of the agency's response or that the response to a given problem may not be strong enough given its seriousness. For example, five drugs were removed from the market in between September 1997 and September 1998, but almost 20 million people had been exposed to their risks before they were removed.[36] Terfenadine was on the market for 12 years, even though researchers earlier identified it as causing deaths; it was removed from the market by the manufacturer only after a substitute was developed.[37]

There have been calls for better methods for obtaining more information about the harm caused by drugs (e.g., greater use of active surveillance systems that look for indicators of problems rather than waiting for reports to be submitted) or for the establishment of an independent drug safety review board.[38] In the fall of 1998, FDA changed the process for follow-up on reported drug problems with the creation of a new Office of Post-Marketing Drug Risk Assessment (OPDRA). Before, incidents were reviewed by a committee, triaged, and sent back to the division that did the original review. This dispersed responsibility for review and follow-up led to variability in response. Now, OPDRA will conduct an analysis of all reported events and develop recommendations that are sent to the manufacturer and the director of the FDA division that conducted the original review. The division director must report to OPDRA in 60 days on the status of the recommendations. OPDRA estimates that approximately half of the causal factors that contribute to adverse events are issues to which it can respond (e.g., labeling problems); the remainder are outside its scope (e.g., bad handwriting) (Jerry Phillips, OPDRA, personal communication, May 4, 1999).

With regard to medical devices, in recent years, FDA has increased its requirements and guidance to manufacturers on designing devices to take into account human factors principles and user testing. Attention to human factors could improve simplicity of use, standardization of controls, and default to a safe setting during failure (e.g., loss of power). For example, intravenous infusion pumps vary markedly in their mode of operation and types of controls. Because they are expensive, hospitals do not replace old pumps when new ones become available, which result in different models being used. The lack of standardization among the models increases the likelihood of error when the pump is set up. Controls on defibrillators can also vary in position, appearance, and function on different machines, leading to errors when they are used rapidly in emergency situations. Although the increased attention to human factors principles does not affect devices already on the market, over time it is expected that manufacturers will become more accustomed to using human factors in the design of medical devices.

With the passage of the Safe Medical Device Act of 1990, FDA was granted the authority to require manufacturers of medical devices to establish and follow procedures for ensuring that device design addressed the intended use of the device and its users.[39] Final rules for this act became effective in June 1997. FDA has continued to emphasize to manufacturers the importance of human factors and is expected to issue a manual of engineering and design guidelines for manufacturers in 1999.

In terms of drugs, the use of human factors principles could reduce confusion of medications that occur because of brand names that look alike or sound alike, labels that are hard to read, and look-alike packaging. Wrong doses also occur frequently because of factors such as the lack of standardized terms in the display of contents. For example, contents displayed by concentration (e.g., 10 mg/mL) rather than total amount (e.g., 100 mg) can result in an overdose. There may also be inconsistent placement of warnings on a label or inconsistent use of abbreviations. Most recently, more than 100 errors have been reported in the use of Celebrex (prescribed for arthritis) and its confusion with Cerebyx (an antiseizure medication) and Celexa (an antidepressant).[40] FDA does not have guidance for using human factors principles in the packaging, labeling, or naming of drugs as exists relative to medical devices.

SUMMARY

The main sources of standards for health care organizations and professionals today are through licensing and accreditation processes. However, medical errors and patient safety are not an explicit focus of licensing and accreditation. Although licensing and accreditation standards do speak to the characteristics of quality improvement programs, and patient safety and error reduction may be part of these programs, many licensed and fully accredited organizations have yet to implement the most rudimentary systems and processes to ensure patient safety. Furthermore, the extent of variation in licensure within and across states suggests that there is no reliable assurance of safety to patients, even for those facilities and professionals covered under current rules.

Although current standard-setting authorities in health care are not devoting adequate attention to patient safety issues, the committee considered and rejected the option of recommending the creation of yet another regulatory authority. The recommendations contained in this chapter direct the existing regulatory structures to increase attention to patient safety issues. Licensing agencies and accrediting organizations have to hold health care organizations accountable for creating and maintaining safe environments. Professional licensing bodies should consider continuing qualifications over a lifetime of practice, not just at initial licensure. Standards for approving drugs and devices must consider safety for patients in actual use and real-life settings, not just safe production.

The actions of professional groups and group purchasers in setting standards and expectations are also critical. Professional groups shape professional behavior by developing practice guidelines and identifying best practices and through educational, convening and advocacy activities. All could be enhanced by a sharper focus on patient safety issues. Group purchasers have the ability to consider safety issues in their contracting decisions, and to reinforce the importance of safety by providing relevant information to employees and beneficiaries.

REFERENCES

1. Institute of Medicine, *Clinical Practice Guidelines: Directions for a New Program,* eds. Marilyn J. Field and Kathleen N. Lohr, Washington, D.C.: National Academy Press, 1990.

2. "All About OSHA," OSHA 2056 1995 (revised), Occupational Safety and Health Administration, Department of Labor, www.osha.gov.

3. *"Joint Commission Accreditation,"* http://www.jcaho.org/whoweare_frm.html.

4. "NCQA Accreditation," *Business and Health,* 17(1):21 (January, 1999).

5. "About URAC," http://www.urac.org.

6. General Accounting Office. *Private Health Insurance: Continued Erosion of Coverage Linked to Cost Pressures.* GAO/HEHS 97-122. Washington, DC: July 1997b.

7. Hibbard, Judith H.; Jewett, Jacquelyn J.; Legnini, Mark W., et al. Choosing a Health Plan: Do Large Employers Use the Data. *Health Affairs.* 16(6):172–180, 1997.

8. Washington Business Group on Health and Watson Wyatt Worldwide. *Getting What You Pay For—Purchasing Value in Health Care.* Bethesda, MD: Watson Wyatt Worldwide, 1997.

9. KPMG Peat Marwick. *Health Benefits in 1997.* Montvale, NJ: 1997.

10. http://www.hcfa.gov.

11. "Quality of Care Information, HCFA Contractors, Peer Review Organizations," http://www.hcfa.gov/qlty-56.htm, last updated July 26, 1999.

12. Timothy Cuerdon, Office of Clinical Standards and Quality, Health Care Financing Administration, Testimony to the IOM Subcommittee on Creating an External Environment for Quality, June 15, 1999.

13. "Medicare and Medicaid Survey and Certification," http://www.hcfa.gov/medicaid/scindex.htm.

14. O'Neil, Edward H., and the Pew Health Professions Commission, San Francisco, CA: Pew Health Professions Commission, December, 1998.

15. Finocchio, Leonard J.; Dower, Catherine M., Blick, Noelle T., et al., *Strengthening Consumer Protection: Priorities for Health Care Workforce Regulation,* San Francisco, CA; Pew Health Professions Commission, October, 1998.

16. *Maintaining State-Based Licensure and Discipline: A Blueprint for Uniform and Effective Regulation of the Medical Profession,* Federation of State Medical Boards of the United States, Inc., 1998. http://www.fsmb.org.

17. Sidney M. Wolfe, "Public Citizen's Health Research Group Ranking of State

Medical Boards' Serious Disciplinary Actions in 1998," April, 1999, http://www.citizen.org. Serious disciplinary actions include revocations, surrenders, suspensions and probations/restrictions on licensure.

18. Timberg, Craig, "Virginia's Physician Discipline Board Too Slow to Act, Audit Finds," Washington Post, June 15, 1999, p. A20.

19. Finocchio, Dower, Blick et al., 1998.

20. Finocchio, Dower, Blick, et al., 1998.

21. "What Is ABMS?" http://www.abms.org/purpose.html.

22. Prager, Linda O. Upping the Certification Ante. *American Medical News,* 42(21):1, 1999. Also, American Board of Internal Medicine, *Continuing Professional Development.* September, 1999. See also Norcini, John J., "Computer-Based Testing Will Soon Be A Reality," *Perspective,* American Board of Internal Medicine, Summer, 1999, p.3.

23. "A Definition," http//www.ama-assn.org/med-sci/amapsite/about/defme.htm.

24. Finocchio, Dower, Blick, et al., 1998.

25. *Computerized Clinical Simulation Testing (CST),* National Council of State Boards of Nursing, Inc., 1999. http://www.ncsbn.org.

26. Pierce, Ellison C. The 34th Rovenstine Lecture, 40 Years Behind the Mask: Safety Revisited. *Anesthesiology.* 87(4):965–975, 1996.

27. http://www.acc.org/clinical/guidelines.

28. President's Commission on Consumer Protection and Quality in Health Care. *Quality First: Better Health Care For All Americans.* Final Report to the President of the United States, March, 1997.

29. Food and Drug Administration, "Managing the Risks From Medical Product Use, Creating a Risk Management Framework," Executive Summary, Report to the FDA Commissioner from the Task Force on Risk Management, May, 1999.

30. Additional strategies include field investigations, epidemiological studies, and other focused studies.

31. Food and Drug Administration, "Managing the Risks From Medical Product Use, Creating a Risk Management Framework," Report to the FDA Commissioner from the Task Force on Risk Management, U. S. Department of Health and Human Services, May, 1999.

32. Food and Drug Administration, "Improving Public Health Through Human Drugs," CDER 1998 Report to the Nation, Center for Drug Evaluation and Research, USDHHS.

33. Shatin, Deborah; Gardner, Jacqueline; Stergachis, Andy; letter. *JAMA.* 281(4): 319–20, 1999.

34. Friedman, Michael A.; Woodcock, Janet; Lumpkin, Murray M., et al. The Safety of Newly Approved Medicines, Do Recent Market Removals Mean There is a Problem? *JAMA.* 281(18):1728–1934, 1999.

35. Food and Drug Administration, Managing the Risks From Medical Product Use, Creating a Risk Management Framework. Report to the FDA Commissioner from

the Task Force on Risk Management, U. S. Department of Health and Human Services, May, 1999.

36. Friedman, Woodcock, Lumpkin, et al, 1999. Also Wood, Alastair J.J. The Safety of New Medicines. *JAMA.* 281(18):1753–4, 1999.

37. Moore, Thomas J: Psaty, Bruce M; Furberg, Curt D. Time to Act on Drug Safety. *JAMA,* 279(19):1571–1573, 1998.

38. Moore, Psaty, and Furberg, 1998. See also Wood, Alastair J.J. and Woosely, Raymond. Making Medicine Safer, The Need for an Independent Drug Safety Review Board. *N Engl J Med,* 339(25):1851–1853, 1998.

39. Weinger, Matthew, Pantiskas, Carl; Wiklund, Michael, et al. Incorporating Human Factors Into the Design of Medical Devices. *JAMA.* 280(17):1484, 1998.

40. Look Alike/Sound Alike Drug Names, Ambiguous or Look-Alike Labeling and Packaging. ISMP Quarterly Action Agenda: April–June, 1999, ISMP Medication Safety Alert, July 14, 1999. Institute for Safe Medication Practices, Pennsylvania.

| 11 | Error in Medicine: Legal Impediments to U.S. Reform |

Bryan A. Liang

Errors in medicine are common (Leape 1994; Brennan et al. 1994). Other similarly complex systems, such as aviation and nuclear power, have experienced these levels of error, and efforts to mitigate them have been successful (Kinkade 1988; Maurino, Reason, and Lee 1995; U.S. Nuclear Regulatory Commission 1981). Recognizing this, groups such as the Anesthesia Patient Safety Foundation (APSF), and, more recently, the National Patient Safety Foundation (NPSF), have embarked on large-scale attempts to reduce human error in medicine and thereby increase patient safety in the health delivery system.

However, in addition to considering how medical error occurs and constructing theoretical modes of intervention to reduce it, understanding important legal principles and physician behavior under the law's incentives and obligations is also essential. Such an understanding can help ensure that frontline, community physicians, rather than only academic and other physicians already engaged in this research, will participate in this important work, have knowledge of its results, and implement its findings. Without attention to legal considerations, error reduction research may be left unutilized by the broader medical community, regardless of demonstrated efficacy or efficiency.

Up to this point, the legal system has been seen by providers as an opponent rather than a partner in efforts to reduce medical error. Reassessing the system and its effect on providers may identify a more effective approach using a

Reprinted from *Journal of Health Politics, Policy and Law,* 24, no. 1 (February 1999): 27–58. Copyright 1999. Duke University Press. All rights reserved. Reprinted with permission.

A version of this article was presented at Health and Risk: An International Symposium, a conference at St. Catherine's College, Oxford University, held from 29 June to 1 July 1998.

medical-legal partnership to fulfill the goal of efficiently minimizing patient injury in the health care system.

A PARADIGM OF REDUCING ERROR

Complex systems have a high potential for error. Generally, these errors are a result of several common characteristics that they share: high-level technical requirements, the need for quick reaction times, twenty-four-hour-a-day operations, team coordination in the context of long hours, trade-offs between service and safety, and the fact that only a small fraction of errors leads to adverse events (Foushee and Helmreich 1988; Helmreich 1984; Lauber and Kayten 1988; Maurino, Reason, and Lee 1995; Reason 1990). Indeed, these complex systems, although they provide for a high level of service and tremendous social benefit, also highlight the potential for human error because "no matter how professional they might be, no matter their care and concern, humans can never outperform the system which bounds and constrains them" (Maurino, Reason, and Lee 1995: 83).

Pioneering work in human error research has identified the critical cognitive processes involved in error generation. Briefly, errors arise from two major sources: unintentional actions in the performance of routinized tasks and mistakes in judgment or inadequate plans of action (Reason 1990). The role of humans in this error-generating process appears to be based on active failures, that is, errors and violations of rules, and managerial, or latent, errors, that is, those focused on the organizational or systemic process. Latent errors—those entwined with the design and structure of complex systems—are considered to be the most dangerous types of cognitive failures that lead to human error (Reason 1990).

Successful error reduction in complex systems has taken advantage of the systems nature of error, which allows for interventions reactively to an adverse event and proactively to prevent recurrence (Maurino, Reason, and Lee 1995). The two outstanding instances of this success are the aviation and nuclear power industries. The systems approach for reducing human error in these complex systems can be seen as a continuous process involving several integral stages with the underlying goal of preventing errors ex ante. The stages of this error reduction paradigm are in-process detection, process change/design, and process reassessment. These stages loop continuously for every detected error and intervention.

The foundation of the aviation industry's success is its reporting and analysis system. Indeed, one of the most highly touted error reduction methodologies of any complex industry is the Aviation Safety Reporting Program, which produced the Aviation Safety Reporting System (ASRS). ASRS was created in 1976 in reaction to a TWA crash in 1974 and a near miss by a United Airlines plane six weeks later. The ASRS allows pilots, flight attendants, mechanics, and air traffic controllers to confidentially report incidents that they believe may lead to accidents, including near-miss situations in which no adverse event resulted but human error occurred. Each report to the ASRS is read and assessed for safety hazard implications and analyzed to allow affirmative steps to be taken to remedy the problem (Dornheim 1996). ASRS has been extremely effective: over 300,000 reports have been made since its inception, with no confidentiality breach for reporters. More than 200 issues of the ASRS publication *Callback* have been published reporting safety information trends, and 2,500 ASRS safety alert bulletins have been issued. In addition, at least ninety ASRS "quick response" analyses for specific safety issues and more than ninety detailed, safety-related research studies have been published by the ASRS staff (Gilbert 1996). Further, ASRS allows for external research access, with ASRS staff responding to at least 4,600 requests for data (Gilbert 1996); this access has been extended by the recent release of the ASRS data set on the Internet (ASRS Incident Reports 1998) as well as in CD-ROM format (ASRS on CD-ROM 1995).

Beyond analyzing dramatic events that have led or may lead to injury due to human error, ASRS analysis has also been useful in monitoring and assessing routinized activities to prevent future accidents. For example, although analysis of ASRS data has shown that flight simulations of significant aircraft malfunctions were successful in training crews to both follow appropriate procedures and coordinate communications efforts effectively, these high-level benefits fall off when less significant stressor events are simulated. This information has resulted in recommendations that airlines and other flight simulation organizations upgrade simulation activities in crew resource management training to include less serious malfunction scenarios (Gilbert 1996). Thus, the ASRS system has resulted in detection and continuous analysis of important and subtle systemic patterns that have led to significant safety intervention programs and reforms in aviation (Moore 1998).

Similarly, the nuclear power industry has been able to take advantage of a systems analysis and approach to reduce error. After the Three Mile Island accident, the presidentially appointed Kemeny Commission was formed to investigate and recommend changes in the industry to reduce error and adverse events. The Kemeny Commission recommended that the industry establish and enforce standards for operations with regard to nuclear power plants. In response, the industry established the Institute for Nuclear Power Operations (INPO), which in turn promulgated training regulations for nuclear power personnel (Nuclear Energy Institute 1998). These training efforts include the regular use of control room simulators, a tenfold increase in professional training personnel, and an eightfold increase in nuclear system space devoted exclusively to nuclear power training. As part of the continuous training process, regular meetings are scheduled to assess how process changes have affected the control room operations, whether these interventions have introduced any other sources of human error, and whether there are other process changes that could improve the system (Kinkade 1988; Serig 1996; U.S. Nuclear Regulatory Commission 1981). These efforts have resulted in the improved performance of nuclear power plants in *both* safety and energy output. For example, the average number of unplanned automatic shutdowns due to potentially dangerous conditions was 7.3 in 1980; in 1996, eleven years after INPO began operations, this number was reduced to .8. During this same period, the power capability rose from 62.7 percent to 82.5 percent, equivalent to adding sixteen nuclear units for power use (Nuclear Energy Institute 1998). Thus, through a systems approach using continuous evaluation and feedback, the nuclear power industry has reduced error and improved function in its energy-generating capacity.

This approach has also been demonstrated in medicine in certain specialties, such as anesthesia (Cooper, Newbower, and Kitz 1984; Gaba and DeAnda 1988; Schwid and O'Donnell 1992). For example, efforts to reduce human error in anesthesia have included ex ante prevention through simulator training; in-process error detection through checks during surgery using electronic and human monitoring systems; error analysis through assessment of human factors that may have contributed to reported and identified errors; design changes through an alteration of both simulator training and monitoring in response to this analysis; and reassessment of this changed process by determining whether the identified error has been minimized and, just as important, by determining if any new sources of error have been created. However, although these efforts have significant promise, these activities in medicine are currently on a smaller scale and certainly have not achieved the level of an established industry standard for continuous safety and monitoring, as in the aviation and nuclear power industries.

Thus, there are established systems methods that would be beneficial for medicine and that would promote the related goals of reducing error in medicine and improving patient safety. However, at critical points, legal difficulties could reduce participation in research on medical error and implementation of its findings and thus stop the error reduction process before it has begun.

LEGAL SYSTEM

The legal system defines theoretically the socially acceptable level of human error that leads to patient injury and thus plays an important role in shaping behavior (Moray 1994). Further, apart from specific statutory requirements that dictate how much care is to be provided (e.g., mandated postpartum hospital stays), the legal system theoretically supplies a personal incentive for each physician to act to minimize patient injury (Liang 1996). Thus, the actual function of law and the responsibilities imposed by its doctrines can significantly affect efforts to reduce error in medicine.

TORT LAW CONSIDERATIONS

Clearly one component of the legal system that has a tremendous impact on providers is the tort system. The tort system is the longest running legal deterrence structure applied to medical practice. Understanding its function and effect on physicians can provide some guidance in designing an effective and efficient system that can induce providers to change their behavior appropriately and incorporate error-reducing activities into their clinical practice. Beyond this, an understanding of how physicians react to the tort system is of paramount importance in error-reduction activities, since potential legal liability often overrides any other incentives to reduce error.

At the outset, it appears that the malpractice tort system has a significant, self-reported effect upon practicing physicians, who believe it alters their behavior in rendering clinical care (American Medical Association 1985; Charles, Wilbert, and Frankie 1985; Havighurst 1991; Kapp 1996; Lawthers et al. 1992; U.S. OTA 1994; Shapiro et at. 1989; Weisman et at. 1989). Investigating and understanding this potential legally based behavior alteration is essential because the reasons underlying it may also block attempts to research and implement error reduction and error-reducing activities (Kapp 1997; Moray 1994).

The effects of the tort system on physician behavior are complex, and the empirical data conflict. On the one hand, it has been reported that the legal system has minimal impact on how physicians actually practice and that defensive medicine responses (i.e., increased or decreased care provided due to malpractice concerns) are limited. For example, Glassman et al. (1996) report that on the basis of responses to case scenarios and claims history, a physician's personal malpractice experience is not related to defensive clinical practice. In malpractice case scenarios designed to elicit a potential positive defensive medicine response (i.e., cases that had the potential to induce additional tests or procedures), physician management and testing recommendations did not vary between physicians who had a significant malpractice history and those who did not. Similarly, defensive medicine actions did not seem predominant in a study of the use of low-osmolar contrast agents (Jacobson and Rosenquist 1996). In this case study, the authors found that physician actions relating to the use of the marginally safer but much more expensive low-osmolar contrast material were based more on clinical appropriateness and less on legal concerns. Somewhat in the middle, the Office of Technology Assessment (OTA) concluded that the incidence of defensive medicine is overstated, while still reporting that between 4.9 and 29 percent of physicians order a particular test or procedure primarily (but not necessarily solely) for malpractice reasons (Klingman et al. 1996; U.S. OTA 1994).

However, the conclusion that the malpractice system does not affect physicians and that medical appropriateness rather than the legal system seems to be the motivating factor for clinical behavior (Jacobson and Rosenquist 1996; Klingman et al. 1996; U.S. OTA 1994) is somewhat specious. Generally, all medical tests provide some relevant clinical information; this factor and physician responses indicating that legal considerations are not the sole or primary reason for a particular clinical action, then, should not imply that physicians are not substantively affected by the legal system. Indeed, medical appropriateness as determined by respondent physicians may now take into account what is legally defensible in the "collective anxiety" of physicians in medical practice (Glassman et al. 1996). As well, clinical factors such as patient safety and comfort (e.g., Jacobson and Rosenquist 1996) may not simply be medical appropriateness issues but should be considered legal ones, because physicians may act to ensure a low probability of an adverse patient event and/or a high level of comfort in an effort to avoid a malpractice suit. In any event, even assuming that the legal system has no effect on the behavior of physicians and other providers, this conclusion highlights the possibility that perhaps its resources might he better allocated to a system that does in fact change physician behavior to minimize patient injury on the basis of data from relevant patient safety studies.

In addition to case study assessments of the factors involved in clinical care activities, other empirical research on the medical malpractice tort system has shown that physicians, who have a strong incentive to learn about the system, have incomplete (and in fact affirmatively incorrect) knowledge of its rules and dictates (Liang 1996, 1997a). These legal misperceptions can lead directly to the practice of both positive and negative defensive medicine, paradoxically increasing the risk of patient injury. For example, if physicians believe that an act of omission will result in malpractice liability, as has been reported by Liang (1996), these physicians may act so that they can never be accused of an act of omission. They will, for example, order excessive tests and procedures, a classic form of positive defensive medicine. Of course, this additional care is not without cost; beyond the pecuniary costs of care, there are the nonpecuniary costs associated with the risk of patients incurring iatrogenic injury, regardless of the "best" method of practice that would minimize patient injury. On the other hand, if physicians believe that a poor outcome is enough to sustain malpractice liability (Liang 1996), they may simply forgo providing the service (e.g., obstetricians-gynecologists deciding not to provide obstetrical care after being sued [Sloan et al. 1989]), or act to limit exposure by performing a potentially less risky procedure (Localio et al. 1993). This negative defensive medicine thus creates access costs for the patient and, again, an increased risk of injury. Consequently, it appears that physicians may act to avoid potential liability by subjecting patients to additional care with additional risks of harm on the basis of their legal misperceptions or by forgoing the provision of care altogether (Liang 1997a), irrespective of the actual rule of law and, potentially, what the results of error reduction research would indicate to be appropriate.

Hence, even in the face of personal liability and the greatest pecuniary risk of loss affecting their practices, physicians are still not well informed about the tort system and its rules and may not act to minimize patient injury. Learning about and implementing error reduction strategies, areas that may not command as much attention from the community physician, may be subject to a similar fate if the reasons underlying physicians' limited knowledge of tort law and their actions in response to it are not assessed.

Beyond physicians' misperceptions of the formal tort system rules, it has also been reported that neutral physicians do not appear to evaluate the actions of defendant physicians in actual malpractice cases as juries do and that they disagree significantly with jury verdicts (Cheney et al. 1989; Liang 1996, 1997a). Indeed, nonphysicians with no medical or legal knowledge have assessed these same cases as well as or better than physicians (Liang 1997a). Generally, nonphysicians would be expected to do poorly and certainly worse than physicians, who have knowledge of medical appropiateness through their clinical training. Thus, exacerbating the independent problem of physician ignorance of legal rules, medical knowledge alone may not assist physicians in understanding what kind of error is culpable in the legal system and what kind is not, again leading to misperceptions that may drive behavior in directions that do not minimize patient injury or take advantage of the results of error reduction research.

Furthermore, in malpractice cases with uncertain or contradictory clinical data, it has been reported that when physicians and nonphysicians were asked to guess jury verdicts, physicians have continued to do poorly, only guessing correctly approximately half the time; however, nonphysicians guessed these verdicts almost perfectly and their guesses are reported to have been statistically identical with actual juries' verdicts (Liang 1997a). These findings raise the possibility that juries composed of laypersons may assess liability on some basis other than or in addition to the legal standard of medical appropriateness, or that they simply misunderstand the law (Charrow and Charrow 1979; Ellsworth 1989; Elwork, Sales, and Alfin 1977; Forston 1975; Hastie, Penrod, and Pennington 1983; Kagehiro 1990; Reifman, Gusiek, and Ellsworth 1992; Strawn and Buchanan 1976).

These findings have significant implications for how error reduction activities will be viewed by the lay agents of the legal system. If the lay agents of the legal system assess physician behavior differently from the way legal rules dictate (for example, by assigning negligence simply on the basis of the presence or severity of patient injury [Brennan, Sox, and Burstin 1996]), physicians will act in accordance with their understanding of that assessment, whatever error reduction research indicates is best. This effect will tend to retard participation in and adoption of appropriate error reduction activities by physicians. Overall, both physician misunderstanding of the tort system and the tort system's function in practice raise significant issues that must be addressed before medical error reduction research can be effectively implemented.

In further clinical assessments, when neutral physicians review malpractice insurance claims of negligence, it appears that there is significant disagreement between them as to relative provider negligence. Cheney et al. (1989) found that in reviewing charts provided by insurance claims records (including jury verdict damages and settlements) although approximately 80 percent of patients provided with "inappropriate" (i.e., negligent) care received payment, over 40 percent of patients who were deemed to have been provided with appropriate, nonnegligent care also received payment. Assuming a single standard of negligence, this 40+ percent error rate for nonnegligent care seems quite high.

Sloan and Hsieh (1990) have also performed an empirical analysis of malpractice, focusing on predictors of payment based in part on physician reviews. They found that claims are generally paid when the defendant physician appears liable according to physician experts who evaluated the cases. However, they also found that the probability of a patient winning at trial was significantly related to the severity of injury; indeed, severity accounted for up to 40 percent of the variation in payments (Sloan and Hsieh 1990: 1025). Yet this result may raise the question of whether the legal rule of negligence has been appropriately applied; unless there is a significant bias for negligence and a high level of severity of injury, jury and settlement awards should not necessarily be correlated with severity. Similarly, Daniels and Andrews (1989) found that in assessing obstetrical eases, "success" rates (i.e., rates for plaintiff wins) were somewhat higher in obstetrical malpractice cases compared with malpractice cases generally (note that this study did not attempt to determine if the care provided was in fact negligent). Further, success rates were related to the class of injury, with high award classes of injury involving labor and delivery and cancer having both high success rates and high injury severity, including permanent injury and death (Daniels and Andrews 1989). Again, however, the issue for the malpractice system is simply whether there was negligence—that is, did a breach of a preexisting duty cause injury or death (Epstein 1990: 128; Keeton et al. 1984: 164–165)? The degree of plaintiff success should not depend on progressive harshness or type of injury, particularly in studies that assess both settlements and trials. These results again may indicate that the malpractice system is not functioning according to its own rule of negligence; perhaps the system is looking simply at causation in these cases (Calfee and Craswell 1984: 987 n. 50). Furthermore, it bears noting that high award amounts may simply be a function of the medical specialty involved rather than the presence of negligence (Liang 1996: 76 n. 43; Sloan et al. 1989).

In contrast, Vidmar (1995) has claimed that the tort system for medical malpractice functions well. He indicates that "juries do not favor claimants over doctors . . . based on . . . the severity of patient injuries. In fact, their verdicts are remarkably consistent with doctors' ratings of negligence" (Vidmar 1995: 265). However, the complexity of the tort system's function is evident here. In addition to studies that seem to show severity effects (Daniels and Andrews 1989; Sloan and Hsieh 1990), Brennan, Sox, and Burstin (1996), using data from the Harvard Medical Practice Study, concluded that severity of injury is the only factor predicting payment of a malpractice award; damage payments were unrelated to the negligence of the treating physician, or, in fact, to the presence of an adverse event or an adverse event due to negligence. Further, Vidmar's claim (1995) that there is no systematic evidence that juries grant higher damages for similar injuries due to malpractice compared with other tort cases is also in conflict with other work, which finds that malpractice cases do result in higher damage awards (Bovbjerg et al. 1991).

Complicating matters further, there are other difficulties beyond data conflict in much of the empirical work in medical malpractice. Most empirical studies of malpractice implicitly assume that there is a single acceptable standard of clinical care (Cheney et al. 1989; Brennan, Sox, and Burstin 1996; Sloan and Hsieh 1990; Vidmar 1995). However, when neutral physicians have assessed clinical case scenarios, there is significant discordance between evaluating physicians as to the relative negligence of the defendant physicians in each case (Liang 1996, 1997a; Localio et al. 1996; Posner, Caplan, and Cheney 1996). Thus, although each physician may fervently believe that there is a single standard of care, there is significant disagreement between physicians as to what that standard should be. This variability phenomena is common in medicine (see, for example, Eisenberg 1986; Liang, Austin, and Alderson 1991; Wennberg and Gittlesohn 1982). In addition, there is a further difficulty: variations in clinical care are not to be considered negligent even if a majority of physicians deem them so; as long as the practitioner follows a school of thought to which a "respectable minority" of practitioners adhere, the provider is not negligent (Keeton et al. 1984: 187). Hence the tort system may once again not be following its own rules when assessing the actions of physicians and other providers in tort and may not be inducing optimal provider behavior.

Highlighting these concerns, research in the psychology literature has indicated that assessment of medically related injury is extremely subject to hindsight bias (Kamin and Rachlinski 1995; LaBine and LaBine 1996). Studies that utilize expert reviewers ex post (Brennan, Sox, and Burstin 1996; Cheney et al. 1989; Liang 1996, 1997a; Sloan and Hsieh 1990; Vidmar 1995) thus are directly subject to this difficulty. Consequently, beyond a misunderstanding of the legal rules by physicians and/or inappropriate application of them by juries, ex post patient and physician perception of error may itself bias research efforts to understand physician actions and reduce human error (Caplan, Posner, and Cheney 1991; Hawkins and Hastie 1990; Hoch and Loewenstein 1989). And again, physicians may act on the basis of these erroneous perceptions, even though they are contrary to effectiveness or efficiency studies relating to error reduction.

Education may be a positive approach in correcting tort misperceptions and the activities so generated. An obvious problem, however, is that it is difficult to imagine how busy physicians and/or medical students would have the time to substantively learn legal rules from nonmedical sources (Liang 1996, 1997a), particularly since medical school curricula do not generally include this information. Further, on a risk management level, it has been reported that active medically based efforts to reduce legal liability and patient injury through risk management seminars have only a limited effect on office-based physicians (Frisch et al. 1996). Indeed, in an interesting complement to the study of Glassman et al. (1996), these seminars appear to provide no beneficial effect for physicians who have not had a claim made against them, and, in fact, risk management efforts may have a *negative* effect on these physicians—that is, those who participate have a *higher* probability of incurring a malpractice suit (Frisch et at. 1996). These results may indicate that current "medical" efforts to educate providers about "legal" information regarding the tort system may be ineffective, and even detrimental, in efforts to reduce human error and patient injury. Clearly, these communication approaches must be studied in more detail to avoid similar results when communicating patient safety error reduction paradigms.

Clinical practice guidelines may also be an effective approach in assisting clinical and patient safety efforts in the context of the tort system. However, there are difficulties with this methodology. First, clinical practice guidelines are not recognized legally as the standard of care in a medical malpractice suit (Anderson, Hall, and Steinberg 1993; Brennan 1991). Second, clinical practice guidelines are not appropriate for setting the standard of care for the current state of medical practice. These guidelines reflect the uncertainty regarding outcomes for particular practice methodologies and are limited by the agenda of the source from which they emanate (U.S. GAO 1991). Certainly, since most guidelines are arrived at by consensus processes rather than by the gold standard of the double-blind study, they are significantly influenced by the value judgments of those whose consensus is being assessed and thus would be expected to vary considerably (Hong and Liang 1996). Third, these guidelines, as well as related clinical outcomes measures, are weak because they inappropriately attempt to use population data to treat individual patients (Kelly and Liang 1997). Fourth, and finally, these guidelines may be outdated when they are published or soon thereafter (Hong and Liang 1996) and they are often manipulated by local physicians before acceptance (Hall and Dadakis 1996).

Thus, at present, there are significant and complex difficulties in assessing how physicians react to the malpractice system. Lack of an effect, too much of an effect, or a misdirected effect seem to indicate that the resources allocated to the tort system, a system "charged . . . to provide an optimal level of injury deterrence" (Sloan and Hsieh 1990: 997), may not prevent error in medicine or minimize patient injury (Brennan, Sox, and Burstin 1996). Further, because one of its other functions, providing patients with compensation, may not be functioning well due to the paucity of "negligently" injured patients being compensated (Weiler et al. 1993: 75 report that only one of sixteen valid negligence claims was paid), the billions of dollars spent annually (Weiler 1991) on the malpractice system may be better allocated elsewhere to more effectively and efficiently reduce medical error and patient injury.

LEGAL ISSUES IN ERROR REPORTING

Another potential source adversely affecting error reduction research is the law and its interface with the reporting process. Reporting errors is the first and most critical step in safety research and implementation so that problematic areas can be identified and addressed; indeed, this is a fundamental need for all error reduction systems (Lucas 1991: 134). But physicians with tort liability concerns may be hesitant to report adverse events and medical errors for fear that plaintiffs' attorneys will have access to this information, thus exposing physicians to liability. Under the current legal rules of discovery, this is a legitimate concern. Indeed, at the present time, only peer review/quality assurance committee proceedings enjoy some form of limited immunity from legal discovery (Cepelewicz et al. 1998; Frantz 1997). Although this privilege historically covers discovery in malpractice cases, it has been used in challenges to peer review staff privilege decisions (Cepelewicz et al. 1998: 588; Frantz 1997: 945).

At the outset, it should be noted that all privileges against discovery are to be construed very narrowly, as indicated by the Supreme Court (*Trammel v. U.S.,* 445 U.S. 40, 100 S.Ct. 906, 63 L.Ed.2d 186 [1980]). Thus, although they are sometimes protected, a variety of peer review and quality assurance records have been admitted in actions involving medical providers. Several recent cases are instructive. For example, broad requests for quality assurance information have been granted by the court over an objection based on the peer review immunity. In *State of Missouri, ex rel., Dixon v. Darnold,* 939 S.W.2d 66 (Mo.Ct.App. 1997), a patient brought a medical action against a hospital and several physicians. The patient requested discovery of an extremely long laundry list of documents including "quality assurance/quality management flow sheet[s] . . . ; infection data . . . ; written documentation by the infection control nurse . . . ; any quality assessment (QA) . . . abstract forms . . . utilized by the quality assessment and/or quality management [QM] department . . . ; any trend sheet prepared from any QA and/or QM abstract form or work sheets . . . ; transmitted sheets or memos generated to or from the infection control nurse or infection control department . . . ; written minutes from an Infection Control Committee meeting . . . ; any transmittal written to the Infection Control Coordinator or nurse . . . ; any transmittal written to the Risk Management Department from any member of the QA department . . . ; the 1994 Semi-Annual Reports of the nosocomial infection rates of [defendants] Drs. Wakeman, Kerber, and Gibson compiled by the Infection Control Coordinator" (*Dixon v. Darnold,* 69–70).

This extensive discovery request was resisted by the defendants on the basis of protected peer review; however, the appellate court disagreed, ordering the trial court to require that the defendants produce the plaintiff-requested documents. Of obvious interest here is that such broad discovery of quality-related documents, including physician-specific nosocomial infection rates, would have a tendency to chill such reporting if litigation could be supported by these data. Indeed, the problem is deeper; even lack of document admissibility in the ultimate adjudication does not support any document privilege exclusion. The court may still order production of the documents, for "it is not grounds for objection that the information may be inadmissible at trial, if the information sought appears reasonably calculated to lead to the discovery of admissible evidence" (*Dixon v. Darnold,* 70).

Further, and very important with regard to patient safety research, there is the issue of discoverability of incident and occurrence reports. These reports have generally been held to be discoverable and outside peer review privilege protection. For example, in *Columbia/HCA Health Care Corp. v. Eighth Judicial District Court,* 936 P.2d 844 (Nev. 1997), the parents of a child who died after being treated for an arachnoid cyst filed a medical malpractice action against the hospital and physicians involved in the child's care. The parents-plaintiffs requested discovery of "any incident report arising out of the treatment of [the child] . . . [and] transcriptions of oral statements about or written statements about any Hospital employee or from any physician with staff privileges at Hospital involved in the care of [the child]" (*Columbia/HCA Health Care Corp.,* 846).

The defendant hospital claimed that these reports were protected from discovery under the peer review privilege. However, the court rejected this argument, indicating that since the reports were prepared in the ordinary course of business—that is, since the hospital required incident and occurrence reports to be filed—it was not protected by the privilege, even though these reports were prepared "to improve 'the quality of care given' " at the hospital (*Columbia/HCA Health Care Corp.,* 848). The court noted that only formal proceedings by peer review committees were privileged, not documents submitted or generated without the peer review committee's impetus (*Columbia/HCA Health Care Corp.*, 849). Unfortunately, this result bodes poorly for error research efforts because reports of error as represented by incident reports are precisely the type of information that is required to begin and build systemic patient safety efforts. Treating incident reports as discoverable will provide little impetus for providers to engage in this reporting.

This result may also occur when providers attempt to invoke another privilege: the attorney-client privilege. For example, in *State of West Virginia, ex rel., United Hosp. Ctr., Inc. v. Bedell*, 484 S.E.2d 199 (W. Va. 1997), a deceased patient's estate brought a personal injury action against a hospital emergency room. The patient had fallen in the emergency room and the estate requested discovery of the incident report that described the event. The hospital refused to supply the report, arguing that the incident report was within the attorney-client privilege because it was submitted to the hospital's general counsel. The court again disagreed. First, the court noted that incident reports were filed for "any event that occurs during the hospital stay of a patient, visitor, or volunteer which is non-routine (i.e., an accident or mistake) . . . [and that] the purpose of incident reporting is not to place blame on individuals. [Reporting] is designed to enhance the care provided and to assist in providing a safe environment" (*United Hospital Center,* 204). This recognition of the document's specific patient safety use notwithstanding, the court held that the information was not privileged. The court noted that the attorney-client privilege is to be narrowly construed like other privileges. The court then held that the incident reports at issue were not protected since the hospital neither showed that the nurse who filed the report with the hospital's general counsel believed that an attorney-client privilege existed, nor did the nurse seek legal advice from the general counsel. Thus, in this case of direct assessment of safety reporting issues, the court still indicated that the materials were discoverable by plaintiffs. Again, this result has a tendency to chill substantive participation in reporting medical error.

In a related matter, staff privilege application documents are also discoverable. For example, in *Harper v. Cadenhead,* 926 S.W.2d 588 (Tx.Ct.App. 1995), the plaintiffs in a medical malpractice action requested discovery from a hospital of "all documents (including applications, inquiries, and recommendations) concerning the credentialing committee's consideration of [defendant physician's] being given staff privileges" at the hospital (*Harper v. Cadenhead,* 588). The hospital refused, claiming that the peer review privilege rendered these documents undiscoverable. However, the appellate court rejected this argument, indicating that because these documents are kept within the regular course of the hospital's business, the credentialing committee was not acting as a peer review committee, and since the committee was only assessing whether the physician was qualified to practice at the hospital, the peer information was not immune from discovery and was thus discoverable by plaintiffs.

This legal result also creates significant difficulties for patient safety efforts. If information regarding a physician's application for staff privileges is generally discoverable, information regarding the physician's error reporting at other hospitals, participation in error reduction training for remedial purposes, and so forth will all be subject to discovery by plaintiffs. Participation in these activities would hence be limited because the plaintiff's lawyers could construe such activities as being indicative of potentially poor medical practice.

Similarly, aviation reporting systems such as the ASRS, which have often been seen as a potential paradigm for reporting medical errors, are not immune from legal discovery (Battelle Group 1995; Commentary 1996). In addition, internal "confidential" safety audits performed by individual airlines have also been ruled as discoverable, placing a significant damper on participation in these error reporting activities (*In re Air Crash at Charlotte, NC on 2 July 1994,* MDL Docket No. 1041 [D.S.C. 1995], review of court order denied sub nom, *In re USAir, Inc.,* 65 U.S.L.W. 3221 [U.S. 8 Oct. 1996]; Commentary 1996). Although there has been some argument for a qualified privilege for this information akin to the psychotherapist-patient privilege, plaintiffs may challenge this qualified privilege if they make the appropriate showing to the court (*In re Air Crash near Cali, Colombia on 20 Dec. 1995,* 959 F.Supp. 1529 [S.D.Fla. 1997]). Indeed, new and innovative proactive programs for detecting possible systemic conditions that might lead to error have limited participation due to concerns regarding discovery. For example, the Flight Operational Quality Assurance program, a federal program that would monitor and use flight data to identify important trends to reduce aviation system errors, has run into this impediment (U.S. GAO 1997). Thus, without attention to the effects of the legal system, medical reporting systems and programs attempting to employ similar methods may have a paucity of participation by physicians and other providers.

An additional reason why the ASRS and other aviation reporting systems may be less readily applicable to medical reporting efforts is that discoverabilitv of this information may have less impact on individual pilots and other reporters since the airlines are the "deep pockets" of interest to plaintiffs and their attorneys. However, in medical tort cases, often it is precisely the individual physician provider (and his or her malpractice insurance carrier) who is considered the deep pocket party. Consequently, physicians currently have a justified hesitancy to report critical incidences for fear of personal liability and increased legal scrutiny of their practices, fears not faced by reporters in the airline industry.

Beyond these provider fears, reporting may also create problems from a managed care organization's perspective. Physicians who engage in error-reporting activities may be undesirable because of their perceived "high" error rate if other groups do not report (or engage in only limited reporting). This is particularly important from the point of view of a potential liability suit against a managed care organization. If a managed care organization's provider group participated in error reporting while others did not, and a patient were injured by one of these group physicians, plaintiff attorneys may claim that the managed care organization had been negligent in credentialing and/or supervising its providers. Because the managed care organization would have had actual knowledge of the provider's "high" error rate as compared to the other groups but had not deselected or required him or her to take special and specific remedial action, the managed care organization could be on the liability hook even if the physician or physician group were an independent contractor (see, for example, *Darling v. Charleston Community Mem. Hosp.,* 211 N.E.2d [Ill. 1965], *cert. denied* 383 U.S. 946 [1966]; *Harrell v. Total Health Care,* 1989 WL 153066 [Mo.Ct.App.], *aff'd* 781 S.W.2d 58 [Mo. 1989]; *McClellan v. Health Maintenance Organization of Pennsylvania,* 604 A.2d 1053 [Pa.Super.], *appeal denied* 616 A2d 985 [Pa. 1992]). Thus, in addition to the reticence of providers to participate in reporting errors, the managed care organizations with whom they contract may also want providers to limit disclosure of errors in their health delivery activities.

TORT LIABILITY OF ORGANIZATIONS

From a different perspective, liability rules on the organization level may also impede error reduction activities in medicine. For example, legal system rules often shield organizations from liability at the expense of the individual provider, even though the organization has designed the incentive structure (e.g., an HMO paying a physician using capitation, a managed care organization using withhold arrangements, or a managed care organization conditioning payments on following denial, authorization, and utilization review requirements). This is a direct result of a physician's independent contractor status; since the physician is not considered to be under the control of the organization and has significant discretion over the performance of his or her responsibilities, the organization, which "merely" pays for services, is generally not liable for the actions of the independent contractor physician except under the caveat noted earlier (Keeton et al. 1984: 501–508).

This result is reinforced by the federal Employee Retirement Income Security Act (Employee Retirement Income Security Act of 1974, 29 U.S.C. §1001 et seq.), which has preempted many (although not all) malpractice actions against managed care organizations while allowing these claims to go forward against the physician (compare *Corcoran v. United HealthCare, Inc.,* 965 F.2d 1321 [5th Cir. 1992], *cert. denied* 113 S.Ct. 812 [1992], and *Dukes v. U.S. Healthcare,* 57 F3d 350 [3d Cir.], *cert. denied* 116 S.Ct. 564 [1995]; see Liang forthcoming). Under this legal rubric, providers may be reluctant to engage in innovative error reduction activities without some form of immunity, or at least indemnity, of the process changes inherent in these efforts.

Further, because managed care organizations do not generally shoulder liability associated with patient injury, they have no incentive to engage in or fund the significant administrative and clinical costs associated with error reduction research and implementation. Indeed, physicians are generally not reimbursed for administrative duties required by managed care organizations (Page 1997) and managed care administrators' and managers' compensation and bonus schemes are tied to financial performance rather than to quality of care, patient satisfaction, or reductions in morbidity or mortality (Desmond 1997).

These considerations indicate that at least on a preliminary level, the tremendous resources allocated to the tort system and the possible physician behavior that it does (or does not) induce should be closely assessed to determine whether these resources can be put to better use when attempting to reduce patient injury and error in medicine. The impediments of misperception and selective liability in a world of managed care also point toward reevaluation of the current tort system as the arbiter of appropriate levels of patient safety and as the optimal source of incentives to minimize patient injury.

CONTRACT LAW CONSIDERATIONS

The legal system also provides the basis for the contractual structure of provider rights and responsibilities in the health delivery system. In the current era of managed care, this includes pecuniary incentives for providing (or not providing) patient care. It has been shown that capitation, withholds, and other financial incentives relating to provider productivity indeed influence physician behavior (Pauly, Hillman, and Kerstein 1990; Haines 1996). These financial incentives may be at odds with activities that could reduce patient injury, particularly if the incentives represent a large proportion of the physician's income and if error-reduction activities consume significant time and resources.

Further, in addition to the carrot nature of payment in these contracts, the stick of enforcement must also be taken into account in assessing their effects on efforts to reduce medical error and patient injury. Research on the most common and standard contractual arrangements between health care delivery organizations and independent contractor physicians—exclusive and nonexclusive contracts with bilateral termination-without-cause clauses—has shown that provider challenges to summary terminations under them have been rejected by the courts, even where there has been no allegation of poor quality of care against the provider (Liang 1997b, 1997c). Thus, at the outset, the potential high turnover of providers and/or unchallengeable dismissal by administrators and other managers may impede efforts to engage in a sustained and coordinated medical error reduction program.

In addition, because these research activities take significant time and energy and are not reimbursed, providers who are potentially terminable at will without recourse may be concerned that their productivity will suffer as a result of engaging in such activities. Thus, providers may refuse to participate in this research due to employment concerns.

These difficulties are exacerbated by a reverse prisoner's dilemma–type problem raised by an error reporting system. A physician group that reports error for the purpose of error reduction research may be prejudged by a managed care organization as being a poor quality provider compared to others who do not report; they may thus be deselected or never selected at all. Providers would, consequently, have no incentive or a negative incentive to report. This catch-22 can only be ameliorated if all groups report, because then all groups will show at least some level of error. But because there is a significant benefit from not reporting, it is unlikely that, without more, a cooperative mode of collective action would occur, at least in the current health delivery climate. Thus, beyond the simple possibility of deselection, the fundamental requirements of error reduction research in combination with the present health care market reality may make providers shy away from participating in these error reduction efforts.

Finally, even simple implementation of established error-reducing processes may be avoided due to the initial time and effort necessary to put such methodologies into place, again due to providers' short-term employment considerations. This effect may be magnified if error reduction systems' postimplementations take more time than previous standard treatment modalities, if they render provider clinical knowledge obsolete, and/or if they do not have the support of the managed care or other health care organization administration. In the intensely competitive market of health care delivery, physicians' and other providers' participation in a research effort that takes significant time, that could change the standard practice patterns, that is unsupported by the organization, and that will most likely provide implementable and visible results only in the long term will be limited.

POLICY RECOMMENDATIONS

The broad goal of error reduction research is to prevent errors ex ante that could lead to adverse events including human injury and death. Like complex industries such as aviation and nuclear power, this goal in medicine can be achieved through increasing knowledge of where error occurs, how it occurs, and what interventions are effective to reduce it. In this effort, patients, physicians, payers, accreditors, and government policy makers all have important roles to play.

The first concern is detection through error reporting. At present, this is the most important issue, and it must be addressed before any other aspect of the error reduction system can substantively have an impact on patient safety. Detection will only occur if the reporting of medical error is widespread and becomes a culturally accepted activity within the medical delivery system. Therefore, physicians, nurses, managed care organizations, hospitals, and others involved in patient care must participate in the error reduction paradigm by reporting all errors and near misses, similar in scope to ASRS reporting and participation. The obvious difficulty in attaining this level of activity is the legally discoverable nature of these reports. Thus, as a first step, policy makers should make these reports privileged from malpractice discovery requests, at least on the level of peer review committee reports if not more so; broader discovery immunity is essential to ameliorate the justified hesitancy of physicians, managed care organizations, and others to engage in the first step of error reduction—identification of where errors occur. Note, however, that this change will not eliminate an injured patient's access to the courts. Like peer review committee information, only the discussions and assessments of the data associated with the event are privileged, not the event itself. Thus, if an injury occurred to a patient due to a medical error and the medical error were reported by the provider to the medical error reporting system, the patient would not be precluded from suing the provider for medical malpractice. The patient would simply be unable to access the medical error report and discussions of it; he or she would have to prove negligence by normal means (i.e., showing a preexisting duty to provide nonnegligent care through an established patient-physician relationship; a breach of that duty by the provider through provision of substandard care as indicated by expert testimony; and causation of injury or damages due to this breach [Epstein 1990]).

However, in addition to addressing the issue of participation, the culture for reporting error, researching it, and implementing error reduction strategies must also be established for the health care industry as it has been for the aviation and nuclear power industries. This cultural goal can be accomplished with the assistance of accrediting agencies such as the Joint Commission for Accreditation of Healthcare Organizations (JCAHO) and the National Committee on Quality Assurance (NCQA), as INPO did for the nuclear power industry after the Three Mile Island incident. As part of their accreditation process, these quality organizations should require error reduction research and implementation participation as a condition for accreditation. This requirement could be implemented as a part of the mandate for quality assurance activities and process and the outcomes measures that these accreditation organizations already use. In this way, the industry standard would be to engage in error reduction research and implementation efforts; thus, information gleaned from reported accidents, near misses, and other errors would be used reactively in the industry to minimize their occurrence and serve as a basis for proactive monitoring that would be broadly integrated into the delivery process.

Similarly, by using the current statutory framework applied to hospitals participating in the Medicare program (U.S. Public Law 89-97, 42 U.S.C.

sec. 1395bb), state and federal governments should mandate that participation in their health programs and licensure of facilities be contingent upon fulfilling the requirements of either JCAHO or NCQA regarding participation in error reduction activities. In this way, all providers would participate in error reduction efforts so that there would be no disadvantage in doing so from physicians', hospitals', or managed care organizations' points of view. As well, patient safety would also become a competitive characteristic, placing further impetus on organizations and provider groups to concentrate on this factor. Since large employer groups are becoming focused on quality and are providing information on the Internet to employees regarding health plans (Employer Quality Partnership 1998), participation in error reduction activities and relative health plan success could be integrated in these efforts to provide a more informed employee choice of health plan.

In addition, by having NCQA and JCAHO participate in the process, data standards would be uniform for collecting information regarding errors, thus facilitating analysis. At a minimum, this information should be in a form that records the physical circumstances of the event, the person injured or potentially injured, the activity that was engaged in during injury or potential injury, deviations from normal or desired procedures, activities, and circumstances, and effective and ineffective technical and procedural controls (Hale et al. 1991). Uniform reporting systems with these characteristics have been used in medical care reporting situations through an interactive computer program (Hale et al. 1991).

It should be noted that JCAHO is currently attempting to mandate medical error reporting and analysis through its sentinel event policy. If a sentinel event occurs (one defined as an unexpected occurrence involving death or serious physical or psychological injury, or risk of it) JCAHO will require the hospital to do a "root-cause" analysis. This analysis is essentially a systems analysis of procedures and activities that may have led to the sentinel event (Moore 1998; Wilder 1998). These events must be reported within five days of the occurrence, and analysis must be provided within forty-five days of the sentinel event;[1] otherwise, the JCAHO may put the hospital on an "accreditation watch," that is, the hospital will be placed on a publicly available list of providers under scrutiny by JCAHO for potential delivery problems not consistent with JCAHO accreditation. Although laudable in the sense that it attempts to use a self-reporting and systems approach in detecting and analyzing error in medicine, the sentinel event system has several significant flaws as an error reduction mechanism. First, there is the ever-present difficulty of legal discovery. Although quality assurance activities for internal analysis of such events may be afforded some protection, this immunity will most likely not extend to reports submitted to JCAHO. Second, there continue to be punitive aspects to the system; potential accreditation watch status and the significant implications of public disclosure of such events will most likely dampen the enthusiasm for program participation (Moore 1998). Third, the reporting deadlines appear to be too ambitious; resources that could be allocated to error reduction activities may be allocated instead to ensuring compliance with the five- and forty-five-day deadlines. Fourth, it is difficult to determine what a thorough and credible root-cause analysis is; JCAHO has not published any guidelines indicating how they will assess these analyses, and thus providers do not have a clear standard to determine how their reports will be evaluated (American Society for Healthcare Risk Management 1998). Therefore, significant alterations to the sentinel event reporting system are required before it can act as an effective component in a larger patient safety effort.

In addition, due to the financial burden of engaging in such research and the current lack of incentive to do so, system changes must be made to provide managed care organizations with an incentive to substantively participate in and implement the findings of error reduction research efforts. If policy makers strip away liability shields of federal law and independent contractor defenses from the managed care organization, the incentives of this actor would be aligned with those of the physician to minimize patient injury and manage care in the best interests of the patient, rather than simply managing costs (Liang forthcoming). Because accreditation as it currently stands is optional and does not involve patient safety research mandates, a legal stick in addition to the possible accreditation carrot is necessary for a sustained effort at medical error research and implementation participation. Note that the shared liability between managed care organizations and physicians would not remove any immunity for reporting or eliminate the right of patients to sue for malpractice. It would simply give both parties involved in the medical decision-making process the incentive to act together to minimize patient injury.

Beyond mere reporting, physicians, other medical personnel, and managed care organizations must also be involved in communications efforts with patients so that all parties are involved in patient safety efforts. Physicians and other personnel must educate themselves in error reduction efforts as well as educate others, including patients, residents, medical students, nursing students, and all who are involved in patient care activities (Christiansen, Levinson, and Dunn 1992; Gosbee and Stahlhut 1996; Warner 1983; Weingart 1996; Wu and McPhee 1996). Like aviation crew training, which attempts to break down communications barriers (Bringelson, Pettitt, and Dunlap 1996; Foushee and Helmreich 1988; Helmreich et al. 1990), these parties could participate in the error reporting process and be active partners in the health care venture. In particular, by becoming members of the error reduction team, patients could take responsibility for their own health, participate in error reporting and outcomes studies, and communicate with health care providers about the potential sources of error at all points along the diagnosis and treatment spectrum. And as a member of the team, the patient could be another observer to identify sources of error in the health care transaction, including identifying effective and ineffective communication strategies, process-based errors, and errors in medical records. In this fashion, an informed alliance between patient and physician could be created for therapeutic and quality improvement purposes.

Once an infrastructure is established to detect medical error, this information must be provided to appropriate research facilities for analysis just as is currently done with ASRS data. Of course, in-house review may be available; however, for broader dissemination, it would be preferable if partnerships between certain academic institutions (e.g., Centers of Excellence) and health delivery organizations were established for data and analysis exchanges. In this way, a uniform data form could be developed (if it has not been already) that would be available for other studies of the same or similar error circumstances (e.g., anesthesia data charts and encounter forms; see Bureau of National Affairs 1997). These data could then be interpreted by the academic organization on a regular basis (e.g., quarterly). Federal regulatory efforts at establishing uniform data forms for electronic transfer purposes are well on their way (Health Insurance Reform 1998) and could be adapted for error reduction analysis in cooperation with JCAHO and NCQA.

Communication of the data and its analyses is the next step. The results of these analyses should be published on the Internet by the government using a cooperative clearinghouse paradigm such as the National Guideline Clearinghouse program, through which the Agency for Health Care Policy and Research is contracting with the American Medical Association and the American Association of Health Plans to list the most up-to-date practice guidelines on the Internet (National Health Lawyers Association 1997). Less preferable, but still useful, would be to have the raw data available on the Internet, as ASRS data are currently (ASRS Incident Reports 1998). In this way, rapid dissemination of the data and the results of error reduction research could be communicated to interested parties for implementation and reconsideration in other research efforts. In addition, other communications mechanisms could be used, such as e-mail, Web pages, and hard copy newsletters like the National Patient Safety Foundation Newsletter, the Anesthesia Patient Safety Foundation Newsletter, the ASRS *Callback* newsletter, and INPO's *Lifted Heads* newsletter, all of which provide anonymous reports of incidents, error control strategies, and error reporting results and analyses.

This extensive dissemination of patient safety research would result in new interventions and new innovations to further reduce patient injury in the health delivery system. These interventions and innovations would then be assessed through the reporting and analysis stages of the process. Thus, as in other complex industries, the error reduction system would continuously be updated, assessed, refined, and updated again so as to result in a continuously improving health delivery system whose research and implementation results are easily obtainable. As well, these efforts and benefits would become standard within the industry and would become an important competitive characteristic that could be of use to patients in deciding which health plan is appropriate for them and their families.

Of course, broader research on physicians, patients, and payers should also be performed to obtain a fundamental understanding of how the interactions between these groups affect patient safety. Interdisciplinary studies on the actual effects of the tort system and other deterrence structures, the impact of organizational delivery differences, and an assessment of communications methodologies would begin to provide a baseline for other investigations that would be important in applying error reduction strategies on a national scale.

CONCLUSION

Research on human error has produced significant insights and has resulted in error reduction in high-risk industries such as aviation and nuclear power. However, such organized and comprehensive methodologies have not yet been broadly applied in medicine. Thus, there is a fundamental need for a concerted effort to establish an investigatory program to determine where human error occurs in medicine, how these causes can be ameliorated, what can be done to continuously improve clinical performance, and how social incentives can be structured to encourage research and implementation of important error reduction activities. Legal considerations, including how physicians understand and react to the law as well as the constraints imposed by it in the context of managed care, must be taken into account in order to effectively induce widespread participation in researching medical error and appropriately implementing its results. As groups stand poised to make a historic effort to comprehensively address issues of patient safety and error in medicine, an agenda of research in medical error coupled with substantive changes in the legal system can bring us closer to the goal of an interdisciplinary, continuously improving health delivery system with a minimal amount of human error and a maximum amount of safe, effective medical care. The consolidation of large numbers of patients into managed care organizations provides a heretofore unparalleled opportunity to study what works in error reduction and what does not. However, platitudes and good intentions are not enough; as Justice Hidden stated in his investigation of the Erebus aviation accident: "The evidence . . . showed the sincerity of the concern for safety. Sadly, however, it also showed the reality of the failure to carry that concern through into action. It has been said that a concern for safety which is sincerely held and expressly repeated but, nevertheless, is not carried through into action, is as much protection from danger as no concern at all" (Maurino, Reason, and Lee 1995: 47). Each of us, as participants in the medical

delivery system, can play an important role in moving this revolutionary health policy endeavor forward. Let us have the courage to join together and begin.

REFERENCES

American Medical Association, Center for Health Policy Research. 1985. *SMS Report.* Chicago: American Medical Association.

American Society for Healthcare Risk Management. 1998. ASHRM to JCAHO: Give Hospitals Game Rules. (Document is available on the Web at www.ashrm.org/JCAHO/jcahopos.htm).

Anderson, G. F., M. A. Hall, and E. P. Steinberg. 1993. Medical Technology Assessment and Practice Guidelines: Their Day in Court. *American Journal of Public Health* 83(11):1635–1639.

ASRS Incident Reports Are Now Available on the Web. 1998. *Business and Commercial Aviation* 82(1):20.

ASRS on CD-ROM. 1995. *Aviation Week and Space Technology,* 13 March, 136.

Battelle Group. 1995 (revision). *The Aviation Safety Reporting System: An ASRS Overview.* Moffett Field, CA: Battelle Group, July.

Bovbjerg, R., F. A. Sloan, A. Dor, and C. R. Hsieh. 1991. Juries and Justice: Are Malpractice and Other Personal Injuries Created Equal? *Law and Contemporary Problems* 54(1–2):5–42.

Brennan, T. A. 1991. Practice Guidelines and Malpractice Litigation: Collision or Cohesion? *Journal of Health Politics, Policy and Law* 16:67–85.

Brennan, T. A., L. L. Leape, N. Laird, L. Liesi, A. Localio, A. Lawthers, J. Newhouse, P. Weiler, and H. Hiatt. 1994. Incidence of Adverse Events and Negligence in Hospitalized Patients: Results from the Harvard Medical Practice Study I. *New England Journal of Medicine* 324(6):370–376.

Brennan, T. A., C. M. Sox, and H. R. Burstin. 1996. Relation between Negligent Adverse Events and the Outcomes of Medical-Malpractice Litigation. *New England Journal of Medicine* 335(26):1963–1967.

Bringelson, L. S., M. A. Pettitt, and J. H. Dunlap. 1996. Reducing Human Error by Increasing Team Effectiveness: Crew Resource Management in Medical Environments. *Proceedings of Examining Errors in Health Care: Developing a Prevention, Education, and Research Agenda.* Oakbrook Terrace. IL: JCAHO.

Bureau of National Affairs. 1997. Information Technology: California Plans, Providers Launch Project to Standardize Data Systems. *BNA Managed Care Reporter* 3(44): 1041–1042.

Calfee, J. E., and R. Craswell. 1984. Some Effects of Uncertainty on Compliance with Legal Standards. *Virginia Law Review* 70(5):965–1003.

Caplan, R. A., K. Posner, and F. W. Cheney. 1991. Effect of Outcome of Physician Judgments of Appropriateness of Care. *Journal of the American Medical Association* 265(15):1957–1060.

Cepelewicz, B. B., L. J. Dunn, D. M. Feltch, L. J. Levin, B. C. Nelson, I. S. Rothschild,

M. E. Rust, and M. J. Zaremski. 1998. Recent Developments in Medicine and Law. *Tort and Insurance Law Journal* 33(2):583–603.

Charles, S. C., J. R. Wilbert, and K. J. Frankie. 1985. Sued and Nonsued Physicians' Self-Reported Reactions to Malpractice Litigation. *American Journal of Psychiatry* 142(4):437–440.

Charrow, R. P., and V. R. Charrow. 1979. Making Legal Language Understandable: A Psycholinguistic Study of Jury Instructions. *Columbia Law Review* 79(7):1306–1374.

Cheney, F. W., K. Posner, R. A. Caplan, and R. J. Ward. 1989. Standard of Care and Anesthesia Liability. *Journal of the American Medical Association* 261(11):1599–1603.

Christiansen, J. F., W. Levinson, and P. M. Dunn. 1992. The Heart of Darkness: The Impact of Perceived Mistakes on Physicians. *Journal of General Internal Medicine* 7(4):424–431.

Commentary:No-Gain Pain. 1996. *Flight International* 150(45–46):3.

Cooper, J. B., R. S. Newbower, and R. J. Kitz. 1984. An Analysis of Major Errors and Equipment Failures in Anesthesia Management—Considerations for Prevention and Detection. *Anesthesiology* 60(1):34–42.

Daniels, S., and L. Andrews. 1989. The Shadow of the Law: Jury Decisions in Obstetrics and Gynecology Cases. In *Medical Professional Liability and the Delivery of Obstetrical Care,* vol. 2, ed. V. Rostow and R. Bulger. Washington, DC: National Academy.

Desmond, K. 1997. Administration: Compensation Gaps Widening between MCOs, Hospitals, Mercer Study Says. *BNA Managed Care Reporter* 3(29):672–674.

Dornheim, M. A. 1996. ASRS Fights to Curb Dangerous Trends. *Aviation Week and Space Technology* 145(19):72.

Eisenberg, J. M. 1986. *Doctors, Decisions, and Cost of Medical Care: The Reasons for Doctors' Practice Patterns and the Ways to Change Them.* Ann Arbor, MI: Health Administration Press.

Ellsworth, P. C. 1989. Are Twelve Heads Better than One? *Law and Contemporary Problems* 52(4):205–224.

Elwork, A., B. D. Sales, and J. J. Alfin. 1977. Juridic Decisions: In Ignorance of the Law or in Light of It? *Law and Human Behavior* 1(2):163–189.

Employer Quality Partnership. 1998. Navigating the Health Care System. (Document is available on the Web at www.eqp.org.)

Epstein, R. A. 1990. *Cases and Materials on Torts,* 5th ed. Boston: Little, Brown.

Forston, R. F. 1975. Sense and Non-Sense: Jury Trial Communication. *BYU Law Review* 1975(3):601–637.

Foushee, H. C., and R. L. Helmreich. 1988. Group Interaction and Flight Crew Performance. In *Human Factors in Aviation,* ed. E. L. Wiener and D. C. Nagel. San Diego, CA: Academic Press.

Frantz, L. B. 1997. Discovery of Hospital's Internal Records or Communications as to Qualifications or Evaluations of Individual Physicians. In *American Law Reports,* 3d ed. (Suppl.). San Francisco: Bancroft Whitney.

Frisch, P. R., S. C. Charles, R. D. Gibbons, and D. Hedecker. 1996. The Role of Previous Claims and Specialty on the Effectiveness of Risk Management Education for Office-Based Physicians. In *Proceedings of Examining Errors in Health Care: Developing a Prevention, Education, and Research Agenda.* Oakbrook Terrace, IL: JCAHO.

Gaba, D. M., and A. DeAnda. 1988. A Comprehensive Anesthesia Simulation Environment: Recreating the Operating Room for Research and Training. *Anesthesiology* 69(3):387–394.

Gilbert, G. A. 1996. ASRS at 20. *Business and Commercial Aviation* 79(5):103.

Glassman. P. A., J. E. Rolph, L. P. Petersen, M. A. Bradley, and R. L. Kravitz. 1996. Physicians' Personal Malpractice Experiences Are Not Related to Defensive Clinical Practices. *Journal of Health Politics, Policy and Law* 21:219–241.

Gosbee, J., and R. Stahlhut. 1996. Teaching Medical Students and Residents about Error in Health Care. *Proceedings of Examining Errors in Health Care: Developing a Prevention. Education, and Research Agenda.* Oakbrook Terrace, IL: JCAHO.

Haines. R. 1996. Are You Getting Good Physician Productivity? *Hospital Managed Care Strategies,* October, 115.

Hale. A. R., J. Karczewski, F. Koornneef, and F. Otto. 1991. IDA: An Interactive Program for the Collection and Processing of Accident Data. In *Near Miss Reporting as a Safety Tool,* ed. T. W. van der Schaaf, D. A. Lucas, and A. R. Hale. Oxford: Butterworth-Heinemann.

Hall, M. A., and D. S. Dadakis. 1996. A Model Process and Statute for Medical Practice Guidelines. *Proceedings of Examining Errors in Health Care: Developing a Prevention, Education, and Research Agenda.* Oakbrook Terrace. IL: JCAHO.

Hastie, R., S. D. Penrod, and N. Pennington. 1983. *Inside the Jury.* Cambridge: Harvard University Press.

Havighurst, C. C. 1991. Practice Guidelines as Legal Standards Governing Physician Liability. *Law and Contemporary Problems* 54(2):87–117.

Hawkins, S. A., and R. Hastie. 1990. Hindsight: Biased Judgments of Past Events after the Outcomes Are Known. *Psychological Bulletin* 107(3):311–327.

Health Insurance Reform: Standards for Electronic Transactions. 1998. *Federal Register* 63:25,272–25,320.

Helmreich, R. L. 1984. Cockpit Management Attitudes. *Human Factors* 26(5):583–589.

Helmreich, R. L., J. A. Wilhelm, S. Gregorich, and T. Chidester. 1990. Preliminary Results from the Evaluation of Crew Resource Management Training: Performance Ratings of Flight Crews. *Aviation, Space, and Environmental Medicine* 61(6):576–579.

Hoch, S. J., and F. F. Loewenstein. 1989. Outcome Feedback: Hindsight and Information. *Journal of Experimental Psychology: Learning, Memory and Cognition* 15(4):605–619.

Hong, D. W., and B. A. Liang. 1996. The Scope of Clinical Practice Guidelines. *Hospital Physician* 32(5):46–59.

Jacobson, P. D., and C. J. Rosenquist. 1996. The Use of Low-Osmolar Contrast Agents: Technological Change and Defensive Medicine. 1996. *Journal of Health Politics, Policy and Law* 21:243–266.

Joint Commission for Accreditation of Healthcare Organizations (JCAHO). 1998. Sentinel Event Policy and Procedures (revised 18 July). (Document is available on the Web at www.jcaho.org/sentinel/se_poly.html.)

Kagehiro, D. K. 1990. Defining the Standards of Proof in Jury Instructions. *Psychological Science* 1(3):194–200.

Kamin, K. A., and J. J. Rachlinski. 1995. Ex Post ≠ Ex Ante: Determining Liability in Hindsight. *Law and Human Behavior* 19(1):89–104.

Kapp, M. B. 1996. As Others See Us: Physicians' Perceptions of Risk Managers. *Journal of Health Care Risk Management* 16:4–12.

———. 1997. Medical Error versus Malpractice. *DePaul Journal of Health Care Law* 1(4)251–772.

Keeton, W. P., D. B. Dobbs, R. F. Keeton, and D. G. Owens. 1984. *Prosser and Keeton on the Law of Torts.* 5th ed. St. Paul, MN: West Publishing.

Kelly, J. T., and B. A. Liang. 1997. Clinical Outcomes Measures. *Hospital Physician* 33(4):26–35.

Kinkade, R. G. 1988. *Human Factors Primer for Nuclear Utility Managers.* NP-5714. Palo Alto, CA: Electric Power Research Institute.

Klingman, D., A. R. Localio, J. Sugarman, J. L. Wagner, P. T. Polishuk, L. Wolfe, and J. A. Corrigan. 1996. Measuring Defensive Medicine Using Clinical Scenario Surveys. *Journal of Health Politics, Policy and Law* 21:185–217.

LaBine, S. J., and G. LaBine. 1996. Determination of Negligence and the Hindsight Bias. *Law and Human Behavior* 20(5):501–516.

Lauber, J. K., and P. J. Kayten. 1988. Sleepiness, Circadian Dysrhythmia, and Fatigue in Transportation System Accidents. *Sleep* 11(6):503–512.

Lawthers, A. G., A. R. Localio, N. M. Laird, S. Lipsitz, L. Hebert, and T. A. Brennan. 1992. Physicians' Perceptions of the Risk of Being Sued. *Journal of Health Politics, Policy and Law* 17:463–482.

Leape, L. L. 1994. Error in Medicine. *Journal of the American Medical Association* 272(23):1851–1857.

Liang, B. A. 1996. Medical Malpractice: Do Physicians Have Legal Knowledge and Assess Cases as Juries Do? *University of Chicago Law School Roundtable* 3(1):59–110.

———. 1997a. Assessing Medical Malpractice Jury Verdicts: A Case Study of an Anesthesiology Department. *Cornell Journal of Law and Public Policy* 7(1):121–164.

———. 1997b. An Overview and Analysis of Challenges to Medical Exclusive Contracts. *Journal of Legal Medicine* 18(1):1–45.

———. 1997c. Deselection under *Harper v. Healthsource:* A Blow for Maintaining Patient-Physician Relationships in the Era of Managed Care? *Notre Dame Law Review* 72(3):799–861.

———. Forthcoming. Patient Injury Incentives in Law. *Yale Law and Policy Review.*

Liang, B. A., J. H. M. Austin, and P. O. Alderson. 1991. Analysis of the Resource-Based Relative Value Scale for Medicare Reimbursements to Academic and Community Hospital Radiology Departments. *Radiology* 179(3):751–758.

Localio, A. R., A. G. Lawthers, J. M. Bengston, L. Herbert, S. L. Weaver, T. A. Brennan, and J. R. Landis. 1993. Relationship between Malpractice Claims and Cesarean Delivery. *Journal of the American Medical Association* 269(3):366–373.

Localio, A. R., S. L. Weaver, J. R. Landis, A. G. Lawthers, T. A. Brennan, L. Hebert, and T. Y. Sharp. 1996. Identifying Adverse Events Caused by Medical Care: Degree of Physician Agreement in a Retrospective Chart Review. *Annals of Internal Medicine* 125(6):457–463.

Lucas. D. A. 1991. Organizational Aspects of Near Miss Reporting. In *Near Miss Reporting as a Safety Tool,* ed. T. W. van der Schaaf, D. A. Lucas, and A. R. Hale. Oxford: Butterworth-Heinemann.

Maurino, D., J. Reason, and R. Lee. 1995. *Beyond Aviation Human Factors.* Aldershot, U.K.: Avery Press.

Moore. J. D. 1998. JCAHO Urges "Do Tell," in Sentinel Event Fight: Aviation's Lesson: Learn from Experience. *Modern Healthcare,* 2 March, 60.

Moray. N. 1994. Error Reduction as a Systems Problem. In *Human Error in Medicine,* ed. M. S. Bogner. Hillsdale, NJ: Lawrence Erlbaum, Associates.

National Health Lawyers Association. 1997. New Clearinghouse Envisioned for Clinical Practice Guidelines. *Health Lawyers News,* July, 44.

Nuclear Energy Institute. 1998. Keeping It Safe: Industry Achievements: Comprehensive Training Programs, Improved Plant Performance. (Document is available on the Web at www.nei.org/safe.)

Page, L. 1997. Doctors Want Extra Pay for Managed Care Paperwork. *American Medical News,* 14 July, 6.

Pauly, M. V., A. L. Hillman, and J. Kerstein. 1990. Managing Physician Incentives. *Medical Care* 28(11):1013–1024.

Posner, K., R. A. Caplan, and F. W. Cheney. 1996. Variation in Expert Opinion in Medical Malpractice Review. *Anesthesiology* 85(5):1049–1054.

Reason, J. 1990. *Human Error.* New York: Cambridge University Press.

Reifman, A., S. M. Gusick, and P. C. Ellsworth. 1992. Real Jurors' Understanding of the Law in Real Cases. *Law and Human Behavior* 16(5):539–554.

Schwid, H. A., and D. O'Donnell. 1992. Anesthesiologists' Management of Simulated Critical Incidents. *Anesthesiology* 76(4):495–501.

Serig, D. I. 1996. Translating a Human Factors Process from Nuclear Power Plants to Health Care. *Proceedings of Examining Errors in Health Care: Developing a Prevention, Education, and Research Agenda.* Oakbrook Terrace, IL: JCAHO.

Shapiro, R. S., D. E. Simpson, S. L. Lawrence, A. M. Talsky, K. A. Sobocinski, and D. L. Schiedermayer. 1989. A Survey of Sued and Nonsued Physicians and Suing Patients. *Archives of Internal Medicine* 149(10):2190–2196.

Sloan, F. A., and C. R. Hsieh. 1990. Variability in Medical Malpractice Payments: Is the Compensation Fair? *Law and Society Review* 24(4):997–1039.

Sloan, F. A., P. M. Mergenhagan, W. B. Burfield, R. R. Bovbjerg, and M. Hassan. 1989. Medical Malpractice Experience of Physicians: Predictable or Haphazard? *Journal of the American Medical Association* 262(23):3291–3297.

Strawn, D. U., and R. W. Buchanan. 1976. Jury Confusion: A Threat to Justice. *Judicature* 59(16):478–483.

U.S. General Accounting Office (U.S. GAO). 1991. *Practice Guidelines: The Experience of Medical Specialty Societies.* Pub. no. GAO/PEMD-91-11. Washington, DC: U.S. GAO.

————. 1997. *Aviation Safety: Efforts to Implement Flight Operational Quality Assurance Programs.* Pub. no. RCED-98-10. Washington, DC: U.S. GAO.

U.S. Nuclear Regulatory Commission. 1981. *Guidelines for Control Room Design Reviews.* Pub. no. NUREG-0700. Bethesda, MD: U.S. Nuclear Regulatory Commission.

U.S. Office of Technology Assessment (U.S. OTA). 1994. *Defensive Medicine and Medical Malpractice.* Pub. no. OTA H-602. Washington, DC: U.S. Government Printing Office.

U.S. Public Law 89-97. 89th Cong., 1st sess., 30 July 1965. Health Insurance for the Aged and Disabled [Medicare Act], Effect of Accreditation. 42 U.S.C. sec. 1395bb.

Vidmar, N. 1995. *Medical Malpractice and the American Jury: Confronting the Myths about Jury Incompetence, Deep Pockets, and Outrageous Damage Awards.* Ann Arbor: University of Michigan Press.

Warner, E. 1983. Telling Patients about Medical Negligence. *Canadian Medical Association Journal* 129(4):366–368.

Weiler, P. C. 1991. *Medical Malpractice on Trial.* Cambridge: Harvard University Press.

Weiler, P. C., H. H. Hiatt, J. P. Newhouse, W. G. Johnson, T. A. Brennan, and L. L. Leape. 1993. *A Measure of Malpractice.* Cambridge: Harvard University Press.

Weingart, S. N. 1996. Finding and Fixing Errors: The Role of Physicians-in-Training. *Proceedings of Examining Errors in Health Care: Developing a Prevention, Education, and Research Agenda.* Oakbrook Terrace, IL: JCAHO.

Weisman, C., L. Morlock, M. Teitelbaum, A. C. Klassen, and D. D. Celentano. 1989. Practice Changes in Response to the Malpractice Climate: Results of a Maryland Physician Survey. *Medical Care* 27(1):16–24.

Wennberg, J. E., and A. Gittlesohn. 1982. Variations in Medical Care among Small Areas. *Scientific American* 246(4):120–134.

Wilder, T. 1998. Accreditation: Hospitals Fear JCAHO's Sentinel Event Policy Could Create Added Legal Exposure. *BNA Health Law Reporter* 7(7):261–263.

Wu, A. W., and S. J. McPhee. 1996. Education and Training: Needs and Approaches to Handling Mistakes in Medical Training. *Proceedings of Examining Errors in Health Care: Developing a Prevention, Education, and Research Agenda.* Oakbrook Terrace, IL: JCAHO.

NOTE

Thanks to Shannon M. Biggs, F. Ronald Feinstein, Mark Peterson, and two anonymous referees for helpful comments on this article. Thanks also to Matt Miller for information on the Joint Commission for Accreditation of Healthcare Organizations sentinel events policy and its updates, and to David M. Gaba for information on the anesthesia medical malpractice studies. In addition, the assistance of Barbara Hicks and John Peele in locating reference materials is gratefully acknowledged.

1. As of 18 July 1998, JCAHO will allow for on-site review of an institution's root-cause analysis for the sentinel event or on-site interviews that include review of relevant documentation regarding the sentinel event. The cost of this visit, which has varied several times, has been set at "a charge sufficient to cover the direct costs of the visit" (JCAHO 1998). Of course, such a visit and payment does not guarantee that JCAHO will deem the institutional root-cause analysis as adequate. In October 1998, JCAHO also introduced a twelve-month pilot project that would allow the hospital to release only its pre- and postsentinel event policies and procedures, rather than information relating to the root-cause analysis itself. This alternative would only be available if the CEO signed an affirmation that state law would not protect the root-cause analysis from legal discovery (JCAHO sentinel event policy hotline, Ann Kobs, Accreditation Operations, phone conversation with author, 2 October 1998).

12

Strengthening Consumer Protection: Priorities for Health Care Workforce Regulation

Leonard J. Finocchio,
Catherine M. Dower,
Noelle T. Blick,
Christine M. Gragnola
and the Taskforce on Health
Care Workforce Regulation

PROLOGUE

THE WORK OF THE PEW HEALTH PROFESSIONS COMMISSION

This latest work on professional regulation by the Pew Health Professions Commission began in early 1997. This report builds upon the Commission's 1995 report of the Taskforce on Health Care Workforce Regulation, *Reforming Health Care Workforce Regulation: Policy Considerations for the 21st Century*. That report proposed ten broad recommendations for improving workforce regulation in the public's interest (Finocchio et. al., 1995). Over a year of

Reprinted from Finocchio, Dower, Blick, Gragnola and the Taskforce on Health Care Workforce Regulation, *Strengthening Consumer Protection: Priorities for Health Care Workforce Regulation* (San Francisco,1998) with permission of the Pew Health Professions Commission.

debate and discussion followed with responses to the recommendations and policy options. Formal responses were captured in *Considering the Future of Health Care Workforce Regulation* (Gragnola and Stone, 1997).

The Pew Commission encouraged the second Taskforce to be bold and visionary, producing work that would be a catalyst for change. Specifically, the Pew Commission charged this taskforce to:

> *Envision a future health professions regulatory system that meets consumers' reasonable expectations of access to comprehensive, appropriate, cost-effective and high quality health services and to explore ways to move the current system toward this future system.*

Here, the Pew Commission focuses on three of the ten issues identified in the 1995 report: professional boards and governance, scopes of practice authority and continuing competence. These critical issues generate the most controversy and present the most challenge to crafting improvement in professional regulation. This report presents these three issues in light of current social, economic and political realities, offers recommendations and rationale for future improvement, and reviews relevant activities and examples from around the country.

INTRODUCTION

THE CHALLENGE OF CONSUMER PROTECTION

The Pew Commission believes that an improved regulatory future will be built on the existing strengths of state-based professional regulation. However, regulation's many weaknesses must be diminished or removed in order to strengthen consumer protection. The overall purpose of this report is to improve professional regulation's role in meeting consumers' expectations for expanded choice of high quality and safe practitioners. Specifically, this report focuses on professional regulatory boards, continuing competence and scopes of practice authority, areas that the Pew Commission believes present the most challenges to, and most promise for, improving professional and occupational regulation.

Consumers expect access to high quality, affordable, effective and safe health care from a range of providers and competent practitioners. The epic changes in the health care marketplace present new challenges for purchasers, consumers and regulators to meet these expectations. As market-based approaches to managing the health care system predominate and continue into the future, government will continue to enact laws that set minimum standards for public safety and remedy market failures. This tension between market and regulatory forces is reshaping consumer protection laws and agencies, fostering an expanded use of information, and promoting the role of the consumer in making choices about health care.

In the marketplace, purchasers of care are using their buying power to promote cost-effectiveness. Both purchasers and consumers are relying on empirical measures to judge health plans and practitioner quality and performance. In the regulatory arena, laws shaping the health care system are rapidly changing. Federal lawmakers are debating and passing legislation on access to and quality of care in managed care organizations. Consumer "Bills of Rights" have been introduced in many state legislatures and in Congress (Moran, 1997). State governments are also working to integrate the regulation of managed care corporations, health insurance and health facilities (Health Policy Tracking Service, 1998).

Another state regulatory institution—health professional licensure—plays a critical role in consumer protection. Licensure is a state privilege bestowed upon a profession that enables it to self-regulate through educational standard setting and peer discipline. For most of this century, state regulation of health care occupations and professions has established minimum standards for safe practice and removed the egregiously incompetent.

This ostensible goal of professional regulation—to establish standards that protect consumers from incompetent practitioners—is eclipsed by a tacit goal of protecting the professions' economic prerogatives. This dichotomy of goals has created serious shortcomings that weaken the states' effectiveness as strong and unbiased consumer protection advocates. These weaknesses have been well documented and analyzed in reports and studies over the past 25 years (*please see the chronological bibliography in the references section*). A brief summary of these shortcomings is provided here:

- Although the professions need to guide their respective boards, professional dominance on boards limits public accountability and can promote self-interest in policy making;
- Some scopes of practice conferred upon licensed occupations and professions are unnecessarily monopolistic, thereby restricting consumers' access to other qualified practitioners and increasing the costs of services;
- Although a practitioner's competence is evaluated upon initial entry into a licensed profession, current state requirements do not assess or guarantee continuing competence;
- Although several professions and states have made progress, national standards for entry to practice, professional mobility, scopes of practice, continuing competence, and discipline are limited;
- Consumers' efforts to make informed decisions about practitioner competence are hindered by the poor quality and limited quantity of information that boards release regarding licensees; and
- Professional regulation is not sufficiently integrated or coordinated with other public and private consumer protection structures and processes.

Because the current changes in health care have exacerbated these short-comings, many state agencies and individual boards are building upon existing strengths to remedy weaknesses. As market forces shape the future of health care, the structures and functions of state professional regulation, and the importance of professionalism, will continue to provide consumers with important protections from unsafe, unethical and ineffective practitioners. However, to become a viable element of consumer protection in health care, professional regulation must demonstrate that it unequivocally serves the interests of the public over those of the professions.

The Pew Commission believes that professional regulation in every state must evolve at the same rate as the economic, political, intellectual and technological environments in which its licensees work. In the paragraphs that follow, this changing environment is briefly described.

PROFESSIONAL REGULATION IN A CHANGING ENVIRONMENT

The way health services are provided by practitioners is being transformed by health plans and hospitals concerned with controlling costs (Hafferty and Light, 1995). Schneller and Ott (1996) note that, "Hospitals, HMOs, and those who represent patients are in a position to shift the balance of power and clinical roles among the different health care occupations and professions." These efforts result in substitutions between similar professionals, demands for multi-skilled workers, and the use of alternative and complementary treatments and practitioners. In addition, the increasing use of information technologies is reducing the hierarchical relationships between professions. The often exclusive privilege of specific professions to diagnose, treat and perform procedures is opening up and being shared by several professions.

Technologies are continually changing care delivery. Telehealth or telepractice, the interaction between provider and patient across distances using an electronic modality, is used by many health professions, particularly medicine and nursing (Brineger and McGinley, 1998). Currently, telepractice is limited in scope to "virtual" office visits, consultations between practitioners, and some minor procedures, but the future may expand its use in other settings (such as school clinics or long-term care facilities), locations (across the entire continent or world) and in other forms (such as diagnostic software where no practitioner is actually involved).

Each state uses different criteria to delineate who can provide health services within its boundaries, resulting in a patchwork of 50 slightly different standards for each licensed profession. Telepractice has no geographic boundaries and therefore interstate electronic practice must contend with a dizzying array of rules and regulations. Although some states and professions have made headway in standardizing regulations, no national standards address interstate practice, information exchange, or discipline. Legislators and regulators must address the inevitability of electronic practice—in all of its potential forms—in a way that maximizes access for consumers, ensures quality practice, and provides redress for substandard care and products.

Biomedical research has vastly expanded the understanding of disease but today's practitioner can be overwhelmed with new knowledge, procedures and treatments such as gene therapies, microsurgery, and thousands of new drugs. The current regulatory system does not ensure consumers that practitioners have kept up with the rapidly changing medical literature and are competent to use these new technologies and treatments. Regulators, purchasers and the professions are grappling with appropriate means to assess and ensure that practitioners can safely and effectively utilize their knowledge, judgment and skills over their practice lifetime.

Finally, consumers want the freedom to select their health plans, practitioners and treatment options based on quality and personal beliefs. Already, consumers are purchasing health care from a range of places and practitioners including nutrition stores, weight management services, complementary therapies, and spiritual healing. Information about practitioner competence and treatment options is essential to enable consumers to make safe and effective choices about their care. In a market system where informed decisions are crucial, legislators and regulators will have to focus on collecting and providing relevant practitioner information to consumers. This will require public and private sector collaboration.

PRINCIPLES FOR HEALTH CARE WORKFORCE REGULATION

The Pew Commission's first Taskforce on Health Care Workforce Regulation articulated five principles upon which state-based regulation should be based to serve the public good (Finocchio et al., 1995). In its continuing work, the Pew Commission and second Taskforce have used the same principles to inform and direct their deliberations. The Pew Commission believes that state-based health care workforce regulation will best serve the public by:

- Promoting effective health outcomes and protecting the public from harm;
- Holding regulatory bodies accountable to the public;
- Respecting consumers' rights to choose their health care providers from a range of safe options;
- Encouraging a flexible, rational and cost-effective health care system which allows effective working relationships among health care providers; and
- Facilitating professional and geographic mobility of competent providers.

The Pew Commission acknowledges that states do not regulate all health care professions and occupations, and those that are regulated are not done so in a consistent manner across states. The principles above should also apply to unregulated professions and occupations and how they are educated, certified and utilized across delivery sites and states. While this report does not directly address the private-sector contributions to standard setting and competence certification it encourages future cooperation between the public and private sectors.

A FUTURE VISION OF HEALTH CARE WORKFORCE REGULATION

Determining the exact nature and structure of health care workforce regulation in the future is indeed a challenge, and many outcomes are possible. Options for regulation in the next century range from continuing our state-based, professionally dominated system to one where licensed private institutions would be responsible for deciding who may provide what services. Other possibilities include a "title protection" system, in which titles are separated from scope of practice authority as has been done in Ontario, Canada.

The future might even see initial state licensure based on broad core competencies shared by several disciplines, with specialized private certifications added to individual scopes of practice throughout one's professional career.

Each of these models has its own strengths and weaknesses and the Pew Commission doubts that any one of them alone will concretely describe regulation in the future. The different elements of regulation—individual licenses, practice authority, continuing competence, and discipline—will undoubtedly be shaped by several tensions as regulation transforms to meet a changing environment. These tensions are illustrated in the sidebar below.

The Pew Commission expects to see an approach to regulating health care professionals that combines various elements into a system that is part governmental, with increasing participation of private sector institutions and of consumers. This emerging system is likely to support national standards in some arenas of health professions regulation (practice authority for example) while remaining at the state level for others (complaint and discipline processes

---

Tensions Shaping State-Based Professional Regulation

Public / governmental ↔ Private / market-based

Licensing individuals ↔ Licensing institutions

State standards & control ↔ National standards & control

Isolated from other consumer protection ↔ Integrated with other consumer protection

---

that can best be administered and responsive to consumer needs locally). Key components of this transformed system include:

A move towards national standards—Health care workforce regulation, along with education and credentialing, is moving in the direction of national standards. This national uniformity may be led by the federal government, agreements among the states or national professional associations. For regulation, the most dramatic effect will be standard scopes of practice authority and continuing competence requirements for each profession across the country.

Significant overlap of practice authority among the health professions— Driven by the professions, new information and technologies, and innovation in the workplace, traditional boundaries—in the form of legal scopes of practice— between the professions have blurred. This trend will continue to pressure the regulatory system to accommodate the demand for flexibility while ensuring that the public's safety is protected. Decisions regarding scopes of practice and continuing competence requirements therefore must be based on comprehensive evidence regarding the accessibility, quality and cost-effectiveness of care provided to the consumer.

New venues and participants for regulatory policy-making—The representation of various parties at health care decision-making tables is changing. Legislatures may not be the best venue to decide technical professional matters as lobbying, campaign contributions and allegiance to constituents often distort rational policy development. A more impartial venue with increased representation of interested parties, particularly consumers of health care services, will better support regulatory policy-making that is accountable, balanced and based on empirical evidence.

Integration of regulatory systems that protect health care consumers— Efforts to regulate health care plans, care delivery sites and health care professionals historically have been independent, both within and across states. This lack of coordination and integration among systems has resulted in inefficiencies and inadequate protection of the public. For example, poor coordination restricts practitioners who might competently provide care, particularly across state borders. Poor coordination also allows incompetent practitioners to move from health plan to health plan and from state to state. Today's market trends to integrate the various regulatory and delivery systems will mean that health professions regulation will be scrutinized and evaluated for its strengths and weaknesses with an eye toward consolidating systems where appropriate to better serve the public.

Increased regulatory focus on quality of care and competence assurance— Concerns over market forces in health care illuminate the need to strengthen all means of ensuring consumer protection. The resulting integration of regulatory entities and increased consumer participation in policy making will contribute to regulations that emphasize quality assurance, continuing competence demonstrations, and cooperation among the professions.

HOW LEGISLATORS CAN USE THIS REPORT

The Pew Commission acknowledges the challenge of reforming a complex system. With this report it hopes to provide legislators and regulators with a tool and resource to understand and shape professional regulation so that it meets evolving consumer protection needs. The report outlines a future vision of the fundamental structures and processes of state-based professional regulation: boards and governance, scopes of practice and continuing competence requirements. The coverage of topics in this report should not be interpreted as an implication that other topics, such as professional discipline, are any less important today than when identified in the 1995 report. The Pew Commission encourages and applauds efforts to improve disciplinary processes and all other aspects of health professions regulation. The recommendations presented here are the building blocks for a transformed regulatory framework.

It is the Pew Commission's expectation that the recommendations targeting state legislators and regulators will be considered and implemented before those targeting the Federal government, such as the establishment of a national public-private policy body. In Appendix A of the Pew Commission's full report, the Pew Commission offers legislative implementation templates for several of their recommendations in key state policy areas as a stimulus and blueprint to move the regulatory system toward the envisioned future. Legislators and their staff should consider and shape these legislative templates in the context of their own state's existing health policies, health care needs and consumer expectations. Appendix B of the Pew Commissions's full report includes an overview of recent activity exemplifying the volume of regulatory reform efforts in the ten areas identified by the Pew Commission in the 1995 report as important.

REGULATORY BOARDS AND GOVERNANCE STRUCTURES: ORGANIZING THE STRUCTURE AND FUNCTIONS OF REGULATORY BOARDS TO BETTER SERVE THE PUBLIC

CURRENT ISSUES

In December 1995, the Taskforce on Health Care Workforce Regulation wrote that regulatory boards were neither sufficiently accountable to the public nor equipped to accomplish their broad objectives. The Taskforce recommended structural changes in board membership, public oversight and increased financial support from the legislature (Finocchio et al., 1995). This recommendation and its accompanying policy options generated considerable controversy among professional associations and regulators (Gragnola and Stone, 1997). Some legislative activity also occurred over the past three years (*see sidebar*).

Activity Addressing Professional Board Governance Structure

- Oregon—Proposed legislation would have required each licensing board to have at least three (out of seven) public members (H 2296, 1997).
- Colorado—Five newly created mental health professional boards—psychology, social work, marriage and family therapy, professional counselors and one for unlicensed psychotherapists—all have public member majorities (Colorado Revised Statutes, article 43 of title 12. 1998).
- California—In its 1997 sunset report, the California Board of Podiatric Medicine recommended that it have a majority of public members (California Board of Podiatric Medicine, 1997). Although the effort did not succeed, the president of the board, a former California Assemblyman, and the former executive director of the California Board of Medicine, support public majorities (Arnett and Presley, 1998).
- Minnesota—Senate File 2380 would create a temporary Occupational Regulatory Coordinating Council to recommend how a permanent council would address issues of new occupations, structural reforms for existing regulation, and state practice acts (Minnesota Board of Examiners for Nursing Home Administrators, 1998). An existing but informal Council of Boards may take on this charge from the Senate Subcommittee on Occupational Regulation.
- Allied health—The National Commission on Allied Health recommended that states increase public representation on individual licensing boards to at least 50 percent (U.S. Department of Health and Human Services, 1995).
- Maine—A report to the Governor and Legislature recommended the establishment of an advisory federation of boards (Kany and Janes, 1997).
- Florida—Although it did not pass, the Senate Committee on Health Care voted to introduce legislation (Senate Bill 256, 1998) to create five new disciplinary boards in five health service areas. There would have been at least three consumer members on each board. The function of these boards would have been to make a determination of the existence of probable cause in health care professional disciplinary cases and to advise the Secretary of the Department of Health on disciplinary matters (Florida Senate Health Care Committee, 1997).

Since that recommendation was made, the health care environment continues to present significant challenges to boards. These include new health care delivery and reimbursement structures, telemedicine and other emerging technologies, and innovative use of health professionals. Regulatory structures and functions must transform to address issues of limited public participation and professional accountability, information management and accessibility, and policy coordination among professions and among states.

The piecemeal and narrowly focused nature of state professional boards may marginalize them in today's health care evolution. For example, determinations about practitioner competence, quality assurance, and consumer protection policy are evolving without the collaboration of boards. Board insularity can be attributed, in part, to a structure of professional dominance and limited effective participation from public members. Despite open meeting laws, board processes are generally unknown to the public. Many state legislatures and boards have recognized the importance and positive contribution of public membership and participation, but efforts to increase public membership remain limited.

In an era when information is crucial for public safety and effective markets, boards are insufficiently staffed and financed to collect and manage information on behalf of the public. Complete information about practitioners, particularly substandard ones, is still not easily available to the public in all but a few states. Moreover, boards have not made much progress enforcing laws requiring hospitals to report sanctioned practitioners (Cohen and Swankin, 1997). In California, for example, the medical board has characterized hospitals' lack of compliance on reporting as a near crisis" (Medical Board of California, 1995).

Collaboration among individual boards in most states remains minimal. This lack of coordination produces discordant results such as underused profession-als, competition for scopes of practice, and restricted access to care (*see the chronological bibliography in the references section*). Such matters of broad state health policy—cost, quality, safety and accessibility of care—tend to be outside the purview of individual boards but few, if any, states have examined the overall impact of regulating each profession separately. While some states have developed mechanisms for inter-board cooperation and policy development, they are limited in number and strength. In addition to this limited *intrastate* coordination, there is little *interstate* coordination in key policy areas. These areas include sharing disciplinary information, scope of practice consistency and continuing competence standards. The increasing presence of multi-state integrated delivery systems and telepractice and other technologies have made political boundaries obsolete. Poor interstate regulatory coordination limits the mobility of competent practitioners and access to care through technology.

At a time of public concern over consumer protection in managed care, some fear that professional boards may become relegated to a sideline role in shaping health policy that serves consumer interests, particularly in the areas of practitioner competence and quality assurance (Andrew and Sauer, 1996). An important role remains for state-based licensure boards but they must evolve in responsive and innovative ways. The recommendations presented below offer an opportunity for professional boards to make meaningful contributions to consumer protection, and to shape a high quality, cost effective and accessible health care system.

RECOMMENDATIONS FOR REGULATORY BOARDS AND GOVERNANCE STRUCTURES

Recommendation 1

Congress should establish a national policy advisory body that will research, develop and publish national scopes of practice and continuing competency standards for state legislatures to implement.[1]

Brennan and Berwick (1996) contend that regulation is disconnected from the best available scientific knowledge about quality and its sources because, "An empirical, scientific foundation for the improvement of regulation does not yet exist." This disconnect with empirical rigor is exacerbated by the multiplicity of practice acts, continuing competence requirements and other rules and regulations that exist in each state for each profession.

A national policy advisory body established by Congress would focus on developing an unbiased empirical rigor in two areas of professional regulation that suffer the most from poor standardization, lack of evidence and turf battles between the professions. These two areas are scopes of practice authority and standards for continuing competence determination. Other policy issues on which this body might perform research and analysis would include professional mobility, data collection, sharing and transfer of data and standards, and public access to the National Practitioner Data Bank.

This policy advisory body would examine and compare education and training standards between the professions, compare practice acts across the states, and collect and analyze evidence about quality of care and practitioner competence (*see recommendation seven*). With this, and potentially other evidence and expert testimony, the advisory body would write practice authority acts for each profession. These standard practice authority acts would be disseminated as templates for use by state legislators and ultimately become recognized and adopted by all the states.

The structure of this new national policy advisory body may resemble the now-defunct Office of Technology Assessment and might be sited in a currently existing agency of the federal government (such as the Agency for Health Care Policy Research or the Bureau of Health Professions). Alternatively, it may be contracted under charter with a private non-profit organization such as the Institute of Medicine in the National Academy of Sciences. In either scenario, it should have representation and input from relevant stakeholders such as hospitals and health plans, health professional associations, consumer organizations, health services researchers, federations of state regulatory boards, and the state and federal governments.

It is important to note that this body will only function in an advisory capacity to Congress, to relevant Federal agencies such as the Health Care Financing Administration, and to state legislators, regulatory agencies, and professional boards. It would not be empowered to promulgate regulations.

Recommendation 2

States should require policy oversight and coordination for professional regulation at the state level. This could be accomplished by the creation of an oversight board composed of a majority of public members or it could become the expanded responsibility of an existing agency with oversight authority, This policy coordinating body should be responsible for general oversight of that state's health licensing boards and for assuring the integration of professional regulation with other state consumer protection regulatory efforts (e.g., health facility and health plan regulation). [See legislative implementation template in Appendix A of the Pew Commission's full report.]

The laws governing the professions are not coordinated around any explicit health policy or consumer protection objectives. Currently, most states have not established forums for such policies—the cost, quality, safety, and accessibility of health care—to be decided in a broadly interdisciplinary and accountable manner. Individual professions now operate with separate governance structures and standards even though they practice together in the same state, at the same health care institutions, and serve the same populations of patients. The current regulatory system is perceived to protect and promote professional self-interest rather than advancing a strong consumer agenda.

Furthermore, the regulation of people and the regulation of institutions have developed autonomously and remain poorly coordinated. Effective working relationships are needed between all public regulatory agencies and private oversight mechanisms such as the Joint Commission on Accreditation of Healthcare Organizations and the National Committee for Quality Assurance. In today's environment of heightened scrutiny of market and regulatory forces and their impact on consumer protection, an opportunity is afforded to legislators to coordinate lawmaking.

A collective and unbiased policy making forum is needed to examine broad health and consumer protection policy issues and establish policy in the context of current health care, economic, political and social realities. For example, an unbiased oversight forum would make decisions on collaborative practice issues where two or more professions are involved. A coordinated approach to consumer protection would also assure that boards standardize their programs and performance objectives in areas such as information dissemination, investigation and discipline, and demonstrations of continuing competence. Regulatory oversight and coordination would also integrate professional regulation with other public and private consumer protection institutions and activities.

Establishing effective and accountable oversight and coordination will be challenging. The Pew Commission proposes two means: 1) a publicly dominated oversight board or council; or 2) centralized administrative oversight by an executive agency branch or office. Legislators in each state will weigh the advantages and disadvantages of each option and decide which would be most effective. In either case, oversight and coordination in the public interest will need to meet the following objectives:

- Establishing, measuring and evaluating performance objectives for individual professional boards, particularly in the areas of continuing competence assessments, investigation of complaints and discipline;
- Ensuring consistency and uniformity of regulatory processes and outcomes by centrally reviewing and approving rules, regulations and other initiatives by individual boards that may affect more than one profession;
- Ensuring policy coordination between individual licensing boards that is not addressed by the work of the national policy advisory body;
- Ensuring coordination between licensing boards and other state and federal agencies, particularly consumer protection agencies;
- Establishing criteria for the appointment of board members and implementing effective education and training programs for all members and staff;
- Establishing programs and criteria for releasing practice-relevant information about licensees to the public; and
- Establishing incentives for effective enforcement including budget review and approval.

States may chose to accomplish these objectives by establishing a new board. This body should be consumer-dominated and include representation from care delivery organizations, payers, consumer advocates, legislators, and other state consumer protection agencies. Representatives of the professions would hold a minority of seats. The chairperson should be a consumer member of the board.

Some states already have centralized administrative agencies for licensure or consumer protection but rarely do they have the powers described above. States that wish to accomplish these oversight and coordination functions through an existing agency will need to enact laws expanding the powers and responsibilities of centralized licensing agencies or other agencies such as state departments of health.

States will face a number of challenges when establishing a new oversight board or empowering an existing centralized agency. In both scenarios, the legislature will have to delegate policy making to this entity. An oversight and coordination body that is solely advisory will not have the power to accomplish the functions set forth above. This delegation of powers from the legislative to the executive branch of government may be complex. Legislators should look to successful examples of such power delegation between branches for guidance.

Also in both scenarios, legislators should ensure that the oversight entities are not assigned authority over boards' day-to-day operations and should not serve as an appeals venue in the investigation and discipline process. An oversight body or agency should not "micro-manage" or duplicate the work of individual boards, but rather establish and enforce overall policy goals. Additionally, any new body or centralized agency will need to have adequate resources and experienced staffing to carry out its responsibilities (*see recommendation five*).

Finally, legislators face the challenge of establishing oversight leadership that is representative and unbiased. In those states where an oversight board is established, the board membership and chairperson selections will be subject to the same appointment process politics as individual boards. While oversight by a centralized agency will have qualitatively different and less direct consumer stewardship than the oversight board (by virtue of its membership and chairperson), its accountability will be similar to the operation of any state cabinet-level department whose leader is appointed by the governor. See the template in Appendix A of Pew Commission's full report for more information and guidance for writing relevant legislation.

Recommendation 3

Individual professional boards in the states must be more accountable to the public by significantly increasing the representation of public, non-professional members. Public representation should be at least one-third of each professional board.[2]

State licensure boards have struggled with the fact that the professions themselves dominate regulation's public purposes. Yessian and Greenleaf (1997) write that, " . . . professionals, because of their expertise and political influence, exert continuing influence in ways that bias the efforts towards their own interests, with little countervailing influence by consumer-biased interests."

If professional regulation is to objectively serve consumer protection and broader health policy goals, participation from those stakeholders with public safety, health policy and economic interests must be included. Moreover, structural changes and external incentives are needed as self-regulating professions rarely initiate improvements in consumer protection that threaten their economic interests and professional sovereignty (Brennan and Berwick, 1996).

To ensure this credibility with the public, the membership structure of individual professional boards must include increased public, non-professional membership with no close familial or fiduciary connections to any regulated licensee. Public representation should comprise at least one-third of members on any board. Legislators should ensure that all board members undergo training before their tenure begins to prepare them for their role as consumer protection regulators. Public members, in particular, must have training to allow them to be as effective as possible in a highly technical and complex environment (Citizen Advocacy Center, 1995). The appointment process for professional and public members to all boards must be as free as possible of politics and cronyism to ensure better objectivity and accountability (Relman, 1997).

Recommendation 4

States should require professional boards to provide practice-relevant information about their licensees to the public in a clear and comprehensible manner. Legislators should also work to change laws that prohibit the disclosure of malpractice settlements and other relevant practice concerns to the public.

For regulation to support the market's strengths and remedy its failures, consumers need information. This requires creating, processing and providing the information necessary to facilitate an efficient and safe marketplace (Jost, 1997). For example, the reporting of sentinel events (such as adverse outcomes) in hospitals is an increasingly important measure of performance used by administrators, regulators, purchasers and consumers. Currently, there is little coordinated management and dissemination of information about professional practice and safety from discrete sources.

The public purpose of boards will be strengthened only if public representation is combined with significant public access to information about licensees. All boards should make publicly available licensee profiles that include such information as education, private certifications, continuing competence assurances, disciplinary actions and sanctions taken by the board, hospital or workplace, criminal convictions and malpractice settlements.

For this to happen, legislators will have to rescind other laws that restrict boards from revealing information such as criminal convictions and malpractice settlements. Without such legislation, consumers may not have critical information they need to determine a practitioner's competence. At the same time, reasonable protections of practitioner confidentiality (as in some cases of chemical dependency) should be respected.

These profiles should be made readily available through multiple means, such as the Internet, toll-free numbers and annual summary reports in public libraries. Furthermore, information about practitioners, particularly their malpractice settlements, should be explained both in a context of malpractice generally, and by specialty group specifically. For example, in Massachusetts, physician profiles that include any malpractice payments are put in statistical context of "below average, average, and above average" (Massachusetts Board of Registration in Medicine, 1998).

Recommendation 5

States should provide the resources necessary to adequately staff and equip all health professions boards to meet their responsibilities expeditiously, efficiently and effectively.

Boards have not been provided the resources, personnel nor technologies to meet their responsibilities effectively (Relman, 1997). Compared to Medicare Physician Review Organizations (PRO) that focus on only a subset of physicians, state medical boards have far fewer resources with which to accomplish their objectives. In Georgia, for example, the medical board's budget in 1995 was $819,000 (Federation of State Medical Boards, 1995). The same state's PRO budget (in 1997) was over $3 million (Health Care Financing Administration, 1997). This ratio—almost four to one—is similar in eight other states.

Board members themselves are poorly compensated given the amount of challenging work they are expected to perform. In Colorado, each board member receives only $50 per meeting, hearing or examination attended. The original act establishing this compensation amount has not changed in over 18 years (Colorado Revised Statutes, subsection 13 of section 24-34-102, 1998). Moreover, it has been estimated that board members spend twice as much uncompensated time preparing for the actual compensated time they spend in meetings and hearings (Douglas, 1998). And, some states do not pay boards members at all.

The funding challenge for boards revolves around two important issues: 1) licensing fees; and 2) boards' control over these fees. Boards generally rely on licensing and relicensing fees to carry out their duties and in many states, these licensing fees are insufficient to support all of a board's activities. Typically, a board spends the lion's share of its resources on disciplinary investigations and legal services for prosecution.

These fees are established by legislatures and influenced by professional associations and societies. For example, when the Medical Board of California proposed a fee increase to expand investigations and discipline, the California Medical Association successfully lobbied to have the measure abandoned (Bernstein, 1998).

The amount of resources provided to boards by legislative appropriation may be less than the amount generated by fees. Legislators may direct collected fees initially to a state's general fund that is then subject to budget battles, appropriations and spending caps. Consequently, a board may be given fewer resources than it could have collected and spent directly as cash fees from licensees.

For boards to better serve the public, states should appropriate and authorize a sufficient amount of funds if fees are routed into the general fund. This may require that legislators exempt professional boards from budget spending caps. Legislators may also allow direct collection and spending of licensing fees, allowing boards to raise fees and spend additional revenues as approved by an oversight entity. Additionally, states should consider alternative funding sources such as a health plan per capita assessment to increase the amount of resources at their disposal.

Recommendation 6

Congress should enact legislation that facilitates professional mobility and practice across state boundaries.

As health care markets become national, a federal role in consumer protection is more warranted. Federal involvement in professional regulation (such as PROs and re-certification proposals) have been justified when state governments or private initiatives have not offered satisfactory public protection or controls on cost increases (Yessian and Greenleaf, 1997).

Telepractice is a compelling justification for a more centralized and better integrated regulatory system as practitioners can "virtually" practice across physical and political boundaries and may pursue a career in several states. Current state licensure laws do not facilitate interstate movement or telepractice; nor do they offer sufficient redress to consumers in the event of substandard telepractice from outside their jurisdiction (Western Governors' Association, 1998).

Recently, the National Council of State Boards of Nursing endorsed a mutual recognition model for interstate nursing practice (National Council of State Boards of Nursing, 1997). This will involve a complex interstate compact that allows a nurse's license to be recognized by participating states. Although encouraging, this undertaking only deals with mobility at a multi-state state level for one profession.

A federal law would preempt state laws that erect barriers to effective telepractice and mobility across political boundaries within the United States. State laws that restrict practice by those from another state generally serve narrow economic interests of the professions to limit competition from other practitioners. This federal law should respect the states' rights to license and discipline individual practitioners while ensuring that a license from one state is recognized in another.

There is legitimate concern, however, that telepractice could make it difficult for a consumer to file a complaint and pursue disciplinary recourse in the event of substandard care. Tort law in the state where the practitioner engaged in telepractice—in other words, where the patient receiving services resides—should apply even when the practitioner resides in another state. State boards should be equally vigilant in taking disciplinary action against their licensees regardless of where the harmed patient resides. The federal government could play an instrumental role in holding individual states accountable for accessible, fair and expeditious complaints and disciplinary structures and processes.

PROFESSIONAL PRACTICE AUTHORITY: DETERMINING WHICH HEALTH CARE PRACTITIONERS ARE PERMITTED TO PROVIDE WHAT SERVICES

CURRENT ISSUES

The recommendation regarding practice authority in the 1995 report, *Reforming Health Care Workforce Regulation* generated considerable controversy. Based on the formal responses submitted regarding the report, this recommendation received one of the highest scores for level of concern and was also one of the most challenged (Gragnola and Stone, 1997).

Despite the 1995 recommendation, the processes by which professional practice authority acts are determined have not changed. Legislative calendars across the country continue to be flooded with bills that would regulate emerging health professions or change the practice authority of currently regulated professions. In 1995, over 800 such bills were considered and approximately 300 laws passed (Fox-Grage, 1995). Two years later, 1600 bills were introduced and about 300 laws enacted (Health Policy Tracking Service, 1997).

This legislative activity is just one component of "turf battles," the apparently inevitable fights between the professions over who can provide what services. Often lost in the battles between the professions is consumer protection, regulation's ostensible primary purpose. The potential benefits and dangers to the public from any proposed change are difficult to determine as each party brings to the dispute arguments that embrace the "public's interest."

State legislators seeking to answer the health care consumers concerns may begin by asking two questions before addressing the merits of any proposed change: First, *who* should determine professional practice authority? Second, *how* should the decision-making be accomplished? In other words, are state legislators the most appropriate experts and are state legislatures the best setting for resolving such technical questions as whether optometrists should be allowed to treat glaucoma; or whether nurse practitioners are qualified to prescribe pharmaceuticals?

An inherent clash of values frames these questions. State legislation values local representation and accountability to constituents, public debate and political compromise. In contrast, today's consumers and providers are operating in regional or national health care markets that increasingly value customer access and choice, collaboration among practitioners, cost-effectiveness and quality grounded in evidence. The challenge to state legislators is to incorporate— or at least acknowledge—these contemporary values and standards into their decision-making about practice acts.

Consumer access and choice—At a minimum, consumers want access to competent health care practitioners and the ability to choose among many types of health care practitioners. Consumers also want to be assured that their choices are at least safe, and preferably effective as well. The public has a reasonable expectation that their health care practitioners, whether selected by the consumer or assigned by the health care provider or plan, are competent to provide the care that they are providing. Finally, consumers and purchasers are increasingly aware of health care costs and demanding value for their dollars, while at the same time wary of health care systems that substitute less expensive workers for their higher paid counterparts.

Balancing these tensions between free choice and protection from harm forms the core of the legislator's charge. State legislators try to achieve this balance by establishing and revising practice acts through normal legislative processes. Practice act decisions benefit from the strengths of state legislative activity and suffer under the shadows of partisan politics, campaign contributions and professional lobbying. Critics charge that the outcomes may not always be in the public's best interest:

> Narrow scope of practice, restrictive reimbursement standards, and other legal barriers may limit access to care for large numbers of Americans. In the absence of a national commitment to universal health insurance, the potential for non-physician practitioners to supply much-needed, general health services at reasonable costs should not be ignored (Sage and Aiken, 1997).

Sharing practice authority among the health professions—It is not only the interests of the public that the state legislator must consider when facing a bill to establish or change a practice act. Health care professionals themselves have additional and conflicting interests. While the professions have an interest in minimal restrictions, they also benefit from the anti-competitive aspects of regulation. It is always the professions—never the public or consumer advocates—who request regulatory changes to practice acts.

However, the health professions do not act in concert in this arena. Partly because of the current regulatory scheme itself, with its separate and often exclusive scopes of practice, each profession sees itself as proprietary owner or manager of a given territory. Some of the grants of authority have been extremely liberal, resulting in expansive practice acts such as that for physicians; others are extremely restrictive. Requests for changes by one profession are viewed as expansions, encroachments, and infringements by another. Every proposal must end in a win for one side and a corresponding loss for the other. In recent years, increased competition, driven by workforce oversupply and by new employment models within managed care systems, has exacerbated these inter-professional practice battles.

Due to different educational and regulatory histories, the various professions are uniquely situated and view regulation and potential changes differently. Medicine is the only profession with state practice acts that cover *all* of health care services. With this exclusivity, little or nothing exists that can be added to the medical act and medicine has no incentive to delete anything. From this position, medicine can see every request for regulatory change from any other profession or occupation as a challenge or confrontation. With all-inclusive practice authority, the profession also has the credentials, expertise and political influence to comment on potential impacts of changed laws on patients, clients, and consumers.

A number of professions that provide some or many of the same services as physicians (for example, nurse practitioners, physician assistants, certified nurse midwives, certified nurse specialists, certified registered nurse anesthetists and optometrists) have spent considerable amounts of time and money in recent years bolstering requests to change their practice acts to permit them to provide care that is consistent with their education and training. Virtually every request has been opposed by organized medicine, often by state medical licensing boards, and sometimes by other professions as well. The outcomes of these requests vary by profession, by year, and by state.

Some of the allied health professions and occupations, and some of the previously unregulated "alternative" and "complementary" professions, have pursued regulation and accompanying subsets of the medical practice acts. Virtually every pursuit has been opposed by at least one other profession. The outcomes of these pursuits vary by profession, by year and by state. Other professions and occupations have declined to pursue regulation.

This fragmented, competitive, and adversarial regulatory activity ignores the fact that clinical practice is no longer based on exclusive professional or occupational domains. Collaborative teams of health care practitioners who often share some elements of practice authority are more the rule than the exception in today's health care systems.

Today's practitioners, administrators, and consumers are increasingly comfortable with the principle that if someone is competent to provide a health service safely, and has met established standards, then he or she should be allowed to provide that care and be reimbursed for it, even if that care was historically delivered by members of another profession (*see sidebar*). Nurse practitioners, physician assistants, pharmacists and midwives for example are providing health care that was in the exclusive domain of physicians a few years ago.

Scope of Practice Decision-Making Activity

Colorado—With the enactment of House Bill 1072 (1998), the State of Colorado recreates and restructures its mental health boards and the practice laws that apply to unlicensed psychotherapists and to licensed psychologists, social workers, marriage and family counselors, and professional counselors. With the new law, title protection is afforded to the licensed groups but none has an exclusive practice authority. No part of the law creating one profession can be construed to prevent members of the other professions from rendering services within their defined scope of practice. Nothing in any of the licensing laws for the four licensed professions can restrict the practice of unlicensed psychotherapists from practicing as long as they are "listed" with the State Grievance Board. Moreover, all five professions are subject to uniform requirements in terms of 23 prohibited acts, such as sexual contact with patients (Colorado Revised Statutes Title 12, Article 43, 1998).

The adversarial system for determining practice authority also ignores the natural evolution of professions, and individuals within the professions, as they develop their education, training, and accreditation standards to meet the changing needs of patients and clients.

Uniformity among the states—Individual state legislators in separate state legislatures are at a disadvantage in a world increasingly driven by regional, national, and global economies and information systems. This is no less true for decisions regarding health care practitioners than for decisions regarding telecommunication, commerce, and aviation industries. With recent developments in telepractice and widespread use of the Internet, the contrast between technological evolution and the relative stagnation in health professions regulation has been sharpened.

Many of the professions have adopted national standards for examination, certification, and accreditation. For example, medical specialty board credentials are national and can be carried with one upon moving to a new state. However, practice acts are still decided at the state level with little or no coordination. The differences among practice acts for single professions vary in magnitude. Some are trivial; others are significant (Dower et al., 1998). For some professions, practice is legal and recognized in some states but illegal in others (Cooper and Stoflet, 1996).

The benefits and necessity of many aspects of state policy-making and policy-enforcement are numerous. However, differences from state to state in practice acts for the health professions no longer make sense.

Finding the evidence to support changes in practice authority—Few would oppose the idea that if certain professionals are found to be competent to provide a service, they should be allowed to do so. Legislators considering practice authority laws must face the following and more challenging question: how must a profession, or a subset of a profession, demonstrate competence?

Mindful of ensuring that the quality of health care is not compromised, decision-makers would optimally look to empirical evidence, and evidence alone, when considering the establishment or change in any practice authority legislation. This evidence would consider objective data regarding outcomes, quality, cost-effectiveness and access. It would be relied upon to determine whether the petitioning profession had demonstrated that its members were competent to provide the health care services in question.

However, evidence of competence in today's legislative activities is only one of many factors that influence the debate. Campaign contributions and lobbying efforts are also part of legislative reality. The inherent conflict of interest for legislators to accept campaign contributions from the very groups about whom they will be making decisions needs to be acknowledged and addressed (*see sidebar*). In a turf battle between two professions, differences in political and financial strength often allows one profession to "out-gun" the other with factors unrelated to competence and empirical evidence. Practice authority decisions made in this environment do not necessarily answer the question of which professionals are qualified to provide safe, competent, and accessible health care.

Estimating the Costs of Battling for Turf: Eye Care in California

A four-year dispute between ophthalmologists and optometrists over who could treat certain eye diseases with what medication in California reportedly cost over $1.8 million in campaign contributions alone to state legislators (Lucas, 1996).

Regardless of these external factors, appropriate and complete evidence is not always available or easy to find, and relevant standards may change over time. For example, the rationale relied upon by the early advocates for all-inclusive medical acts for physicians at the turn of the century may not be viewed as favorably by today's experts in empirical evidence. Nonetheless, no state practice act today prohibits any licensed physician from performing surgery even though surgical competence may vary tremendously depending on training and specialty. Furthermore, the range of possible sources of evidence is large and the data collection techniques and methodologies differ. Research is expensive, time-consuming, and constantly evolving. This can be perceived by those seeking change as a relentless "raising-of-the-bar." The "gold standards" of one profession's research philosophy may run counter to another profession's. Consideration of non-Western therapies and disciplines may be particularly challenging when evidence may come from other countries or in other languages.

Complicating the matter of evidence and competence is the issue of burden of proof. Consensus is far from reached on whom the burden should fall. Many would argue that the profession seeking new or changed practice authority should bear the burden of demonstrating to the decision-makers that its members are competent to provide the care in question. However, from hearing records, written testimony, and lobbying efforts, it appears that other organized professions that might also be affected by the proposed changes often assume the duty of "proving" that the petitioning profession is not competent to provide the services in question. It is unclear whether this shifted burden was the intent of legislators and whether it serves the best interests of the public.

Keeping these issues in mind and intending to offer guidance to legislators facing the challenges of reforming the process for determining professional practice authority, the Pew Commission offers the following recommendations for states to consider today and to work to implement over the coming years.

RECOMMENDATIONS FOR PROFESSIONAL PRACTICE AUTHORITY

Recommendation 7

The national policy advisory body recommended above should develop standards, including model legislative language, for uniform practice authority acts for the health professions. These standards and models would be based on a wide range of evidence regarding the competence of the professions to provide safe and effective health care.

A national policy advisory body (*see recommendation one*), composed of members not captured by the interests of state regulatory agencies or state health professions associations, would be able to develop evidence-based models and standards for professional practice authority in a non-political forum.

While this policy body needs to be established at the national level, and possibly within the Federal government, the Pew Commission emphasizes that it does not make this recommendation lightly or with the intent of creating new and unnecessary bureaucracy. The goal is to address the shortcomings of the decision-making process regarding practice authority and to limit the negative aspects of turf battles. The intended outcomes would be evidence-based practice authority acts that are uniform across the states.

In carrying out its mandate, the national policy advisory body would start by establishing guidelines that define, for example, the types of evidence permissible for consideration (*see sidebar*). By setting up guidelines in advance that are based on consensus and advice of experts, some of today's problems might be avoided. For example, it is not unusual for one profession to testify that the research techniques, methodologies or data analyses relied upon by a profession seeking changes in their practice act are substandard. It is difficult for state legislators to know the validity of such statements when the criticizing profession has an interest in the outcome.

The range of potential sources of evidence is broad. The national policy advisory body might consider educational standards, outcomes data and expert testimony. It would also consult with the states to identify existing models and practice acts and consider using the least restrictive practice acts for each profession as models for the rest of the states, unless there is any indication that a given act was enacted on grounds other than evidence of competence of a profession. In addition, it would look to model practice acts developed by the professions, controlled clinical trials, customary usage, surveys, natural experiments, data from demonstration projects, and meta-analyses. It would decide which of these sources and methodologies were acceptable, and if necessary, weight them.

Once the guidelines were in place, this national-level body would review the evidence available. It would then develop and disseminate models (examples to

Examples of Evidence that Have Been or Could Be Relied upon by Nurse Practitioners Seeking Changes in Practice Authority Through State Legislation

States' laws and experiences regulating nurse practitioners

- Legislative and regulatory tracking by professional associations and services such as Health Policy Tracking Service at the National Conference of State Legislatures
- Questionnaires sent to the states

Research about nurse practitioners, their practices, and outcomes of services provided

- Meta-analyses (e.g. Brown and Grimes, 1992; Office of Technology Assessment, 1986)
- Survey articles (e.g. Mundinger, 1994)
- Office of the Inspector General reports (1993)
- Agency for Health Care Policy and Research bibliography (Weston, 1990)
- Individual studies (contained in meta-analyses) addressing cost, access, quality
- Pilot and demonstration project descriptions and outcomes (e.g., Freudenheim, 1997)

Individual state studies of practice

- For example: Prescribing of Controlled Substances by Advanced Registered Nurse Practitioners, A Report to the Governor of Florida and the Florida Legislature, 1997

Educational curricula, training and accreditation standards
Data collection from state and federal agencies

- U.S. Drug Enforcement Agency rules and regulations regarding prescriptive authority for controlled substances (Code of Federal Regulations, Title 21, 1998).
- State regulatory boards and national databanks regarding malpractice payments and disciplinary actions

Opinion pieces—from the professions, health care leaders, foundations, health policy advocates, elected officials

emulate) and standards (for comparison and measurement) to the states, which would choose to implement them. The models and standards would be updated regularly as appropriate to acknowledge new evidence about the evolution of health care practice. Throughout its work, the advisory body would assume that professions would share practice authority when appropriate and justified by the evidence at hand.

Recommendation 8

States should enact and implement scopes of practice that are nationally uniform for each profession and based on the standards and models developed by the national policy advisory body.

The Pew Commission recommends that the individual states maintain responsibility for enacting and implementing practice authority legislation for the health professions as necessary. Unlike today's system however, the states should adopt the models and standards developed by the national policy-making body so that the practice acts are uniform among the states, more grounded in evidence and demonstrations of competence and less influenced by the current shortcomings of state-based "turf battles."

Although a national policy advisory body is better suited to develop evidence-based standards and models for professional practice authority, the states are well positioned to implement those standards and models. The individual states have the flexibility to create boards as required, to site the regulated professions under appropriate boards, and to delegate licensing and disciplining authorities to the regulatory boards. The focus of the national policy advisory body in this arena would be limited to establishing the range of services and categories of care the professions should be allowed to provide.

Recommendation 9

Until national models for practice authority acts can be developed and adopted, states should explore and develop mechanisms for existing professions to evolve their existing practice authority and for new professions (or previously unregulated professions) to emerge. In developing such mechanisms, states should be proactive and systematic about collecting data on health care practice. These mechanisms should include:

- *Alternative dispute resolution processes to resolve scope of practice disputes between two or more professions;*
- *Procedures for demonstration projects to be safely conducted and data collected on the effectiveness, quality of care, and costs associated with a profession expanding its existing scope of practice; and*
- *Comprehensive "sunrise" and "sunset" processes that ensure consumer protection while addressing the challenges of expanding existing professions' practice authority and regulating currently unregulated healing disciplines.*

[*See legislative implementation template in Appendix A of Pew Commission's full report.*]

The establishment of a functioning national policy advisory body responsible for collecting, researching, and disseminating models and standards of practice authority acts will take time. The Pew Commission proposes that the states proactively lay the foundations for the national policy advisory body in the interim. Specifically, states should find reasonable and safe ways for the health professions and disciplines to evolve their practice authority. The first step in the process would be for the states to employ mechanisms for the collection of data on health care practice.

Underlying this activity should be the following themes: health care professions and disciplines should be able to evolve and expand their practice domains to incorporate safe and effective practices; a number of professions and disciplines that use non-mainstream therapies safely and effectively should be recognized and regulated as appropriate; and any change in practice authority should be done with the interests of the patients, clients and consumers foremost in the mind of the decision-makers.

Three possible mechanisms for states to employ as they expand the collection and analysis of evidence regarding health care practice are described below in general and in the legislative implementation appendix in more detail.

Alternative Dispute Resolution Processes

Alternative dispute resolution (ADR) mechanisms have been tested in a number of arenas as methods to settle conflicts where the formalities, costs or adversarial framework of the legal system is not appropriate. Following Hawaii's lead, states should explore the use of ADR to resolve conflicts between the health professions over practice authority (*see sidebar*). State legislators familiar with the current battles between optometrists and ophthalmologists concerning laser surgical procedures and conflicts over prescriptive privileges for psychologists would rely on the "fact-finding" model of ADR to assist them in making the decisions required in the public's interest.

With a fact-finding charge from legislators, a body of interested parties facilitated by an ADR expert would be convened to collect and review all the evidence presented on the question at hand. This group would then come to consensus on the quantity, quality, and relevance of the available evidence and submit their findings to the legislature. The legislators would then rely on that document to make their decision regarding the request to establish or change a practice authority act. See the template in Appendix A for more information and guidance for writing relevant legislation.

Guidelines and parameters for demonstration projects—As health professions and disciplines evolve to meet the needs of their patients and clients and to incorporate new knowledge and technologies into their practices, they may face significant hurdles. One of these challenges is in designing and conducting research that will accurately reflect their competence to provide services that have not traditionally been within their practice authority.

While innovation and evolution within the health professions is a necessity, legislatures must safeguard against potentially unreasonably inappropriate,

Alternative Dispute Resolution as a Mechanism for Resolving a Scope of Practice Dispute

For more than three years, the Hawaii state legislature considered numerous bills and passionate (yet often conflicting) testimony in a scope of practice authority battle between psychologists and psychiatrists over prescriptive privileges. Psychologists sought authorization to prescribe drugs to their patients, arguing that this authority would improve access to mental health care in rural under-served communities. Psychiatrists argued that psychologists did not have the proper training to prescribe safely and that there were less costly and more efficient ways to meet the needs of this population.

In 1990, the legislature used a unique process to resolve the battle. The legislature turned to Alternative Dispute Resolution (ADR) which uses a neutral third party to facilitate resolving the dispute. The legislature called upon The Hawaii State Judiciary Center for ADR and charged it with facilitating this dispute by compiling a "single text" document which contained all of the arguments, data, citations, and sources from testimony offered by both sides.

During a six-month period, The Center for ADR convened three roundtable sessions that were open to anyone who wished to testify. Between 25 and 30 people attended each roundtable, and although there were many representatives of professional associations, consumers and individual professionals also participated. Center facilitators successfully carried out their charge and returned a single text document to the legislature. The legislature determined that the psychologists had not adequately proved their competence to prescribe and the proposed bill did not pass (Chandler, 1997; Kent, 1997, 1998; American Psychiatric Association, 1996).

unsafe, and ineffective care. Balancing the need for valid data on changed practice authority with the need to protect the public, legislatures should develop the guidelines and parameters necessary to conduct safe and informative demonstration projects for professions seeking changes in their practice authority acts. Without such guidelines, it is difficult, if not impossible, to conduct research safely that compares outcomes of practitioner care.

These demonstration projects would allow practitioners to *safely* provide care that lies beyond their current statutory authority with the goal of collecting data on the quality and costs of care so delivered. Legislative guidance should be available to groups of professionals and health care delivery organizations so that they may design and implement pilot programs for controlled innovation and experimentation of more flexible use of health care providers. See the template in Appendix A for more information and guidance for writing relevant legislation.

Comprehensive "sunrise" and "sunset" processes—In some states, legislators can rely on standard "sunrise" processes when reviewing requests for new or changed practice authority acts. These processes, when comprehensive, include criteria for review, allowances for public participation and recommendations for evidence-based decision making. The Pew Commission recommends that all states employ such processes that facilitate the work of legislators and professionals while ensuring that the public is protected.

Similarly, some states have enacted sunset laws to use for periodic review of existing professions and their regulatory structures. The value of such laws, when written and implemented correctly, is significant in their effect to hold self-regulatory entities accountable to the public. Optimally, these laws would provide a mechanism for evaluation to assure that regulatory bodies are operating effectively and efficiently and that professional practice acts are kept current and relevant. See the template in Appendix A of Pew Commission's full report for more information and guidance for writing relevant legislation.

CONTINUING COMPETENCE: THE STATE REGULATORY ROLE IN ENSURING THE CONTINUED COMPETENCE OF HEALTH CARE PRACTITIONERS

CURRENT ISSUES

Of the ten issue areas identified in the 1995 report *Reforming Health Care Workforce Regulation: Policy Considerations for the 21st Century,* the call for requiring continuing competence assessments of health care professionals has likely generated the most action in accord with the recommendation (*see sidebar*). In the formal responses to the 1995 report, this recommendation received the highest score for level of concern and one of the highest scores for level of support (Gragnola and Stone, 1997). The high level of activity may be due to tremendous tension between consumer anxiety over quality of care and practitioner anxiety over being asked to demonstrate their competence more than once.

While continuing education and life-long learning have numerous benefits, the Pew Commission agrees with the assessment that continuing education credits do not guarantee competence (Relman, 1997). Continuing education simply is not sufficient to ensure quality throughout a practitioner's career. Additionally, few if any regulatory boards require their licensees to *demonstrate* their competence at any point after initial licensure and current systems for detecting incompetence are imperfect. Perhaps most pressing is the fact that the monumental shift to new reimbursement and delivery structures in this country has highlighted the need to pay attention to quality of care. Underlying managed care's critics and legislative restraints is the concern that high quality health care—and a professional's competence to provide it—may suffer from too much attention on reducing costs. Requiring demonstrations of competence

Recent Activities Regarding Continuing Competency

- The Interprofessional Workgroup on Health Professions Regulation held a two-day "Continued Competency Summit" in July 1997. Attended by representatives of many different health professions, the conference focused on methods of assessment and other issues related to continued competency (Interprofessional Workgroup, 1997).
- Citizen Advocacy Center, a training, research, and support network for public members of health care regulatory and governing boards, held a two-day conference in December 1996 entitled, "Continuing Professional Competence: Can We Assure It?" (Citizen Advocacy Center, 1997).
- The National Council of State Boards of Nursing has developed Personal Accountability Profiles to serve as a framework for licensed nurses to document learning needs, learning plans and goals/objectives and strategies for development and evaluation as to whether goals/objectives have been achieved (Sheets, 1997).
- The State of Washington's Department of Health has established an interdisciplinary task force to look at continuing competency efforts, and to examine the feasibility of continuing competency requirements for health care professionals (Ehri, 1998).
- The Colorado Personalized Education for Physicians is a model program for individualized competency assessment along with a personalized learning plan. It is used by physicians from around the country on a self-referral basis; referrals can also be made by employers or the Board of Medical Examiners (Colorado Personalized Education for Physicians, 1998).
- California's SB 1981, if enacted, will require persons licensed to practice podiatric medicine to demonstrate their competence throughout their careers at regular intervals via a number of different options (1998).

during professionals' careers could shift attention to the quality of care delivered to patients and clients.

Regulators could be involved in competence requirements at the four junctures identified by the National Council of State Boards of Nursing: entry to practice, for continued authority to practice, reentry to practice, and after disciplinary action (Citizen Advocacy Center, 1997). To date, however, legislatures have largely declined to require that regulatory boards insist that their licensees demonstrate competence for continued authority to practice.

Historically, the challenge has been in defining and measuring competence in ways that meet the needs of consumers for safe and effective care without unreasonably burdening the individual practitioner. For more than a century, policy makers and consumers have used a complex assortment of methods to indirectly evaluate competence and quality. Both preventive measures and punitive interventions serve as proxies for demonstrations of competence.

Consumers rely largely on "positive" or preventive mechanisms such as education at accredited institutions, licensing examinations, character checks, and continuing education requirements to protect them from incompetent practitioners. The system is then bolstered with "negative" or punitive interventions to deal with problems after they have arisen. These interventions include regulatory departments for complaints, enforcement and discipline, as well as extra-regulatory bodies—peer review bodies, criminal justice, malpractice and tort actions—that serve as post-occurrence safety nets to further protect the public and provide avenues of redress.

Despite all these efforts, significant numbers of patients, clients and consumers continue to suffer the consequences of health professional incompetence (Leape, 1994). A RAND Corporation study for the National Coalition on Health Care found that, "there are large gaps between the care that people should receive and the care they do receive." This is true for preventive, acute and chronic care (Schuster et al., 1997). While Public Citizen's Health Research Group reports that 16,638 doctors were disciplined (primarily for: criminal convictions; substandard care, incompetence or negligence; mis-prescribing or over-prescribing drugs; substance abuse; and professional misconduct) by either state medical boards or federal agencies as of January 1997, the group also estimates that this makes up only a small percentage of the total number of incompetent physicians (Wolfe, 1998).

Partly in response to these indicators of low quality care, external factors—ranging from the evolution of public expectations and demands for accountability to market-driven rationalization of health care costs—have already changed the way competence is assessed and enforced. Currently, competence is often better determined by private sector assessments and employer evaluations than by the self-regulating boards. Efforts by the National Committee for Quality Assurance to privately regulate health plans are beginning to include attention to the individual practitioner. Total quality management or continuous quality improvement endeavors that include individual practitioners as well as systems of care may be shifting the level of quality of health care upward. Some of the medical specialty boards and other private sector professional boards, also have developed continuing competence requirements.

The potential for collaboration between public regulators and private sector credentialing bodies is significant but the professions are not in agreement on the prospect. Representatives from medicine have voiced their preference that public regulators and private certifying agencies keep their distance, whereas a collaborative relationship between regulation and private specialty credentialing is developing in nursing. This split in perspective may be due in part to different histories of the professions; the medical license is all-inclusive and state boards of medicine have not traditionally recognized specialties. Nursing regulation, on the other hand, recognizes professional specialization (Citizen Advocacy Center, 1997).

Whether done by the private or the public sector, or by a partnership of the two, the challenges of better assessing and assuring continuing competence are significant but not insurmountable. They include coordinating efforts between establishing competence at the entry-to-practice level with ongoing assessment throughout a practitioner's career; identifying and researching the links among practitioner competence (at initial licensure and relicensure), high quality care, and consumer expectations for accountability; and knowing when concerns over quality and competence must include looking at the broader systems of care in which individual professionals practice. In addition, regulators must address the question of how often practitioners must demonstrate their competence. These periods between demonstrations will likely vary from profession to profession and depend on the practice circumstances of individual practitioners.

Requirements that practitioners demonstrate competence throughout their careers must also be supported by meaningful ways of ensuring that practitioners meet those requirements. When requirements are not met, enforcement mechanisms might include sanctions, restriction of privileges, revocation of license or public or private censure. Positive incentives for meeting requirements might include licensing fee reductions and public acknowledgments.

Given the current social, political and economic environment, the regulatory system may have a small window of opportunity to commit itself to answering these questions and assuming the responsibility for requiring continuing competence of its licensees. Although the professions, private sector testing and practice institutions may all be involved, the role of the state is critical. One entity must be capable of, and responsible for, collecting and coordinating the information from the various sectors, including tying continuing competency requirements to the disciplinary process.

RECOMMENDATION FOR CONTINUING COMPETENCE

Recommendation 10

States should require that their regulated health care practitioners demonstrate their competence in the knowledge, judgment, technical skills and interpersonal skills relevant to their jobs throughout their careers. [See legislative implementation template in Appendix A of Pew Commission's full report.]

In addition to being responsible for setting competence standards for individuals wishing to enter professional practice, state regulatory boards should expand their responsibilities to include requiring regulated health care practitioners to demonstrate their competence throughout their careers. Legislators also should encourage unregulated health professions and disciplines to establish standards regarding continuing competence.

The current system that relies on continuing education and disciplinary action is insufficient. And, although the private sector has begun to ensure practitioner competence, it is unlikely that it alone can or will be accountable

The Federal Aviation Administration: A Nationally Unified Regulatory System

The Federal Aviation Administration (FAA) is an example of a nationally unified system of professional, facility and equipment regulation. The Air Commerce Act of 1926 charged the Secretary of Commerce with fostering air commerce, issuing and enforcing air traffic rules, licensing pilots, certifying aircraft, establishing airways, and operating and maintaining aids to air navigation (Federal Aviation Administration, 1998).

For all pilots, initial licensure for competence, continuing competency requirements, testing and discipline are administered by one federal agency. Through the Federal Aviation Requirements, all pilots at all levels are qualified for flying based on physical condition (medical certificate), aeronautical experience (logbook), knowledge (written tests) and skill (flight tests).

The pilot certification and re-certification process becomes more rigorous as a pilot's responsibility increases (e.g. larger aircraft, larger passenger loads, flying using instruments/technology, night flying, and permission to captain an aircraft). The two examples below illustrate the process:

- Student Pilot License is restricted to flying without any passengers, within twenty-five miles of the home airport, and in good flying conditions. The FAA requirements are for a third-class medical certificate (lowest grade), 40 hours of flight time (half of which with a certified instructor), no written test and a single flight test administered one time.
- Air Transport Pilot is necessary for any pilot flying a turbojet with more than ten-seat capacity. Requirements include passing the first class medical certification (highest level), having 1500 hours of flight time (broken into a variety of categories including night flying, instrument time, pilot-in-command time, etc.), and having completed testing for Instrument Certification. An Air Transport Pilot must re-test as often as every six months, depending on job requirements, at both flight and medical levels (Code of Federal Regulations, Title 14, 1997).

ultimately for developing and sustaining an effective system. State legislators and regulators can provide the necessary support, incentives, and accountability lacking in the private sector. Moreover, the states, as protectors of the public's health, safety and welfare, can no longer ignore the implications of *not* addressing the issue of health professions competence beyond initial licensure.

With the goal of working in conjunction with the private sector, states would take the lead in defining competence to include basic knowledge, skills and judgment and also specialized knowledge, skills and judgment. Definitions should eventually include less clinical competencies such as communication skills, ethics, concepts of continuous quality improvement, the capacity to admit errors, and the ability to empathize.

States should also develop criteria by which private sector competence assessments would be deemed to have satisfied state requirements. For example, states might develop mechanisms by which regulatory bodies can accept voluntary certification by private sector entities as evidence of public sector requirements for demonstrating continuing competence.

With the establishment of the national policy advisory body (*see recommendation one*), definitions, models and standards for continuing competence assessment would be researched, developed, and disseminated by that body to the states to implement. States and private sector entities would in turn provide the national policy advisory body with their findings on the effectiveness and benefits of the models they have employed. Of particular importance will be the need to relate continuing competence assessments to practice performance and scope of duties or services provided. This may lead to reevaluations of practice acts that are particularly broad, if it becomes evident that continuing competence should be linked to areas of specialty or expertise.

Ultimately, national standards for continuing competence assessments would complement the national standards for practice authority acts. Differences from state to state in requirements for continued licensure within any given profession cannot be justified any more than differences in scope of practice acts. One relevant model that might be considered is the Federal Aviation Administration (*see sidebar*), which requires the same periodic demonstrations of competency from specified categories of licensed pilots (Leape, 1994).

Alternative models for determining whether practitioners are competent throughout their careers need to be tested and evaluated for effectiveness, costs, and benefits. Currently, a number of different tools are being used to measure education and knowledge, experience and demonstrated ability (*see sidebar*). These measurements include standardized examinations, computer simulations, standardized patients, objective structured clinical examinations, office record reviews, practice evaluations and peer review. Patient satisfaction may also serve as an adjunct to assessment tools by confirming observations. All of these tools need to be evaluated for validity, reliability, and fairness (Citizen Advocacy Center, 1997).

The actual assessment of competence may best be left to the professional associations, private testing companies and specialty boards that would continue their current efforts to develop and offer continuing competence assessment tools that are meaningful (empirically-based, valid and reliable), effective (psychometrically sound) and cost-efficient.

College of Nurses of Ontario Quality Assurance Program

Among other things, Ontario, Canada's Regulated Health Professions Act requires that the professional colleges (akin to the professional boards in the United States) develop and maintain programs and standards to promote the continuing competence of members. In accord with this requirement, the College of Nurses of Ontario (CNO) has taken a comprehensive approach to ensuring continuing competence throughout practicing nurses' careers. The College's Quality Assurance Program has three parts, all of which can be tailored to meet the needs of individual practitioners:

- Reflective practice;
- Competence assessment; and
- Practice setting consultation.

As of 1998, only the first part—reflective practice—has been implemented as a requirement of practicing nurses. The practice setting component will be implemented in 1999 and the competence assessment component is in development.

Nurses in the province must complete five steps and submit relevant documentation to satisfy the reflective practice component: complete a self-assessment; get feedback on his or her practice; create a learning plan; learn (i.e., do the activities identified in the individual's learning plan); and evaluate the learning. Although all nurses must complete all five steps, they may choose from among several options for actually meeting the requirements. These options include using a professional development system at their workplace; using their own or a CNO-produced self-assessment tool; or using formal education programs.

Future requirements will include the competence assessment and practice setting consultation components of the Quality Assurance Program. When in place, these will require that nurses: 1) complete a self-directed competence assessment tool, an interview with an assessor and/or observation of practice by an assessor; and 2) participate in the Practice Setting Consultation Program, which is designed to encourage nurses and other members of multidisciplinary teams to work with their employer to ensure that the key attributes of a quality practice environment are in place. These attributes include care delivery processes, communication systems, facilities and equipment, professional development systems, leadership, organizational supports, and response systems (College of Nurses of Ontario, 1998).

To encourage market strengths while protecting consumers from market failures, parameters should be set around this potentially lucrative business. The states should establish the assessment standards they expect their licensees to meet, thereby stimulating private sector responsiveness and minimizing the chance of inappropriate, irrelevant, or unreasonable standards being set. States might begin this process by cataloging and analyzing continuing competence requirements of private accreditors.

Finally, there will always be health care professionals whose competence, for a number of reasons, might not be assessed by private sector institutions. To address the limitations of the private sector, states would also be responsible for focusing on the practitioners who "fall through the cracks" or are outliers. State governments would have to address this reality and be responsible, for example, for establishing relevant triggers that would link private quality assurance mechanisms with state boards to identify outliers. See the template in Appendix A of Pew Commission's full report for more information and guidance for writing relevant legislation.

REFERENCES

CITATIONS USED IN THE REPORT

Prologue and Introduction

Brinegar P and McGinley M. Telepractice and Professional Licensing: A Guide for Legislators. The Council on Licensure, Enforcement and Regulation. Lexington, KY. 1998.

Finocchio LJ, Dower CM, McMahon T, Gragnola CM and the Taskforce on Health Care Workforce Regulation. Reforming Health Care Workforce Regulation: Policy Considerations for the 21st Century. Pew Health Professions Commission. San Francisco, CA. December 1995.

Gragnola CM and Stone E. Considering the Future of Health Care Workforce Regulation. UCSF Center for the Health Professions. San Francisco, CA. December 1997.

Hafferty FW and Light DW. Professional Dynamics and the Changing Nature of Medical Work. Journal of Health and Social Behavior, Extra Issue: 132–153. 1995.

Health Policy Tracking Service. Issue Brief: Comprehensive Consumer Rights Bills. National Conference of State Legislatures. Washington, DC. May 1998.

Moran DW. Federal Regulation of Managed Care: An Impulse in Search of A Theory? Health Affairs 16(6):7–21. November/December 1997.

Schneller ES and Ott JB. Contemporary Models of Change in the Health Professions. Hospital and Health Services Administration 41 (1):121–136. Spring 1996.

Regulatory Boards and Governance Structures

Andrew G and Sauer H. Do Boards of Medicine Really Matter? The Future of Professional Regulation. Federation Bulletin 85 (4):228–236. 1996.

Arnett D, former Executive Director, Medical Board of California and Presley R, President, Board of Podiatic Medicine. Letter to The Honorable Leroy F. Greene, Chairman, California Joint Legislative Sunset Review Committee. February 23, 1998.

Bernstein D. Doctors' group heads off fee hike: Objects to cost of malpractice prosecutions. The Sacramento Bee. August 1,1998.

Brennan T and Berwick D. New Rules: Regulation, Markets and the Quality of American Health Care. Jossey-Bass. San Francisco, CA. 1996.

California Board of Podiatric Medicine. Sunset Report in Brief. November 3, 1997.

Citizen Advocacy Center. Public Representation on Health Care Regulatory, Governing, and Oversight Bodies: Strategies for Success. Washington, DC. May 1995.

Cohen RA and Swankin DA. Hospital Reporting to State Regulators and to the National Practitioner Data Bank: What Can Be Learned To Improve Compliance with Mandatory Reporting Requirements? Citizen Advocacy Center. Washington, DC. March 1997.

Colorado Revised Statutes: article 43 of title 12. 1998.

Colorado Revised Statutes: subsection 13 of section 24-34-102. 1998.

Douglas, Bruce. Director, Division of Registrations, Department of Regulatory Agencies, State of Colorado. Personal communication. July 29, 1998.

Federation of State Medical Boards of the United States, Inc. The Exchange, 1995–96. Section Three: Licensing Boards, Structure and Disciplinary Functions. Euless, TX. 1995.

Finocchio LJ, Dower CM, McMahon T, Gragnola CM and the Taskforce on Health Care Workforce Regulation. Reforming Health Care Workforce Regulation: Policy Considerations for the 21st Century. Pew Health Professions Commission. San Francisco, CA. 1995.

Florida Senate Health Care Committee. Interim Project Report 97-P-42. Superboard for Disciplining Health Care Practitioners. August 1997.

Florida SB 256, 1998.

Gragnola CM and Stone E. Considering the Future of Health Care Workforce Regulation. UCSF Center for the Health Professions. San Francisco, CA. December 1997.

Health Care Financing Administration. Office of Clinical Standards and Quality. Unpublished Data. 1997.

Jost TS. Introduction—Regulation of the Healthcare Professions. In: Jost TS (ed.), Regulation of the Healthcare Professions. Health Administration Press. Chicago, IL. 1997.

Kany JC and Janes SD. Improving Public Policy for Regulating Maine's Health Professionals. Medical Care Development, Inc. Augusta, ME. October 1997.

Massachusetts Board of Registration in Medicine. Website for Massachusetts Physician Profiles. (http://www.docboard.org/ma/ma_home.htm) 1998.

Medical Board of California. Action Report vol. 52. January 1995.

Minnesota Board of Examiners for Nursing Home Administrators. Letter to Licensees. February 9, 1998.

National Council of State Boards of Nursing. Boards of Nursing Adopt Revolutionary Change for Nursing Regulation. National Council Issues (18)3. 1997.

Oregon H 2296, 1997.

Relman AS. Regulation of the Medical Profession: A Physician's Perspective. In: Jost TS (ed.), Regulation of the Healthcare Professions: 199–210. Health Administration Press. Chicago, IL. 1997.

U.S. Department of Health and Human Services, Public Health Service, Health Resources and Services Administration, Bureau of Health Professions, Division of Associated Dental and Public Health Professions. Report of the National Commission on Allied Health. Rockville, MD. 1995.

Western Governors' Association. Telemedicine Action Update. Denver, CO. June 1998.

Yessian MR and Greenleaf JM. The Ebb and Flow of Federal Initiatives to Regulate Healthcare Professionals. In: Jost TS (ed.), Regulation of the Healthcare Professions. Health Administration Press. Chicago, IL: 169–198. 1997.

Professional Practice Authority

American Psychiatric Association. Hawaii Psychiatrists Again Victorious Over Psychologists. Psychiatric News (31)9. May 3, 1996.

Brown SA and Grimes DE. A Meta-Analysis of Process of Care, Clinical Outcomes, and Cost-Effectiveness of Nurses in Primary Care Roles: Nurse Practitioners and Nurse-Midwives. Prepared for The American Nurses' Association, Division of Health Policy. June 1992.

Chandler, David. Professor of Sociology, University of Hawaii; former Director, Hawaii State Judiciary Center for Alternative Dispute Resolution. Personal communication. Nov. 3, 1997.

Code of Federal Regulations. Title 21, Parts 1300–1301, 1304. Drug Enforcement Administration, Department of Justice. Definitions; Registration of Manufacturers, Distributors, and Dispensers of Controlled Substances; Records and Reports of Registrants. 1998.

Colorado Revised Statutes: Title 12, Article 43, 1998.

Cooper RA and Stoflet SJ. Trends in the Education and Practice of Alternative Medicine Clinicians. Health Affairs (15)3: 226–238. Fall 1996.

Dower CM, Gragnola CM, Finocchio LJ. Changing Nature of Physician Licensure: Implications for Medical Education in California. Western Journal of Medicine 168: 422–427. 1998.

Fox-Grage W. An Overview of 1995 State Legislative Activity: Scopes of Practice. Intergovernmental Health Policy Project, George Washington University. Washington, DC. December 15, 1995.

Freudenheim M. Nurses Working Without Doctors Angers the Medical Establishment. New York Times. September 30, 1997.

Gragnola CM and Stone E. Considering the Future of Health Care Workforce Regulation. UCSF Center for the Health Professions. San Francisco, CA. December 1997.

Health Policy Tracking Service. National Conference of State Legislatures. Info@hpts.org, www.hpts.org. Washington, DC. December 1997.

Kent, Elizabeth. Director, Hawaii State Judiciary Center for Alternative Dispute Resolution. Personal communications. October 6, 1997, March 13, 1998.

Lucas, Greg. Eye Care Compromise Reached. San Francisco Chronicle. February 15, 1996.

Mundinger M. Advanced-Practice Nursing—Good Medicine for Physicians? New England Journal of Medicine (330)3: 211–214. January 20, 1994.

Office of Technology Assessment. Nurse Practitioners, Physicians' Assistants and Certified Nurse Midwives: A Policy Analysis. Health Technology Study 37. OTA-HCS-37. Government Printing Office. Washington, DC. 1986.

Office of the Inspector General. Enhancing the Utilization of Nonphysician Health Care Providers. U.S. Department of Health and Human Services. May 1993.

Prescribing of Controlled Substances by Advanced Registered Nurse Practitioners. A Report to the Governor of Florida and the Florida Legislature pursuant to chapter 96-274, Laws of Florida. December 1997.

Sage WM and Aiken LH. Regulating Interdisciplinary Practice. In: Jost TS (ed.), Regulation of the Healthcare Professions. Health Administration Press, Chicago, IL: 71–101. 1997.

Weston JL. Annotated Bibliography of AHCPR Research on Nonphysician Primary Care Providers 1969–1989. U.S. Department of Health and Human Services. Public Health Service. July 1990.

Continuing Competence

California SB 1981, 1998.

Citizen Advocacy Center. Continuing Professional Competence: Can We Assure It? Washington D.C. May 1997.

Code of Federal Regulations. Title 14, Part 61. Aeronautics and Space. Federal Aviation Administration, Department of Transportation. Certification: Pilots, Flight Instructors, and Ground Instructors. 1997.

College of Nurses of Ontario. The Quality Assurance Program: Your Guide for 1998. CNO Quality Assurance Program. Toronto, Ontario. 1998.

Colorado Personalized Education Program for Physicians. Aurora, CO. 1998.

Ehri, Diana, Acting Executive Director, Health Policy & Constituent Relations, Health Professions Quality Assurance Division, State of Washington Department of Health. Personal communication. February 9, 1998.

Federal Aviation Administration Web Page (http://www.faa.gov/). U.S. Department of Transportation. 800 Independence Avenue, SW, Washington, DC. July 27, 1998.

Gragnola CM and Stone E. Considering the Future of Health Care Workforce Regulation. UCSF Center for the Health Professions. San Francisco, CA. December 1997.

Interprofessional Workgroup on Health Professions Regulation. Continued Competency Summit: Assessing the Issues, Methods, and Realities for Health Care Professions. Course Materials: A Compendium of Conference Handouts. 1997.

Leape L. Error in Medicine. JAMA (272)23:1851–1857. December 21, 1994.

Relman AS. Regulation of the Medical Profession: A Physician's Perspective. In: Jost TS (ed.), Regulation of the Healthcare Professions. Health Administration Press. Chicago, IL: 199–210. 1997.

Schuster MA, McGlynn EA, Brook RH. Why the Quality of U.S. Health Care Must Be Improved. RAND. Santa Monica, CA. October 1997.

Sheets VR. What's Out There? A Critical Look at Two Paradigms: Markers Model vs. Continuous Quality Assurance Model. In: Continued Competency Summit: Assessing the Issues, Methods, and Realities for Health Care Professions. Course Materials: A Compendium of Conference Handouts. Interprofessional Workgroup on Health Professions Regulation. 1997.

Wolfe S, et al. Questionable Doctors Disciplined by State and Federal Governments 1998 Edition, Public Citizen's Health Research Group. Washington, DC. 1998.

BIBLIOGRAPHY

A chronological selection of key reports, books and articles discussing the strengths and weaknesses of professional regulation.

Council of State Governments. Occupational Licensing Legislation in the States. Chicago, IL. 1952.

U.S. Department of Health, Education and Welfare, Public Health Service, National Center for Health Statistics. State Licensing of Health Occupations. DHEW Publication No. 1758. Washington, DC. 1967.

U.S. Department of Health, Education and Welfare, Office of Assistant Secretary for Health and Scientific Affairs. Report on Licensure and Related Personnel Credentialing. DHEW Publication No. (HSM) 72-11.Washington, DC. 1971.

Shimberg B, Esser BF, Kruger DH. Occupational Licensing: Practices and Policies. Public Affairs Press. Washington, DC. 1972.

U.S. Department of Health, Education and Welfare, Public Health Service, Health Resources Administration, Bureau of Health Manpower. State Regulation of Health Manpower. DHEW Publication No. (HRA) 77-49. Washington, DC. 1977.

Cohen HS. On Professional Power and Conflict of Interest: State Licensing Boards on Trial. Journal of Health Politics, Policy and Law. 5(2) Summer 1980.

Shimberg B. Occupational Licensing: A Public Perspective. Educational Testing Service. Princeton, NJ. 1980.

Starr P. The Social Transformation of American Medicine: The Rise of a Sovereign Profession and the Making of a Vast Industry. Basic Books. New York, NY. 1982.

Abbott, A. The System of Professions: An Essay on the Division of Expert Labor. University of Chicago Press. 1988.

Cox C and Foster S. The Costs and Benefits of Occupational Regulation. Bureau of Economics of the Federal Trade Commission. Washington, DC. October 1990.

Maryland Department of Fiscal Services. Sunset Review: State Board of Physician Quality Assurance. October 1991.

State of Tennessee, Comptroller of the Treasury, Department of Audit, Division of State Audit. Performance Audit of Health-Related Boards. March 1992.

Texas Sunset Advisory Commission. Health Care Licensing Boards: A Staff Report to the Sunset Advisory Commission. October 1992.

Begun J and Lippincott R. Strategic Adaptations in the Health Professions: Meeting the Challenges of Change. Jossey-Bass. San Francisco, CA. 1993.

Friedson E. Professionalism Reborn: Theory, Prophecy and Policy. University of Chicago Press. Chicago, IL. 1994.

Gross SJ. Of Foxes and Hen Houses: Licensing and the Health Professions. Quorum Books. Westport, CT 1994.

Shimberg B and Roederer D. Questions a Legislator Should Ask. Kara Schmitt (ed). Second edition. The Council on Licensure, Enforcement and Regulation. Lexington, KY. 1994.

State of Arizona, Office of the Auditor General. Performance Audit of The Board of Medical Examiners. Report to the Arizona Legislature. November 22, 1994.

Finocchio LJ, Dower CM, McMahon T, Gragnola CM and the Taskforce on Health Care Workforce Regulation. Reforming Health Care Workforce Regulation: Policy Considerations for the 21st Century. Pew Health Professions Commission. San Francisco, CA. December 1995.

State of Arizona, Office of the Auditor General. Special Study of The Health Regulatory System: Report to the Arizona Legislature. December 1, 1995.

Brennan T and Berwick D. New Rules: Regulation, Markets and the Quality of American Health Care. Jossey-Bass. San Francisco, CA. 1996.

Jost TS. Regulation of the Healthcare Professions. Health Administration Press. Chicago, IL. 1997.

NOTES

The Pew Health Professions Commission is a program of The Pew Charitable Trusts. The Pew Charitable Trusts support nonprofit activities in the areas of culture, education, the environment, health and human services, public policy and religion. Based in Philadelphia, the Trusts make strategic investments that encourage and support citizen participation in addressing critical issues and effecting social change. In 1997, with more than $4.5 billion in assets, the Trusts awarded $181 million to 320 nonprofit organizations.

1. Commissioner Graham abstained from voting on this recommendation.

2. While all of the Commissioners support this recommendation, some Commissioners also support these configurations for boards: 1) 50 percent public membership; 2) public member majorities; or 3) one-third public members, one-third health care professionals, and one-third other representatives (e.g. other licensed health care professionals, hospital and health plan administrators, health services researchers).

13

The Changing Nature of Health Professions Education

John Naughton

For most of the twentieth century, health professions education has experienced unprecedented growth, development, expansion, importance, influence, and acceptance in America.

As we entered the second decade of the century, for example, medical schools started to evolve from proprietary teaching institutions into complex structures responsible for the education of medical students, graduate biomedical scientists, and graduate medical education (GME) trainees; the conduct of biomedical research; and direct involvement in patient care and community health. Most medical schools became colleges in universities that either owned or were affiliated with hospitals.

Then, with the end of World War II, the relationships of a medical school to its teaching hospitals, community, and university changed gradually, but dramatically. Many medical and health professions schools are now aggregated around the common theme of health education and organized as academic health centers.

Today, medical and other health professions education must deal with the dilemma posed by an excellent and superb medical education and health care system that exists side by side with a society that desires increased access to health care, reasonable cost of care, and a high level of consumer satisfaction.

Academic health centers include, at a minimum, a medical school and one or more other health professions schools and one or more teaching hospitals. A recent report by Blumenthal (1997) on the role of academic health centers

Reprinted from Elaine R. Rubin (ed.), *Mission Management: A New Synthesis*, pp. 93–128 (Washington, D.C., 1998) with permission from the Association of Academic Health Centers.

TABLE 13.1

Academic Units by Schools of AHC Members (1996)

Academic Unit	AHC Member with Academic Unit
Medical	105
Allopathic	(99)
Osteopathic	(6)
Nursing	64
Allied health	57
Graduate studies	50
Dental medicine	45
Pharmacy	30
Public health	24
Social work	4
Veterinary medicine	4
Optometry	2

in providing public goods indicates that 125 centers have met these minimum criteria. More typically, however, an academic health center comprises a number of associated health professions schools that work collaboratively with each other and with hospital and ambulatory facilities to conduct clinical training.

Table 13.1 reflects the diversity of health professions schools among members of the Association of Academic Health Centers (AHC). In addition to medical schools, approximately one-half of the academic health centers also have schools of nursing, allied health, graduate studies, and dental medicine; almost one-quarter have schools of pharmacy and public health; and less than one-twentieth have a school of social work, veterinary medicine, optometry, or law. Approximately one-half of the academic health centers own or apparently control a teaching hospital; those remaining are affiliated only with one or more hospitals or health care systems. Sixty-seven are affiliated with a major Veterans Administration Health Center (VAHC). Approximately 100 VAHCs, in turn, are affiliated with one or more of the nation's allopathic medical schools.

The important role played by academic health centers in our nation was clearly recognized during the recent health care reform debate (Clinton 1994) when the Administration recommended universal, unified health care financing for the United States. Critics of the proposal suggested that the Administration's proposed amendment to the Health Security Act did not sufficiently appreciate the intricate dependence of health science schools and teaching hospitals on Federal funding to support and conduct health-related education and research. Because major cost-shifting across multiple institutions occurs in any academic health center, the case presented to the President and Congress for fiscal support was often made under the guise of academic health centers, in general, rather than for individual schools or other health care organizations.

The failure of the amendments to the Health Security Act dramatically changed the situation for academic health centers. Rather than develop a national health care system that was both more regulated and also limited to one universal payor, as proposed by the President, the nation chose to maintain optimal autonomy and choice, with health care financing and education determined by competitive market forces.

This paper summarizes the activities reflecting the nation's support and commitment to advances in health professions education during the period 1910–1994, sometimes known as The Golden Era, and the changing health care scene since 1994. In the paper, I also speculate on health care changes that most medical and health professions schools will experience with the coming of the twenty-first century. Although it is too early to conclude unequivocally, it appears that a trend is emerging for Federal and state governments to purchase increased amounts of health care through commercial insurers. Under this approach, the share of funds allocated to health care is negotiated competitively through contracts between the public and private sectors with the providers of care.

An additional major approach to medical care that will become widespread before the Year 2000 is that of managed care, a mechanism designed to manage and reduce the cost of health care. Its introduction, combined with the effects of Medicaid, Medicare, and welfare reform, already reflects an acceleration in hospital mergers, the formation of integrated vertical systems of care, the onset of medical school mergers, and the start of downsizing the number of medical school enrollees and graduate medical education trainees.

THE GOLDEN ERA (1910–1994)

The modern era of medical education has its roots in the Flexner Report (1910). This scathing document condemned the dominance of proprietary medical schools and an excess in the number of physicians, most with minimal formal education, and recommended a reduction in the number of proprietary medical schools as part of an approach to planned obsolescence. Table 13.2 summarizes the number of medical schools that were operating in California, Illinois, Indiana, New York, and Pennsylvania in 1910, together with the number Flexner recommended as ideal for 1910 and the number in existence in 1997. (Note that at the time of the Flexner Report, a half school was one limited to preclinical education. Two states, New York and Illinois, each had four postgraduate schools, probably the forerunners of today's graduate medical education.) California, Illinois, and Pennsylvania had fewer full schools in 1997 than they did in 1910; Indiana had the same number; and New York had more.

TABLE 13.2

**Examples of Flexner's Recommendations for Reducing
Allopathic Medical Schools Compared with Current Situation**

	Number of Schools		
State	*In 1910*	*Recommended by Flexner*	*In 1997*
California	9.0 (1 half)	1.0 (1 half)	7.0
Illinois	14.0	7.0	7.0
Indiana	1.0 (2 half)	1.0 (1 half)	1.0
New York	11.0	2.0	12.0
Pennsylvania	9.0	2.0	6.0

Note: In addition, California, Illinois, New York, and Pennsylvania have a total of five osteopathic medical schools.

The nation in 1910 apparently was ready for the Flexner Report because, in short order, extensive changes took place. They included the following events:

- Approximately two-thirds of existing medical schools merged or closed.
- Commercial (proprietary) allopathic medical schools became unacceptable to the profession and the public.
- States established accreditation and licensing standards.
- Medical education became more standardized and access to medical education became highly competitive.
- The quality and status of the medical profession were enhanced.
- Medical schools either became intrinsic units within a university or closely aligned to a university. (Even in 1910, universities were willing to include medical schools, but unwilling to commit many resources to finance them.)

The Flexner Report reflected attitudes still relevant for contemporary educational and societal concerns. Flexner, for example, emphasized that a quality medical education required students to be well educated in the sciences basic to medicine. A strong scientific faculty did not yet exist. Although Flexner's interest was education, not research per se, subsequent generations of faculty did go on to help medical schools become more research intensive, especially as the post–World War II partnership developed between the National Institutes of Health (NIH) and the nation's universities and medical schools.

WOMEN IN MEDICINE

Flexner did not see a need to establish medical schools solely to serve women, as three schools were then doing. His conclusion that, in general, access for women to medical careers need not be a concern, based on an enrollment in the years 1904 through 1909 of 1,264 women (5.7 percent), turned out to be faulty because it failed to perceive the important role that women could and would later contribute to the profession.

In addition, the Flexner Report evaluated the seven traditionally black medical schools. Total enrollment from 1904 through 1909 was 750 medical students. Flexner concluded that these graduates would remain in the South to treat African-Americans living primarily in rural environments. He recommended that five of the seven schools be closed, which did take place, and that two, Meharry and Howard Universities, remain open and be upgraded. Despite the socioeconomic and cultural issues that faced African-Americans in 1910, he thought two schools sufficient to attract qualified African-American students to serve the South's minority population. He was apparently unaware of a need for minority physicians in the North.

Influenced by the Johns Hopkins Medical School, Flexner also stated unequivocally that every medical school must control at least one hospital. Ultimately, Flexner's report achieved the Carnegie Foundation's intent to move medical education, the medical profession, and health care to a standard previously not achieved in society. Those aspects of the report that served school and university interests, especially the improvement of education and developing research programs, were successfully implemented; those that were not implemented remain largely unattended even to this day.

TRANSFORMATION (1910–1945)

The period from 1910 through 1945 can be described as one of significant transformation for the medical profession. The American Medical Association (AMA) and the Association of American Medical Colleges (AAMC) fostered medical school accreditation. Medical schools required collegiate preparation for medical education and became more selective in accepting students. Licensure boards were established in every state, national standardized examinations evolved, and formal approval of internships was implemented (AMA 1923). Ultimately, every allopathic physician performed at least one year of internship after graduation before entering medical practice. Medical schools, with rare exception, continued a mission limited to educating students prepared to practice clinical medicine. Although a limited number of outstanding hospitals initiated additional training opportunities, the expansion of graduate medical education began in earnest only after World War II. In the first list of approved residencies, published by the American Medical Association (1928), the ratio of interns to residents was 3 to 1.

The impact of World War II on medical schools and the medical profession was tremendous. The entire nation was mobilized for the war effort, with all medical students expected to enter military service after graduation. Education for the medical student was compressed to three consecutive calendar years compared with four years in the past. A large proportion of the existing practicing physician base was called to military service. These physicians, together with the recent medical school graduates, built on their experience in battlefield situations to expand the professional capacity and skill of the medical profession on a scale never before achieved.

THE POSTWAR YEARS (1945–1960)

Medical education experienced numerous profound changes in the postwar years. These included increases in the number of applicants to medical school; many, as veterans of the war, were, of course, older and more mature than applicants in the past. However, medical school enrollments increased from 6,000 students per graduating class in 1945 to only 7,300 in 1964 (Coggeshall 1965), even though the nation's population had increased rapidly in number.

By 1960 new missions and increased professional opportunities, which limited the size of a medical practice as each new scientific and technological advance came on the scene, resulted in a trend to the increased specialization and fragmentation of education and the profession. Thus, the number of medical school graduates available to enter general practice was gradually and consistently depleted.

In addition, in contrast to 1910, the nation now had too few medical schools and too few physicians. The Federal and state governments responded by providing funds to construct additional medical schools and provide incentives, leading to an increase in annual class enrollments from 7,500 to more than 16,000 students. Once this goal was achieved, the number of publicly supported schools exceeded that of private schools. But direct government involvement in medical education and health care was limited to supporting the Veterans Administration Health System (VAHS), the Public Health Service, the Department of Defense, the NIH, and a few other smaller Federal programs.

INCREASED GOVERNMENT INVOLVEMENT (1960–PRESENT)

The Federal government became increasingly involved in all aspects of medical education and health care from 1960 on. The VAHS had been formed in 1929. Until the end of World War II, its mission was limited to serving the medical and health care needs of veterans. Dr. William Middleton, who served as chief medical director from 1955 to 1963, advocated increased VAHS involvement in biomedical and rehabilitation research, and Congress formally approved the VAHS role in medical and health professions education in 1955. By 1996, the system was supporting 8,910 approved residency training positions, or 12 percent of the nation's pool of the Accreditation Council for Graduate Medical Education (ACGME) (Knapp 1997).

The Ransdell Act of 1930 had formally established the National Institutes of Health, which had its origins on Staten Island, New York, in 1889. In 1960, the Omnibus Medical Research Act mandated that NIH establish disease-related institutes and fund research grants to medical schools and universities. The impact of this legislation was the development by medical schools of a cadre of outstanding basic science and clinical investigators, most of whom were faculty members who also taught medical and graduate students. The NIH made the United States the unchallenged leader in biomedical research throughout the world and achieved a number of enunciated national priorities, especially the eradication of numerous preventable diseases.

Selected governmental involvements in the areas of medical and health professions education, biomedical research, and health care are summarized in Table 13.3. Each legislative initiative had a major purpose and focus, and the integration of the intended activities into health education and health care facilitated the development of academic health centers.

At least nine major laws provided increased funding to medical schools from 1958 through 1976. These early initiatives encouraged an increase in medical student enrollments and in the number of medical schools, particularly in the South and West, the two regions in the United States rapidly gaining population. The Health Professions Educational Assistance Act of 1963 provided funds specifically to support other health professions, especially nursing and dental medicine; offered financial assistance to students in need; and established a loan forgiveness program for students whose debt levels exceeded a capacity to repay loans in a timely fashion.

The Health Professions Educational Assistance Act of 1976 provided special incentives to medical schools in the form of capitation related to the continued promulgation of needed public goods. Particular emphasis was again placed on encouraging more medical students to enter primary care, and funds were appropriated to construct educational ambulatory care centers.

Termination in 1973 of special appropriations to schools was accompanied, as could have been predicted, by annual escalations in tuition fees paid by students enrolled in these and other privately supported schools. In discontinuing the distress financing, the assumption was that medical students could assume higher debt levels because their professional incomes would be sufficiently high to repay them. Unforeseen was the possibility that the continued rise in physician income could cease (which, indeed, it has), thus limiting the rate at which students' loans could be repaid. As a result, students with large debts often choose more lucrative, higher-paying specialties in preference to a generalist career (Colwill 1992). An even greater concern is that many highly indebted students may bring an attitude of personal deprivation and professional unhappiness to the practice of medicine that can interfere with developing an optimal physician-patient relationship.

TABLE 13.3

**Federal Iniatives Designed to Affect Change in the Nation's
Health Through Medical Research and Education**

Year	Initiative	Recommendation
1930	Executive Order 53-95	Reorganize three agencies to establish national network for veterans' health care
1930	Ransdell Act	Fund National Institutes of Health
1958	Bayne-Jones Report	Increase physician output; increase number of medical schools; advance medical research and education
1959	Bayne Report	Increase physician output; institute Federal program of student financial aid
1960	Omnibus Medical Research Act	Provide Federal support for biomedical sciences
1960	Boisfiuillet Jones Report	Increase Federal support of medical research; provide direct Federal support to medical schools and medical education
1962	Kerr-Mills Act	Fund health care for elderly poor
1963	Health Professions Educational Assistance Act	Expand enrollment in medical, dental, and other health professions schools by funding construction of medical schools and grants for school loans
1965	Medicare and Medicaid	Fund graduate medical education
1966	Health Professions Educational Assistance Amendments	Support construction for new medical schools; provide special grants to improve curricula and provide loan forgiveness
1968	Health Manpower Act	Continue to expand medical schools; assist schools in financial distress
1970	Health Training Improvement Act	Offer special project grants; provide emergency assistance to medical schools in financial distress
1971	Comprehensive Health Manpower Training Act	Provide capitation grants; continue and expand medical school construction; expand enrollment; support GME in family medicine
1971	National Cancer Act	Establish National Cancer Institute; provide funds to support free-standing comprehensive cancer centers

continued

TABLE 13.3 *continued*

Year	Initiative	Recommendation
1976	Health Professions Educational Assistance Act	Fund capitation in relation to number of primary care residents; increase third-year enrollment to accommodate American students enrolled in foreign schools; construct ambulatory care and primary care teaching facilities; expand primary care training grants
1983	Tax Equity and Fiscal Responsibility Act	Change Medicare to prospective payment system; help teaching hospitals meet costs of complex health care; indirectly fund medical education costs
1994	White House health care reform proposal (fails)	Move toward less government funding and control of health care; encourage market forces and negotiated rates

The Kerr-Mills Act of 1962, enactment of Medicare and Medicaid in 1965, and subsequent revised Medicare legislation in 1984 appear in table 3 even though the principal focus of these legislative acts was providing patient care. Kerr-Mills, the forerunner of Medicaid, provided funds for the elderly poor. Califano (1993) has reported that despite this intent, the vast majority of the funds were absorbed by five states with lower-than-average numbers of the elderly population. Medicaid succeeded Kerr-Mills and extended coverage to more of America's poor and to nursing homes. In terms of medical education, the enactment of Medicare was most significant because it provided funds to support supervising physicians in teaching hospitals and for GME. In 1983, according to reports prepared for the House Ways and Means Committee and the Senate Finance Committee, the Medicare legislation changed the reimbursement system from a cost-plus methodology to a prospective payment system; it also added a source of reimbursement—indirect medical education (IME) reimbursement—to help teaching hospitals absorb the costs related to providing the complex medical and health care typical of teaching hospitals. (The actual costs for education were not determined.) Today, the combined budget for Medicare's share of GME support approximates 6.6 billion dollars annually, one-third to support supervising physicians and residents and two-thirds for IME.

This movement toward providing health care financing for the nation's poor and elderly provided medical schools with additional resources for funding medical education and full-time faculty. The new influx of money to teaching hospitals to support patient care and graduate medical education provided the impetus for schools to become directly involved in patient care and to develop faculty practice plans.

Thus, over a span of more than fifty years, Congress enacted major legislation that, in the aggregate, gradually enunciated a comprehensive, multifaceted public policy in support of medical and health professions education, biomedical research, and health care for the nation's poor, veterans, and elderly. Medical schools, universities, teaching hospitals, and academic health centers benefited significantly from these important developments.

Diversity in Funding

The diverse activities required to support a modern-day health professions school places a tremendous burden on its leaders to develop a cohesive strategy that protects its primary mission—education. Table 13.4 depicts the sources of mean funds, by category, that support the expanded missions of 125 allopathic medical schools in 1996 (AAMC 1995), 54 dental schools in 1994 (ADA 1995), and 63 academic health center-related nursing schools in 1992 (AACN 1993). State-appropriated funds primarily flow to publicly supported schools for educational programs. Hospital funds are developed through the allocations that support GME, from direct operating funds to other institutional resources. Grants and contracts flow primarily from NIH and the National Science Foundation (NSF), pharmaceutical organizations, and private industry to faculty investigators. Faculty practice funds are generated through direct patient care and consultations. Of the 54 dental schools, 35 are publicly supported, 13 are private, and 6 are state assisted.

The data also give an indication of the importance of research grants, contracts, and faculty practice plans to the current operational support of medical and dental schools. If budgetary allocations are related to an institution's mission, it is important for institutional administrators to determine how the research and service missions relate to a primary mission of education and what boundaries (if any) should be placed on developing these resources in relation to the funds necessary to provide an outstanding educational experience. The clinic revenue includes fees generated by faculty practice and the rendering of care by supervised students. The item "other" includes gifts and other sources of dental education support. Clearly, most dental schools are more dependent on tuition and state-approximated funds than are medical schools.

In contrast, nursing schools are supported primarily by institutional funds. The American Association of Colleges of Nursing (AACN) classifies 63 of its members as academic health center-related and 165 as nonrelated. In 1992, AACN reports, academic health center-related schools had a median annual budget approximately fourfold that of nonacademic health center-related nursing schools. The specific distribution of research funds was not reported, but

TABLE 13.4

Sources of Mean Funds Currently Supporting
Allopathic Medical, Dental, and Nursing Schools

Funding Source	Medical School (1996) $000 (mean)	%	Dental School (1994) $000s (mean)	%	Nursing School (1992) $000s (mean)	%
Tuition	9.2	5.6	56.2	30.5	—	—
State	22.6	13.3	76.2	40.4	2.9	81.0
Hospital	31.7	14.1	—	—	—	—
Grants, contracts	50.2	18.5	3.4	1.6	0.7	19.0
Faculty practice	78.2	32.0	43.4	23.8*	—	—
Other	32.0	16.5	6.9	3.7	—	—
Total	235.0	100.0	186.1	100.0	3.6	100.0

*Also reflects clinical income earned from student supervision and teaching.

an extrapolation of the information available suggests that the median for an academic health center school was approximately $690,000. A total of 255 schools, 63 academic health center-related and 192 nonrelated, permit nurses to earn additional salary through faculty practice. No fiscal data were available to evaluate the impact of practice revenue on the conduct of the educational programs (AACN 1993).

Significant Reports on Medical Education

The increased participation of the Federal government in biomedical research, medical schools, and medical and health care since 1960 was stimulated by the interests of educational advocates, their representative organizations, and the perceived needs of the American public. Three major reports, published in the mid- to late-1960s, for example, provided direction to academic medicine. They were the reports of the Citizens Commission on Graduate Medical Education for the AMA (Millis 1966); the Planning for Medical Progress Through Education Report (Coggeshall 1965); and the report on the Role of the University in Graduate Medical Education published by the AAMC's Council on Academic Societies (Smythe et al. 1968).

The Millis Report. The AMAs Citizens Commission was made up of ten prominent members from the public and professional sectors, three of whom were physicians. Among AMA's charges to the commission were two particularly pertinent to academic health centers. One was "the preponderance of the narrow specialty viewpoint in decisions affecting the pattern of graduate medical education." The other was that "the general nature of graduate medical education is based largely on the same fundamental concepts that determined the essential characteristics of graduate training programs as initially devised more than thirty years ago."

The commission forwarded fourteen recommendations to the AMA Board of Trustees. In so doing, the commission:

- Recognized the interaction between medical education and patient care that was required for GME to be successful, and recommended that GME be treated as a corporate, not a programmatic, responsibility.
- Acknowledged the important role of medical specialty societies and residency review committees, but saw a need for a single national accreditation organization comparable to the Liaison Committee on Medical Education (LCME).
- Expressed concern about the erosion of primary care medicine, and emphasized the need to nurture and encourage generalism.

The commission also forwarded additional recommendations supporting the following objectives:

- Termination of rotating and mixed internships and establishment of specialty residencies that medical school graduates can enter immediately after graduation from medical school.
- Provision by medical schools of the necessary foundation to be generalists.
- Involvement in—but not control of—the GME process.

Had all of the commission's recommendations been implemented, the existing situation with medical student and graduate medical education might be vastly different. Although a national consensus is gradually evolving that GME be governed corporately, it was not until 1980 that the ACGME (1982) promulgated guidelines requiring a sponsoring institution for programs conducted in multi-institutional settings. The recommendation that rotating and mixed internships be discontinued was readily implemented even though it was inconsistent with the two charges involving academic health centers presented to the commission by the AMA. Predictably, the commission's recommendations served to strengthen and accelerate the increased specialization and fragmentation that continue to erode generalism as a value in education and health care.

The Council of Academic Societies. In 1968, the Council of Academic Societies sponsored a conference on medical education. The core leadership committee included a dozen major academic leaders; the working conference was attended by approximately 155 other academic leaders (Council of Academic Societies 1968). Its recommendations on two matters differed considerably from those of the Millis Report, as follows:

- University medical school faculty should provide the same leadership for GME that it provides to medical student education.
- Universities should be encouraged to introduce educational innovations in GME.

The report also emphasized the need for a single accreditation organization, but did not explore in detail the issues of generalism and specialization.

The Coggeshall Report. The Coggeshall Report should be required reading for every academic leader and policymaker. Developed by the AAMC executive council, it is cohesive, inclusive, and visionary. Indeed, it largely accounts for the events that subsequently transpired in medical education and health care. However, the AAMC moved in a different direction. Rather than move more closely to the university, as recommended by the executive council, AAMC added two other units, the Council of Teaching Hospitals and the Council of Academic Societies, to its organization.

Coggeshall grouped the vast array of social change occurring in the United States and estimated the future impact of such change on medical education and health care. Table 13.5 shows the arbitrary level of importance that the Coggeshall report accords to social changes and the implications for medical education in 1965, and the level of importance accorded by the author of this paper on the 1995 implications. The greater the number of plus signs, the more important the change. "Scientific growth," for example, receives three pluses for 1965 and two for 1995. The differences in these two ratings do not suggest that growth would not occur in 1995, or that science was less important in that year. The rating system does indicate, however, that in 1965 the knowledge explosion was in its fundamental stages of growth and that scientific advance was developing rapidly. This same degree of change was not anticipated to occur in 1995 and beyond.

The nation's academic health centers have done an admirable job of educating more and better-prepared physicians and other health professionals. The number of physicians in 1995 and projected for the future will probably decrease to a yet undetermined level. However, as the health care industry continues to grow, personnel requirements will call for more people with less, rather than more, professional education. The immediate impact is on medical education, but over a period of a few years, the need for other highly educated health professions will also diminish.

Of special note is the council's emphasis on medical schools devoting more attention to the nation's needs. In many ways, helping meet the nation's needs should be regarded as an as-yet unmet goal, and one to which academic health centers and their professional organizations must give increased emphasis.

In 1965, the AAMC was the sole organization speaking on behalf of academic medicine. Thus, Coggeshall's vision appeared realistic and achievable.

TABLE 13.5

**Implications of Emerging Social Changes
for Medical Education in 1965 and 1995**

	*Relevance**	
Changes	*1965*	*1995*
1. Scientific growth	+++	++
2. Population changes	++	+++
3. Individual expectations for health	+	++
4. Increased demand for health care	+	++
5. Increased specialization	+	+++
6. Technological achievement	+	+++
7. Institutionalization of health care	++	+
8. Team approach for health care	+	+++
9. Increased number of physicians	+++	+
10. Increased number of health personnel	+	+++
11. Expanded government role	+++	+
12. Rising costs	+	+++

	*Relevance**	
Implications	*1965*	*1995*
1. Scientific growth	+	+++
2. Population changes	+++	+++
3. Individual expectations for health	+	+++
4. Increased demand for health care	+	+++
5. Increased specialization	+	+++
6. Technological achievement	+	+++
7. Institutionalization of health care	+	+

*Coggeshall (1965)

It is regrettable that organized medicine today, especially its academic components, often does not speak with a single voice. There is reason to be optimistic
that this situation might change; in 1997, for example—and for the first time
in recent history—six major professional organizations signed a joint letter to
the House Ways and Means Committee supporting the Institute of Medicine's
position on establishing a GME Trust Fund. The six organizations are the AMA,
AAMC, AHC (Association of Academic Health Centers), AOA (American
Osteopathic Association), AACOM, and the National Medical Association.

Medical schools and health manpower.   Medical education is always at
the core of discussions on the development of medical and health professions
manpower. Even in the early 1960s, many skeptics were expressing concern

that the nation's efforts to increase medical personnel were overzealous. In recent years, a number of studies have consistently indicated that by the Year 2000 there will be a substantial excess of physicians. The Graduate Medical Education National Advisory Committee (GMENAC 1980) has estimated the excess at 145,000, Weiner (1994) projects an excess of 163,000, and the Federal Council on Graduate Medical Education has estimated the surplus at 105,000. In general, there was not sufficient information to predict the effect of managed care; if such estimates could have been made, the surpluses would have been much larger.

Most health-policy experts agree that, to improve the health care system, the nation should be educating more generalists and fewer specialists. Whitcomb (1995) and Cooper (1994) have alerted the medical-education community to the fact that the projected physician excess is not limited solely to an excess number of specialists but to a projected excess of all types of physicians; the actual depletion in the number of available generalists will be less than originally projected by health analysts. However, Cohen and Whitcomb (1997) indicate that despite earlier projections, the emphasis on educating an increased number of generalists per graduating class must continue well into the next century.

The Pew Report. The Pew Health Professions Commission Report (1995) also addressed critical challenges to revitalizing the health professions for the twenty-first century. The Commission recommended the following actions:

- Decrease the number of medical student enrollees by 20 to 25 percent by the year 2005.
- Close some medical schools.
- Reduce the number of ACGME-approved resident positions to 110 percent of the number of American medical student graduates (the Canadian model).
- Distribute GME positions: fifty percent to generalist disciplines and fifty percent to specialty disciplines.
- Conduct at least twenty-five percent of the training experience at off-site locations.
- Develop an all-payor system to finance GME.

The Institute of Medicine Report. The recommendations of the Pew Commission were further amplified by the Institute of Medicine's (IOM 1997) report submitted to the House Ways and Means Committee. This report contained the following recommendations:

- Stop establishing new allopathic medical schools. (The report is mute on the issue of closing existing schools and the roles of osteopathic medical schools.)

- Do not increase medical school enrollment. (It was mute about the possibility of reductions in enrollment.)
- Reduce the number of funded GME positions provided that substitution funds are available to support alternative care providers.
- Improve career advice for medical students and GME trainees.
- Determine the relationship of physician supply to other workforce issues.
- Expand the definition of GME fields.

ON TO THE 21ST CENTURY

As health professions educators enter the twenty-first century, the need to restructure most educational programs will grow. The task will be more challenging and difficult than it was in 1910. Medical student education and GME do not relate to, and interdigitate with, one another as well as many people seem to believe. A recommendation to decrease the number of medical students and to close or merge medical schools precipitously may aggravate rather than solve the GME problem.

At present, almost 16,000 students are enrolled in allopathic medical schools, and approximately 2,000 students in osteopathic medical schools. In 1995, there were 84,968 ACGME-approved residents funded in the United States (Table 13.6) or about 12,000 to 14,000 more trainees per year than graduate from American allopathic and osteopathic medical schools (ACGME 1982). The excess numbers of GME trainees either represent American students enrolled in foreign medical schools or immigrants to the United States. Of the latter, approximately half immigrate from India, Pakistan, or the Philippines. Any public policy that is developed must relate the GME pool to the production of future physicians by American medical schools. The public-policy community and the medical-education community must work cooperatively and constructively to determine whether GME should continue to be a surrogate for the care of the poor as well as the final professionalization phase of a physician's education.

Medicine and other health professions remain attractive careers for many of the nation's brightest and most creative youngsters. We should have learned a valuable lesson in the 1970s when alternative solutions were developed for qualified students who couldn't gain access to American medical schools. Medical education and policymakers may understand the relationship of medical education to physician personnel, but it is of utmost importance that we take into account the political and public confusion that people have about these issues. Most citizens simply don't understand the rationale for maintaining medical school enrollments at levels almost 35 percent below the number of available ACGME-approved GME positions. At some point, medical school enrollments and GME programs must be reconciled and coordinated, replacing the disparate efforts of today. Throughout the nineteenth century, even when

TABLE 13.6

Number of Programs and Residents, 1981 and 1995, Compared to White House Goals for 1997

	1981		1995		Projected 1997	
	Programs	*Residents*	*Programs*	*Residents*	*Programs*	*Residents*
Allergy and immunology	73	203	84	254	50	166
Anesthesiology	161	2,930	154	4,681	92	3,128
Colon and rectal	26	40	31	53	17	31
Dermatology	99	814	105	850	60	508
Emergency medicine (1982)	63	885	112	2,812	56	1,249
Family medicine	385	7,004	455	9,261	551	9,783
Internal medicine	443	17,537	416	21,071	585	26,916
Neurology	123	1,236	121	1,536	71	772
Neurosurgery	93	608	99	846	57	415
Nuclear medicine	93	197	82	154	50	111
Obstetrics-Gynecology	304	4,705	272	5,007	383	6,793
Opthalmology	155	1,543	137	1,602	80	935
Orthopaedics	180	2,667	158	2,872	95	1,679
Otolaryngology	112	995	108	1,211	62	632
Pathology	314	2,413	185	2,788	113	1,428
Pediatrics	245	5,961	215	7,354	300	9,369
Physical medicine and rehabilitation	65	605	81	1,129	44	573
Plastic surgery	105	389	101	461	60	260
Preventive medicine	33	166	89	434	15	69
Psychiatry	223	4,336	201	4,919	116	2,881
Radiation oncology (1988)	85	470	83	506	48	288
Radiology	221	3,135	206	4,090	122	2,365
Surgery	331	8,105	269	8,221	161	4,721
Thoracic surgery	98	281	92	346	54	186
Urology	153	1,027	122	1,094	74	592
Transitional year (1983)	197	1,377	167	1,416	101	861
TOTALS	4,380	69,629	4,146	84,968	3,417	76,711

GME was not related intrinsically to basic medical education and licensure, there were an excess of GME positions. In 1964, for example, 60 percent of all GME trainees in New York City were of foreign origin (DHHS 1997).

The Federal government, through the Council on Graduate Medical Education, has attempted to analyze the complex issues surrounding medical and health professions education, health personnel issues, and the availability of health care. Many states have developed advisory bodies devoted to GME, and leadership on this concern has emerged from organizations such as AHC and AAMC. Still, a sufficiently coordinated and cohesive approach has yet to evolve. Although a single all-payer system at the Federal level may not come into being, it is conceivable that, if they so desire, individual states might be able to achieve this goal on their own.

As the twenty-first century approaches, public attitudes toward medical and health professions education will probably change greatly. The age of unfunded mandates will be replaced by voluntary choices made at regional or state levels. More important, political and economic forces will coalesce to prevent the seemingly paradoxical behaviors characterized by differences in the stances taken by Congress, professional societies, medical schools, and teaching hospitals.

Medical and health professions education exert important influences on many aspects of American life that earn academic health centers and their professionals enormous credibility, acceptance, and respect for their leadership and contributions to the well-being of society. The largesse provided to academic health centers by many different programs and agencies has helped develop a world-renowned infrastructure.

Can academic health centers redefine and restructure themselves as individual institutions tied into a network of academic health centers still valuable to American society? A few years ago, economist Eli Ginzberg (1995) and the Macy Foundation conducted a conference to determine how medical schools and academic health centers planned to respond to changes.

At the Macy Conference, held in the midst of the health care reform debate in 1994, participants believed that a universal payor system and increased Federal regulation would become the law of the land. Whatever the outcome of the ongoing debate on health care, however, conference participants held that the perpetuation of fee-for-service medical practice would diminish and be replaced by a system of managed care designed to negotiate rates based on community health outcomes rather than episodic care rendered to individual patients.

To determine both the current status of fiscal support and the outlook for the future if this scenario came to pass, case statements for twelve representative medical schools from throughout the United States (eleven allopathic and one osteopathic) were presented. The assumptions were as follows:

- Public fiscal support of medical and health sciences education, GME, biomedical research, and patient care will decrease.
- Fiscal control for the above functions will be shared by the Federal government, state governments, and the business community.
- Physicians, hospitals, health insurance payers, and large investors will vie for control of health care.
- Academic health centers, through their unique roles related to provision of patient-related services, will begin to work more directly with payors in addition to the affiliated teaching hospitals.

Three schools were heavily dependent on practice plan income. Three were using a public hospital as the principal teaching hospital. Three had a major research program. Three had a predominantly regional role. Regardless of classification and current resource base, each school saw its major future strategy to be that of securing of larger and larger amounts of patient revenue.

In analyzing the twelve case statements, conference participants were impressed by the lack of attention the institutions had directed to their core missions and functions. Accordingly, the Macy Commission recommended that medical schools give the highest priority to strategic plans that reexamine and redefine the institution's missions, and align activities to support the mission.

An institutional mission statement, by definition, must reflect the mission's individual sense of being and worth. But it must also emphasize its relationship to patients and community. It is here that institutions have the opportunity to establish a charter that aligns an institution's spirit to the needs of the nation as well as to other constituents and consumers. In today's chaotic situation, the charter should define the institution's relevance and commitment to the concept that education is a required public good: It helps people become independent thinkers and learners, and more important, to become servers of society. The mission can also be an instrument that defines its providers and elucidates what students, patients, and community represent its consumers.

Mission statements become meaningless and ineffective unless accompanied by a statement of values that represent the commitment to attaining the mission and a statement of vision that can empower, and define the role of, its leadership. And, of course, the institution, at all levels, must lay out an annual work plan designed to meet mission, vision, and value.

In his review of thirty operational multidisciplinary GME consortia for the Council on Graduate Medical Education (COGME), Cox (1997) recognized that many of these organizations were conducting operational affairs unrelated to their mission statements. Such incongruity may exist in many other academic health centers in the United States.

In *Academic Medicine as a Public Trust* (Schroeder et al. 1989), the authors recognized the significant contributions of academic medicine to scientific discovery, new knowledge, medical technology and pharmaceuticals, and de-creased death rates, particularly those from cardiovascular disease and stroke. However, the authors suggest that academic medicine was not fulfilling one of its missions, namely, to improve the health of the public. They single out five areas of failure, as follows:

- Failure to influence a reduction in cost of medical care.
- Failure to eradicate the nation's substandard indexes of public health.
- Failure to eliminate the maldistribution of the uneven quality of care among our citizens.
- Failure to help correct the unfavorable geographic and specialty distribu-tion of physicians.
- Failure to minimize needless disability from long-term medical and psy-chiatric problems.

Ginzberg and Schroeder each emphasize that academic medicine is the beneficiary of very generous amounts of public funding, given in part to carry out a mission that benefits society, expended with an extraordinary degree of institutional autonomy.

MEETING THE NATION'S NEEDS

Throughout the past fifty years, the nation, through Congress and multiple commissions, has consistently and repeatedly identified a common set of na-tional needs and expectations. Some of these needs and expectations have been identified by Schroeder et al. (1989); others are identified according to Congressional intent. At least three of these show how a disconnect can occur among the intent of providers, the stated mission of an academic health center, and the values and vision necessary to implement the missions. The disconnect occurs with the need to (1) promote increased commitments to generalism, (2) join basic science and clinical education with preventive medicine and community health, and (3) ensure increased access, retention, and graduation of students from underrepresented and socially disadvantaged populations.

Generalism—The nation has expressed its need for generalist physicians consistently and repeatedly since 1960. The rationale was affirmed by the Coggeshall Report of 1965, the Millis Report of 1966, and numerous subsequent reports. The Federal government and many state governments provide generous fiscal incentives to encourage medical schools, GME programs, and teaching hospitals to support generalism. The advent and pervasiveness of managed care organizations in recent years is a new stimulus that heightens the need.

Despite the emphasis placed on developing more generalists, in 1997, 8 of the 125 allopathic medical schools in the AAMC still do not offer a required clerkship or its equivalent in Family Medicine. Three of these schools are in New York City, a region with the largest ratio of physicians and medical specialists to population in the United States (and perhaps with the largest proportion of medically underserved consumers).

Twenty-two medical schools require a clerkship in Primary Care, but not in Family Medicine. Although a Primary Care clerkship may fulfill some of the desired elements of generalism, one should not assume this is always the case. In the Millis Report, the assumption was made that medical schools would provide an integrated experience in generalism that would spawn several disciplines—simultaneously, it was hoped but, more important, in a coordinated manner.

In many schools, a Primary Care clerkship may be limited to one of the identified primary care specialties, and fail to integrate the many desired elements suggested in the Millis Report and the report by the New York State Council on Graduate Medical Education. Seven medical schools require an educational experience in Ambulatory Care but not in Family Medicine. A broad-based, comprehensive Ambulatory Medicine clerkship that requires continuity of care may be a preferable educational experience to one limited to a single primary care discipline, depending on its organization and curricular content.

The findings suggest that the value system necessary to implement a mission of generalism effectively does not yet exist in many of the nation's academic health centers.

Preventive medicine—Another area in which there is likelihood for incongruity between mission and value is that of preventive medicine and community health. Institutions that do not nurture generalism are the least likely to support these efforts. Because preventive care and community health are identifiable national priorities for providing alternative forms of care and improving the health status of communities, academic health centers must work more closely with other health professional programs such as those in schools of public health.

Educational opportunities for the socially disadvantaged—Unfortunately, Flexner missed an important opportunity to report correctly on the status of medical education for minority and socially underrepresented citizens in 1910. The important matter was not addressed further until the civil rights movement of the 1960s. Despite tremendous social and fiscal support to increase the access for a growing minority population, medical schools still do not enroll sufficient numbers of minority students. This problem provides an example of how an academic health center's commitment to an educational mission must be extended to work with primary and secondary schools and community groups in a way that promotes the flow into and through the educational pipeline. It also illustrates how leaders in GME, in particular must work to secure a continuum of academic growth and development for a defined constituency. Ginzberg has concluded that a serious dilemma for medical schools in the future will be the need to reduce faculty size and student enrollments while, at the same time, providing opportunities for faculty and students from socially disadvantaged populations.

TABLE 13.7

How Much Do Constituents Value Academic Health Centers?

Major functions	Students, families, parents	Parent university	Region	State	Nation
Education	1	1	1	1	3
Research	1	1	1	3	4
Patient care	2	1	2	5	5
Leadership	2	1	1	2	4
Public service	3	3	2	1	3

Note: Rated on a scale of 1 to 5, with 5 the lowest rating.

In the changing world, where accountability and negotiation will determine the availability of fiscal support and stability for academic health centers, new concepts of evaluation will be required to implement viable strategies. Well-defined missions, vision, and value statements are vital. But there also must be a process to determine to which constituents an institution is of value. Table 13.7 illustrates the concept of value for a hypothetical academic health center. The value of each academic health center function for each constituent group is stated, with 1 representing a high score and 5 a minimal, or low, score.

Looking at Ginzberg's analysis of the four groups of medical schools that served as case studies at the 1994 Macy Conference, it appears that the schools with major research programs should achieve a higher value score to the nation than a school largely dependent on faculty practice revenues for research. On the other hand, the latter school should be of higher value to the more immediate constituents for functions such as education, patient care, and community service. It seems feasible to suggest that this evaluation can help academic health centers reconcile missions, vision, and values with operations, and further define how their resources should be consistently allocated. It can also be used by departments and other program units as well as academic health centers.

RELEVANT MODELS FOR ACADEMIC HEALTH CENTERS

The past fifty years have witnessed the development of large centers in which the functions of education, research, and patient care were coordinated.

This concept promulgated the perception that all of the needs of medical and health professions education could be met in such centers. Because health education is so closely related to health care and health service delivery, the formation of centers to which all required sources would flow was eventually subject to change. In the past decade, hospitals have come to realize a need to expand beyond existing structures and locations and to form systems of care rather than centers of care.

It is obvious that medical and health systems education must now move from a centralized to a systems approach. Under this scenario, tertiary patient care would remain in a limited number of highly technically specialized facilities while basic science research would be concentrated around expensive, technically oriented laboratory settings. All other elements of care would be provided throughout the community and region. Although masked under the concept of "managed care," the real goal would be to manage the cost of care, make access to care easier and more efficient, and promote the concept of comprehensive, continuous care. It is imperative that health science education be reformed so it can adapt to a new learning environment.

Although it is foolhardy to think that any academic health center has yet accommodated to the required changes, we can evaluate some relevant models to determine how each center might position itself to cope more readily to changes that will continue to occur. Some examples follow:

Indiana. The University of Indiana had one complete medical school in 1910; its current model maintains a single medical school rather than a number of additional independent schools. (Its neighbor, Ohio, has seven allopathic and one osteopathic medical schools, having added the allopathic schools during the expansionist period.) When Indiana increased its medical school enrollment, it developed a program in which preclinical education was conducted at a number of university and college campuses throughout the state, and clinical education was conducted at facilities in Indianapolis and in the physician and hospital community throughout the state. As the years went on, the relationships between the University of Indiana and Purdue University strengthened to the point where an educational consortium was formed to provide a seamless education for all of its students at the two institutions.

Washington, Alaska, Montana, and Idaho. A novel situation exists in the relationship between these partner states and the University of Washington to form the four-state program known as WAMI. In this model, these four components serve as an interstate educational organization managed by the university. Educational activities extend into the partner states. Despite the wide range of educational responsibility, the university continues to also be a major national leader in biomedical research.

Illinois. The University of Illinois at Chicago has always had a relatively large number of medical schools. Its response to the era of expansion was to develop a single new public medical school, the Southern Illinois University Medical School. The University of Illinois medical school, located in Chicago, developed an expanded single institution with additional campuses in Urbana, Peoria, Rockford, and Champaign-Urbana.

Texas.　A more ambitious model is one developed by Texas Tech University in Lubbock. Representing a regional health professions education institution serving West Texas, its program extends northward from Lubbock to Amarillo and southward to El Paso; programs are also located in the Permian Basin region, which includes Midland and Odessa.

New York.　The educational network of the New York Medical College located in Valhalla (Westchester County), New York, includes approximately thirty-five hospitals and other training sites extending south to Staten Island, New York, and to its north to Kingston, New York.

Oklahoma, Kansas, New York, and Florida (clinical campuses).　Several states have opted to maintain a single centralized health science campus joined to clinical campus training sites at distant locations. They include the University of Oklahoma with a clinical campus in Tulsa; the University of Kansas in Wichita; the SUNY Upstate Medical Center in Binghamton, New York; and the University of Florida in Jacksonville. Grafting clinical campuses onto the well-established medical schools mentioned above proved to be more of a challenge than did the models developed in Indiana, Washington, and Illinois.

New York, Tennessee, Illinois, and Ohio (GME consortia).　A recently introduced alternative model for the governance of GME that could be extended to include other components of academic health centers educational programs is that created through the establishment of consortia. This type of organization falls midway between an educational program operated by multiple, independent organizations, on the one hand, and a program operating as a single, merged fiduciary entity. As such, a consortium provides the unique opportunity to manage and coordinate merged institutional interests without a need to surrender total institutional integrity and autonomy. Today, there are thirty identifiable multidisciplinary GME consortia in the United States. A recent report by Malcolm Cox (1997) on behalf of the Federal COGME, indicates that consortia have the following attributes:

- They are better positioned than any national organization to deal with local or regional GME training needs.
- They provide a framework for examining GME from the perspective of all interested constituencies.
- They possess the inherent flexibility and potential for inclusiveness needed to organize a fragmented GME system.
- They can be effective when given appropriate levels of authority.

- They can focus on the content and quality of programs.
- They can serve as models of shared governance.

The prospect for consortial governance has been evaluated by a number of organizations. In New York State, both the state's Commission on Graduate Medical Education and its successor, the Council on Graduate Medical Education, encouraged the development of GME consortia. The Macy Foundation (Morris and Sirica 1993) also encouraged GME governance by consortia. Cox's report strongly recommended that educational consortia become the coordinators and facilitators for medical student education and GME.

The most comprehensive GME Consortium developed thus far is in Buffalo, New York (Rosenthal et al. 1997). This organization was formed in response to the revised standards promulgated by the ACGME in 1980 (GMENAC 1980). Its members include a medical and dental school, nine teaching hospitals, and a representative for each residency program. The organization also joined the views recommended in the reports by Millis and the Council on Academic Societies Reports in 1965 and 1968, respectively. It has fostered and implemented changes in residency and medical student education (ACGME 1982) and served as an important catalyst for institutional cooperation and collaboration.

New York State's recently enacted Health Reform Act, which neither mandates nor denigrates the potential value of consortia, allocates $54 million per year for regional distribution, and encourages teaching hospitals and academic health centers to develop cooperative plans designed to achieve a specific set of public goods. Included are (1) a decrease in the number of GME positions; (2) an increase in the number of primary care resident positions and a concomitant decrease in the number of specialty GME positions; (3) an increase in representation of minority and other socially underrepresented constituents; and (4) development of GME consortia.

The state of Tennessee was the first state to secure a Medicaid Managed Care Waiver. Initially, the rapid change that ensued placed the medical educational system at risk. The four medical schools—East Tennessee State University, Meharry Medical College, Vanderbilt University, and the University of Tennessee (Memphis)—have now formed a single statewide GME consortia. Its effectiveness will not be known for several more years, but it could become another important model to emulate.

An alternative form of educational consortia is being developed by osteopathic medical schools. Osteopathic schools may be fortunate when they develop this model because each one has more management flexibility and is not as tightly joined to health delivery organizations as the allopathic schools. Some examples of approaches undertaken by osteopathic schools follow.

- The New York College of Osteopathic Medicine provides the educational umbrella for its graduates who train in AOA-approved GME programs throughout New York State.

- The Midwestern University School of Osteopathic Medicine in Chicago has added a new school in Phoenix.
- The Ohio University of the College of Osteopathic Medicine and the Michigan State University College of Osteopathic Medicine each has developed statewide GME consortia.

Federal government.   The Uniform Services University of the Health Sciences is a relatively new academic health center that could serve as an ideal model for future organizational structures. The only health science school owned and operated by the Federal government, its affiliates are the well-respected Walter Reed Army Medical Center; the Naval Medical Center in Bethesda, Maryland; the Malcolm Grow Air Force Medical Center; and the Wilford Hall Air Force Medical Center. It is conceivable that, as the Federal government is downsized and reorganized, a broader health education enterprise allied with the Public Health Service and NIH could evolve from this academic health center.

REINVENTING HEALTH PROFESSIONS EDUCATION

Flexner emphasized the need for a sound fundamental educational preparation for physicians that includes the sciences related to medicine. Today, medical schools require not only the basic biomedical sciences but also those sciences related to prevention of disease, behavioral medicine, and community health. It was the need for this type of broader education that led Flexner to believe that medical schools must be intimately joined to universities. Coggeshall also recognized the importance of other academic disciplines to medicine that are not part of the usual biomedical science array.

There are some very relevant priorities that every academic health center should reaffirm with the approach of the new millennium. They are:

- The primary function of a medical and health professions school is to educate the physicians and health professionals of the future.
- Conducting research is important to the development of new knowledge and biotechnical advances, excellence in rendering care, and the proper inculcation of the values of medical practice. In a school, it also serves the needs of the student consumer by providing a proper education that includes breadth of knowledge and fosters curiosity and self-learning, as well as depth of knowledge.
- The focus of a health science education is the patient and the community, not a science or a single specialty. Thus, "the patient" must be returned to medical education and the importance of the health of a community to the well-being of society must be appreciated in proper detail.

Education's importance has been devalued by the tremendous expansion that has occurred in the past half-century and by the relative dominance of the engrafted research and patient care missions. The viability, excitement, and mass of these latter missions have overwhelmed the educational mission to the point where education's professional value and importance are often not recognizable. Abrahamson (1996) ascribed the problem to the enhancement and expansion of the research entrepreneur and the clinical entrepreneur. This assessment is probably correct; increased numbers of faculty are indeed expected to risk their livelihoods through the securing of research grants or practice income, or both. Although this behavior and need probably will not change, they must be seen as tasks that properly value and nourish the educational missions; in addition, all faculty should be rewarded for performance and achievement rather than for the sole ability to generate fiscal resources.

The devaluation of education is evidenced further by at least two observations. The AAMC Survey Report (McInturff 1996), for example, found that the average citizen did not appreciate the role of education in academic health centers but did clearly value the research and patient care missions. And, writes Dr. Edwin Rosinski in a personal communication to this author, when he interviewed medical school deans and other leaders in medical education to determine their perception of advocacy for medical education in America, he found to his surprise that neither the AAMC nor the AHC are recognized as effective advocates for the importance of education.

FUTURE EDUCATIONAL NEEDS

An academic health center must consider the specific learning objectives for each of its student constituencies. Most important, it must separate the differences required for graduate trainees from students seeking a primary degree.

The needs of today's students are vastly different than those of their predecessors. As Coggeshall indicated, this situation is largely due to social change. The United States is now populated by a healthier, wealthier, older population whose medical and health care needs are different from those in the past. Physicians and health care professionals must be better prepared to deal with preventive health care and chronic rather than acute illness and with a larger proportion of people who will live into their nineties. Most important, health professionals must adapt to an environment in which patients will help determine the kind of care desired, and care will be rendered less frequently in hospitals and more often in a decentralized but coordinated manner in ambulatory care sites and other community facilities.

Under the above assumptions, medical and health professions education will also be distributed throughout regions and include utilization of professionals and facilities with little previous involvement in academic health centers. How can academic health centers cope with this situation in which previous defined centers of learning become systems of education?

- Many faculty will develop into facilitators of education rather than functioning solely as teachers.
- Students will be expected to gain more information through self-learning strategies, problem-based learning techniques, simulation, experience with standardized patients, and computerized technologies.
- Curricula will be restructured to facilitate more small-group learning experiences, include measured emphasis on preventive and community health, and better integrate basic science and patient care education.
- Reliance on the hospital setting will be reduced, and use of ambulatory and urban and community sites increased.
- Formal classroom instruction will be reduced, with more emphasis directed toward program development and evaluation, self-learning, and use of technology. The educational center will be a resource for all components of a region's educational partners.
- Educational materials will be distributed through an educational information network with materials available to consumers online twenty-four hours a day. The National Library of Medicine will continue to grow as a major resource.

The Buffalo Consortium has worked cooperatively and collaboratively with New York Telephone (NYNEX) to develop fiber optic connection and routing among its ten partners as inexpensively as possible. The university's Health Science Library and its hospital consortium of libraries provides online transmission of bibliographic, journal, and textbook materials to 7,000 users. The network serves thirty-five to forty organizations that include ambulatory teaching sites and health insurers. This system, HUBNET, will form the foundation for an eventual health information network.

It seems apparent that health science libraries and computer information systems will become the backbone and infrastructure for the conduct of education. If this does indeed occur, the Association of Academic Health Centers should determine if health science libraries should not be more prominently represented and involved.

Distance learning and regional teleconferencing capacity will continue to be developed. They are of particular importance to those educational programs that will be conducted in multiple distant sites and as a decentralized effort.

The community, in addition to the teaching hospital, will be utilized as another classroom. Already, education programs are increasingly being operated outside the teaching hospital in urban, suburban, and rural areas. Accordingly, the education center will have to develop adequate evaluation methodologies for the trainees located in remote, less standard environments. The adequacy of the environments will also have to be evaluated.

FINANCING HEALTH PROFESSIONS EDUCATION

Future strategies to finance very expensive forms of medical and health professions education remain to be determined. It is apparent that the actual costs must be determined and isolated from budgetary strategies that permit cost-shifting. During the past twenty years, two principal sources have been used to replace other sources of insufficient or lost revenues, namely, research funds and faculty practice plans.

Although these sources can be incremented, it is unlikely that the magnitude will sustain the current enterprise. The strategies being developed by the Federal and state governments and by the business community are designed to reduce expenditures in these areas. The 1994 Macy Conference recommended that the Federal government develop and implement a national workforce plan and provide direct financial support to academic health centers in the form of incentives that will address national needs. Such possibilities still exist, but they are unlikely to occur unless these centers individually and collectively agree to take additional fiscal risks, be held accountable, and demonstrate that their productivity is effective in meeting the specified national needs.

CONCLUSION

In a span of less than one hundred years, health professions education moved from a cottage industry to a very sophisticated, complex organization manifesting itself as the academic health center. Today, this concept of maintaining centralized centers that can be perceived as self-reliant is being challenged. The nation has rebelled against the concept of government regulation for health care and, for the next generation, control will be shared by the Federal and state governments and the business community. Competition, driven by cost-reduction and efficiency, quality, and consumer satisfaction will be the major path to success.

The nation's academic health centers are expert at competing with one another to achieve excellence in education, research, and patient care. However, they are not particularly adept at being cost conscious or efficient or at restructuring their organizations to become smaller, leaner, and meaner. However, given their importance to society, there is little doubt that most, if not all, academic health centers will make necessary adjustments to compete and serve society's fulfilled role. However, many treacherous forces can serve to detract academic health centers from their principal missions. Each academic health center, therefore, must select its strategies wisely and make certain they are in keeping with its stated purposes. Perhaps the greatest threat to the future would be to view the new competitive environment as an end rather than a means. The competitive forces that have been unleashed will surely thrive on a profit incentive. Furthermore, when this initial period has passed, competition may have attained the results previously attempted through regulations, and have done so more rapidly. However, the results of the profit incentive may bring about more pain, disruption, and chaos than the regulatory approach. Thus, academic health center leadership must focus on its missions constantly, make appropriate midcourse adaptations, and enunciate those values held important and immutable to the students, faculty, patients, and community.

Academic health centers will continue to provide students with a sound scientific foundation while nurturing values of compassion, caring, and generosity. Another major conflict for many academic health centers will be that of idealism versus reality. The former must be held in high esteem in order to promote the most altruistic health professionals possible. The latter, of course, reflects a restructured environment in which being the best, most productive competitor may be viewed as more important and relevant. Medical professionals in particular are already experiencing a loss of professional autonomy and control of patient care. It is at this interface that the academic health centers must structure new educational strategies designed to prepare their graduates for a vastly different reward system, one in which entrepreneurial behavior is more valued than professional stature. And in this respect, the influence of role models will be even more important than was the situation in the past.

WORKS CITED

Abrahamson, S. 1996. Time to return medical schools to their primary purpose: Education. *Academic Medicine* 71(4).

ACGME (Accreditation Council on Graduate Medical Education). 1996. *Accreditation Alert.* Chicago: ACGME.

———. 1982. *Institutional Responsibility for Graduate Medical Education—The New General Requirements for Residency Training.* Chicago: ACGME.

AACN (American Association of Colleges of Nursing). 1993. *Institutional Resources and Budgets in Baccalaureate and Graduate Programs in Nursing 1992–93.* Washington: AACN.

AAMC (Association of American Medical Colleges). 1995. *Institutional Profile Annual Report 1994–95.* Washington: AAMC.

———. 1997. *Directory of American Medical Education 1996–1997.* Washington: AAMC.

ADA (American Dental Association). 1995. *Survey Center Report.* Chicago: ADA.

AMA (American Medical Association). 1923. *Principles Regarding Graduate Medical Education.* Chicago: AMA.

———. 1928. *Essentials of Approved Residencies and Fellowships.* Chicago: AMA.

Blumenthal, D. 1997. Understanding the social missions of academic health centers. *Report of the Commonwealth Fund Task Force on Academic Health Centers.* New York.

Califano, Jr., J.A. 1993. The last time we reinvented health care we made a mess of it. *Buffalo Evening News* 7(April).

Coggeshall, L.T 1965. *Planning for Medical Progress Through Education.* Evanston, IL: AAMC.

Cohen, J.J. and M.E. Whitcomb. 1997. Are the recommendations of the AAMC's task force on the generalist physician still valid? *Academic Medicine* 72.

Colwill, J.M. 1992. Where have all the primary care applicants gone? *New England Journal of Medicine* 326(6).

Cooper, R.A. 1994. Seeking a balanced physician workforce for the 21st century. *Journal of the American Medical Association* 272.

Council of Academic Societies. The role of the university in graduate medical education. Washington: October 2–5, 1968.

Cox, M. 1997. Graduate medical education consortia: Changing the governance of graduate medical education to achieve physician workforce objectives. Final Report from the University of Pennsylvania Health System to the National Council on Graduate Medical Education (COGME). Washington: U.S. Department of Health and Human Services.

DHHS (Department of Health and Human Services). 1997. (News release) Letter to the editor re appointment of task force (COGME). May 30.

Flexner, A. 1910. *The Flexner Report.* Washington: Carnegie Foundation for the Advancement of Teaching.

Ginzberg, E. 1995. *The Financing of Medical Schools in an Era of Health Care Reform.* New York: Josiah Macy Jr. Foundation.

GMENAC (Graduate Medical Education National Advisory Committee). 1980. *Summary Report to the Secretary. Department of Health and Human Services.* (vol. 1) Washington: GMENAC.

Health Security. The President's Report to the Public. 1994. Washington: U.S. General Accounting Office.

Indirect medical education funds. 1983. (Report prepared for House Ways and Means Committee, no. 98-25.)

———. 1983. (Report prepared for Senate Finance Committee, no. 98-23.)

IOM (Institute of Medicine). 1997. *Implementing a National Graduate Medical Education Trust Fund.* Washington: National Academy.

Knapp, R.M. 1997. Medical school GRR's with a VA affiliation. (memorandum) Washington: AAMC.

McInturff, W.D. 1996. What Americans say about the nation's medical schools and teaching hospitals. *Final Report on Public Opinion Research to the Association of American Medical Schools.* Washington: AAMC.

Millis, J.S. 1966. *Citizens Commission on Graduate Medical Education.* Chicago: AMA.

Morris T.Q., and C.M. Sirica (eds). 1993. *Taking Charge of Graduate Medical Education To Meet the Nation's Needs in the 21st* Century. New York: Josiah Macy Jr. Foundation.

Pew Health Professions Commission. 1995. *Critical Challenges: Revitalizing the Health Professions of the Twenty-first Century.* San Francisco: Pew Health Professions Commission.

Rosenthal, T., R. Hager, M. Noe, and J. Naughton. 1997. A consortium, graduate medical education, and Buffalo: Defining a common ground. *Family Medicine* 29(7).

Schroeder, S.A., J.S. Zones, and J.A. Showstack. 1989. Academic medicine as a public trust. *Journal of the American Medical Association* 262.

Smythe, C. McC., T.D. Kinney, and M.H. Littlemeyer. 1968. *The Role of the University in Graduate Medical Education.* (Proceedings of the 1968 conference) Washington: AAMC.

Weiner, J.P. 1994. Forecasting the effects of health reform on U.S. physician workforce requirements. *Journal of the American Medical Association* 272.

Whitcomb, M.E. 1995. A cross-national comparison of generalist physician workforce data. *Journal of the American Medical Association* 274.

14 | Litigation and Public Health Policy Making: The Case of Tobacco Control

Peter D. Jacobson
and Kenneth E. Warner

We live in an age of litigation. Since roughly the 1960s, many social activists have viewed litigation as not merely a means of seeking redress for individual wrongs, but also as the solution to a myriad of public policy issues. Invited by a welcoming Supreme Court under Chief Justice Earl Warren, liberals used litigation to achieve social goals when other policy solutions, particularly legislative, were blocked by a more conservative establishment. During the Reagan backlash, conservatives began to mount a litigation counterattack before a no less receptive Chief Justice William Rehnquist.

Despite this history of litigation as policy, a salient question remains largely unresolved: what is the appropriate role of litigation relative to the political process (i.e., the legislative and regulatory institutions) in forming public policy? This is a controversial topic that has generated considerable disagreement among legal scholars. To those who believe in a more limited judicial role within the governmental separation of powers, judicial policy making is anathema. Litigation is only designed to resolve disputes between particular parties by applying the law to specific facts, with the democratic institutions of legislatures and regulators better suited to establishing public policy. In this view, the Constitution's framers intended the judiciary to correct wrongs, not make policy.

Reprinted from *Journal of Health Politics, Policy and Law,* 24, no. 4 (August 1999): 769–804. Copyright 1999. Duke University Press. All rights reserved. Reprinted with permission.

Funding for this project was provided by grants numbers 030444 and 026421 from the Robert Wood Johnson Foundation's Investigator Awards in Health Policy Research Program.

Others maintain that it is legitimate to seek policy change through the courts when the democratically elected institutions fail to address pressing social problems. Some scholars, including Stuart Scheingold (1974) and Michael McCann (1994), argue that courts can be forceful and effective movers of social and political change. In many ways, advocates of this approach treat litigation as an opportunity to extend and expand the political process into a forum where powerful interests have fewer inherent advantages.

By the mid-1990s, the use of litigation to formulate public policy once again moved to the forefront of public policy debate with the unprecedented scope of litigation against the tobacco industry. Many tobacco control advocates have long touted litigation as the best hope for overcoming the tobacco industry's historic invincibility and achieving changes in tobacco policy, despite the fact that until mid-1997 the industry had never paid damages resulting from litigation. Even opponents of the lawsuits brought by the state attorneys general to recover smoking-related Medicaid costs regard the litigation as serving a policy-making function. For example, former Arizona Governor Fife Symington, who opposed his state's participation in the suits, was quoted as saying, "This issue has nothing to do with smoking. It has to do with policy by litigation."[1]

In this article, we examine the relationship between litigation and public health policy formulation in the context of the debates over tobacco control policy.[2] We will focus on the evolution of the lawsuits brought by the state attorneys general (the state litigation) from a state-based complaint for monetary damages (to correct for past harms caused by tobacco) into litigation intended to influence public health policy. The public health aspects of the litigation, which were initially subordinated to the economic aspects, have emerged as central to both the litigation and the debate over the litigation as policy.

It is thus important to analyze why the litigation has emerged, what its goals have been, whether these goals can be achieved, what alternative policy approaches should be considered, and whether this model can be applied to other public health objectives. From a public health policy perspective, the fundamental questions are how social policy on the use of tobacco products will be made, and which institutions will be responsible for controlling tobacco use: the market, the political system (i.e., the legislative and regulatory branches of government), or the courts. As a philosophical matter, when, if ever, should public health policy be made through the judicial, and not the legislative, branch of government?

Underlying the debate over which institution is best suited to formulate public policy is the challenge of defining what constitutes optimal social policy in any given area. Defining desirable tobacco control policy obviously depends on one's perspective, with antismoking activists and tobacco industry supporters occupying opposite ends of the spectrum. Whatever optimal policy goals partisans on either side might want, public opinion polls clearly demonstrate support for a variety of stronger tobacco control measures than the political system has provided, hence inviting the use of litigation to shape policy. Yet litigation also has institutional constraints that may limit its ability to achieve the policy goals the public appears to desire. The debate over the proper locus of institutional policy making, we can see, is not an abstract exercise.

In the first section of the paper, we examine the functions of litigation in general and consider its applications in the case of tobacco control litigation. In the second section, we describe the specific policy-oriented objectives and strategy of contemporary tobacco control litigation. In the third, we present a conceptual framework for evaluating the desirability and potential utility of employing litigation as a policy-defining strategy. This section focuses on the roles of the judiciary and the legislative/regulatory system in each of several areas of tobacco-control policy making. In the fourth and concluding section, we offer lessons from this case study about the philosophical and pragmatic rationales for using litigation as a component of public health policy making both in tobacco control and in other areas of public health. We also consider this matter in the context of the perennial challenge that defines so much of public health: balancing the interests of the state in the health of the collective public with protection of the individual's liberty interests.

THE LITIGATION ENVIRONMENT

FUNCTIONS OF LITIGATION

Traditionally, civil litigation serves three basic purposes: compensation, deterrence, and accountability. A fourth function of the civil courts, equity jurisdiction, is also important in the context of the lawsuits the state attorneys general brought against the tobacco industry.

The most obvious function of the tort system is to compensate an injured victim for harm suffered as a result of the defendant's wrongdoing.[3] Compensation includes economic damages (e.g., actual medical expenses), but can also include noneconomic damages for pain and suffering. In the tobacco litigation, the plaintiffs, including the state attorneys general, are suing to recover monetary damages resulting from the costs of treating tobacco-related diseases. This may be thought of as the law's corrective function.

The second function of the tort system is to deter future wrongdoing. In tobacco litigation, the tort system might deter the tobacco industry from producing and marketing harmful products by imposing large damage awards, causing price increases that would lead to significant reductions in youth tobacco use and smoking initiation rates (Daynard 1988; Kelder and Daynard 1996; Hanson and Logue 1998).

A closely related function is accountability. By establishing rules to assess liability, the tort system provides a mechanism for society to hold wrongdoers accountable for their actions. One accountability mechanism in litigation is the assessment of punitive damages, which also serves as a deterrent. Punitive damages may be assessed by a jury for particularly outrageous behavior such as malice, oppression, and fraud (Keeton et al. 1984) if the jury first finds the defendant liable. Plaintiffs' attorneys in the individual and class action tobacco litigation have requested that juries assess punitive damages for the industry's fraud in concealing information about the harms of tobacco. State attorneys general also requested punitive damages in their tobacco litigation.

A function of the courts available to the state attorneys general in the tobacco litigation context is to seek equitable remedies. In general, courts can impose equitable remedies when justice and fairness require relief that cannot be obtained through monetary damages. An injunction is a typical equitable remedy. The benefit of seeking equitable remedies is that if a court so desires, it can go well beyond traditional pecuniary awards in fashioning appropriate relief. In addition to financial compensation, courts can require a range of remedies not generally available to private litigants, such as industry-funded counteradvertising and smoking cessation programs. From a tobacco control policy perspective, the ability to seek equitable relief may be more significant than the available financial awards.[4]

A more controversial use of the courts is the promotion of social goals unattainable through other institutions. The civil rights litigation beginning in the 1950s is one example, as is the ongoing litigation over expanding the right to privacy in areas such as abortion and the right to die. The controversy over this function revolves around whether the courts should focus narrowly on correcting past wrongs or, rather, on resolving policy disputes. We discuss this function, as used by the states, in greater detail below.

TOBACCO CONTROL LITIGATION

The courts have two roles in tobacco litigation. First, they review challenges to regulatory actions for appropriate legislative authority and constitutionality. Second, they serve as a venue for injured litigants seeking to recover damages incurred from tobacco-related diseases.

Regulatory Review

In general, courts have played a limited role in reviewing challenges to tobacco control regulations, usually granting governmental entities wide-ranging authority to regulate tobacco products. The courts' reluctance to overturn laws regulating smoking was succinctly summarized by the U.S. Supreme Court in *Austin v. Tennessee,* 179 U.S. 343 (1900), in holding that the regulation of cigarette sales was within the powers of the states: "Without undertaking to affirm or deny their evil effects, we think it within the province of the legislature to say how far [cigarettes] may be sold or to prohibit their sale entirely . . . and there is no reason to doubt that the act in question is designed for the protection of the public health." As a result, challenges to tobacco control laws or regulations have generally failed. For example, a court recently upheld the constitutionality of cigarette billboard advertising restrictions in *Penn Advertising of Baltimore, Inc. v. Mayor of Baltimore,* 63 F. 3d 1318 (4th Cir. 1995). And the Florida Supreme Court permitted a municipality to require prospective employees not to smoke on the job or at home as a condition of employment in *City of North Miami v. Kurtz,* 1995 Fla. LEXIS 568 (Fla. 1995). However, in *Brown and Williamson Tobacco Co. et al. v. U.S. Food and Drug Administration,* 1998 U.S. App. LEXIS 18821 (4th Cir. 1998), the Fourth Circuit Court of Appeals declined to uphold the Food and Drug Administration's (FDA) jurisdiction to regulate tobacco products.[5]

One reason that the courts have played a limited role to date is that the regulatory system has not enacted strong tobacco control law and regulation, which many tobacco control advocates view as a case of regulatory failure. Tobacco lobbyists have succeeded at the federal level in blocking the regulation of tobacco products as drug delivery systems or of nicotine as a drug. For instance, the agency most likely to oversee tobacco products, the FDA, has until recently exercised only limited jurisdiction over tobacco products (USDHHS 1989). Congress has contributed to the limited federal presence in several ways. Cigarettes have been specifically exempted from coverage under the Fair Labeling and Packaging Act of 1966, the Controlled Substances Act of 1970, the Consumer Product Safety Act of 1972 (establishing the Consumer Product Safety Commission), and the Toxic Substances Act of 1976 (CDC 1989).

At the state level, tobacco lobbyists have successfully blocked strong tobacco control legislation in all but a few states, such as New York, Minnesota, Massachusetts, and California. In many others, including Florida and Illinois, the tobacco industry has successfully promoted weak statewide antismoking legislation that preempts stronger local ordinances (Jacobson, Wasserman, and Raube 1993).

Damages Litigation

For many years, the tobacco industry was invulnerable to tort litigation seeking damages (Schwartz 1993; Annas 1997). Until very recently, juries have been reluctant to hold cigarette manufacturers responsible for the choices an adult smoker makes, and courts have not imposed strict liability on the manufacturers, thus limiting the incidence of litigation (see, e.g., Schwartz 1993). Until 1997, the tobacco industry's defense that the smoker assumes the risk has meant that "tort liability has contributed virtually nothing to the array of strategies employed to control tobacco use" (Rabin 1991: 494).

According to tobacco litigation scholars, there have been three waves of litigation. The first two were dominated by individuals suing the tobacco companies for negligence. In these cases, the litigation was intended to impose damages for the harms caused to individuals by the tobacco industry. The third has also included individual lawsuits, but it has been dominated by class actions and especially by the state litigation to recover states' Medicaid costs for tobacco-related illness.

The legal theories for the first two waves of litigation were based on negligence and strict liability. To succeed under negligence, a smoker needs to show that (1) the industry owed a duty to the smoker, (2) the duty was breached, (3) the breach caused the plaintiff's injuries, and (4) the plaintiff suffered damages. In product liability, the plaintiff needs to show that the product is inherently defective or that the consumer was inadequately warned of the dangers inherent in using the product.

During the first wave of litigation (1954–1973), the industry successfully defended negligence charges by arguing that smokers assumed the risk and should not be able to recover. Even though this wave dealt with smoking that preceded the first Surgeon General's pronouncements on the dangers of smoking (USDHEW 1964), claims of breach of implied and express warranty and failure to warn of the risks of smoking were uniformly rejected by juries and courts (Schwartz 1993; Rabin 1993; Kelder and Daynard 1996). In essence, as Schwartz (1993) noted, juries held that smokers bore responsibility for smoking-related disease, not the tobacco manufacturers.

In the second wave of litigation (1983–1992), attorneys relied on product liability doctrine to argue that cigarettes were defective in design, manufacture, and warning. Courts held, however, that while the product is inherently dangerous, neither design nor manufacturing defects could form the basis for liability. Like the cases in the first wave, these cases also lost, with one exception, *Cipollone v. Liggett Group, inc.*, 893 F. 2d 541 (3d Cir. 1990, aff'd in part and rev'd in part, 112 S. Ct. 2608 [1992]), although the $400,000 jury award was later reversed on appeal.[6]

One consistent theme throughout the first two waves was the tobacco industry's skillful invocation of freedom of choice arguments and an individual rights perspective that invariably convinced juries not to award damages. Indeed, Robert Rabin (1993: 127) concluded that the individual-rights basis of the first two waves was "an instructive lesson in the limits of social control through the tort system." In this context, he argued, the tort system has made a moral judgment that conscious risk taking will not be rewarded.

Considering the almost unbroken streak of tobacco industry victories prior to 1996, the scope, extent, variety, and legal innovativeness of the current, third wave of antitobacco litigation (beginning in 1994) are breathtaking. A partial list of third-wave litigation would include large private class action damage suits by current and former smokers (e.g., *Castano v. American Tobacco Co.*, 160 F.R.D. 544 (E.D.La. 1995), rev'd 84 F. 3d 334 [5th Cir. 1996]), class action litigation by nonsmokers to recover for the damage caused by secondhand smoke (i.e., airline stewardesses in *Broin v. Philip Morris Companies, Inc.,* 641 So. 2d 888 [Fla. 1994]), lawsuits by state attorneys general to recover state Medicaid costs attributable to smoking-related diseases, reimbursement litigation by municipalities, personal injury lawsuits brought by individuals to recover damages from nicotine addiction and other smoking-related injuries, and contribution claims by asbestos manufacturers.

According to some tobacco litigation observers, the third wave has differed from its predecessors both legally and substantively (Kelder and Daynard 1996). Legally, the major component of the third wave, the state litigation, was based not on the facts pertaining to individual smokers' behavior, but on the ability of the state to recoup its Medicaid costs, primarily through the doctrine of unjust enrichment.[7] The underlying theory of this litigation was that the state sued in its own right to recoup the tobacco-related financial costs absorbed by the Medicaid program (Moore and Mikhail 1996; Kelder and Daynard 1997). States were not suing on behalf of injured smokers through subrogation.[8] In essence, the litigation was designed to circumvent the freedom-of-choice and individual-rights strategies that tobacco attorneys had used to win previous litigation. In the state litigation, claims were aggregated at the state level to avoid the blameworthiness problems faced by individual litigants and the need to show individual causation. Consistent with the underlying theory of the case, the state attorneys general attempted to prove their case based on epidemiological studies of the population-based harms caused by tobacco, not by harms to specific individuals. Since the state has no choice but to absorb the Medicaid costs of tobacco-related diseases, and it is the taxpayers, not smokers, who are injured financially, the states argued that the traditional industry defenses raised in individual litigation are irrelevant (Moore and Mikhail 1996).

Substantively, third-wave proponents have argued that the disclosure of tobacco industry knowledge and concealment of tobacco's carcinogenic properties, and the industry's manipulation of nicotine levels (Hilts 1996; Glantz et al. 1996), provide better litigation outcomes. Litigation advocates expected these facts to absolve smokers from blame and place responsibility on the tobacco manufacturers. The third wave also differs in the public's increased knowledge of the tobacco industry's behavior. As a consequence, public attitudes toward the industry have become substantially more negative. Most importantly, the third wave differs from previous litigation strategies in that the state litigation avowedly sought to achieve public health objectives in response to the perceived failures of the regulatory system to control tobacco use. The political system had not attained the policy outcomes that the attorneys general believed were desirable and that they anticipated litigation would provide.

While it is beyond the scope of this article to examine in detail the complex reasons why resorting to litigation became more plausible during 1997, we believe that three primary factors were at work. First, the enormous pressure on the tobacco industry from financial markets to settle the industry's liability exposure produced considerable momentum within the industry to reach an accommodation (Pertschuk 1997). Wall Street's unease over the industry's potential liability suggests that even the threat of continuing litigation was likely to suppress tobacco industry stock values. Second, testimony at previous Congressional hearings, especially in 1994 when the CEOs of the major tobacco companies swore under oath that their product was not addictive, exposed these executives to criminal prosecution for perjury and had a negative influence on public attitudes toward the tobacco industry. Third, this marked the culmination of a larger change in political attitudes about smoking that had been emerging for more than a decade (Jacobson, Wasserman, and Anderson 1997). Litigation explains the first factor, and no doubt contributed to the others as well. In this sense, litigation is both cause and effect of important changes in social trends.

Several recent cases indicate the potential for successful litigation outcomes, while demonstrating that difficulties lie ahead. In 1996, a jury in *Carter v Brown and Williamson Tobacco Corp.*, 95-934-CV-B (Fla. Cir. Ct. Duval Co.) ruled in favor of a plaintiff who had started smoking before warnings were required on packs of cigarettes. This could indicate that, compared to juries in the first two waves, contemporary juries are more willing to consider the industry's culpability in the manufacturing and marketing process. One year later, however, in the case of *Raulerson v. R. J. Reynolds Tobacco Co.*, 95-1820-CV-C (Fla. Cir. Ct. Duval Co.), brought by the same legal team, a jury rejected the plaintiff's claims (supported by information on the industry's mendacity contained in newly disclosed tobacco industry documents) and awarded judgment for the defendant. Most recently, two juries (the first in California, the second in Oregon) awarded plaintiffs damages of more than $51 million and $81 million, respectively. These large awards, primarily for punitive damages, may signal a sea change in the public's attitude toward the industry.

LITIGATION AS TOBACCO CONTROL POLICY MAKING

During the summer of 1997, the tobacco industry settled the first two of the scheduled Medicaid cases, agreeing to pay Mississippi and Florida more than $3 billion and $11 billion respectively over a twenty-five-year period. The industry then settled the third case, with Texas, for $14 billion, reached an agreement in the Broin case to dedicate more than $300 million to tobacco research, and settled the Minnesota case for $6 billion. In November 1998, the industry and the state attorneys general announced a general settlement that covered all of the remaining states, with the industry agreeing to pay $208 billion to the states over the next twenty-five years. Certainly, these unprecedented actions by the tobacco industry constitute success for the third wave.

The state litigation was initiated in 1994 to obtain damages from the tobacco industry, with public health objectives a secondary concern. But, by 1997, as a result of pressure from public health advocates and among the state attorneys general, the focus of the litigation shifted toward securing public health objectives.[9] Many tobacco control advocates have embraced the third wave as the solution to regulatory failure. This contrasts with the first two waves, when advocates did not view litigation as a mechanism for changing public health policy,[10] concentrating instead on conventional legislative and regulatory strategies.

The third wave of litigation thus addresses the issue of whether a public health strategy will fare better than the narrower tort approach. From a policy perspective, the question is what public health goals will be achieved if the new strategy is successful. That is, what are the *ex ante* public health goals inherent in this new litigation, and what might be the *ex post* policy changes?

PUBLIC HEALTH OBJECTIVES OF THE CURRENT LITIGATION

In this discussion, we focus attention on the Medicaid litigation because it is the most explicitly policy-oriented litigation of the current wave.[11] In March 1997, the attorneys general articulated four goals and objectives guiding their Medicaid litigation strategy: (1) to protect children by stopping the marketing of tobacco to minors and reducing youth access to tobacco products; (2) to provide full disclosure of tobacco's adverse health effects (by releasing tobacco industry documents obtained through litigation);[12] (3) to protect consumers by reforming tobacco industry business practices; and (4) to recover the states' tobacco-related health care expenditures. Embedded in these broader goals, the attorneys general enumerated several public health policy objectives for resolving the litigation, such as (1) including tobacco products under FDA regulation and adopting the current FDA rules on tobacco marketing and sales, (2) funding research into teen tobacco use and cessation and meeting certain teen tobacco use-initiation rate targets, (3) funding a public education campaign, (4) improving tobacco labeling to disclose all tobacco ingredients, (5) disclosing all industry documents relating to research, marketing, and nicotine addition, and (6) compensating the states and individuals for tobacco-related diseases and the costs of quitting smoking.

Our review of the initial complaints and subsequent documents filed by the state attorneys general confirms the broad strategic goals outlined above but raises some differences as well. Most important, perhaps reflecting the limitations imposed by pleadings and procedural requirements, the original state complaints focused on recovering monetary damages. Because the basis of the litigation was recovery of the states' Medicaid tobacco-related costs, other objectives were framed in terms of damages. For example, as part of its request for damages, the Kansas complaint alleged that the tobacco industry breached its duty to advance the public's health by failing to disclose accurate information about the risks of tobacco consumption *(State of Kansas v. R. J. Reynolds Tobacco Co. et al.,* Case No. 96-C V-919).

With one exception, however, the initial pleadings contained only limited mention of public policy goals. That exception deals with children. From the beginning, the state attorneys general specified a policy objective in the pleadings to reduce the marketing of cigarettes to minors. In Florida's complaint against the tobacco industry, for instance, the state argued that because of the industry's conduct, children will become addicted to tobacco, some will become Medicaid patients, and they will be treated for tobacco-related diseases paid for by the state. As a result, the state asked the court to order the tobacco industry to fund a corrective public education campaign aimed at preventing the distribution and sale of tobacco products to minors, and to provide other remedies to reduce youth access to cigarettes. To be sure, the state also requested relief for other public health purposes, such as funding for clinical smoking-cessation programs, ending industry misinformation campaigns, and dissolving the industry-sponsored Council for Tobacco Research and the Tobacco Institute, but the primary public health focus was on youth access.

What is most interesting about the pleadings is the extensive reference to industry duplicity, manipulation, and deception. With each subsequent state complaint and each additional disclosure from the tobacco industry about its previous knowledge of tobacco's health hazards, the pleadings become more meticulously detailed. There are four possible reasons for this strategy. First, even though the original basis of the litigation was to recover the states' economic losses, the objective of the litigation shifted over time to public health goals. The increasing detail can be viewed as support for the public health objectives and for the requested equitable relief. This can be demonstrated both in the subsequent pleadings and documents filed by the attorneys general, and, more particularly, in their public statements regarding negotiations with the tobacco industry to settle the litigation. In part as a response to demands from tobacco control advocates, the attorneys general may have included strong public health goals as a condition of settling the litigation. Second, this recitation of industry behavior may be seen as a defense against a tobacco industry motion for summary judgment (a motion that would accept the facts as pleaded and decide the case on the law if there is no dispute of material fact) and to meet state requirements for specific pleading of fraud. Third, this may be viewed as justification for initiating what the attorneys general concede is novel litigation. Fourth, this information may have been part of the strategy to educate citizens about the extent of tobacco industry culpability.

In sum, public health policies are mentioned more explicitly in the relief sought than in the complaints themselves. Despite the ambiguity in specifying the public health goals of the litigation (at least within the court documents), it seems clear that the litigation was intended to achieve certain public health objectives. Contrary to what some critics of the litigation have argued, it does not appear to be just about money. The question thus remains whether the litigation is the best way to achieve broad public health goals relative to alternative policy approaches.

A FRAMEWORK FOR ANALYSIS

ROSENBERG'S MODEL

Several scholars have analyzed the role of the courts in stimulating and achieving social and policy change. The most systematic conceptual approach is Gerald Rosenberg's (1991) analysis of the social change implications of judicial decisions in civil rights and abortion cases. Although we do not necessarily share his conclusions about the role of litigation in civil rights or abortion policy, he has produced a useful model for analyzing litigation-as-policy-making that seems particularly applicable to tobacco litigation. He notes that two very different versions of judicial involvement in social policy disputes motivate scholarly commentary. One is that the courts are effective producers of social change,[13] what he calls the *dynamic view*. In contrast, what Rosenberg terms the *constrained view* holds that inherent constraints inhibit courts from producing social change.[14]

The constrained view postulates that three structural limitations prevent courts from becoming effective social change agents: (1) constitutional limits on creating rights, (2) the lack of independence from other branches of government, and (3) the inability to establish, implement, and enforce policies. In response, proponents of the dynamic view argue that as independent institutions, courts can issue rulings (especially constitutional interpretations) that directly induce policy change when other institutions are politically stymied. The dynamic view postulates that courts can also induce policy change indirectly by educating the public, stimulating public debate, and serving as a catalyst for change (McCann 1996). In this way, the dynamic view takes into account the courts' ability to influence the nature of the policy agenda, if not directly its outcome.

Other observers, including R. Shep Melnick (1983, 1994) and David Horowitz (1977), share Rosenberg's general skepticism about courts as policy makers.[15] In particular, Horowitz (1977: 257) argues from both empirical and conceptual grounds that judicial policy making is undesirable, primarily because "the judicial process is a poor format for the weighing of alternatives and the calculation of costs." Both Horowitz and Melnick argue that judicial capacity to make policy is limited relative to other institutions, especially given judicial limitations on implementation and enforcement, the problem of case-by-case decision making, and constraints on the setting of agendas. Nevertheless, Melnick (1983, 1994) concludes that judicial decisions on statutory interpretation indeed help shape program policy, though not always favorably and not necessarily in the direction expected by Congress or the regulatory agencies.

More broadly, Thomas Stoddard (1997) argues that litigation is capable of "rule-shifting," that is, influencing the behavior of individuals and institutions, but that only the legislative process can induce "culture-shifting" changes that transform society. Thus, Stoddard argues that advocates of social change should focus on legislative action, rather than on litigation, to achieve their goals (in Stoddard's case, greater social acceptance of homosexual rights). To be sure, litigation that succeeds in changing a lot of individual and institutional behavior will also be capable of changing the culture.

COMPARATIVE INSTITUTIONAL ANALYSIS

The policy agenda is rarely determined exclusively by the courts. The courts engage in a dialogue with the other branches of government, but the instances in which the judiciary can unilaterally determine policy are likely to be few. Particularly in the area of public health, the agenda is primarily set by other institutions, especially the regulatory and legislative branches. As such, Neil Komesar (1994) argues that it is misleading to view public policy goals from the perspective of one institution alone. Rather, he postulates, the appropriate analysis must determine which institution, among imperfect alternatives, is best suited to achieve the specified policy goals. In this view, institutional choice is an important determinant of public policy outcomes. For analytical purposes, Komesar defines the relevant institutions as the market, the political process (i.e., the legislative and regulatory branches), and the courts. Since the market has rarely responded to public demands for changes in tobacco control policy,[16] we limit our analysis to the courts and political institutions.

The notion that the system specifically designed to address policy issues—the legislative and regulatory institutions—is sufficient in and of itself fails to account for the well-known phenomenon of regulatory capture, that agencies might be dominated by the interests of the regulated industry (Wilson 1989). Jon Hanson and Kyle Logue (1998) argue persuasively, for example, that the regulatory system has failed to regulate the tobacco industry in part due to capture. Similar deficiencies occur at the legislative level, where legislators have also been dominated by the tobacco and other powerful industries (Arno et al. 1996; Samuels and Glantz 1994; Jacobson, Wasserman, and Raube 1993). Thus, while it is certainly accurate that the regulatory system has not aggressively regulated tobacco products, this situation may be attributable to both regulatory capture and the tobacco industry's influence on Congress. Some dissent from this view, however. James Q. Wilson (1989) has expressed dissatisfaction with the capture theory because it may not apply to those agencies most likely to be involved in tobacco regulation, such as the FDA, where antismoking policy entrepreneurs may be able to offset the tobacco industry's influence. Indeed, William Weissert and Carol Weissert (1996) note that recent empirical studies testing the capture theory have shown continued regulatory vigor, rather than subservience, in overseeing the regulated industry.

One must therefore examine the potential policy influence of the current litigation within a framework that includes the roles of legislatures and regulators at the federal, state, and local levels. To better understand litigation's potential to influence public health policy, we need to ask a series of questions dealing with interactions among the relevant policymaking institutions. First, what are the tobacco control policies that might be influenced by litigation? Second, which institution is best able to set the relevant policy? Third, are there areas where litigation can define the policy agenda? Fourth, are there areas in which litigation complements other institutions in setting public health policy?

To answer these questions, one needs to determine the appropriate public health objectives in tobacco control. We believe that tobacco control policy should be organized to achieve two broad objectives: reducing tobacco-related morbidity and mortality among current smokers (along with the effects of environmental tobacco smoke on nonsmokers) and reducing tobacco-initiation rates among children. Thus, we concur with the state attorneys general that protecting children is a fundamental public health goal. However, we classify the other goals they listed—disclosure of health effects, reforming business practices, and providing financial relief—as policy instrumentalities intended to increase the likelihood of achieving the two basic objectives.

To examine the possible and appropriate tobacco control roles of political institutions and the courts, and to provide a conceptual means of organizing the comparative analysis, we offer Table 14.1. We divide tobacco control policies into three categories: economic (i.e., financial incentives), regulatory/legislative (rules), and information/education (persuasion) (Warner et al. 1990). Although we could separate the legislative and regulatory into two discrete categories, we list them together because they exhibit considerable overlap. Both branches play a role in each of the listed policy instrumentalities because the legislature provides the authority under which the regulators determine the rules. But executive agency interpretations of legislative policy (whether state or federal) may be more expansive or restrictive than the legislature intended. For example, it is not clear that Congress would approve of the current FDA regulations standing alone, even though there are insufficient votes to overturn the FDA's approach.

There is an important distinction between local, state, and federal legislative and regulatory policy. Certain actions, including reducing nicotine and

TABLE 14.1

Tobacco Control Policies

Economic
 Excise taxes
 Damage awards from litigation
Regulatory/Legislative
 Youth access restrictions
 Restrictions on smoking
 Advertising restrictions
 Marketing curbs (i.e., on logos and sporting event scholarship)
 Enforcement activities
Information/Education
 Education about the harms of tobacco products
 Disclosure of tobacco industry documents
 Settlement negotiations with the tobacco industry
 Shifting the public health debate
 Smoking cessation programs
 Research in tobacco control policy or in tobacco-related diseases
 Counteradvertising (i.e., antismoking ads)

producing safer cigarettes, are likely to be an exclusively federal regulatory responsibility, the result of both existing federal law and regulatory tradition. Other activities, such as youth access restrictions, may involve local, state, and federal regulators. For purposes of understanding the policy implications of litigation, however, the probable effects can be viewed as similar across governmental entities.

In the following sections, we assess how the judicial and legislative/ regulatory institutions influence the particular policy instrumentality, either directly or indirectly. One limitation of this analysis is that we do not have complete information on the outcomes of third-wave litigation (since it is still under way). As such, our assessment represents our estimate of the most probable institutional determinants on the tobacco control policy outcomes of interest.

THE ROLE OF LITIGATION

Exclusive Domain

One area in which courts clearly have an advantage over other institutions is in providing financial relief to individuals and to states through the awarding of damages. In certain circumstances, such financial relief can also serve larger policy interests. As noted by the U.S. Supreme Court in *San Diego Bldg. Trades*

Council v. Garmon (359 U.S. 236, 247 [1959]), awarding damages is "a potent method of governing conduct and controlling policy."

For a variety of political and economic reasons, it is difficult for states to raise taxes high enough to substantially reduce the demand for cigarettes, although high taxes can discourage teen smoking initiation rates (Grossman and Chaloupka 1997), an important policy objective. Courts can effectively force the tobacco industry to raise the price of cigarettes significantly if damages are large enough and pervasive enough (i.e.. awarded in multiple jurisdictions). Damage awards would also have the effect of penalizing tobacco industry misbehavior and holding the industry accountable for the harms it has caused. In the extreme, multiple punitive damages awards could cause bankruptcy or force tobacco companies to leave the market altogether, as happened with asbestos manufacturers.[17] Clearly, damages is an area in which courts have exclusive authority. Graham Kelder and Richard Daynard (1997:170) focus on this aspect as being perhaps the strongest and most direct public health policy benefit of the third-wave strategy: "Victory in any of the class actions would result in a partial transfer of costs from injured smokers to the tobacco industry. Victory in any of the cost reimbursement suits would result in a transfer of costs from injured states forced to shoulder the economic burden of tobacco-induced illnesses to the tobacco industry. Such a transfer of costs would likely have the immediate impact of raising cigarette prices, thereby lowering cigarette consumption."

Damages per se do not constitute public health policy. At best, they may have an effect on prices, with that effect likely to be substantial only if truly sizable damages are assessed in multiple jurisdictions.[18] In this sense, damages-induced price increases would mimic a policy of tax increases, but not actually constitute a public policy.

Direct Effects, Nonexclusive Domain

In some instances, courts share with legislatures the ability to define policies. For example, as a corrective measure, the courts could order cigarette manufacturers to mount a public education campaign designed to clarify the dangers of smoking and of nicotine addiction. Legislatures could mandate such an educational effort as well, although they would be more likely to charge a public agency with responsibility for carrying it out. In these instances, courts possess direct policy-defining power, but they share it with legislatures.

Indirect Effects

More often, the litigation has several important indirect effects on tobacco control policy formulation. One lies in forcing the disclosure of incriminating documents showing a pattern of industry deception and duplicity on major issues such as marketing to children and the addictive properties of nicotine.

This disclosure has enhanced the public's perception of the dangers of cigarette smoking and has undermined the industry's credibility. For example, interviews with jurors following the multimillion dollar verdicts for plaintiffs in California and Oregon certainly suggest the importance of the disclosed documents as well as a significant change in public attitudes with respect to industry culpability. The resulting public antipathy toward the industry has certainly encouraged more stringent regulatory restrictions, such as those promulgated by the FDA. In addition, the disclosures clearly influenced the course of the settlement negotiations between the state attorneys general and the tobacco industry, and, in turn, congressional deliberations.

The litigation process also serves a very important educational function that complements regulatory tobacco control strategies. As just one example, consider the extraordinary publicity surrounding the release of industry documents, courtroom testimony, and depositions. The judicial process captivates the public's attention to a degree that the normal regulatory and legislative processes rarely achieve, giving the public additional information with which to make more informed judgments about the use of tobacco. The resulting information disclosure provides an important incentive to use litigation in tobacco control policy. In a democratic society, policy should be made based on the full availability of information to the public. The disclosure of this information will motivate more informed tobacco policy choices.[19]

Perhaps the most important potential indirect influence is to stimulate other policy makers to enact and enforce tobacco control laws and regulations. So far, the third wave of litigation has not prompted such policy responses at the state and local levels, and the tobacco control activity demonstrated during the past ten years occurred despite the unsuccessful outcomes of the first two waves of tobacco litigation (Jacobson, Wasserman, and Anderson 1997).[20] Nonetheless, the states' lawsuits convinced the tobacco industry to accept settlement negotiations in 1997 and grant public health advocates with seats at the negotiating table.[21] A negotiated settlement can obtain creative solutions that may be difficult for regulators to impose or litigators to achieve through formal court proceedings. For example, a settlement proposed in June 1997 included terms that would have imposed fines on the tobacco industry if youth smoking failed to decline by a set amount in a given number of years.

Settlement negotiations of individual litigation may also lead to changes in industry behavior. For example, plaintiffs in *Mangini v. R. J. Reynolds Tobacco Co.*, 875 P. 2d 73 (Cal. 1994) sued to enjoin the Joe Camel advertising campaign as a violation of California's unfair and unlawful business practices laws. After the court allowed the claim to go forward, the parties negotiated a settlement ending the Joe Camel campaign in California. Since the litigation may well have played an important contributing role in the decision to end the Joe Camel regime nationally, we include this as an indirect effect.[22]

Another area in which the states' litigation could indirectly affect public health policy is through the courts' equitable jurisdiction. For instance, marketing curbs, public education, and smoking cessation programs are primary functions of regulatory bodies, but the question of who pays can be answered through litigation. Absent some agreement between the tobacco industry and the government, it is difficult to envision a legislature ordering private industry to pay for smoking cessation programs, although the federal regulatory agencies may have such jurisdiction. Acting under its broad equitable remedial authority, a court could order the industry to pay for such programs as part of the compensation for the public health harms caused by tobacco products.

We characterize these influences as indirect because the potential policy outcomes from these activities are not yet determined. For example, the final net effect of the multistate settlement on retail cigarette prices—and hence the impact on smoking and health—is thus far unknown. In particular, if the financial settlement substitutes completely for a tax increase, that would not result in a net change in public health policy.[23] Likewise, the ultimate importance of shifting the public debate is likely to lie in forcing the legislative and regulatory branches to initiate stronger tobacco control measures. It is somewhat ironic that state court litigation to recover damages formed the basis, in 1997, for proposed federal legislation to control tobacco use.[24]

No Effects (and Negative Effects)

In certain areas, court decisions are likely to have no public health policy implications. For example, courts are unlikely to order lower nicotine levels through their equitable powers, but will tend to defer to FDA. Perversely, as just noted, litigation could indirectly have a negative effect on cigarette excise taxation by discouraging Congress or state legislatures from raising taxes because they conclude that awarded damages raise the price of cigarettes "enough."

It can be argued that settlements and awards resulting from individual litigation, if replicated across a large number of cases, could indirectly affect youth access and public smoking restrictions. For instance, in *Staron v. McDonald's, Inc.,* 51 F. 3d 353 (2d Cir. 1995), the plaintiff sued under the Americans with Disabilities Act (ADA) to ban smoking to accommodate plaintiff's asthma condition. The court ruled that plaintiffs would be allowed, on a case-by-case basis, to show that a smoking ban would constitute a reasonable accommodation under the ADA. In part as a response to this litigation, the defendant created no-smoking sections in its restaurants. The same holds for cases such as *Kyte v. Store 24,* where a chain of convenience stores agreed to check buyers' identification prior to sale. At this point, because these types of cases are limited, with few reported similar settlements, their potential for achieving public policy changes is uncertain.

THE ROLE OF REGULATORY AND LEGISLATIVE INSTITUTIONS

Direct Effects

In theory, adequate tobacco control measures should have been produced by the legislative and regulatory branches of government without the need for litigation. No legal restrictions prevent states from enacting and enforcing more stringent tobacco control laws (except where the federal government has preempted the field). In reality, the legislative process at the state and federal levels, if not at the local level, has traditionally favored the tobacco industry (Jacobson, Wasserman, and Raube 1993; Samuels and Glantz 1991; Arno et al. 1996). Until the recent FDA rules restricting youth access, the federal regulatory process had rarely impeded the tobacco industry's marketing or sales efforts.[25] Arguably, therefore, litigation proceeded by default. Nevertheless, certain aspects of tobacco control can only be addressed by regulatory and legislative bodies. And, in contrast with policy through judicial decisions, no independently initiated litigation is needed to activate the legislative and regulatory system.

Most of the policy instrumentalities that can reduce smoking-related morbidity and mortality and reduce teenage smoking-initiation rates are primarily legislative and regulatory functions. In particular, both states and the federal government can affect the price of cigarettes, and hence discourage teen smoking-initiation rates, through the imposition of higher cigarette excise taxes. Also, through stringent enforcement of current antismoking laws, states can remove vendor licenses for selling tobacco products to minors. Indeed, the development, implementation, and enforcement of youth access restrictions and restrictions on smoking in public places are entirely within the purview of state and local jurisdictions (Jacobson and Wasserman 1997), although federal legislation can certainly influence state and local developments, as shown by the Synar amendment. Equally important, state and federal regulators can develop and fund smoking cessation programs, counteradvertisements, tobacco advertising restrictions, and research into the effectiveness of various tobacco control initiatives, without ceding authority to the courts. Within constitutional limits, states and municipalities can also enact restrictions on the location of advertising billboards and on marketing aimed to induce youths to smoke. States can undertake new initiatives, such as a recent Massachusetts law requiring cigarette manufacturers to disclose all ingredients.

Federal agencies also have the power to directly regulate tobacco products. For example, reducing the nicotine content of cigarettes and requiring the production of less hazardous cigarettes are within the FDA's exclusive regulatory jurisdiction. Similarly, as demonstrated in the recently promulgated FDA regulations, marketing curbs on product logos, prohibition of advertising at sporting events, and development of counteradvertisements are also regulatory strategies that the FDA can undertake.[26] Legislatures can specify what regulatory strategies should be undertaken, but they rarely do so. The congressionally mandated rotating cigarette labels were an exception. Sometimes, also rarely, legislators can overrule regulatory actions.[27]

While courts play an important educational role in exposing the tobacco industry, the primary educational role in discouraging smoking lies with governmental and private institutions. Only they can develop and implement a sustained educational campaign that adjusts to changes in cigarette consumption trends and generates the public support needed to enact stronger tobacco control measures. Educational campaigns range from health education in school classrooms to antitobacco media campaigns ("counteradvertising").

Indirect Effects

Legislative and regulatory agencies have the authority and power to initiate negotiations with the tobacco industry and to alter the nature of the public debate. To date, they have not done so. Indirectly, however, there is a constant dialogue between these groups over proposed legislation and regulations.

DISCUSSION

An ultimate judgment on the desirability and consequences of using litigation to shape tobacco policy rests on a combination of both philosophical and pragmatic considerations. Although arguments favoring and opposing such litigation can be drawn from both spheres, it is predominantly philosophical considerations that militate against litigation as policy making. In contrast, proponents of the litigation can appeal to compelling practical concerns to justify its role in the policy process. The role of the courts in public health policy making must also be considered in the context of institutional choice in formulating policy and in balancing governmental interests in the public's health with protecting individual liberty interests. Except where noted, *litigation* in this section refers to the state lawsuits.

ARGUMENTS FAVORING JUDICIAL INTERVENTION

The principal pragmatic argument in favor of using litigation to seek tobacco control policy objectives emerges from proponents' perceptions that the legislative and regulatory systems have failed. They point to surveys demonstrating clear and often strong support for tobacco control regulations that the nation's legislative bodies continually fail to adopt. This occurs, they say, primarily due to the powerful economic, and hence political, influence of the tobacco companies on state and national lawmakers (Glantz and Begay 1994; Taylor 1984). Secondarily, they argue that the industry has a stranglehold on the

bureaucracies charged with regulating cigarette-related health and safety matters. Proponents of tobacco control litigation as policy thus focus on the potential
of litigation to achieve, or initiate, the policy development that a captured
legislative and regulatory system (see, e.g., Stigler 1971) has failed to produce,
despite widespread public support. It is important to note, however, that agency
or legislative capture need not be permanent. Through the disclosures emerging
from the litigation, the tobacco industry appears to have lost some of its ability
to capture Congress, though its influence remains significant. The litigation may
well have changed the policy agenda in ways potentially favorable to public
health interests.

Litigation proponents also argue that courts have the unique ability to
impose substantial damages on the tobacco industry and that such damages
can substitute for large excise tax increases that, absent the political power of
the industry, would be imposed by Congress and the states. Jurors might well
impose punitive damages on tobacco firms more frequently, given the release
of incriminating industry documents, as they have done recently in California
and Oregon. Further, courts can require measures that will limit the industry's
marketing efforts, again "simulating" a legislative/regulatory function.

Despite concerns about implementing judicial decisions, proponents of litigation can argue that there are no cultural beliefs that would contradict court
rulings. In fact, Rosenberg (1991) concludes that under certain conditions, the
constraints inhibiting the use of litigation to produce social or policy change
can be overcome. Those conditions require political or market support for
implementing court decisions. For example, this could include the willingness
of political actors to provide funds or other inducements to implement judicial
decisions or to impose costs for not complying.[28] In the context of Rosenberg's
analysis, the litigation offers cover for those previously afraid to offend the
tobacco industry and strengthens those who would like to impose additional
regulatory constraints on tobacco products. Proponents can make a strong case
that the constraints no longer apply to tobacco litigation and that the conditions
for litigation as policy are already in place.

Even though movies are once again glamorizing cigarettes and more teens are
smoking cigarettes than a decade ago, the cultural dominance and significance
of smoking have been reduced by changes in civil norms and concomitant legislation limiting smoking in public places (Kagan and Skolnick 1993; Jacobson,
Wasserman, and Anderson 1997). In addition, there is considerable public support for stronger curbs on smoking in public places and for restrictions on youth
access to tobacco products, including pressure from numerous state and local
antismoking coalitions. Regardless of some pronounced political opposition,
many bureaucrats and public officials are likely to welcome judicial rulings favorable to public health. At the state level, although some state officials are likely
to mount considerable opposition to expansive judicial rulings, the emergence

of tobacco control policy entrepreneurs, including antismoking coalitions and other nonsmokers' advocacy groups, may pressure governmental agencies to implement and enforce the courts' decisions.[29] At the federal level, the FDA's recent willingness to promulgate regulations restricting youth access to tobacco products (61 Fed. Reg. 44.396 [1996]) suggests that the regulators will be receptive to judicial rulings imposing additional restraints on tobacco use.

Another reason to believe that litigation as policy might succeed in this area is that the litigation may induce policy changes by virtue of the tobacco industry's desire to avoid other potential outcomes of litigation. Quite clearly, the threat of litigation convinced the tobacco industry to enter into settlement negotiations in 1997 that would not have otherwise occurred, led to the disclosure of damaging internal tobacco industry documents, and induced Liggett Tobacco Co., Inc., to concede the harms from tobacco products (Settlement Agreement 1997). Four states (Mississippi, Florida, Texas, and Minnesota) settled their litigation with large damage awards and public health provisions (including terms negotiated by Minnesota that apply retroactively to the other settlements). The subsequent settlement that covered all of the remaining states also included large financial payments by the industry and modest public health provisions.

These are not trivial accomplishments. Whether these successes will result in driving the policy agenda or even in ordering policy priorities remains to be seen. At a minimum, the environment in which tobacco control legislation and regulation are now being debated is, unarguably, fundamentally altered as a result of the lawsuits.

OBJECTIONS TO JUDICIAL POLICY MAKING

On the philosophical side, there are legitimate objections to the appropriateness of judicial policy making. Opponents of the use of litigation as policy emphasize the conceptual structure of governance in our democracy: the separation of powers, the vesting of policy decision making in an elected and representative legislature, the burden of implementing and enforcing policy falling upon a bureaucracy that answers to the elected legislature. In this conceptual framework, the responsibility for policy clearly belongs within the legislative and regulatory systems, with the role (and use) of the courts focused on ensuring that procedural requirements are closely adhered to, particularly the due process strictures of the Constitution. As unelected officials, courts threaten their legitimacy as impartial arbiters when they attempt to go beyond the dispute resolution functions and impose public policy changes. Many commentators argue that the complex (and value-laden) policy judgments and trade-offs entailed in making tobacco control policy should reside exclusively with the legislative branch. In this view, courts lack the ability to define policy objectives, interpret empirical data, select the "right" parties to the litigation or the "right" cases for policy judgments, understand the policy implications of their decisions, assess the economic impact of various policy choices, and obtain the proper information needed to resolve conflicting policy choices (Schuck 1988; Capron 1990; Horowitz 1977; Melnick 1983, 1994).

An additional problem is that the procedural constraints of litigation, including limits on remedies, circumscribe the extent to which policy changes can be ordered by courts. Courts may be reluctant to impose the requested equitable relief (the remedies most directly affecting public health policy) and may limit the remedies to monetary damages, or they may determine that these cases are not suitable for class action status. Judges generally do not like to usurp regulatory functions, especially when a constitutional violation is not charged. When a perceived political failure is the source of the litigation, courts are less likely to move beyond monetary awards. And there is always the problem of how the court would enforce any policy changes and whether such an order would produce a political backlash. For example, judicial takeovers of prisons have been widely resisted by state officials. An aggressive regulatory enforcement effort would be required to implement any judicial decisions (Jacobson and Wasserman 1997).

The case against using litigation as a means of establishing public policy is not without its own pragmatic considerations. For one thing, because the legal theories being tested by the attorneys general are novel, the litigation promises to be long, drawn out, and expensive, with no guarantee of consistent success. For another, as discussed above, there are certain policy measures that are less likely to be directly affected by litigation, including restrictions on smoking in public places and setting legal barriers to youth access to tobacco products. In fact, litigation could potentially create an impediment to effective tobacco control policy by diverting government attention and resources from policies designed to limit smoking. At least in the short term, litigation will do little to reduce smoking-initiation rates among teenagers, absent substantial price increases resulting from jury awards or settlement negotiations.

As a general proposition, litigation might detract from other policy efforts if the public perceives that the problem has been "solved" through litigation, in part through the allure of money. Public policy might well be distorted by an attempt to extract financial concessions at the expense of public health objectives. The debate over whether the 1997 settlement proposal was justified by its public health outcomes in view of the impressive-sounding financial terms (industry payments totaling $368.5 billion over twenty-five years, raised to more than $500 billion in Congress) should be a warning that litigation can focus attention on financial recovery instead of public health goals. For instance, in Mississippi's settlement with the tobacco industry, the state settled for $3.5 billion, but essentially abdicated its broader public health objectives, and Florida legislators argued over whether to spend that state's settlement money on health-related or other social needs, mainly education. In contrast, the Minnesota settlement did include many important public health provisions. These provisions will be applied retroactively to the previous settlements, since each state was assured that it would benefit from any additional concessions made by the tobacco industry in subsequent settlements. But in the most recent development—the settlement covering all of the remaining states—public health provisions were distinctly secondary to the settlement's focus: the payment of monetary damages.

THE ROLE OF THE COURTS IN PUBLIC HEALTH POLICY

Institutional Choice

We believe that part of the reason for the success in using tobacco litigation to leverage settlement negotiations is that advocates built the moral and political case against the tobacco industry through years of legislative lobbying, grassroots organizing, and savvy use of the media. In doing so, advocates also clearly demonstrated the failure of the political and regulatory systems to respond to popular sentiment. As a result, resorting to litigation to achieve public health goals gained legitimacy. Those preconditions may not currently be present in other public health battles, such as alcohol and gun control.

Of course, legal theoreticians can and do argue about the appropriate level of judicial involvement in policy matters, but a more activist use of the judicial system may be warranted, indeed even required, primarily due to system failures in the other branches of government. Debates then ensue about precisely what constitutes a system failure, and how egregious such failures must be to justify judicial intervention. In theory, a narrow separation of powers approach would argue for a limited role for litigation in tobacco policy, deferring instead to legislative and regulatory prerogatives. In practice, the tobacco litigation has blurred the line between litigation and the politics of public health. The interaction between the courts and the political process often obscures clear policy boundaries, as contentious struggles over civil rights, abortion, breast implants, and auto safety indicate.

From an institutional perspective, therefore, litigation may be a second-best solution; but as a component of a broader, comprehensive approach to tobacco control policy making, litigation has a distinct role given the lackluster performance of the political institutions. Litigation can be viewed as a necessary but not sufficient component, with its necessity dictated by the failure of the conventional policy system to represent the will of the citizenry. Minnesota's recent settlement with the tobacco industry, replete with public health policy measures supported by the public but never adopted by its elected representatives, serves as a vivid illustration of the practical role that can be played by litigation.

Even if one views the use of litigation to pursue policy objectives as legitimate, proponents must be wary of over-reliance on litigation as a substitute for regulation. This could weaken the political organizing efforts and effectiveness of proponents of social change and energize their opponents (Rosenberg 1995).[30] Litigation may be a complement to the more traditional apparatus of policy making and implementation, but it seems destined to fail as an alternative. For one thing, as Judge Osteen's recent opinion overturning the EPA's environmental-tobacco-smoke findings indicates, there is no guarantee that courts will correct political deficiencies; courts can just as easily create confusion as establish desirable policy. For another, the extensive literature on the role of policy entrepreneurs in setting and achieving the policy agenda (see, e.g., Oliver and Paul-Shaheen 1997) argues for public health advocates keeping focused on the political process.

Hanson and Logue (1998) reach a different result. They argue that the probability of effective regulation of the tobacco industry is so low that the status quo, especially the prospect of continuing litigation, is preferable to the negotiated settlement that relies on a regulatory approach. Their preferred options, either an enterprise liability system or a smokers' compensation fund that forces the tobacco industry to internalize the health costs of smoking, are interesting policy alternatives to regulation.[31] Specifically, they contend that their incentive-based system will deter smokers by including the full social costs of smoking in the price of cigarettes and force tobacco manufacturers to compete over safety. But since courts and legislatures have been reluctant to impose enterprise liability, and since attempts to establish a smokers' compensation fund would encounter fierce resistance from the tobacco industry, it is not clear how these reforms could be implemented.[32] In the alternative, Hanson and Logue (1998: 190) argue, without elaboration, that the third wave of litigation is likely to produce public health outcomes superior to the outmoded command and control regulatory strategies motivating the settlement negotiations. Instead, they assert that products liability law in theory and "the growing inevitability of many large civil judgments against the industry" would provide substantial deterrent and other public health benefits not achievable through regulation. Whatever the merits of their proposed alternatives, we find no evidence in their analysis compelling enough to conclude either that litigation will achieve superior public health outcomes or that it is a more appropriate mechanism for formulating public health policy.[33]

Individual Choice and Accountability

While we have framed the argument in terms of the courts as policy makers, it is important to recognize that other functions of judicial involvement remain salient in tobacco and other public health issues. Where the public's health has been harmed, individuals retain the right to seek damages and the political system retains the right to impose appropriate restrictions, subject to judicial balancing between industry culpability and individual responsibility. In any given public health issue, the balance will vary depending on the nature and extent of the abridgment of individual liberties, the nature and costs of the public health intervention, the alternatives to governmental intervention, the voluntariness of the activity, and the extent of harm to third persons in the absence of governmental activity.

In several ways, tobacco is an extreme case. The tobacco industry is highly culpable morally for the harms it has caused and deserves to be held accountable. Moreover, the exercise of the individual choice to smoke is almost always made during childhood, after which addiction plays a defining role. Just as important, a reasonable approach to tobacco control need not tread too harshly on individual liberties. One can imagine protections for children and nonsmokers that still maintain the adult's right to consume tobacco products in circumstances not harmful to others (Warner 1997).

Although it seems unreasonable to completely absolve the tobacco industry to protect the principle of individual choice, one must recognize the possibility that there may be costs to rewarding risk-taking behavior through litigation, even if, as here, it is conditioned by addiction.[34] To us, litigation is an appropriate mechanism for ensuring the tobacco industry's accountability; yet we are concerned that public health advocates might generalize the lesson from this experience, which could well produce undesirable outcomes in other situations. For instance, advocates might apply this example to a situation in which industry culpability is less clear and where the intrusion into individual liberties might be greater. As an example, although motorcycle injuries are a serious public health issue, and motorcycles and helmets warrant regulation, litigation against manufacturers to set public health policy, either through extensive damages or through equitable relief, would not be desirable. There is little of the moral culpability seen with the tobacco industry, and the litigation would distract attention from what should be a matter of individual responsibility and public policy (such as more stringent traffic safety regulations). The same would be true of litigation against the makers of high-fat foods, particularly where the manufacturers also offer consumers low- and no-fat alternatives. In short, the intrusion into individual liberty would be too great. The "slippery slope" argument provides attractive rhetoric to opponents of tobacco control policy precisely because it contains genuinely troubling elements.

Public health advocates and public policy theoreticians need to consider what role a litigation strategy should play in the handful of difficult public health arenas that bear an important resemblance to tobacco control, such as gun control and alcohol abuse. Gun control, particularly, poses strikingly similar challenges and opportunities, as is evident in the recent municipal lawsuits initiated against the gun industry. There, too, public health advocates face what they consider to be a failed regulatory and legislative system that has inadequately addressed the public health harms from gun availability and use. There, too, one encounters the individual-rights versus collective-good debate. One lesson public health advocates can draw from the tobacco control litigation is that the strategic use of litigation can help set the policy agenda by providing essential information to the public and by forcing legislators to confront issues that powerful interest groups would prefer remain unaddressed.

CONCLUSION

To a certain extent, the conclusions reached in this analysis are ambiguous and unlikely to satisfy either proponents or opponents of litigation as policy. Yet democracy is an often untidy and disorderly process where the strengths and weaknesses of the three branches of government collide. The case of tobacco control litigation exemplifies the complex interactions between political theory and the more pragmatic world in which political differences are attenuated through compromise. The resulting policy, although rarely lauded by all stake-holders, is then shaped by the responses of each governmental entity.

Those who believe that litigation should not be used to influence policy must reflect on the failure of the legislative and regulatory systems to confront the public health harms of tobacco. Continued failure to address legitimate public health needs will invite the same type of litigation and potential judicial intervention with the legislative process in other public health domains, as we have seen with tobacco control.

Those who believe that litigation is a legitimate way to make policy need to recognize that there is no guarantee that public health policy will be dramatically altered by the litigation process. Indeed, the experience with the state Medicaid cases provides an instructive example. This litigation appears to have been motivated by a desire to fundamentally alter tobacco control policy. It produced a national settlement proposal in 1997 that was breathtaking in its policy scope. And yet that proposal ultimately collapsed. Its successor, the multistate agreement of 1998, included only very modest policy measures. Like most lawsuits, its outcome focused on awarding monetary damages to the plaintiffs. As this experience demonstrates, policy-making responsibility and power will continue to rest with legislators and regulators. Litigation has stimulated a national debate over the role of smoking in society and eventually may well move the policy agenda. But a sustained legislative and regulatory presence is required to ensure meaningful policy changes.

REFERENCES

Annas, G. J. 1997. Tobacco Litigation as Cancer Prevention: Dealing with the Devil. *New England Journal of Medicine* 336(4).

Arno, P. S.. A. M. Brandt, L. 0. Gostin, and J. Morgan. 1996. Tobacco Industry Strategies to Oppose Federal Regulation. *Journal of the American Medical Association* 275:1258–1262.

Broder, J. M. 1997. Cigarette Makers in a $368 Billion Accord to Curb Lawsuits and Curtail Marketing. *New York Times,* 21 June, Al.

Capron. A. M. 1990. The Burden of Decision. *Hastings Center Report* May/June: 36–41.

Centers for Disease Control (CDC). 1989. The Surgeon General's 1989 Report on Reducing the Health Consequences of Smoking: Twenty-Five Years of Progress. *Morbidity and Mortality Weekly Report* 38(2):1–32.

Cook, P. The Social Costs of Drinking. 1991. In *The Negative Social Consequences of Alcohol Use. Oslo, Norway.* ed Olaf Gjerlow. Oslo, Norway: Aasland.

Daynard, R. A. 1988. Tobacco Liability Litigation as a Cancer Control Strategy. *Journal of the National Cancer Institute* 80(1):9–13.

Glantz, S. A., and M. E. Begay. 1994. Tobacco Industry Campaign Contributions Are Affecting Tobacco Control Policymaking in California. *Journal of the American Medical Association* 272:1176–1182.

Glantz, S. A., J. Slade, L. A Bero, P. Hanauer, and D. E. Barnes. 1996. *The Cigarette Papers.* Berkeley: University of California Press.

Grossman, M., and F. J. Chaloupka. 1997. Cigarette Taxes: The Straw to Break the Camel's Back. *Public Health Reports* 112:291–297.

Hanson, J. D., and K. D. Logue. 1998. The Costs of Cigarettes: The Economic Case for Ex Post Incentive Based Regulation. *Yale Law Journal* 107:1163–1262.

Hilts, P. J. 1996. *Smoke Screen: The Truth behind the Tobacco Industry Cover-Up.* Reading. MA: Addison-Wesley.

Hodgson, T. A. 1992. Cigarette Smoking and Lifetime Medical Expenditures. *Millbank Quarterly* 70(1):81–125.

———. 1998. The Health Care Costs of Smoking. *New England Journal of Medicine* 338:470.

Horowitz, D. L. 1977. *The Courts and Social Policy.* Washington. DC: Brookings Institution.

Jacobson, P. D., and J. Wasserman. 1997. *Tobacco Control Laws: Implementation and Enforcement.* Santa Monica, CA: RAND.

Jacobson, P. D., J. Wasserman, and J. R. Anderson. 1997. Historical Overview of Tobacco Legislation and Regulation. *Journal of Social Issues* 53(1):75–95.

Jacobson, P. D., J. Wasserman, and K. Raube. 1993. The Politics of Antismoking Legislation. *Journal of Health Politics, Policy and Law* 18:787–819.

Kagan, R. A., and J. H. Skolnick. 1993. Banning Smoking: Compliance without Enforcement. In *Smoking Policy: Law, Politics, and Culture.* ed. R. L. Rabin and S. D. Sugarman. New York: Oxford University Press.

Kaufman, J. 1997. Was This Tobacco CEO ahead of His Time? *Business Week,* 4 August 1997, 6.

Keeton, W. P., D. B. Dobbs, R. E. Keeton, and D. G. Owen. 1984. *Prosser and Keeton on Torts.* 5th ed. St. Paul, MN: West Publishing.

Kelder, G. E., and R. A. Daynard. 1996. Tobacco Litigation as a Public Health and Cancer Control Strategy. *Journal of the American Medical Women's Association* 1(1–2):57–62.

———. 1997. Judicial Approaches to Tobacco Control: The Third Wave of Tobacco Litigation as a Tobacco Control Mechanism. *Journal of Social Issues* 53(1):169–186.

Komesar, N. K. 1994. *Imperfect Alternatives: Choosing Institutions in Law, Economics, and Public Policy.* Chicago: University of Chicago Press.

McCann, M. 1996. Causal versus Constitutive Explanations (or, On the Difficulty of Being So Positive). *Law and Social Inquiry* 21:457–482.

McCann, M. W. 1994. *Rights at Work: Pay Equity Reform and the Politics of Legal Mobilization.* Chicago: University of Chicago Press.

Melnick, R. S. 1983. *Regulation and the Courts: The Case of the Clean Air Act.* Washington, DC: Brookings Institution.

———. 1994. *Between the Lines: Interpreting Welfare Rights.* Washington, DC: Brookings Institution.

Moore, M. C., and C. J. Mikhail. 1996. A New Attack on Smoking Using an Old-Time Remedy. *Public Health Reports* 111:192–203.

Oliver, T. R., and P. Paul-Shaheen. 1997. Translating Ideas into Actions: Entrepreneurial Leadership in State Health Care Reforms. *Journal of Health Politics, Policy and Law* 22(3):721–788.

Pertschuk, M. 1997. We've Come a Long Way—Maybe: Assessing the Strengths and Weaknesses of the Tobacco Control Movement Today. Keynote address at Entering a New Dimension: A National Conference on Tobacco and Health, 22 September, Houston, Texas.

Rabin, R. L. 1991. Some Thoughts on Smoking Regulation. *Stanford Law Review* 43:475–496.

———. 1993. Institutional and Historical Perspectives on Tobacco Tort Liability. In *Smoking Policy: Law, Politics, and Culture,* ed. R. L. Rabin and S. D. Sugarman New York: Oxford University Press.

Rosenberg, G. N. 1991. *The Hollow Hope: Can Courts Bring About Social Change?* Chicago: University of Chicago Press.

———. 1995. The Real World of Constitutional Rights: The Supreme Court and the Implementation of the Abortion Decisions. In *Contemplating Courts,* ed. L. Epstein. Washington, DC: CQ.

Samuels, B., and S. A. Glantz. 1991. The Politics of Local Tobacco Control. *Journal of the American Medical Association* 266(15):2110–2117.

Scheingold, S. A. 1974. *The Politics of Rights: Lawyers, Public Policy, and Political Change.* New Haven, CT: Yale University Press.

Schuck, P. H. 1988. The New Ideology of Tort Law. *Public Interest* 92:93–109.

Schwartz, G. T. 1993. Tobacco Liability in the Courts. In *Smoking Policy: Law, Politics, and Culture,* ed. R. L. Rabin and S. D. Sugarman. New York: Oxford University Press.

Settlement Agreement between State Attorneys General, and Brooke Group, Ltd., and Liggett Corp. 1997. *Tobacco Products Litigation Reporter* 12(1):3.1.

Stoddard, T. B. 1997. Bleeding Heart: Reflections on Using the Law to Make Social Change. *New York University Law Review* 72:967–991.

Taylor, P. 1984. *The Smoke Ring: Tobacco, Money, and Multinational Politics.* New York: Pantheon.

United States Department of Health and Human Services (USDHHS). 1989. *Reducing the Health Consequences of Smoking: Twenty-Five Years of Progress. A Report of the Surgeon General.* DHHS Publication No. (CDC) 89–8411. Washington, DC: Government Printing Office.

United States Department of Health, Education, and Welfare (USDHEW). 1964. *Smoking and Health: Report of the Advisory Committee to the Surgeon General of the Public Health Service.* PHS Publication No. 1103. Washington, DC: U.S. Government Printing Office.

Warner, K. E. 1979. Clearing the Airwaves: The Cigarette Ad Ban Revisited. *Policy Analysis* 5:435–450. Reprinted in *Cases in Public Policy-Making,* ed. J. Anderson, 2d ed. New York: Holt, Rinehart and Winston (1982 [1976]).

———. 1997. Dealing with Tobacco—The Implications of a Legislative Settlement with the Tobacco Industry. *American Journal of Public Health* 87(6):906–909.

Warner, K. E., T. Citrin, G. Pickett, B. G. Rabe, A. Wagenaar, and J. Stryker. 1990. Licit and Illicit Drug Policies: A Typology. *British Journal of Addiction* 85:255–262.

Warner, K. E., T. A. Hodgson, and C. E. Carroll. 1999. The Medical Costs of Smoking in the United States: Estimates, Their Validity, and Their Implications. Working paper, Department of Health Management and Policy, University of Michigan School of Public Health, Ann Arbor, MI.

Weissert, C. S., and W. G. Weissert. 1996. *Governing Health: The Politics of Health Policy.* Baltimore. MD: Johns Hopkins University Press.

Wilson, J. Q. 1989. *Bureaucracy: What Government Agencies Do and Why They Do It.* New York: Basic Books.

NOTES

We appreciate the valuable comments we received on a previous draft from Jeffrey Wasserman, Harold A. Pollack, Barry Rabe, Richard A. Daynard, David A. Hyman, and Ruth Roemer. We also appreciate the extremely helpful comments from Mark A. Peterson and three anonymous reviewers.

1. "Symington said that the way to cut down on smoking deaths is through educational programs, such as a statewide advertising campaign, and not through recovering damages in a lawsuit"; *Arizona Republic,* 16 November 1996. Other commentators have been skeptical about the public health aspects of the litigation. Alabama Attorney General Bill Pryor wrote that "this wave of lawsuits is about politics, not law, and money, not public health"; *Wall Street Journal,* 7 April 1997, A14.

2. We will not discuss the legal merits of any of the lawsuits.

3.   Torts (civil wrongs, e.g., negligence) can be either intentional or unintentional. Most of the tobacco litigation has involved alleged intentional torts, thereby increasing the potential for punitive damages.

4.   Truly substantial financial awards could lead to cigarette price increases that would deter smoking far more effectively than the plausible nonfinancial terms of a decision (Grossman and Chaloupka 1997).

5.   As of this writing, the case is under appeal. Even if the appeal is denied, this case is likely to be an exception to the general rule that courts are reluctant to overturn regulatory decisions.

6.   The underlying legal issues and strategies in the earlier litigation have been covered extensively by others, including Robert Rabin (1993) and Gary Schwartz (1993).

7.   An unjust enrichment claim is based on the theory that the tobacco companies are unjustly enriched because the state is forced to absorb the financial costs of tobacco-related diseases through the Medicaid program while the tobacco companies profit without internalizing those costs. See, e.g., Kelder and Daynard 1997. The complaints filed by the various states can be found at www.stic.neu.edu.

8.   Subrogation is the substitution of one party for another regarding a lawful claim, such that the substituted party (the state) sues on behalf of the rights of the other party (the Medicaid recipient).

9.   The private attorneys handling the litigation are motivated to no small degree by potential personal financial rewards. Indeed, all of the private litigation is made possible by the contingency fee system, which allows attorneys to collect a portion of any settlement or jury award. Some tobacco control advocates have charged that the result in the Broin case, where the named litigants will receive little cash remuneration but the attorneys will be highly compensated, appears to have been resolved for financial rather than social policy reasons. Public statements issued by the state attorneys general about their motivations for initiating the litigation suggest a mixture of financial (reducing state Medicaid costs), political (using tobacco litigation as a high-profile campaign tactic), and policy (using litigation to change public health policy) reasons. Without in-depth interviews with a reasonable sample, we cannot further characterize or assess their motivation. However, the relative rapidity with which so many state attorneys general adopted the litigation strategy suggests a perception that the antismoking cause has political appeal, as demonstrated by the outcry when presidential candidate Bob Dole declared that nicotine is not addictive. It seems only fair to point out that state attorneys general may be motivated by potential political rewards in using the visibility of tobacco litigation to run for higher office. The state attorneys general are not a unitary entity; each one may have his or her own policy or political agenda.

10.   As we discuss below, many advocates hoped that a successful barrage of lawsuits would have the same effect as a large cigarette-tax increase: increasing price (to pay judgments against the industry) would discourage tobacco use by children and, to a lesser degree, adults. In lieu of excise tax increases, damages would amount to a policy "substitute." In addition, we note that Daynard (1988) has clearly stated the policy agenda underlying the use of litigation to achieve public health policy objectives.

11.   Michael Moore and Stuart Mikhail (1996), cocounsel in Mississippi's litigation against the tobacco industry, describe their litigation strategy but do not discuss the litigation's policy objectives. Both George Annas (1997) and Daynard (1988) directly address the issue of tobacco litigation as public health policy, but they focus more on

litigation strategy and settlement negotiations than on a systematic analysis of what policy objectives can be achieved through litigation relative to alternative regulatory or legislative approaches.

12. Disclosure in tobacco litigation serves two functions: (1) to alert the public to the lies told by the tobacco industry, thus influencing public opinion and facilitating more stringent regulation; and (2) to provide ammunition for a jury to impose punitive damages. In addition, tobacco litigation fascinates the American public, holding out the promise of continuing exposure of tobacco industry mendacity and public health harms.

13. Rosenberg is primarily concerned with the role of the courts as social change agents, but the model is useful in analyzing the role of litigation in influencing public health policy.

14. A proponent of the constrained view, Rosenberg (1991) argues that the presumed political and social changes stemming from civil rights, abortion, and environmental litigation have been illusory. Instead, Rosenberg (1991, 1995) concludes that changes in public opinion and action by elected officials, rather than court decisions, are required to engender significant social change. These conclusions and this model remain controversial. For example, McCann (1996:472) criticizes the approach for ignoring 'the many more subtle, variable ways that legal norms, institutions, actors and the like do matter in social life." For our purposes, Rosenberg's framework simply provides a useful starting point.

15. Rosenberg studied the effects of judicial decisions in civil rights, abortion, and environmental cases. Horowitz reached similar results in studying the effects of leading cases in police practices, education, juvenile justice, and the Model Cities program. Melnick studied environmental litigation (1983), and welfare, education for handicapped persons, and the food stamp program (1994).

16. There are important exceptions. An obvious example is the provision of non-smoking hotel rooms where not required by law.

17. There are any number of reasons why bankruptcy is not likely to remove tobacco products from the market. Even if bankruptcy were declared, firms would still remain in business for several years under court-ordered reorganization protection. Furthermore, new companies, unencumbered by liability for past actions, would emerge to replace older ones driven out of business.

18. Following the multistate settlement in late 1998, the major cigarette manufacturers raised wholesale prices 45 cents per pack, announcing that this move was necessitated by settlement payment obligations. Clearly, this was a desirable outcome for the attorneys general. There is some question, however, as to how much of a real price increase took effect, since the companies apparently also increased special purchase offers that have the effect of reducing listed price increases (e.g., three packs sold for the price of two).

19. Indeed, the debate over disclosing documents in the Minnesota case led House Commerce Committee Chairman Thomas Billey, a tobacco industry ally, to demand the release, first, of over eight hundred industry documents that the state of Minnesota was trying to obtain through litigation, then of another thirty-nine thousand documents.

20. To be sure, new ideas have emerged, such as the Massachusetts tobacco ingredients disclosure law, and the pace of antismoking activity has increased during the third wave. While it can be argued that the popularity of the third-wave approach

contributed to these initiatives, we believe they would have occurred anyway, given the amount of antismoking activity already under way.

21.   *Business Week* reported on 4 August 1997 that a former tobacco industry executive, Michael Miles, had wanted to initiate similar negotiations in 1994 but was unable to identify a powerful group with whom to negotiate (Kaufman 1997).

22.   This situation illustrates the difficulty of labeling effects as exclusively direct or indirect, since one might well categorize the Mangini experience as a direct policy outcome at the state level. R. J. Reynolds's fear of similar lawsuits in other states may well have hastened the demise of Joe Camel nationwide, but some observers have argued that the Joe Camel campaign had run its course anyway, and hence died a near-natural death. Ironically, the replacement campaign has been criticized as a more sophisticated form of pandering to both teens and the original cohort of "Joe's kids" now in their twenties.

23.   As an example, the Balanced Budget Amendment of 1997 included a provision that would have credited the industry, in the event of a settlement, for the 15 cents in additional cigarette excise tax included in the bill as a revenue-generating measure. After the provision was brought to the public's attention. Congress repealed it.

24.   This is an irony not lost on Congress itself. Senator John McCain (R-AZ), a leader in the congressional effort to enact comprehensive tobacco control legislation, said, "There was institutional reluctance—resentment, even—that a handful of attorneys general and plaintiffs' lawyers would come to us with such a detailed agreement, even divvying up the spoils. Who do these people think they are? That's a legislative and executive branch prerogative" (Broder and Meier 1997). Despite this sentiment, Congress embraced the settlement as the starting point for legislative deliberation.

25.   An exception to this was the ban on television and radio advertisements, effective in 1971, which clearly impeded the industry's marketing effort by prohibiting it from using what was then its principal mode of marketing. However, the legislation had the felicitous effect for the industry of eliminating the need for broadcasters to donate airtime to antismoking messages, demonstrated during that era to have suppressed smoking more than the prosmoking ads increased it. The tobacco industry recognized this and therefore supported the legislation banning broadcast advertising of cigarettes (Warner 1979).

26.   To be sure, regulatory authority is not unbounded. In *Coyne Beahm, Inc., et al. v. U.S. Food and Drug Administration* (CA No. 2:95CV00591, M.D. N.C., 27 April 1997) the court overturned some of the FDA's restrictions on advertising and promotion of tobacco products, saying they went beyond the agency's statutory authority.

27.   A compelling example occurred when the Consumer Product Safety Commission considered investigating the safety of cigarettes. Congress responded by specifically exempting cigarettes from the commission's purview (USDHHS 1989).

28.   According to Rosenberg, courts may produce social change when the three constraints discussed earlier are overcome and when one or more of the following conditions is also present: (1) when other actors offer positive incentives to induce compliance; (2) when other actors impose costs to induce compliance; (3) when judicial decisions can be implemented by the market; and (4) when judicial decisions provide cover or leverage for implementers to act.

29.   A recent study found that smoking control advocates have been slow to engage in the implementation and enforcement process (Jacobson and Wasserman 1997).

30.   However, McCann (1996) argues that judicial decisions can just as easily motivate advocates to organize to secure the social changes made possible by the litigation. While the evidence suggests that the tobacco litigation has not yet weakened the engagement of the tobacco control movement, it is undeniable that tobacco control advocates were seriously split over whether to accept the negotiated settlement (Pertschuk 1997).

31.   Enterprise liability holds the manufacturer or other entity (such as a managed care firm) liable for the harms it or its products cause.

The issue of the health costs of smoking is complicated, and largely beyond the scope of this article. It revolves around whether and how one should adjust smoking-related health care costs to reflect smokers' shorter lives, and hence reduced later-life health care costs. Although there is reason to believe that the net health care costs of smoking are positive (Hodgson 1992, 1998; Warner, Hodgson, and Carroll 1999), the magnitude of the net costs is not well established. In addition, there is considerable disagreement as to which health care costs should be considered "social" and hence subject to internalization as part of a compensation fund or through taxation. The general distinction between the economic and public health views of social costs is nicely articulated in Cook's (1991) discussion of the social costs of alcohol abuse. These issues have been raised by the tobacco industry in defending itself against the state litigation, but have not yet played a discernible role in case outcomes.

32. Other public administrative compensation schemes, such as the federal vaccine compensation fund, and similar private litigation settlement mechanisms, such as the asbestos claims settlement fund, have mixed track records.

33. Without engaging in an extended discussion, it is important to note that regulation can be a successful, if imperfect, strategy. For example, automobile safety, pharmaceuticals, and even environmental regulations have had some success. There is also evidence to suggest that tobacco control regulations are effective (Jacobson and Wasserman 1997).

34. One of the possible ironic, potentially tragic, unintended consequences of the 1997 tobacco settlement proposal was that, by establishing an annual fund of $4 billion to compensate smokers who sue, some smokers might have chosen to continue smoking, rather than quitting, rationalizing that if they were killed by smoking, they might be able to leave a financial inheritance to their children.

15

Social Movements as Catalysts for Policy Change: The Case of Smoking and Guns

Constance A. Nathanson

The United States is unique both historically and today in the major role played by health-related social movements in changing health policies and health be-haviors (Nathanson 1996; Mechanic 1993). With a few notable exceptions (e.g., Gusfield 1963; Staggenborg 1991), these movements have received relatively little attention from social movement scholars. This article employs an analytic framework drawn from social movement and related sociological theories to account for the relative success of the United States' campaigns against smoking and guns in bringing about change in the policies and behaviors targeted by these movements.

While the article's primary focus is on the smoking/tobacco control move-ment, the analytic strategy is comparative. Aspects of the movement that may account for its relative success (as well as for the pitfalls it may still face) are best identified through comparison with the experience of another contemporary health-related social movement. Gun control was selected because it has certain initial similarities with smoking/tobacco control. Cigarettes and guns were both widely used "democratic" consumer products accessible to and enjoyed by

Reprinted from *Journal of Health Politics, Policy and Law,* 24, no. 3 (June 1999): 421–488. Copyright 1999. Duke University Press. All rights reserved. Reprinted with permission.

Preparation of this article was supported by the Association of Schools of Public Health and the Centers for Disease Control and Prevention; by a Health Policy Research Award to Dr. Nathanson from the Robert Wood Johnson Foundation; by a Visiting Scholar Award from the Russell Sage Foundation; and by the Hopkins Population Center (NICHD grant no. 5 P30 HD06268).

millions in all walks of life, romanticized in film and (in the case of cigarettes) advertising. Movements against these products were initiated in the late 1960s and early 1970s. Both movements confronted well-connected, well-financed opponents. Based on a detailed comparison of the two campaigns I argue that the success of the smoking/tobacco control movement may be accounted for by an ideologically persuasive construction of the relevant health risks, by grassroots mobilization for nonsmokers' rights, and—in the end—by important weaknesses in the movement's opposition.

Sources for the analysis presented include interviews with movement activists and observers, participant-observation in movement-related activities, archival materials, and published books and articles by advocates, journalists, and scholars.[1] Research was largely completed by the end of 1996, but some reference is made to later events.

The choice and definition of variables to be examined as well as the analysis of research materials were guided by two bodies of theory: social movement theory as elaborated by sociologists and political scientists (e.g., Gamson 1990; Tarrow 1994; Kriesi 1995; McAdam, McCarthy, and Zald 1996) and work on the social construction of public problems and perceptions of risk by Joseph R. Gusfield (1981), Mary Douglas and Aaron Wildavsky (1982), and others (Kunreuther and Linneruth 1983; Wynne 1987). Where quantitative measures of particular variables were available and appropriate, they have been used. However, for the most part the method used was qualitative and comparative (see, e.g., Glaser and Strauss 1967; Lofland 1996).

The analytic framework employed includes three sets of variables. These are, first, movements' supporting ideologies; second, each movement's capacities for mobilizing potential constituencies and organizational resources; and, third, political opportunity structures, defined to include a broad range of opportunities and threats external to the movements themselves. Each variable is more fully described in the context of analysis of the movements themselves.

The article is organized in four sections. The first section consists of brief historical overviews of each movement. Measures of movement success are described and then the movements' relative success by these criteria are compared in the second section. The third section is devoted to a comparative analysis of the two movements, and in the fourth and concluding section I reflect on what can be learned from this analysis.

HISTORICAL OVERVIEW

Movements have histories. The content and relative importance of each of the elements I have identified—ideologies, organization, and political opportunities—shift over time. Aspects that appear highly important at an early stage of movement evolution may become much less important and, indeed, change their character altogether as the movement either declines or becomes institutionalized. Political opportunities, in particular, are subject to marked change as elites more or less friendly to the movement's cause gain or lose power. What Charles Tilly (1986) has labeled "repertoires of contention"—the sit-in, the protest march, the courtroom battle—shift over time in popularity and in value as vehicles of expression and influence. Particularly in the case of movements that attract substantial media attention, immediate drama (or what the media defines as drama) tends to obscure the complex reality of how change comes about. This complexity is illuminated by close attention to each movement's history.

On 11 January 1964, less than two months after President John F. Kennedy's assassination, the Commission on Smoking and Health that Kennedy had appointed two years earlier issued its report. The assassination and the report each generated substantial pressure for change toward greater control, respectively, of guns and smoking, and produced corresponding opposition to the changes proposed. Here I present a summary and highly selective account of these events.

U.S. TOBACCO WARS, 1950–1996

The history of smoking control over the past half-century is one of almost continuous struggle—for much of this period a very lopsided struggle—between the tobacco industry and its allies on one side and a disparate array of antismoking forces on the other. I have divided these "tobacco wars" into three partially overlapping phases, outlined in Tables 15.1–15.3. These are "Phase 1: Making the Health Connection," which runs from 1950 to 1964; "Phase 2: The Struggle for Regulation," running from 1965 to 1996; and "Phase 3: The Discovery of Innocent Victims," which runs from 1971 to 1995.[2]

The critical events of Phase 1 are the scientific reports that appeared primarily but not exclusively in the medical press and that established cigarette smoking as a significant hazard to human health.[3] The culminating event in this series was the 1964 Surgeon General's Report on Smoking and Health (U.S. DHEW 1964). Serious congressional attention to smoking and health (initiating Phase 2, the struggle for regulation) was triggered less by the Surgeon General's report itself than by its political fallout: actions taken in several state legislatures to pass package labeling laws and an administrative initiative taken by the Federal Trade Commission (FTC) within a week of the report's public unveiling to require package warning labels.[4] With much huffing and puffing about chaos in the states and administrative encroachment on legislative authority, Congress took back its turf and in 1965 passed the Federal Cigarette Labeling and Advertising Act. This bill was regarded by contemporary smoking control advocates as considerably stronger in its protection for the tobacco industry than the "remedial action" recommended by the Surgeon General (Pertschuk 1986; Fritschler 1989). The warning label was far milder and less certainly

TABLE 15.1

U.S. Tobacco Wars, 1950–1964

Phase 1: Making the Health Connection

1950	Wynder and Graham. Tobacco Smoking as a Possible Etiologic Factor in Bronchiogenic Carcinoma: A Study of 684 Proved Cases. *Journal of the American Medical Association.*
1952	Doll and Hill. A Study of the Aetoiology of Carcinoma of the Lung. *British Medical Journal.* Norr. Cancer by the Carton. *Reader's Digest.*
1954	Hammond and Horn. The Relationship between Human Smoking Habits and Death Rates: A Follow-up Study of 187,766 Men. *Journal of the American Medical Association.*
1956	Doll and Hill. Lung Cancer and Other Causes of Death in Relation to Smoking. *British Medical Journal.*
	First official involvement by U.S. Public Health Service: Scientific study group on smoking and health.
	S. G. Burney publishes statement in JAMA: "The weight of the evidence at present implicates smoking as the principal factor in the increased incidence of lung cancer" (2104).
1962	Royal College of Physicians of London: "Cigarette smoking is a cause of lung cancer and bronchitis and probably contributes to the development of coronary heart disease" (S7).
1964	Surgeon General's Report on Smoking and Health: "Cigarette smoking is a health hazard of sufficient importance in the U.S. to warrant appropriate remedial action" (33).

legible than advocates would have preferred; adding insult to injury, the bill prevented individual states from imposing their own (possibly stricter) labeling requirements. Less noted at the time, but of overriding importance in the long run, was the bill's language mandating annual reports by the Surgeon General on the health consequences of smoking.[5] The continuing drumbeat of these reports throughout the 1970s and 1980s played a critical role in fueling the antismoking movement.

The pattern established in 1965 of minimal regulation in response to public pressure, combined with significant protection for the tobacco industry, has continued to characterize the congressional approach to regulation in the smoking/tobacco arena.[6] After many years of disclaiming authority over tobacco, the federal Food and Drug Administration (FDA) took up the regulatory banner in the 1990s, labeling nicotine as a drug "within the meaning of the Federal Food,

TABLE 15.2

U.S. Tobacco Wars, 1965–1996

Phase 2: The Struggle for Regulation

1965	Federal Cigarette Labeling and Advertising Act passed 1. Mandates annual SG reports and legislative recommendations. 2. Requires warning label: "Caution: Cigarette Smoking May Be Hazardous to Your Health." 3. Preempts more restrictive state action.
1966–1976	Congress specifically excludes tobacco from regulation under: 1. Fair Packaging and Labeling Act (1966). 2. Controlled Substances Act (1970). 3. Consumer Product Safety Act (1972). 4. Federal Hazardous Substances Act (1976). 5. Toxic Substances Control Act (1976).
1970	Public Health Cigarette Smoking Act of 1969 passed. 1. Renews SG report mandate. 2. Requires warning label: "Warning: The Surgeon General Has Determined That Cigarette Smoking Is Hazardous to Your Health." 3. Bans tobacco advertising on radio and TV. 4. Continues preemption.
1984	Comprehensive Smoking Education Act passed. Requires four rotating warning labels preceded by "SURGEON GENERAL'S WARNING."
1996	FDA issues regulations of tobacco products.

Drug, and Cosmetic Act" (U.S. DHHS 1995: 41455) and proposing regulation, aimed primarily at the protection of children. The first phase of these regulations went into effect on 1 March 1997.[7]

On 11 January 1971—the seventh anniversary of the Surgeon General's report—Jesse L. Steinfeld (then Surgeon General) used the opportunity of an address to the Interagency Council on Smoking and Health to urge the adoption of a Bill of Rights for the Nonsmoker to include a ban on smoking in "all confined public places" (Steinfeld 1983: 1258).[8] Independently, but almost simultaneously, the nonsmokers' rights movement was launched. As documented in Table 3, these actions on behalf of smokers' "innocent victims" inaugurated a period of gradually intensifying legislative activity to regulate smoking in public places.

DOWNS AND UPS OF GUN CONTROL, 1963–1996

A chronology of recent struggles over gun control is presented in Table 15.4. Public attention to this issue has a marked cyclical character, driven by violent

TABLE 15.3

U.S. Tobacco Wars, 1971–1995

Phase 3: The Discovery of Innocent Victims

1971	Country's first Group against Smokers' Pollution (GASP) formed in Maryland.
1972	First reference in SG report to potential dangers of involuntary smoking.
1973	Civil Aeronautics Board requires no smoking sections in all commercial airline flights.
	Arizona is the first state to ban smoking in some public places due to dangers of involuntary smoking.
1975	SG report contains entire section on involuntary smoking.
1976	Madison, WI, is the first municipality to restrict smoking in restaurants.
1983	National Institute on Drug Abuse declares smoking to be the nation's "most widespread form of drug dependency."
1986	SG report: The Health Consequences of Involuntary Smoking.
1988	SG report: The Health Consequences of Smoking: Nicotine Addiction.
1993	EPA declares that environmental tobacco smoke (ETS) is a human lung carcinogen (Class A).
1995	*Consumer Reports* article: Hooked on Tobacco: The Teen Epidemic.
	FDA finds that "nicotine . . . is a drug" and that cigarettes are "drug delivery devices" (U.S. DHHS 1995: Table 3).

acts against individual public figures or by a spectacular mass slaughter of "innocents."[9] The first significant piece of gun control legislation, New York State's Sullivan Law (requiring a police permit for possession of a handgun), was passed in 1911 in response to an attempted assassination of the mayor of New York City. The first recorded instance of NRA lobbying against gun control was in opposition to the Sullivan Law (Sugarmann 1992: 27). The history of gun control, like that of smoking/tobacco control, is one of ongoing struggle with an implacable foe.

Regulatory Action, 1968–1994

It took five years of legislative wrangling to pass the Gun Control Act of 1968; the end result was substantially watered down from the more sweeping legislation (including firearms registration and licensing of gun owners) proposed by President Lyndon Johnson.[10] Despite its relatively modest advance over

TABLE 15.4

The Downs and Ups of Gun Control, 1963–1994

1963	Assassination of President John F. Kennedy.
1968	Assassination of Rev. Martin Luther King, Jr.
	Assassination of Senator Robert Kennedy.
	Congress passes Gun Control Act of 1968.
1972	Congress excludes guns from regulation under the Consumer Product Safety Act.
1975	National Coalition to Ban Handguns (NCBH) founded.
	Handgun Control Inc. (HCI) founded.
1977	HCI splits from NCBH.
1980	John Lennon shot, killed.
1981	President Ronald Reagan shot.
	Pope John Paul shot.
	Morton Grove, IL, passes a ban on handgun possession.
1983	CDC labels gun violence a threat to public health.
1985	Sarah Brady joins HCI board.
1986	Congress passes Firearm Owners Protection Act (McClure-Volkmer Bill).
	Police split with National Rifle Association (NRA).
1988	Maryland bans Saturday night special.
1989	Stockton, CA, schoolyard killing of five children with an assault weapon.
1991	Killeen, TX, killing of twenty-two people in a cafeteria with an assault weapon.
1993	Congress passes Brady bill.
1994	Congress passes assault weapons ban.

previous federal efforts to regulate guns, Robert J. Spitzer notes that "the gun act was one of the most controversial and contentious bills that was considered by Congress" during the twenty-year period between 1954 and 1974 (1995: 146).

Gun regulation in the United States is predominantly local, not federal: the NRA estimates that there are 20,000 local, state, and federal firearms laws, nearly all of which exist at the state and local level.[11] Thus, in June 1981, shortly after the shootings of President Reagan and the Pope, the village trustees of Morton Grove, Illinois, banned the private possession of handguns by town residents. The NRA had been active in opposition to the ban; its passage was nationally publicized and was treated as a watershed event by the NRA and by gun control advocates (Davidson 1993: 133). The Supreme Court refused to hear appeals from two federal court rulings upholding the ban. An equally significant regulatory event at the local level was the Maryland state legislature's passage in 1988 of a ban on the manufacture and sale of "Saturday night specials" (small inexpensive handguns). The ban was petitioned to a state referendum by the NRA and upheld by a margin of 58 percent to 42 percent.[12]

The 1968 Gun Control Act had little apparent impact on the U.S. stock of guns in private hands (see Figure 15.6). It was, nevertheless, anathema to the NRA and its congressional supporters, who began work to overturn the act as soon as it had passed (Spitzer 1995: 147). Their efforts culminated in the Firearms Owners Protection Act of 1986, also known as the McClure-Volkmer Act after its principal House and Senate sponsors. As enacted, the bill eased a number of provisions of the 1968 act but retained the ban on interstate sale (but not transport) of handguns. Despite the latter concession to gun control advocates, the McClure-Volkmer Act is regarded by most observers as a victory for the NRA (Davidson 1993; Spitzer 1995). A significant consequence of the bill, however, was that it "solidified the split between the NRA and police organizations" (Spitzer 1995: 151). McClure-Volkmer had been actively opposed by a newly organized coalition of police groups.

After a fallow period of over twenty-five years, two pieces of federal legislation strengthening gun restrictions were enacted in quick succession in 1993 and 1994. Neither of these measures was particularly draconian; both include exemptions and other provisions favored by gun supporters. Nevertheless, both took over five years to pass from the time of their first introduction in Congress and both were the subject of virulent debate between supporters and opponents.

Emergence of the Gun Control Movement

Josh Sugarmann reports that gun control became an issue for some women's groups in the early 1930s (1992: 29). However, there is little evidence of an organized gun control movement in the United States before the mid-1970s. The National Coalition to Ban Handguns (NCBH) (renamed the Coalition to Stop Gun Violence in 1990) evolved out of church groups' response to the assassination of President John F. Kennedy. Following a period of dormancy between 1968 and 1974, the group reorganized in 1975 as the NCBH. Handgun Control, Inc. (HCI) was founded at about the same time by a Republican businessman whose son had been shot and killed with a handgun (Spitzer 1995: 115).

Beginning in the early 1980s, the NRA found itself in a series of high-profile political conflicts with the police around the regulation of "cop killer bullets" and plastic guns and around the McClure-Volkmer bill.[13] Important outcomes of these conflicts were independent mobilization by the police to advance their own interests in gun control and a political realignment of sorts, with the Democrats on the side of the police against the Republicans and the NRA.

A final important development in this brief history is the redefinition of guns and gun control as issues in the domain of public health as well as, or in addition to, the domains of crime and law enforcement. Among the proponents of this definition have been the federal Centers for Disease Control and Prevention (CDC), which established a violence prevention unit in the mid-1980s, and former Surgeon General C. Everett Koop (Koop and Lundberg 1992). Medicalization of the gun question has important consequences for how the problem is characterized and into whose province it falls. This redefinition has triggered a new wave of gun control organization, and in the last few years several gun control groups led by health professionals and by lawyers with training in public health have emerged. Not surprisingly, medicalization of guns has been heavily contested by the NRA and by some members of Congress.

MEASURES OF MOVEMENT SUCCESS

While scholars' interest in social movements "stems from their belief that movements represent an important force for social change" (McAdam, McCarthy, and Zald, cited in Burstein, Einwohner, and Hollander 1995: 275), the measurement of change and its causal attribution present considerable methodological problems (see, e.g., Diani 1997).

For example (following Diani), the adoption of a restaurant smoking ban may be due to nonsmokers' rights activism; the activism may have been generated by politicians in support of the ban; or both activism and the ban may result from other social forces (e.g., increased consumer sensitivity to health threats and accompanying media hyperbole around these threats). The problems of causal attribution are somewhat alleviated when (as in the present case) attention is narrowly focused on specific campaigns and the time span over which movements are observed is fairly long. Nevertheless, while I will argue that nonsmokers' rights activism played a causal role in bringing about change in smoking-related policies and behaviors in the United States, this argument does not preclude the existence of additional causes and causal paths that I may not have fully considered.

Conceptualizations of movement success generally begin with William Gamson's two-dimensional criteria of "new advantages" for its constituency and/or "acceptance" of the movement by its targets or by the public as the legitimate spokesperson for the interests it represents (1990: 31–34; e.g., Amenta, Dunleavy, and Bernstein 1994; Burstein, Einwohner, and Hollander 1995). Beyond this reference point, there is little consensus. For example, Paul Burstein and colleagues state that "assessing a movement's success involves determining whether it has achieved its goals" (1995: 281), while Edwin Amenta and colleagues argue that achievement of "new advantages" not anticipated by the movement should also count as success (and that new advantages are more "meaningful" than acceptance as a measure of success) (1994: 681). An additional problem arises in the case of ongoing social movements: how successful the movement appears depends on at what point in the movement's trajectory (unknowable, except in retrospect) success is measured.

The long-range goals of the smoking/tobacco and gun control movements are to bring about a decline in the relevant parameters of mortality and morbidity. In the short run, both movements advocate behavior change in, respectively, patterns of cigarette smoking and in gun ownership and use. Beyond these generalities, smoking/tobacco control movement representatives have from the beginning been quite explicit in their aims of stigmatizing cigarettes and the smoker and, more recently (in the words of one activist), of "getting the bully [the tobacco industry] off the block." There is less consensus among gun control advocates, in part because of disagreement on the meaning of the word *control*. In the following paragraphs I evaluate the extent to which each movement has achieved its goals.[14]

SMOKING

Mortality

On 14 November 1996, the *New York Times* reported an overall decline in cancer death rates "for the first time since 1900" (Brody 1996). Philip Cole and Brad Rodu (1996), whose work was the basis for the *Times'* report, attributed about half of the reduction in cancer mortality to declines in smoking since 1965 and anticipate continued reduction "as the now rising lung carcinoma mortality rates among women stabilize and then decline," a consequence, presumably, of declines in women's smoking. Their work was foreshadowed in several earlier reports. *Morbidity and Mortality Weekly Report* (MMWR) noted in November 1993 that "the declines in smoking prevalences have resulted in a stabilization or decline in the lung cancer death rate for men aged <55 years and for women aged <45 years, respectively" (CDC 1993). Cardiovascular disease (CVD) is responsible for nearly twice as many deaths as lung cancer and it is clear that cigarette smoking plays a substantial role in CVD mortality. Cardiovascular disease mortality, however, has been declining for the past three decades among both women and men and the relative part in this decline played by changes in smoking behavior is difficult to determine with precision (see, e.g., Hunink et al. 1997).

Behavior

Change over the last three decades in the behaviors targeted by tobacco advocates are presented in Figure 15.1. Two measures of change are employed:

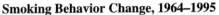

FIGURE 15.1

Smoking Behavior Change, 1964–1995

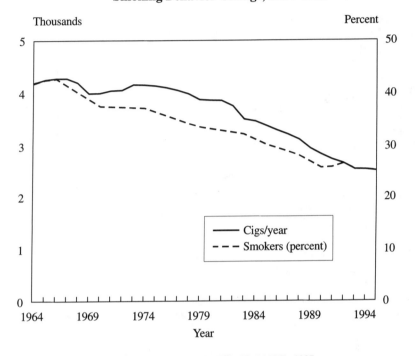

Sources: Giovino et al. 1994; USDA 1995–96, 1998; CDC 1996b, 1997.

cigarette consumption per capita per year (in numbers of cigarettes) and smoking prevalence (percent of the population age eighteen and over who are current smokers).

Both cigarette consumption and the reported prevalence of smoking have declined substantially since 1964. Despite these declines, there are a number of reasons for caution in evaluating changes in cigarette smoking. First, both of the aggregate measures employed in Figure 15.1 have recently plateaued. Second, as shown in Figure 15.2, by far the sharpest declines in cigarette smoking have occurred in that proportion of the population with a college or graduate school education. Among individuals with less than a high school education, the percentage who smoked in 1994 was about the same as the percentage of the highly educated who smoked in 1966. Furthermore, absence of recent change— even increase—in the percentage of smokers is most evident among the least well educated. In contrast to its democratic pattern in the 1960s, smoking is now concentrated in the lower socioeconomic strata.[15] A third basis for caution,

FIGURE 15.2

Percent Current Smokers by Education, 1966–1995

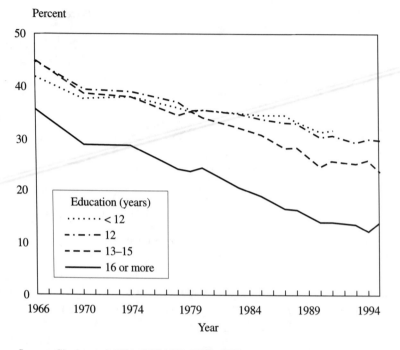

Sources: Giovino et al. 1994; CDC 1994, 1996b, 1997.

one that has received a great deal more public attention, are recent increases in the percentage of smokers among high school students. These data are presented in Figure 15.3. Smoking prevalence among high school seniors declined steadily until the mid-1980s, rose and fell erratically until around 1992, and since then has sharply increased.

Attitudes and Beliefs

Attitudes and beliefs about cigarettes and guns may be compared using two dimensions: beliefs about the degree and nature of the danger that these products represent, and responses to that danger in the form of support for or opposition to legal restrictions on their use.[16] Data on changes over the past several decades in attitudes and beliefs about cigarettes are presented in Figures 15.4 and 15.5. Two dimensions of belief about the danger of cigarettes are included in Figure 15.4: first, the belief that cigarette smoking causes harm to the smoker, and second,

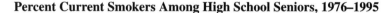

FIGURE 15.3

Percent Current Smokers Among High School Seniors, 1976–1995

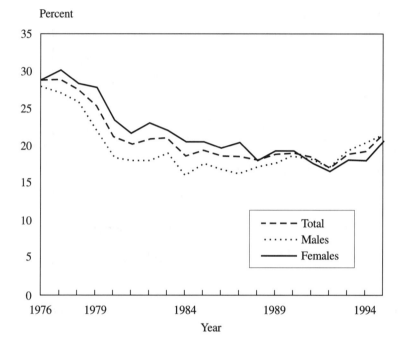

Source: Giovino et al. 1994.

the belief that cigarette smoking causes harm to (or at the very least) incommodes individuals in the smoker's environment. The former belief stigmatizes the cigarette; the latter belief stigmatizes the smoker as well. All of these beliefs increased markedly during the period of observation. Particularly notable is the near doubling between 1974 and 1987 (from 46 percent to 81 percent) of the proportion of the survey sample who believed that smoking is hazardous to the health of nonsmokers.

Public support for legal restrictions on smoking, advertising, and sales of cigarettes is described in Figure 15.5. While support for limitations on where people could smoke clearly increased over the period between 1964 and 1987, support for more draconian policies was considerably weaker. Neither a ban on cigarette sales nor even a ban on smoking in restaurants was ever supported by more than 23 percent of those surveyed.

Among the goals articulated most clearly by early antismoking activists was to make smoking so unpopular that smokers would be forced to quit. The data

FIGURE 15.4

The Stigmatization of Cigarettes, 1964–1987

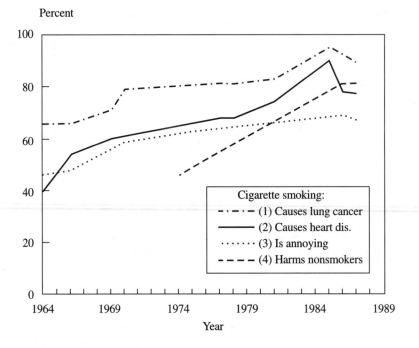

Percent

Year

Source: U.S. DHHS 1989.
Note: Survey items (percent agree): (1) Cigarette smoking causes lung cancer; (2) cigarette smoking causes heart disease; (3) it is annoying to be near a person who is smoking cigarettes; (4) smoking is hazardous to nonsmokers. Item wording varied.

presented in Figure 15.4 are evidence of how successful the effort has been to stigmatize smokers as harmful to themselves and to others. Translating this stigmatization into public policy consensus has proved more difficult.

Public Policies

Stronger local, state, and federal regulation has been among the major goals of the smoking/tobacco control movement (and of the gun control movement as well). Major regulatory achievements at the federal level were noted in Table 15.2. However, the antismoking movement has had its greatest success at the local and state levels. By 1993, over 500 local communities had enacted some form of smoking regulation, almost all since 1980 (U.S. DHHS 1993). By 1995, all but ten states regulated smoking in state government work sites; all but twenty restricted smoking in restaurants (CDC 1996a).

FIGURE 15.5

Public Support for Legal Restrictions on Cigarettes, 1964–1987

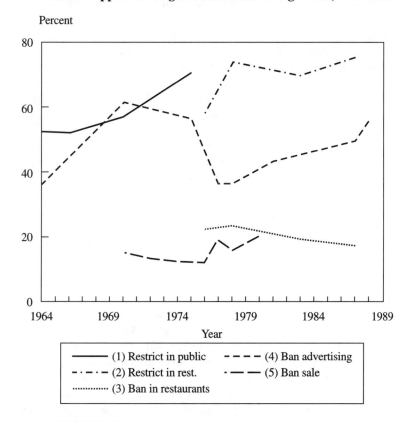

Source: U.S. DHHS 1989.
Note: Survey items (percent agree): (1) Smoking should be allowed in fewer public places; (2) smoking should be limited in restaurants; (3) smoking should be banned in restaurants; (4) cigarette advertising should not be permitted; (5) selling cigarettes should be stopped completely. Items varied.

GUNS

Mortality

Gun-related deaths fall into three categories: homicide, suicide, and accidents. Homicide and suicide account for approximately equal numbers of deaths (in 1994, 17,527 and 18,765 respectively); accidents are a distant third (1,356) (Anderson, Kochanek, and Murphy 1997). Of these categories, only accidental deaths have shown a consistent decline over several decades (Spitzer 1995:

74). Since the early 1960s, age-adjusted death rates for firearm homicides have doubled and such rates have increased by half for firearm suicides (Karlson and Hargarten 1997: 1). The age-adjusted homicide firearm death rate declined slightly in 1994 (and the crude rate has continued to decline, along with the total homicide rate).

Half of all homicide victims are minorities (double their representation in the total population); the highest rate is among African Americans: "For African Americans, the risk of being killed in a homicide is nearly seven times greater than for whites and more than twice as great as for Hispanics" (Karlson and Hargarten 1997: 6). Firearms are the leading cause of death for adolescent black males.

A recent increase in suicide rates appears to be associated with the increased use of guns: "From 1968 through 1985, the rate of suicide involving firearms increased 36 percent, whereas the rate of suicide involving other methods remained constant" (Kellerman et al. 1992: 467). In contrast to the pattern for homicide, the risk of suicide is greatest for young white males. However, the largest recent increases in suicide rates have been among young black males, coming close to convergence with those of their white peers (CDC 1995).

Behavior

Change in gun-related behaviors is described in Figure 15.6. The three measures of change employed are the cumulated stock of firearms per 10,000 population, the percent of households owning at least one gun, and the percent of adults personally owning a gun. The reported percentage of households owning at least one gun shows a "slow, but notable, decline . . . over the last twenty-three years" (National Opinion Research Center [NORC] 1997: 13); however, the percentage of individuals owning guns has changed very little.[17] Continuing a long-term trend, the estimated cumulated stock of firearms in the U.S. increased sharply between 1964 and 1978. More recent data from the 1994 National Survey of Private Ownership of Firearms (NSFOP) suggest that the gun stock may have plateaued; Philip J. Cook and Jens Ludwig (1997) estimate that approximately 192 million guns are in private hands, for a rate of 7,373 per 10,000 population, close to Gary Kleck's (1984) estimate for 1978.

Gun ownership is more prevalent among men than women, more prevalent among whites than blacks, and highest among "middle-aged, college-educated people of rural and small-town America" (Cook and Ludwig 1997).[18]

Attitudes and Beliefs

Data on beliefs about the harm associated with guns are not directly comparable over time, due to differences in question wording. However, surveys conducted by Gallup, AP/Media General, Yankelovich, and NORC between 1986 and 1996

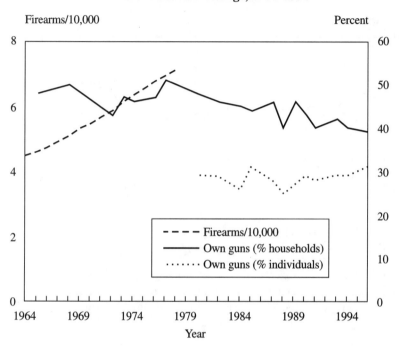

FIGURE 15.6

Guns: Behavior Change, 1964–1996

Sources: McAneny 1993; Kleck 1984; NORC 1997.

show the extent to which public opinion is split on the basic question of whether or not guns are, in fact, harmful (NORC 1997; Newport and Saad 1993). In 1993, the Gallup poll presented respondents with the following question: "Suppose a law were passed making it illegal for all citizens other than the police to have a gun. Would you feel *more* safe or *less* safe, or wouldn't it make a difference?" Twenty-five percent of respondents would feel more safe, 39 percent less safe, and for 34 percent it would make no difference. A second question was worded as follows: "Which of the following comes closer to your view: having a gun in the house makes it a *safer* place to be because you can protect yourself from violent intruders, or having a gun in the house makes it a *more dangerous* place to be because you increase the risk from gun accidents and domestic violence?" Forty-two percent of respondents stated that having a gun in the house makes the house safer (Newport and Saad 1993). Forty-one percent of respondents to the 1996 NORC survey believed that having a gun made the house safer (NORC 1997: 7).

FIGURE 15.7

Public Support for Legal Restrictions on Guns, 1959–1996

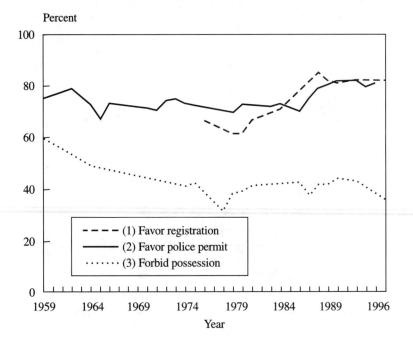

Source: NORC 1997.
Note: Survey items: (1) Do you favor or oppose mandatory registration of handguns or pistols?
(2) Do you favor or oppose police permits for gun purchase? (3) Do you think there should/should
not be a law to forbid handgun possession except by police or other authorized persons?

Data on patterns of change between 1959 and 1996 in public support for
legal restrictions on guns are presented in Figure 15.7. Percentages of the U.S.
population in favor of mandatory handgun registration and of police permits for
gun purchase increased sharply during the 1980s. Consistent with these data,
Gallup polls carried out between 1988 and 1993 demonstrated strong support
for the Brady bill (ranging from 88 to 95 percent) (McAneny 1993: 3). At the
same time, as Figure 15.7 demonstrates, support for a ban on the possession of
handguns "except by police or other authorized persons" declined during the
1960s and 1970s and has changed very little since 1980. Advocates of more
restrictive gun laws confront the public's belief that guns—unlike cigarettes—
not only have harmless uses but may, indeed, be protective. There is little
evidence in these data that the gun control movement has as yet been successful

in making gun ownership unpopular; personal ownership of a gun has increased in recent years. Support for restrictive gun control policies has increased as well, but in a selective and somewhat inconsistent fashion.[19]

Public Policies

Legislative action to strengthen gun regulation has occurred primarily at the federal rather than at the state or local levels. With the important (and very recent) exception of California (Gorovitz 1996), there has not been an upsurge of local regulation comparable to what has taken place in the tobacco arena.[20] Indeed, many states "are passing laws that make access to guns easier" (Karlson and Hargarten 1997: 121; Gorovitz 1996).

SUMMARY

The antismoking campaign in the United States has made remarkable progress toward achieving its goals. Declines in lung cancer death rates, a marked shift toward stigmatizing the cigarette and the cigarette smoker, the passage of significant legislation to limit smoking in public, and a substantial reduction in the overall prevalence of smoking qualify as "new advantages" for the movement's beneficiaries. The gun control movement is arguably at an earlier point on the same trajectory. While the movement has achieved some important changes in public policy, guns remain relatively unstigmatized, and trends in gun ownership are inconsistent, depending on how ownership is measured. It is too early for firm conclusions about the sustainability of recent declines in gun-related mortality rates.[21]

COMPARATIVE ANALYSIS OF THE SMOKING/TOBACCO AND GUN CONTROL MOVEMENTS

CONSTRUCTIONS OF RISK

Guns and cigarettes are hardly newcomers to the American scene. Spitzer describes "the long-term sentimental attachment of many Americans to the gun" grounded in cultural myths about the role of the gun in the struggle for independence and the taming of the frontier (1995: 8). During the early part of the twentieth century cigarettes became powerful symbols of sexuality, power, autonomy, and modernity (Brandt 1992). The two symbolic traditions merge in the Marlboro man, the fiercely independent, (possibly) gun-toting cowboy smoker. Mobilization against these powerful cultural symbols demanded that their meanings be transformed so as to legitimate and guide protest activity (McAdam 1994: 37).

Central to this transformation has been the construction of credible risks. Dangers abound. Whether or not these dangers rise to a community's threshold of awareness and become defined as risks to the public's health, much less elicit responsive action, depends on the active intervention of human agency, on what I have called "constructions of risk" (Nathanson 1996: 614–615). The first element essential to this construction is the existence of groups or individuals with the authority to define and describe the danger that threatens. The second element is the assertion of a causal framework to account for the danger.

THE MAKING OF A CREDIBLE THREAT

Smoking

The consequences of smoking for health and morality have been argued at least since James the First wrote his famous polemic in 1604 (Kluger 1996: 15). Progressive Era antivice campaigns encompassed cigarette smoking, along with drinking and sexual adventurism, as immoral, unhealthful, and a corrupter of youth. States passed restrictive legislation, setting the age at which cigarettes might be legally purchased, or in some states, prohibiting the sale of cigarettes altogether. The Progressive Era antismoking movement petered out in the 1930s, along with the other campaigns against vice, only to reappear in new guises more suitable to the tenor of the times.

The late-twentieth-century construction of cigarette smoking as a credible risk was the work of the Surgeon General's Advisory Committee on Smoking and Health.[22] The committee brought together the large body of existing evidence that cigarette smoking was a danger to human health, summarized that evidence in a scholarly fashion, and put the imprimatur of the federal government on its central conclusion, that "cigarette smoking is *causally related* to lung cancer in men" (U.S. DHEW 1964: 31, emphasis mine). The committee did not collect any new data or make any new discoveries. Its report did, nevertheless, construct new knowledge. It transformed scattered evidence into official authoritative knowledge, providing "power and legitimacy to the epidemiologic findings" (Brandt 1992: 67).[23]

Gusfield argues that public consensus on the dangers of smoking "represents the hegemony of medical science over the culture of health: . . . by the time the Surgeon General issued the report of 1964, social conditions had become favorable to the transmission and credibility of medical science and the position of the federal government as a source of authoritative advice and activity in the promotion of health" (1994: 54–55). Perhaps. Medical authorities have, indeed, made substantial inroads as arbiters of personal conduct; the latest scientific reports are carried on television and the public is highly attentive (but substantially more skeptical, I would argue, than it was in 1964).[24] Nevertheless, the smoking story is more complex than Gusfield allows.

The federal government did not embrace ownership of the smoking and health issue in the 1950s and 1960s. A reluctant executive branch had ownership thrust upon it by the efforts of the health voluntaries (principally by the American Cancer Society [ACS]) and by a small minority of dissident members of Congress who believed that the authoritative voice of the federal government was essential to confer legitimacy on their cause. Further, while Congress in 1965—with its mandate for annual reports on the health consequences of smoking—awarded continuing ownership to the Surgeon General, it was a limited-purpose ownership. The Surgeon General was given authority to define and describe the problem—to assert the risks of smoking—but very little power to limit those risks. Location of political responsibility for the smoking and health issue was and is controversial within the federal government as well as without.[25]

Second, the "hegemony of medical science" was fragile at best. The most prominent representative of medical science in the United States, the American Medical Association (AMA), actively disowned the smoking and health issue: in 1965, the AMA House of Delegates refused to endorse the 1964 Surgeon General's report (Wolinsky and Brune 1994: 152). The AMA's emergence as an active player on the side of the anti-smoking forces is of very recent vintage (Friedman 1975; Wolinsky and Brune 1994). Less surprisingly, ownership of the cigarette smoking issue by government and medical science was hotly contested by the tobacco industry and its political allies. A stated objective of the Tobacco Institute, founded by the industry in 1958, was "to secure recognition for the Tobacco Institute, Inc., as the central source of authoritative information concerning all aspects of the industry with which the Institute is concerned" (cited in Friedman 1975: 26). The Surgeon General's report was as much a political as a scientific document—a salvo, powerful and effective as it was— in the ongoing tobacco wars.

GUNS

The challenge to tobacco industry authority over the portrayal of cigarettes was based on a high level of scientific consensus on the dangers of smoking. Each Surgeon General's report includes a long and impressive list of the names and affiliations of the physicians and scientists whose work has contributed to the report's findings. The gun control movement enjoys no such scholarly or scientific consensus. Not only is there disagreement on the existence and nature of a causal relationship between guns and injury or death, there is also disagreement on who is qualified to speak about these dangers. Health professionals are relative newcomers to this debate. They were preceded by and have continued to share the "gun scholarship" stage with criminologists, political scientists, sociologists, historians, and lawyers. These scholars disagree on fundamental

issues of conception and fact, as evidenced, for example, by a recent exchange
between scholars at the University of Chicago and Johns Hopkins University
concerning whether or not recently enacted state laws granting the right to carry
a concealed weapon reduce violent crime (Lott and Mustard 1997; Webster et
al. 1997). Further, they have notably little respect for each others' ideas (see,
e.g., the exchange between Gary Wills and his critics in the 16 November 1995
issue of *New York Review of Books* and published comments by Franklin E.
Zimring and Gordon Hawkins [1987: 99] and William R. Tonso [1984]).

Law enforcement agencies have recently become an additional competitor
for ownership of the gun control issue, pushing some movement activists toward
the promotion of gun control for the purpose of crime prevention rather than as a
response to danger inherent in the gun itself.[26] The identification of gun control
with law enforcement has been politically effective. Nevertheless, competition
for ownership of the gun issue continues internally as well as with the NRA.
Advocates disagree on the construction of gun control as crime prevention
(Sugarmann 1992) and on the promotion of "safe" guns (Glick 1998). The NRA
campaigns to have the CDC's firearms research program (premised on the public
health construction of guns) defunded (Lewis 1995) and attacks police organizations and the Bureau of Tobacco, Alcohol, and Firearms (LaPierre 1994).

The question arises as to whether these disagreements may be explained
by inherent differences between guns and cigarettes. Clearly, widespread public *perception* of inherent differences is part of the gun control movement's
problem, particularly when it comes to framing guns as a danger to health. I
would argue, however, that the differences are not in fact inherent, any more
than, say, the differences between marijuana and nicotine are inherent. Guns
and cigarettes do not have essences; they have histories and cultural baggage
with which social movement entrepreneurs must contend.

THE FRAMING OF RISK

Public health policies are adopted in response to perceived danger. The framing
of danger (or risk, in modern parlance) is culturally patterned. Societies vary
in the things or events considered dangerous, in ideas about the sources of
danger, and in conceptions of who or what is endangered and these cultural
presuppositions are remarkably consistent over time and place (Douglas and
Wildavsky 1982; Douglas 1992; Dobbin 1994; Nathanson 1996). In the U.S.,
we concern ourselves with dangers to the individual, not (e.g., as in France)
to the state. Furthermore, the dimensions of risk are highly predictable. In any
given case, risks may be portrayed as acquired deliberately or involuntarily
(and the victims as correspondingly culpable or innocent), as universal (putting
us all at risk) or as particular (only putting *them* at risk), as arising from within
the individual or from the environment, as visible or invisible.[27] The most

acceptable risks are universal, are attributable to the external environment, and are incurred involuntarily by innocent victims.

Smoking

The remarkable transformation of the cigarette and smoking from symbols of "modernity, autonomy, power, and sexuality" to symbols of weakness, irrationality, and addiction (Brandt 1992: 70) was accompanied and driven by shifts in underlying constructions of risk. The initial construction of the cigarette as a danger to the health of the male smoker did not disappear, but has been added to and elaborated over time. Throughout the period in question, advocates for the dangers of smoking were aided and abetted by a highly interested and attentive news media.

During the first phase of the tobacco wars, the messages conveyed to the U.S. public were that the hazards of smoking are attributable to the risky choice of the person who smokes and that the individual is responsible for risk reduction by making the necessary changes in his or her behavior. The most consistent advocate of this perspective, the American Cancer Society, was also the dominant player in the early stages of the smoking and health drama. The following is from the society's 1957 annual report: "The society believes that at our present state of knowledge, the question of whether to start smoking or to give it up must be left to the judgment of individuals. For intelligent decisions everyone should know the facts: There is a definite association between cigarette smoking and cancer" (19). The ACS approach is striking in two respects: first, in its validation of individual choice and, second, in the limitation of its own responsibility to "just the facts."

Knowledge of the association between cigarette smoking and cancer as well as other diseases accumulated, but the posture of the ACS as articulated in the cited quotations did not, in fact, begin to change until the early 1980s. Lest it be thought that the ACS was unique in its individualization of the smoking and health issue or in the timidity of its recommendations, federal health officials took much the same tack. Their approach to the preparation of the Surgeon General's report was that of an individual physician advising an individual patient: "What do we [that is, the Surgeon General of the United States Public Health Service] advise our patient, the American public, about smoking?" (cited in Brandt 1992: 66). Implicit in this question is not only, as Allan Brandt points out, "a particular model of public health and the role of the state," but also a particular model of where the hazards of smoking are socially located. Themes of personal responsibility for health (and the limits of government intervention) were echoed in influential publications throughout the 1970s: cigarette smoking became the quintessential exemplar of lifestyle change within the individual's control (Lalonde 1974; Knowles 1977; U.S. DHEW 1979).[28]

There is a striking disjunction between the Surgeon General's 1964 procla-
mation of smoking as "a health hazard of sufficient importance in the United
States to warrant appropriate remedial action" (U.S. DHEW 1964: 33) and the
actions that were, in fact, taken by the major players at the time. While there
is a strong libertarian bias in Americans' approach to health protection, early
constructions of smoking and health were driven as much by political as by
philosophical concerns. In an interview, an ACS official who had worked in
the national office from 1960 through 1990 described the society's internal
struggles:

> I was there when the great debates were held on how far the American Cancer
> Society should go as an organization in taking up an antitobacco position. And
> you could well realize that there was tremendous resistance within the American
> Cancer Society in the late 1950s and early 1960s, because here you have tobacco-
> growing states and here you have divisions, North Carolina, South Carolina,
> Kentucky, Tennessee, that said, "You are going to destroy us. We are not going
> to be able to raise money in these states. We are not going to get any media
> attention," et cetera. . . . Then the question came up, how shall we deal with the
> tobacco companies? Shall we openly debate them? Shall we condemn them? In
> the early 1960s a position was taken that there should be no open debates with the
> tobacco companies. The villain is the cigarette. The victim is the cigarette smoker.
> So we will condemn the cigarette. We will help the smoker quit, but there will be
> no attacks on the Philip Morris Company, R. J. Reynolds, et cetera. (ACS files)[29]

Not until the late 1980s did it become fashionable and politically safe to
openly attack the tobacco companies.

Between 1954 and 1970, the percentage of the U.S. public who agreed
that cigarette smoking causes lung cancer increased from 41 to 70 percent
(U.S. DHHS 1989: 189). An authoritative case for the hazards of smoking
had been made. The most significant consequences of this successful claims-
making were not, however, federal legislation but the legitimation of smoking
and the cigarette as actionable targets by aggrieved nonsmokers and a marked
change in where and by whom the tobacco wars were fought. The Group against
Smokers' Pollution (GASP) was founded in early 1971. From its inception,
GASP's mission was twofold: first to "get nonsmokers to protect themselves"
against the immediate, irritating effects of cigarette smoke, and second "to
make smoking so unpopular that smokers would quit" (Gouin 1995). In the
first paragraph of the first number of its newsletter *The Ventilator,* published in
March 1971, GASP called on innocent nonsmokers, the "involuntary victims
of tobacco smoke," to rise up and assert their "right to breathe clean air [that]
is superior to the right of the smoker to enjoy a harmful habit" (1971: 1).

This new construction of smoking and health as an issue not of smokers'
health but of nonsmokers' rights represented a radical shift in the assignment
of risks and responsibilities: it literally turned the old rhetoric on its head. The

hazards of smoking were relocated from the individuals' risky behavior to the behavior of his smoking neighbor; exposure was no longer a matter of choice but of involuntary victimization; and, finally, the responsibility for risk reduction was shifted away from the individual at risk to the "polluting" smoker and to the regulatory agencies of government. The importance of this reconstruction is hard to overstate. Suddenly, libertarian ideology—Mill's notion that "the only purpose for which power can be rightfully exercised over any member of a civilized community, against his will, is *to prevent harm to others*" (cited in Beauchamp 1988: 90; emphasis added)—was available to be deployed against the act of smoking. Further, and equally important, movement founders framed their appeals in the language of the civil rights and environmental movements, connecting nonsmokers' rights with the most powerful ideologies of the time.[30]

Both Brandt (1995) and Gusfield (1993) date the emergence of passive smoking as a central theme in the smoking and health debate from the appearance of authoritative scientific reports (i.e., by the Surgeon General and the National Academy of Sciences) in the mid-1980s.[31] Based on the data collected for this project, I would date its emergence much earlier. The construction of the cigarette as harmful to the nonsmoker and of the smoker as pariah came to public attention in the early 1970s. As early as October 1973, the tobacco industry (among the more attentive members of this public) warned that "the most potentially dangerous threat to the future of the tobacco industry is not so much legislative smoking advertising bans . . . but the developing psychological attitude that smoking is somehow socially unacceptable" (cited in Gouin 1975: 55).[32]

Earlier observers of the tobacco control movement have tended to focus on "the softness of the scientific case against secondhand smoke" prior to the 1980s, assuming that a strong scientific case was essential to the nonsmokers' rights movement (Kluger 1996: 375). It was not, for two reasons. First, the level of scientific certainty required to reject risks we perceive as imposed on us by others is relatively low.[33] Second, the dangers of the cigarette to smokers had been well established by the early 1970s. Little more in the way of scientific evidence was required for movement entrepreneurs to persuasively argue that involuntary exposure to this deadly product was dangerous to nonsmokers as well.[34]

Powerful as this argument has been, it has been more persuasive to some segments of the public than to others. The early nonsmokers' rights activists were well-educated members of relatively affluent (often university) communities. While they were notably successful in persuading groups like themselves that smoking in others' presence was socially unacceptable,[35] they have been less successful among blue collar workers. Data were presented earlier showing sharp differences in the decline in smoking prevalence by level of education. The meaning and persistence of these differences is suggested in recent statements by a representative of the AFL-CIO, commenting on the fact that many union members smoke: "Well, there has been a change in the culture, but there are still a lot of people who smoke who think that they should be able to smoke in workplaces. They think they should be able to smoke in bars and restaurants. And so I would say that there has been a change in the culture, but I think that it is not evenly distributed and that there are a lot of places in this country where the culture is not the same as it is in Washington, DC, or in southern California" (U.S. OSHA 1995: 12281).[36]

Prevention of harm to others is, of course, a legitimate responsibility of government. Characterizing its members as the "involuntary victims of tobacco smoke" allowed GASP to call on government for redress: "Surgeon General suggests ban on public smoking" was headlined in the first number of its first newsletter. Over the past twenty-five years, "innocent victims" rhetoric has proved to be a powerful force in obtaining local, state, and some federal smoking regulation. Alternative constructions of smoking—as an issue of personal habits, individual rights, even of cultural differences—continue however, to be readily available and are deployed in opposition to regulation when occasion requires.

The most recent phase in the cigarette's downward spiral is the discovery that smoking is addictive. The 1964 Surgeon General's report analogized smoking to drinking coffee, tea, and cocoa (U.S. DHEW 1964: 350). Today it is more likely to be linked with heroin and cocaine (U.S. DHHS 1988).[37] This linkage does not reflect new scientific knowledge—the addictive properties of nicotine "have been common knowledge in medical and public health circles for years" (Slade et al. 1995: 225)—so much as it reflects the increased vulnerability of the tobacco industry and the shifting political and legal strategies of its opponents.[38]

The addiction label allows opponents to make the identical argument employed on behalf of nonsmokers' rights: exposure is not a choice. *"The Health Consequences of Smoking: Nicotine Addiction* provided a comprehensive review of the evidence that cigarettes and other forms of tobacco are addicting and that nicotine is the drug in tobacco that causes addiction. These two factors refute the argument that smoking is a matter of free choice. Most smokers start smoking as teenagers and then become addicted" (Koop 1989: v). This construction has a number of consequences, some of which may be less predictable than others. It is the basis for FDA efforts to regulate cigarettes as drug delivery devices; it gives plaintiffs' lawyers a counterargument against the industry's long-standing claim that smokers assume the risk of their behavior; it enables opponents to characterize tobacco industry executives as drug dealers and to play on deep-seated American fears of adolescent vulnerability to seduction by unscrupulous predators.[39]

Insofar as the addiction label results in increased government regulation of access to and advertising of cigarettes, it may act to further decrease the prevalence of smoking. On the other hand, there is little reason to believe that the label itself will change behavior—indeed, it could lead adolescents to prefer smoking as the cheapest, least dangerous form of addiction and it is unclear why judges and juries would find addicted smokers more sympathetic plaintiffs than risk-assuming smokers.

Inherent in the attribution of risks is the designation of potential victims. Who, precisely, is at risk? Citing limitations in the available data, the 1964 Surgeon General's report focused on men: "Cigarette smoking is causally related to lung cancer *in men*" (U.S. DHEW 1964: 31; emphasis added). As early as 1957, however, the American Cancer Society began to develop educational programs targeted at adolescents (ACS 1957: 47) and by 1997, forty years later, children dominated the roster of victims.[40] In the interval, nonsmokers, women, minorities, pregnant women, the fetus, and residents of third-world countries have received attention as designated victims. This is not, of course, a random selection. In varying degrees, these categories lend themselves to portrayal as innocents, deserving of government protection and control.

In the foregoing scenarios, the tobacco industry was virtually invisible.[41] The most striking recent shift in constructions of cigarette risk has been the explicit attribution of causal responsibility to the industry itself. The government's rhetoric, initially veiled in the bureaucratic language of the FDA, has become increasingly explicit; the language employed by private health organizations is unambiguous. Slogans like "protect our children from the tobacco companies" and "tobacco lawyers versus America's kids" appeared in public service announcements in major media outlets (CNN, the *New York Times*) in 1996 and 1997, sponsored in the first case by the American Cancer Society and in the second by the American Heart Association, the American Lung Association (ALA), the Association of State and Territorial Health Officials, and other health, religious, and educational organizations.

The ACS official quoted earlier explained the ACS's change of course:

> In the 1970s when the laws went into effect banning cigarette advertising from broadcasting, putting tougher warning statements on cigarette packages and in advertising (1984), when more and more congressmen became articulate on this subject, we began to see that we could now openly criticize not just the cigarette but the manufacturer of the cigarette. And I'll never forget when I ended up on a MacNeil/Lehrer show one day (7 April 1988) with a representative from the Tobacco Institute and I was able to say tobacco companies are merchants of death. (ACS files)

As political opportunities change, so do constructions of risk.

Guns

Every element in the construction of risk—claims of danger, attributions of causality, and designation of victims—has proved more problematic for the gun control movement than for the smoking/tobacco control movement. First, as I noted earlier, claims of danger are disputed. Second, even when the existence of danger is admitted, causal attributions vary widely between and among the different groups who claim ownership of the gun question. Third, different causal attributions are associated with different categories of victims.

For those to whom guns are a problem only insofar as they are associated with crime (a category that includes not only the NRA but also many criminologists and representatives of the criminal justice system), the cause of gun-related mortality and morbidity is not guns as such, but guns in the hands of bad people. The public health community casts a wider net. First, crime-associated injuries and death are often conflated with gun-related injuries and death generally (e.g., from suicide or accidents) and labeled as gun violence. Second, causal attributions cover a broad range: criminogenic circumstances, inappropriate use of guns, poorly designed guns, guns in the home, and so on.[42] An idea of the relatively easy task of smoking/tobacco as compared with gun control advocates can be gained by comparing the faintly oxymoronic sound of "safe cigarette" and "responsible smoker" to the widespread use—even by many advocates—of parallel characterizations in the world of gun control. Risks are most persuasive when they can be portrayed in black and white. Guns come in shades of gray.

Lay and public health advocates of gun control have tended to characterize the risks of guns as universal—everyone is at risk—or to focus on risks to children. In a forum at the Johns Hopkins School of Hygiene and Public Health, Martin Wasserman, Secretary of the Maryland Department of Health and Mental Hygiene, invoked universality: "This is a statewide problem, not just [a problem in] Baltimore City and Prince George's County [subdivisions with high crime rates]. It is urban and rural." Calling attention to the health care costs of gun injuries is another universalizing construction, intended to address the public as taxpayers.

Children, however, are central figures in current discourse on guns, just as they are at the center of discourse on smoking/tobacco control. Statistically, the most likely victims of gun violence are young black men living in the inner city and suicides (Fingerhut, Ingram, and Feldman 1992; Spitzer 1995: 71). Children are, however, a substantially more appealing risk group, so much so that in the article cited Lois A. Fingerhut and colleagues characterize black male homicide victims aged fifteen to nineteen as "children" (3058).[43] As a rallying cry, "protect our children" is politically safe. Whether or not it is effective remains to be seen.[44]

In smoking/tobacco control rhetoric, the "innocent victimization" of non-smokers and their "right" to clean air are two sides of the same coin: innocence and rights are conflated. Rights discourse has been effectively employed to empower the movement's adherents and to agitate for government regulation. By contrast, rights discourse in the gun control arena has been almost entirely controlled by the NRA and its adherents, as in their selective recitation of the Second Amendment to the U.S. Constitution, "the right of the people to keep and bear arms shall not be infringed." In public debate, Spitzer observes, this right is "constantly invoked" by gun control opponents: "To pick a single example from publications of the National Rifle Association (NRA), its October 1993 issue of *American Hunter* contained thirty-four references to the Second Amendment or the ownership of guns as a constitutionally protected right. Its November 1993 issue of the *American Rifleman* contained fourteen such references" (1995: 25). Mary Ann Glendon has called attention to what she characterizes as "our increasing tendency to speak of what is most important to us in terms of rights, and to frame nearly every social controversy as a clash of rights" (1991: 3–4). The NRA's successful appropriation of this frame, which resonates not only with the American individualist tradition but also with the powerful late-twentieth-century ideologies associated with civil rights and women's rights, has severely limited the gun control movement's rhetorical maneuvering room.[45] Predictably, the tobacco industry experimented with the rights framework as well (taking out full page ads in major newspapers to advocate "smokers' rights") with little evident impact on public opinion.

MOBILIZATION AND ORGANIZATION

Critical to the emergence of social movements are, first, mobilizing structures, preexisting formal and informal social networks through which individuals with common grievances are brought together (the role of black churches in initiation of the civil rights movement is a classic example) and, second, the command of resources, including tangible assets such as financing, space, and mailing lists as well as intangible assets—organizational experience, scientific expertise, and social and political contacts (McCarthy and Zald 1977; Jenkins 1983; McAdam 1982; McAdam, McCarthy, and Zald 1996). From this perspective, a critical difference between the movements against smoking and guns is that the former was sparked by an innovative and highly energetic grassroots movement, while the latter not only lacked a strong grassroots base itself, but confronted (and continues to confront) a powerful, well-financed, and well-organized grassroots movement already in the field.[46]

THE SMOKING/TOBACCO CONTROL MOVEMENT

Until very recently, the core of the smoking/tobacco control movement consisted of three sets of players: the health voluntaries (American Cancer Society, American Lung Association, American Heart Association), Action on Smoking and Health (ASH), and the nonsmokers' rights groups.[47] These groups have varied in relative importance over time and have played different and, arguably, complementary roles in advancing the overall tobacco control agenda.[48]

The American Cancer Society

The ACS was started in 1913 by "a group of public-spirited physicians and laymen" (1950: 7). The society did not, however, begin to move toward its present size until after World War II; it underwent a major reorganization in 1945, bringing "a group of influential (and wealthy) businessmen" onto the ACS Board of Directors (ACS 1950: 7).[49] Among the results of this reorganization were a substantial commitment to cancer research (consistently just under 30 percent of the ACS budget), a major expansion in volunteers (ranging in number between one and three million), and extremely effective fund-raising. The ACS total budget grew from $14 million in 1950 to $347 million in 1990, a twenty-five-fold increase.[50]

The ACS's role in the smoking/tobacco control movement began to take shape in the late 1940s. In 1948, the ACS Annual Report noted that lung cancer mortality was "increasing"; in 1951 a National Lung Cancer Committee was created and the society issued its first public warning of the rise in lung cancer. In 1952 the ACS began its population-based follow-up study of smoking and death rates in "white men between the ages of fifty and sixty-nine" (Hammond and Horn 1954).[51] In an interview published in 1965, E. Cuyler Hammond stated that "only an institution like the American Cancer Society" could have carried out this study (Pfeiffer 1965: 12). Not only did the ACS have the necessary political independence and sufficient financial resources; it was able to draw on its huge network of volunteers to do the actual fieldwork and on its "goodwill among physicians and hospital authorities" to assist in obtaining follow-up information on men who had died (Pfeiffer 1965: 12). The ACS committed its substantial resources to this project despite considerable skittishness on the part of some of the society's officials, who were perfectly aware of the study's potential political sensitivity (Kluger 1996: 146). Many observers have described and commented upon ACS's reluctance to act on the study's striking results (Jacobson, Wasserman, and Raube 1992; Pertschuk 1986: 53; interview with ACS official, ACS files).

From the perspective of the larger smoking/tobacco control movement, the ACS played its most important role in the 1950s and 1960s, using its substantial resources and authority to help create and then to promote the problem of smoking and health within and outside the government. Conservative leadership and an unwillingness to risk other interests for the sake of the smoking/tobacco control movement prevented the society from going much beyond its self-defined role as health educator until the early 1980s.[52] Indeed, during the 1970s the ACS virtually disappeared as a public advocate on behalf of smoking and health (Troyer and Markle 1983: 68). The banner was taken up by a proliferation of single-issue groups, resource-poor relative to the ACS but unburdened by its conservative baggage.

Action on Smoking and Health

ASH was founded in 1967 by John Banzhaf, a professor of law at Georgetown University in Washington, D.C., with the sole purpose of engaging in legal action at the federal level. ASH's initial focus was on cigarette advertising, but it soon branched into additional arenas including public transportation, birth control package inserts, and others. By far the largest part of ASH's activities have been actions before the various regulatory commissions involved with tobacco (FCC, FTC, FDA, etc.). ASH's organization and mode of operation during the 1970s were well described by Ronald J. Troyer and Gerald E. Markle (1983: 80–86). In no sense was (or is) ASH a grassroots organization. It was a small (eight staff members in 1979), professionally operated, public interest group with a paid staff and no organization or activities at the local and state levels (indeed, ASH members were not allowed to engage in local action under the ASH banner). ASH's income in 1979 was approximately $366,000, well below that of any of the health voluntaries, of course, but far above the income (at that time) of any local nonsmokers' rights group.

There is evidence (from interviews and the GASP newsletter) of occasional ASH cooperation with its relatively near neighbor, the Maryland GASP. However, it was clear from interviews with other participants in the smoking/tobacco control movement that ASH is perceived as an independent operation, closely identified with its founder and not on the whole a collegial member of the larger movement.

The Nonsmokers' Rights Movement

By 1971, deaths of white males from lung cancer had reached a critical threshold of visibility: fathers and uncles of the generation that came of age in the late 1960s and early 1970s—an activist generation profoundly influenced by the example of civil rights, antiwar, and environmental movements—were dying of lung cancer.[53] The activists I interviewed identified a latent constituency composed of two groups: individuals who had lost loved ones to smoking and a much larger group who were profoundly irritated by tobacco smoke. The latter could be induced to come out of the closet, so to speak, by persuading them first that their irritation was legitimate and, second, that it was shared.

Clara Gouin, the founder of GASP, had been active in a local environmental movement. She attributed her father's death from lung cancer at the age of fifty-seven to cigarette smoking and friends complained to her about cigarette smoke in their hair and clothes.[54] In her own words. "You suddenly get an inspiration. That's what it was. I convened a meeting of my friends. There were several friends in the neighborhood, and several friends at church, and some mothers of young children my girls' age, and we had a meeting in our living room and said let's start this group and see what we can do" (Gouin 1995).

Gouin contacted local branches of the health voluntaries and the interest of the local lung association's program director made possible the combination of her "inspiration" with certain critical resources: space, a mimeograph machine, and—of inestimable importance—a mailing list. The first issue of *The Ventilator,* published in March 1971, went out to local lung associations (then the TB and Respiratory Disease Association) throughout the country. Buttons (reading "GASP—nonsmokers have rights, too") and posters were offered, plus a subscription to the newsletter for $1 per year. The response was far beyond the group's anticipation. Chapters were quickly formed in Berkeley and San Francisco. By 1974, the newsletter listed fifty-six local chapters in the U.S. and two in Canada. At least twenty-two (and probably more) of these chapters were unofficially associated with their local lung associations; in 1973, Clara Gouin and Willard Morris (the program director mentioned above) received the Public Relations Award of the American Lung Association on behalf of GASP and the Lung Association of Southern Maryland.[55]

From the beginning, GASP chapters were locally organized autonomous groups, staffed almost entirely by volunteers. "Once we got a bunch of chapters going we organized all the names we had by states and localities and mailed those names out to local Lung Associations and local GASP groups around the country, saying these are people who have written to us from your area. Contact them, get them active in your group. . . . We actually sent them envelopes with just stacks of little mailing labels" (Gouin 1995). Although Gouin mailed the first issue of the newsletter to members of Congress and federal officials were aware of GASP's existence, the group's initial tactics were almost entirely local and on a small scale, focused on getting smoke-free meeting rooms (particularly meeting rooms of obvious groups, like environmental groups and the Lung Association itself), doctors' offices, hospitals, natural food stores, and the like. Funding requirements for these activities were minimal (Gouin's budget never went above $10,000 per year) and came from contributions and from the pockets of the organizers themselves.

Although GASP struck a responsive chord in some quarters, nonsmokers' rights were by no means immediately popular with the general public: "When I started getting up there on my soapbox, it was a very unpopular issue . . . they thought who was this crackpot telling us we shouldn't be smoking in public" (Gouin 1995). The media, nevertheless, were very interested and "we got a lot of free publicity," at first locally and then nationally and internationally. Exposure brought new recruits.

By the mid-1970s, the focus of nonsmokers' rights activists began to shift from "passing out leaflets and buttons" to the passage of state and local anti-smoking regulations (Hanauer, Barr, and Glantz 1986: 2). Seventeen of the fifty-four GASP groups listed in 1974 were in California. These groups incorporated as California GASP in 1976 and focused increasingly on regulatory action,

FIGURE 15.8

**Grassroots Organizations and Nonsmoking Ordinances,
1964–1992: Number of Nonsmokers' Rights Groups and
Passage of Local Restaurant Nonsmoking Ordinances**

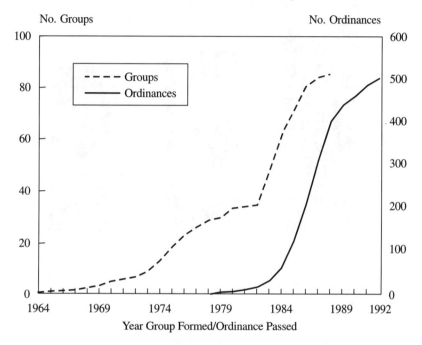

Sources: U.S. DHHS, NIH 1993; U.S. DHHS 1990.

first at the state and later (after narrow defeats in 1978 and 1980) at the local level.[56] These activities brought additional groups and individuals into the movement: the California chapter of the ACS in particular played "a very crucial role" in the initiative campaigns (interview with smoking/tobacco control activist, 1995). Data presented in Figure 15.8 on the timing of grassroots organization in relation to the passage of local restaurant nonsmoking ordinances (the first type of ordinance to be widely adopted) suggest that organization at the local level played a critical role in subsequent regulatory action.

There are no published surveys of nonsmokers' rights activists. However, some idea of the population groups to whom their activities had most appeal can be gained from an analysis of the relationship between the average family income of California counties and the timing of smoking control ordinance adoption. These data are shown in Figure 15.9. Counties that adopted smoking

FIGURE 15.9

**Smoking Ordinance Adoption and Wealth: Timing of Smoking Control
Ordinance Adoption and Family Income (California Counties)**

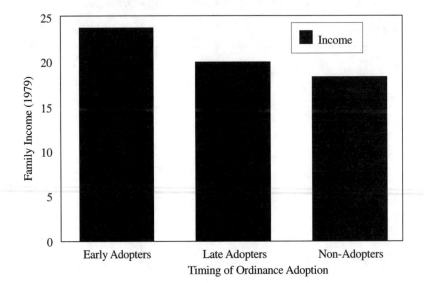

Sources: U.S. DHHS, NIH 1993; U.S. Department of Commerce 1980.
Note: Significance of difference between income means (ANOVA): $F = 14.91$, $p < .0000$.

control ordinances in 1985 or before are defined as early adopters, counties that
adopted ordinances after 1985 are late adopters, and the remaining counties
are nonadopters. Wealthier counties are substantially more likely to be early
adopters: the difference in mean income levels across the three adopter groups
is highly significant. It is a reasonable inference from these data that individuals
active in the nonsmokers' rights movement were also likely to be above average
in education and wealth.

As the nature and scope of their activities changed, funding requirements
increased and GASP groups became somewhat more professionalized (although
they were still largely voluntary); drafting legislation and engineering its passage demanded legal experience and organizing a statewide initiative campaign
(i.e., in California) was expensive. Along with these changes came greater
bureaucratization, concerns about incorporation and tax exemption and, ultimately, paid staff. The early activists I interviewed remarked on the movement's
evolution with evident nostalgia for an earlier time: "Maybe part of the secret of
[GASP's] success was that it was never thoroughly organized. Sometimes you

have a good idea and in the beginning stages there is great enthusiasm, and then once the idea gets structured into rules, regulations, formal dues, offices, and all of that, it loses a bit of its initial impetus. . . . [People in the movement now] didn't have to join a group and carry a banner. When you feel you're alone, have to join a group. Don't need little organizations when everybody's doing it" (Gouin 1995). The transformation Gouin describes is a classic process of organizational change, the price a social movement pays for public acceptance and success.[57]

A significant characteristic of the smoking/tobacco control movement has been the shifting participation over time of several groups with quite different goals, resources, and constituencies. Although these groups have often appeared antagonistic, I would argue that their roles were, in fact, complementary and contributed in important ways to the movement's relative success.

The Gun Control Movement

The gun and smoking/tobacco control movements have certain things in common: both movements have reformist goals of health-related social change through public education and political advocacy, both draw on largely white, middle-class constituencies, and both have a clearly identifiable, large, well-financed, and politically well-connected opponent. At the time of our research, however, there were major differences with implications both for the mobilization potential and for the organizational resources of the gun control movement.

First, not only the smoking/tobacco control movement but other social movements that have achieved substantial success in the latter half of the twentieth century—the civil rights, gay rights, and feminist movements, as well as health-related movements (e.g.. breast-cancer survivors, Mothers against Drunk Driving)—have been in a position to draw heavily on self-defined victims with the personal and social resources to engage in social movement activity. Among the leaders of the gun control movement we interviewed, almost all had direct experience with gun violence. However, large sectors of the gun control movement's potential constituency—victims of gun violence or individuals in fear of victimization—are unlikely candidates for mobilization by a white, middle-class reform movement.[58] Half of all victims of homicide are minorities, as I have pointed out. A high proportion of these victims are inner-city black youth.[59] Fear of victimization is as much or more likely to result in the purchase of a gun than in joining Handgun Control, Inc. Police are perhaps the most obvious potential middle-class victims of gun violence, and the gun control movement received a major boost when police organizations came to its support in the mid-1980s.

Interest in gun control among the larger population is driven, in Spitzer's terms, by a "cycle of outrage, action, and reaction usually [beginning] with the sensational and the horrific" (1995: 13). This point was eloquently made by a gun control activist we interviewed:

> From 1975 [when his group was founded] to 1980 we were a very small, basically inconsequential organization. We were just a voice out there in the wilderness. . . . In 1980–81, the Pope, John Lennon, and the president were all shot . . . . Suddenly, the issue became hot. We were one of the few sources that people had to go to for information, especially the news media. So in 1980, we grew rapidly. And then, it died. The president took that "aw shucks, it didn't hurt" approach, the Pope didn't say anything about the issue, and all we were left with were John Lennon fans. The other folks disappeared.[60]

The problematic character of its recruitment base may be responsible for what another movement activist described as "probably the greatest shortcoming of the gun control movement: even though we have strong public support, we have no organized grassroots."

Grassroots support for the gun control movement has been sporadic and difficult to sustain, and the movement has only recently begun to attract support from established organizations comparable to that of the health voluntaries for smoking/tobacco control. Further, while both movements have experienced and continue to experience conflict between more conservative and more radical factions, the impact of this conflict on the movement's ability to present a united front may be more serious in the case of gun control.[61]

In the mid-1990s, the national stage was shared by two gun control organizations. Handgun Control, Inc. (HCI) and the Coalition to Stop Gun Violence (CSGV). Spitzer gives a concise summary of the groups' background, beginning with HCI: "[HCI] began in partnership with the National Coalition to Ban Handguns (NCBH), formed at about the same time. The groups soon parted ways. The NCBH was renamed the Coalition to Stop Gun Violence in 1990. It has generally pursued a tougher stand on gun regulation than HCI, and has been overshadowed by HCI's greater size and visibility, especially since Sarah Brady has become a prominent HCI figure" (1995: 115). Only two state-level gun control advocacy groups were identified by our respondents, in Maryland and Illinois. One activist described most other organizations as consisting of "dedicated people with a hunk of letterhead."

A range of low-profile groups do exist, however. Missing Peace, for example, is a primarily educational rather than political advocacy group (although it has employed direct action occasionally, e.g., a candlelight vigil in front of the White House). The group was founded by a suburban Maryland woman after a twelve-year-old brought a gun to her son's school; its director would like to expand nationally and pointed to affiliates in eighteen states. At the same time, she suggested that she might quit if additional funds were not forthcoming soon. Missing Peace has much in common with the original GASP: it is small, with meager funds, and is staffed almost entirely by volunteers. A major (and,

I believe, critical) difference is the absence of anything comparable to the American Lung Association's support for GASP.

A standard question in the interviews we conducted asked respondents to comment on the relationship of their own group with other groups working on the gun control issue. The level of perceived competition, even conflict, elicited by this question was striking. Reactions ranged from strongly negative— extending to an unwillingness to share mailing lists and to uneasiness about appearances on the same platform—to expressions of competition over financial resources, to more thoughtful analyses:

> There are a couple of splits in the gun control movement. One is between the controllers and the banners. The controllers who want to control handguns through licensing, registration, things like that, tend to view the banners as radicals who give them a bad name. The controllers also tend to see gun violence as a crime issue versus gun violence as a public health issue. The banners, we're talking handguns here, tend to be public health people, those who take a public health perspective and one of the problems with the public health argument is that it points out many of the limitations and internal flaws of the gun control's control argument! Which doesn't lead to good relations. I think that's one of the problems in this movement in that whereas in most movements certainly you have differences of opinion, differences in approach, but there's a recognition that for the greater good, you should work together on specific issues you can agree upon. That had never really happened in the gun control movement. And that's been one of our big failings. (Gun control activist, 1995)

While smoking/tobacco control groups have had their share of conflict as well, these remarks suggest that conflict within the gun control movement has been more profound and has contributed to movement fragmentation.

It must be emphasized that both the smoking/tobacco and gun control movements are moving targets, shifting their character as different actors move onto and off the stage. The recent wholesale entry of lawyers into the smoking/tobacco control arena and of health professionals and lawyers with public health training into the gun control arena will inevitably change how these movements are organized and the constituencies to whom they appeal.

POLITICAL OPPORTUNITIES

THE SMOKING/TOBACCO CONTROL MOVEMENT

A full analysis of the role of shifting political opportunities—in particular, analysis of critical actions of relevant elites with the power to push or block the smoking/tobacco control agenda—would require a level of data gathering and insider access that was beyond the scope of this project. Thus, my account depends primarily on interpretation and inference from published sources and may be incomplete.

The Permeable American State

The purpose of social movements is to "force their targets and public decision makers to recognize their concerns and to commit institutional resources to implement movement goals" (Oberschall 1993: 32). Recognition by public decision makers is substantially easier in a nation-state with many different points of access: "The chaos [in the American system] allows citizens to utilize *multiple cracks* to gain their ends" (Morton Grodzins, cited in Friedman 1975: 170; emphasis in the original).

A. Lee Fritschler argues that the "normal relationship" among institutions of government (including outside interest groups) was typified by pre-1964 tobacco politics. Policies were made "in a spirit of friendly and quiet cooperation" among members of what Fritschler calls the "tobacco subsystem": "The tobacco subsystem included the paid representatives of tobacco growers, marketing organizations, and cigarette manufacturers; congressmen representing tobacco constituencies; the leading members of four subcommittees in Congress—two appropriations subcommittees and two substantive legislative committees in each house—that handle tobacco legislation and related appropriations; and certain officials within the Department of Agriculture who were involved with the various tobacco programs of that department" (1989: 4). The 1964 Surgeon General's report was the opportunity that threw a monkey wrench into this system by creating openings for dissident individual members of Congress, federal agencies unconnected with the tobacco subsystem (the FTC, DHEW, FCC), the health voluntaries, and not least, the states, by virtue of their traditional responsibility for public health. There was no grassroots antismoking movement in 1964.

Of course, opportunities must be grasped, and these entities varied substantially in the aggressiveness with which they took advantage of the openings that the Surgeon General's report offered. The FTC and certain states (e.g., New York) were prepared to take action quickly, until they were slapped down by Congress in the form of the 1965 cigarette labeling act. The DHEW was relatively timid, perhaps due to an absence of presidential support for aggressive antismoking measures, and the health voluntaries, although they had played a major role in initiating government action that led to the report, were less than enthusiastic in their endorsement of government action in response to the report's findings.[62]

Jill Quadagno has hypothesized that "the permeability of state agencies to social movement demands depends on their autonomy from the targets of social movement goals" (1992: 631). Kenneth Michael Friedman and Fritschler, political scientists who have studied the smoking and health controversy, both emphasize the critical role played by independent regulatory agencies in initiating policy and in sustaining public attention to smoking as a public health problem: "The FCC and the FTC have been able to act because their relative independence in the present situation has protected them from economic and political pressures. . . . The importance of independent actors, including the regulatory commissions, in spurring governmental action [against smoking] in the United States has been crucial. Without them consideration of the issues and governmental action would have been at least postponed if not precluded" (Friedman 1975: 56). The creation of the Consumer Products Safety Commission in 1973 offered a further opportunity for outside groups (in this case the American Public Health Association [APHA] and Senator Frank Moss [D-UT]) to demand regulatory action against cigarettes that, even though unsuccessful, kept the problem in the public eye: "In a large pluralistic system, there are many ways to keep an issue alive" (Fritschler 1989: 118).

Among the most important of those ways, as I pointed out earlier, was action at state and local levels. Many northern states had little dependence on the tobacco industry and clean-air legislation was consistent with traditional state responsibilities. When the tobacco industry became aware of this threat to their interests and began to exert its influence successfully at the state level, nonsmokers' rights groups turned to the local level where the industry was substantially less effective. Of course, the industry has found ways to counter this latter strategy as well (e.g., by state preemption of local clean-air regulations) and the struggle continues. However, without the multiple venues for action offered by the U.S. state, the struggle would have been even more one-sided.

The potential importance of federal agencies with authority independent of Congress, if not (in the case of the FDA) of the executive branch, was demonstrated again in 1980, when the FTC, under Michael Pertschuk, an activist commissioner appointed by President Carter, was instrumental in reviving the cigarette labeling issue, leading to eventual congressional passage of a somewhat stronger system of rotating labels; and, more recently, this was also illustrated in the critical role played by the FDA under another activist commissioner, David Kessler, in labeling nicotine as a drug and cigarettes as devices for drug delivery. Published accounts of these events are relatively silent about the role of interest group pressure—for example, from the coalition of health voluntaries newly organized in 1981—in initiating action by the FTC and/or the FDA. If John W. Kingdon's (1995) work is any guide, however, the pressure was there, waiting for the right moment to make its presence felt.

Elite Allies

Pertschuk recounts that in 1965, when the first cigarette labeling bill was under consideration in Congress, President Lyndon Johnson personally "called FTC Chairman Paul Rand Dixon and excoriated him for persecuting the tobacco industry" (1986: 37). President Clinton, by contrast, was "the first avowedly antismoking president in the White House" (Kluger 1996: 549). Allies (or their absence) in the federal government have played a significant role in the smoking/tobacco control movement. Probably of most importance, Surgeons General and Secretaries of the Department of Health and Human Services friendly to the movement (Terry, Steinfeld, Califano, and Koop) have been able to use the annual Surgeon General's reports on smoking and health as vehicles to direct public attention to the problem of smoking and health and to lend the power of scientific legitimacy to smoking's opponents. Indeed, Fritschler credits the 1964 report with dealing the tobacco "subsystem a blow that was to prove fatal" by providing "the Federal Trade Commission with an opportunity to make its move" (1989: 43). Allies in the executive branch and, of particular importance, in Congress, have played vital roles in the recent past as well: hearings and the introduction and shepherding of legislation (even legislation that does not pass) contribute to the legitimization of smoking/tobacco control as public policy issue and, of course, keep the issue in the public eye.

Depending on one's perspective, the health voluntaries and the major organizations of health professionals may be regarded as elite allies, rather than as part of the smoking/tobacco control movement itself, and I have already described the shifting roles these groups have played.[63] Another important potential ally whose leadership has not, on the whole, been supportive of the movement are trade unions. As the director of the AFL-CIO Department of Occupational Safety and Health stated in opposing federal regulation of environmental tobacco smoke (ETS), "we have a lot of individuals who smoke and don't think this is the kind of thing the government should be involved with" (U.S. OSHA 1995: 12217–12218). Since 1991, twenty-eight states and the District of Columbia have passed laws protecting smokers from discrimination in the workplace (McKenzie 1998), and OSHA's proposed regulations have stalled, possibly as a consequence of trade union opposition.

Target Vulnerabilities

The avowed target of the smoking/tobacco control movement has shifted over time between potential smokers (children, adolescents), smokers (first as victims, later as perpetrators), and the tobacco industry itself. The health voluntaries were extremely reluctant to confront the tobacco industry, as I have noted, and it is only in the very recent past that the industry itself has been isolated as a target, if not the major target. While it is evident from hindsight that the industry has become more vulnerable over time, objective indicators of vulnerability are difficult to come by: that is, vulnerability tends to be judged by results (e.g., legislation passed or failed, court cases won or lost) rather than by predictive measures. However, I will suggest a few changes that may have made a difference.

First, congressional representation of southern states that grow tobacco as a major crop has shifted over time from predominantly Democratic to predominantly Republican. For most of the period in question, the majority party in Congress and thus the chairs of congressional committees have been Democrats, and the Democrats with the greatest seniority (and consequently most likely to occupy those chairs) were from the tobacco-growing South. As the South began to send more Republicans than Democrats to Congress, the occupants of committee chairs shifted from southern to northern Democrats, who are less sympathetic to tobacco interests. The change in party representation from tobacco states may have played a role in President Clinton's relative willingness as compared with (for example) Lyndon Johnson's to speak out on issues of smoking/tobacco control.

Cigarette manufacturers have benefited from their ability to present a united front with tobacco growers. However, not only have there been changes in the political representation of tobacco-growing states, but changes have occurred in the circumstances of the growers themselves to make them a less certain ally. Both the number of tobacco farmers and the acreage devoted to tobacco have declined since 1964 and manufacturers' use of tobacco imported from outside this country has substantially increased. The latter issue appears to have played an important role in eroding congressional support for the industry in the course of debate on what became the 1984 cigarette labeling bill: Pertschuk quotes North Carolina Democrat Charles Rose, then chair of the House Tobacco Subcommittee, as remarking to the staff director of the Coalition for Smoking or Health, "Your concern is health. What really concerns me is imports. They're ruining my farmers, destroying them!" (1986: 67: see also Kluger 1996: 546).[64]

Finally, the industry's posture of denying either that cigarettes cause disease or that they are addictive was powerfully undermined by the 1994 discovery of company documents dating hack to the early 1950s in which these properties were clearly acknowledged (Glantz et al. 1996; Hilts 1996). While this information was hardly new, hard evidence of the industry's knowledge substantially increased its vulnerability not only in the court of public opinion, but (and possibly of even greater long-run importance) in the courts of law. Lawyers on behalf of clients who claim injury from smoking can now, as the *New York Times* pointed out, "rely on industry documents to portray smoking as part of a lethal conspiracy on the part of cigarette makers" (Collins 1997).

The increasing political and legal vulnerability of the tobacco industry is part of a downward spiral, inseparable from concomitant changes in the number, composition, and social position of smokers. Thus, as the number of smokers in the population has declined to under 30 percent, as their composition has shifted toward younger and less affluent groups, and as adult smoking has become more and more stigmatized, it has become that much easier to attack the industry that supports the smoking habit.[65]

THE GUN CONTROL MOVEMENT

Many of the external conditions confronted by the gun control movement— a lack of public (or scholarly) consensus about the dangers of guns, a high prevalence of gun ownership among ordinary citizens, and a well organized and implacable foe—have stayed relatively constant over time. Consequently, the gun control movement has been more than usually dependent for recognition in the public and political arenas, as well as for the successes it has so far achieved, on its ability to take advantage of often transient political opportunities. The most obvious of these opportunities have been the high-profile assassinations and wholesale killings of young children and other innocent victims that have marked the last three decades. These events have led to brief openings of opportunity, resulting in temporary increases in recruitment to the gun control movement and in gains to the movement's financial resources. The impact of these events on the movement's success in achieving its regulatory goals is less clear: the first piece of federal gun legislation passed after the 1981 shootings of Reagan, John Lennon, and the Pope was the McClure-Volkmer Act, which was explicitly intended to weaken the 1968 Gun Control Act.

Whether and how the gun control movement has been able to take advantage of the opportunities offered by public outrage, indeed the existence of *any* opportunities for action in the gun control arena, has been almost wholly dependent on the National Rifle Association.

The National Rifle Association

Both the tobacco industry and the NRA are well organized and well funded, with powerful political allies. There is a critical difference, however, in the constituencies each of these entities represent. The tobacco industry is a business (in reality, of course, several businesses allied largely in response to external threat). The NRA is an interest-group organization of firearms users, described by one observer as "the prototypic single-issue interest group in America" (cited in Spitzer 1995: 99). Several thousand local sporting and gun clubs came under its umbrella during the NRA's early years, and for most of its history the group's primary focus was marksmanship and (particularly after World War II) hunting (Spitzer 1995: 100). The NRA has long benefited from a range of government subsidies (e.g., donations of surplus guns, permission for target ranges on federal land) and has close ties to the gun industry. "The key to the NRA's [political] effectiveness," however, "lies in its highly motivated mass membership and the organization's ability to bring pressure from that membership to bear at key moments and places" (Spitzer 1995: 108).

Smokers' rights groups in this country were organized in reaction to the antismoking movement, but they have never been more than barely disguised window dressing for the tobacco industry and have never been taken seriously.

The gun control movement, by contrast, has had to confront a powerful organization already on the ground, one that included among its members not only past presidents of the United States and influential members of Congress, but a large and extremely loyal following of ordinary citizens.

Given the NRA's perceived power, it comes as little surprise that observers of recent gun control politics attribute the gun control movement's legislative successes (the Brady bill, the assault weapons ban) less to movement influence than to NRA missteps.[66] Spitzer (1995), Osha Gray Davidson (1993), and others have described in some detail the series of events leading to the NRA's alienation of important allies, including not only major political figures (former President George Bush resigned in 1995), but the police. Beginning in the late 1970s, the NRA took an increasingly hard and uncompromising line toward all forms of regulation, both of guns and of ammunition: "One of the most highly publicized consequences of this unyielding approach has been the alienation of most national police organizations" (Spitzer 1995: 114). The NRA's split with the police and its rigidity on other issues have resulted in isolation from its natural allies among conservative groups and from the gun industry as well (Spitzer 1995: 115; Wayne 1997).

Among the consequences of the NRA's increased vulnerability was that it lost the ability to keep legislation it disliked off the congressional agenda (Spitzer 1995: 170). And, in further parallel with the tobacco industry, having lost in Congress once, the NRA's vulnerability the next time around increased: "People realized that there's life after voting against the NRA" (Representative Charles E. Schumer [D-NY], cited in Spitzer 1995: 162).

The NRA's vulnerability should not be exaggerated, however. Like the antiabortion movement and the smoking/tobacco control movement, the NRA responded to loss on the federal level by turning to state and local venues, and it has been reasonably successful. Since 1986, twenty-two states have adopted what are known as right-to-carry or shall-issue laws, laws that "[require] authorities to issue, without discretion, concealed weapon permits to qualified applicants" (Lott and Mustard 1997: 4). In contrast to cigarettes, guns are easily concealed. These laws are strongly opposed by gun control advocates (see, e.g., Webster et al. 1997, commenting on the Lott and Mustard study). The NRA has become active on the international stage as well. It obtained observer status at the United Nations in 1997 and joined with gun groups and firearms manufacturers from other countries to oppose international firearms regulation (Seelye 1997).

Following (often consciously) in the footsteps of the smoking/tobacco control movement, some within the gun control movement have begun to target the manufacturers of what the movement defines as a dangerous product (Teret and Wintermute 1993). That this did not happen earlier may be due to the manufacturers' lack of visibility on the public stage. While it supports (financially and otherwise) the NRA's goals, the NRA's aggressive tactics have allowed the firearms industry to adopt a very low profile in gun control debates: "Many firearms manufacturers have chosen to remain in the background of the raging debate over tighter restrictions on the sale and possession of guns, preferring to leave their public talking to the National Rifle Association" (cited in Spitzer 1995: 104).[67] However, reluctance to target manufacturers is also due to some movement leaders' ambivalence about "safe guns": "On the one hand, [safer guns] could help reduce fatal accidents, unintentional injuries . . . On the other hand, if you make the 'safe handgun' are you giving the industry a whole new marketing tool? Where they can go back and re-sell [guns to] every handgun owner in America—hey, this is new, this is safe. . . . I have very strong concerns about that—I'm not really sure where I come down on it" (gun control activist, interview, 1995). These remarks are, of course, highly reminiscent of smoking/tobacco control advocates' opposition to the promotion of "safe cigarettes" as a public health measure.[68] From the advocates' perspective, these are halfway measures, diluting and potentially compromising the purity of their cause.

Elite Allies

Open support by the police was accompanied by a significant expansion of the gun control movement's organizational resources. In interviews, the leaders of HCI and Missing Peace made clear their close affiliation with police groups. Asked what other organizations she worked with, an HCI leader responded, "I'd say over the last ten years we worked probably for the most part with law enforcement." Long-time gun control activists (as well as observers like Spitzer and Davidson) credit police organizations with a principal role in passage of the Brady bill: "We got the Brady bill passed because they made it a police issue. . . . we're just liberal preachers out there talking about this subject and nobody cares. But [when] a local cop says this is something I'm concerned about . . . people start caring" (gun control activist, interview. 1995). Recently, several well-established interest group organizations—the Children's Defense Fund (CDF) and the Consumer Federation of America (CFA)—have also begun to take action on behalf of gun control primarily through dissemination of educational materials and, in the case of CDF, through mobilization on a local level through church groups. Our interview with a representative of CFA was striking in the expression of concerns almost exactly parallel with the concerns reflected in interviews with ACS officials.[69] On the one hand, gun control was a good cause ("preventing consumer injuries and deaths") and would clearly benefit from association with a "mainstream" (the CFA representative's term), conservative organization like the CFA. On the other hand, many of the groups under CFA's umbrella were skittish about jeopardizing their "reputation" in a fringe cause, about being associated with "people who want to take away people's rights," and about taking on "the big bad NRA." These groups' actual level of involvement in gun control is unclear—in both cases, it forms a small part of much broader agendas—and their effectiveness remains to be seen.[70]

DISCUSSION

I address four issues in this discussion: the methodological questions of movement outcome and causal attribution, the substantive reasons for the relative success of the antismoking campaign, implications of this comparison for the relationship of social movements to social change, and, finally, the implications for public policy.

MOVEMENT OUTCOMES

I have elected to judge the success of the smoking/tobacco and gun control movements based on the goals articulated by movement activists and have concluded on this basis that the antismoking campaign has been relatively more successful than the campaign against guns. It is important to note, however, that the very use of this criterion favors the smoking/tobacco control movement. First, the greater consensus among smoking/tobacco control activists made their goals easier to identify. Second, the public attitude change that they accomplished so successfully was an explicit goal of the nonsmokers' rights movement from its initiation. The focus of gun control activists was more exclusively on change in public policies, and both movements have encountered resistance in that arena.

The question of a causal relationship between the nonsmokers' rights movement and decline in cigarette consumption in the United States during the 1970s was addressed directly by Kenneth Warner in an article published in *Science* in 1981. Warner used multiple regression techniques to take account of changes in media attention to smoking's health effects and in taxation and concluded that "both declining consumption and growth in legislation (restricting smoking in public places) probably reflect a prevailing nonsmoking ethos" induced by the movement for nonsmokers' rights (1981: 730). This article is particularly interesting and important for the time period to which it refers, when the nonsmokers' rights movement was virtually the only game in town.

ACCOUNTING FOR SUCCESS

The initial circumstances confronting the smoking/tobacco and gun control movements were quite similar. Differences emerged over time and consisted both in advantages enjoyed by the smoking/tobacco control movement and in disadvantages it avoided.

The smoking/tobacco control movement benefited enormously from the "good cop/bad cop" combination of the conservative, highly respectable and respected health voluntaries with the initially radical (or perceived as radical) nonsmokers' rights movement. When the American Cancer Society dropped the ball in the late 1960s, it was taken up by movement activists, aided and abetted by the silent partnership of another health voluntary, the American Lung Association. The movement's grassroots base enabled it to engage in local actions beyond the capacities (or inclinations) of the health voluntaries, actions that the tobacco industry found it difficult to contain. Gun control has been weak at the grassroots level, and until the adherence of police organizations in the mid-1980s, the movement had no allies comparable in size and respectability to the health voluntaries. The recent refraining of guns as a public health problem has attracted a new set of allies, however, and these groups have had considerable success in California (Gorovitz 1996). Their impact nationally remains to be seen.

Of greatest importance both to the smoking/tobacco control movement's initial mobilization and to its enduring impact has been the constriction of credible risks. The authority of medicine and science in the smoking/tobacco control arena was well established before the organized movement emerged; the movement drew on this authority and on a culturally powerful discourse of innocence and rights both to transform public perceptions of cigarettes and smoking and to create a new collective identity, that of the nonsmoker.

A second critical difference between the smoking/tobacco and gun control movements is a negative one: the absence of a credible or effective counter-movement to nonsmokers' rights (or to the larger movement that it spawned). Opposition to gun control, by contrast, has been orchestrated by a grass-roots organization with substantial elite support, the ability to mobilize its constituency at every level of government, and command of an ideologically resonant cultural frame.

SOCIAL MOVEMENTS AND SOCIAL CHANGE

Doug McAdam has written that "given the entrenched political and economic opposition movements are likely to encounter, it is often true that their biggest impact is more cultural than narrowly political or economic" (1994: 49). This article has described a striking case of movement-created cultural change. What can be learned from the comparison between smoking and guns about the conditions under which cultural change is more or less likely to occur? With few exceptions, discussion of outcomes in the social movement literature (and in the partially parallel political science literature on interest groups) assume that movements' targets are political elites and that the outcomes of interest are policy and political change. Findings presented here are consistent with this work: movements benefit from elite allies (particularly allies who can play roles complementary to that of the movement proper) and from being positioned to take advantage of political windows of opportunity (Shapiro 1985; Walker 1991; Tarrow 1994; Kingdon 1995; McAdam, Mc-Carthy, and Zald 1996). Organizational advantages, however, are no guarantee of movement impact on the larger society (see, e.g., Schwartz and Paul 1992).[71]

McAdam's comments suggest that one reason for the smoking/tobacco control movement's relative success is that cultural change is easier to accomplish than social and economic change. While the relative success of the two movements considered here is consistent with this proposition, I doubt its universal truth: in France, for example, laws were passed in 1976 and 1990 regulating tobacco advertising and smoking in public places, but there has been relatively little change in the French culture of smoking. I advance two factors to account for the cultural impact of the smoking/tobacco control movement in the United States: first, the construction of credible risks already described at length and second, the culturally receptive climate into which this risks discourse was inserted.

Moral crusades—and the nonsmokers' rights movement is, in many respects, a moral crusade—are a recurring feature of American life. The timing of this particular crusade, however, contributed to its success. In the 1970s, the United States was characterized by an increasing demand for health as an individual right (see, e.g., Fox 1979; Freeman 1983) and, at the same time, there was increasing concern about the costs of medical care, disenchantment with the value of medical care in improving health, and a "growing reaction against liberalism and government" (Starr 1982: 380). Across the political spectrum, from Ivan Illich to John Knowles, critics argued that greater access to medical care was not the path to better health. In this context the crusade against smoking appealed both to middle-class liberals concerned about the environment and generally sympathetic to rights-based movements and to conservative advocates of "individual responsibility" (as opposed to government responsibility) for health. This compatibility with ideologies of both the left and right may partially explain one of the enduring puzzles of the smoking/tobacco control case: why no credible or effective countermovement developed. David S. Meyer and Suzanne Staggenborg have proposed that the "likelihood that opposition to a movement will take the form of a sustained countermovement is directly related to the opposition's ability to portray the conflict as one that entails larger value cleavages in society" (1996: 1639). Neither proponents of smokers' rights nor the tobacco industry have been successful in making that case.[72]

POLICY IMPLICATIONS

The power of social movements in the health policy arena raises a number of questions. First, what is the role of science in the construction of health risks?

Second, what is the movements' class-based impact? And third, what are the risks to the movement of its own success?

Health-related movements must invoke credible risks. However, whether those risks are perceived as credible by the audience addressed has more to do with ideology than science. In the case of passive smoking, credibility was present far in advance of scientific knowledge; in the case of nicotine addiction, knowledge long preceded either public or institutional acceptance. The lesson from these observations is that there may be little correlation between the scientific grounding of health-related social movements and their success in the policy or public arenas. Publications in the *Journal of the American Medical Association* or the *New England Journal of Medicine,* however sound, are seldom persuasive on their own. Movement success in reaching the policy agenda may be only tangentially related to the scientific importance of its public health message, and movements with important messages may fail.

Individuals with the interest, resources, and network connections to initiate health-related social movements tend to be white and middle class. Unlike many reform movements, the first targets of the nonsmokers' rights movement were people much like themselves: white, middle-class professionals and business people who smoked. These efforts were successful to the point where smoking has become a status marker. The shock we feel when a professional colleague lights up a cigarette is due to the contradiction between his or her perceived high status and the low status we now attach to the act of smoking. The other side of this coin, however, is that as smoking becomes increasingly concentrated among people unlike movement activists—blue collar workers and adolescents— behavior change efforts will, almost inevitably, be less successful. The social gulf between reformers and those whom they would protect or reform is a problem generic to reform movements (including the gun control movement). The smoking/tobacco control movement was unique in its ability to avoid this problem for so long.

A last reflection has to do with the shifting target of the smoking/tobacco control movement. As the movement has changed from one of citizen activists to one that is professionalized and, to a large extent, lawyer-dominated, it has experienced some level of what might be called goal displacement— from smoking and smokers to the tobacco industry. The wealth, visibility, and political clout of the smoking/tobacco control movement's opponents makes them easy for advocates to demonize: struggles between David and Goliath have an obvious romantic appeal and there is satisfaction in mounting attacks on greedy corporations. However, the degree to which these attacks serve movement advocates' long-term goals is unclear. Declines in smoking prevalence occurred because smoking was made socially unacceptable, not— or at least not directly—as a result of pressure on the industry itself. If they are to be successful, health-related social movements need to keep their long-term goals in mind.

REFERENCES

Amenta, E., K. Dunleavy, and M. Bernstein. 1994. Stolen Thunder? Huey Long's "Share Our Wealth," Political Mediation, and the Second New Deal. *American Sociological Review* 59(5):678–702.

American Cancer Society (ACS). 1948, 1950, 1957. *Annual Report.* New York: ACS.

———. ACS Files. Atlanta: ACS.

Americans for Nonsmokers' Rights (ANR). 1996. *ANR Update* 15(1): 1.

Anderson, J. 1996. *Inside the NRA: Armed and Dangerous.* Beverly Hills. CA: Dove Books.

Anderson, R. N., K. D. Kochanek, and S. L. Murphy. 1997. Report of Final Mortality Statistics, 1995. *Monthly Vital Statistics Report* 45 (11, suppl. 2):97–1120.

Apple, R. W. Jr. 1998. For Tobacco Growers, a Changing Life. *New York Times.* 14 September 1998, A12.

Barnes, D. E., and L. Bero. 1998. Why Review Articles on the Health Effects of Passive Smoking Reach Different Conclusions. *Journal of the American Medical Association* 279(19): 1566–1570.

Beauchamp, D. E. 1988. *The Health of the Republic.* Philadelphia: Temple University Press.

Brandt, A. 1992. The Rise and Fall of the Cigarette: A Brief History of the Antismoking Movement in the United States. In *Advancing Health in Developing Countries,* ed. L. C. Chen, A. Kleinman, and N. C. Ware. New York: Auburn House.

———. 1995. Blow Some My Way: Passive Smoking, Risk, and American Culture. Paper presented at a Symposium on the History of Smoking and Health. Wellcome Institute for the History of Medicine, London, 26–27 April.

Brody, J. 1996. Decline Seen in Death Rates from Cancer as a Whole. *New York Times,* 14 November, A21.

Burney, L. E. 1959. Smoking and Lung Cancer: A Statement of the Public Health Service. *Journal of the American Medical Association* 171(13): 1829–1837.

Burstein, P., R. L. Einwohner, and J. A. Hollander. 1995. The Success of Political Movements: A Bargaining Perspective. In *The Politics of Social Protest: Comparative Perspectives on States and Social Movements,* ed. J. C. Jenkins and B. Klandermans. Minneapolis: University of Minnesota Press.

Butterfield, F. 1998. Chicago Is Suing over Guns from Suburbs. *New York Times,* 13 November, A18.

Centers for Disease Control and Prevention. 1993. Mortality Trends for Selected Smoking-Related Cancers and Breast Cancer—United States, 1950–1990. *Morbidity and Mortality Weekly Report,* 12 November, 865.

————. 1994. Health Objectives for the Nation: Cigarette Smoking among Adults—United States, 1993. *Morbidity and Mortality Weekly Report,* 23 December, 925–930.

————. 1995. Suicide among Children, Adolescents, and Young Adults—United States, 1980–1992. *Morbidity and Mortality Weekly Report,* 21 April, 289.

————. 1996a. *State Tobacco Highlights—1996.* Centers for Disease Control and Prevention Publication No. 099-4895. Atlanta: Centers for Disease Control and Prevention, National Center for Chronic Disease Prevention and Health Promotion, Office on Smoking and Health.

————. 1996b. Cigarette Smoking among Adults—United States, 1994. *Morbidity and Mortality Weekly Report,* 12 July, 588.

————. 1997. Cigarette Smoking among Adults—United States, 1995. *Morbidity and Mortality Weekly Report,* 26 December, 1218.

Cole, P., and B. Rodu. 1996. Declining Cancer Mortality in the United States. *Cancer* 78(10):2045–2048.

Collins, G. 1997. Lawyer Is in Round No. 2 against Tobacco Industry. *New York Times,* 14 April, A12.

Consumers Union. 1995. Hooked on Tobacco: The Teen Epidemic. *Consumer Reports* 60(3):142–147.

Cook, P. J., and J. Ludwig. 1997. Guns in America: National Survey on Private Ownership and Use of Firearms. *Research in Brief* [National Institute of Justice] May, 1–11.

Davidson, 0. G. 1993. *Under Fire.* New York: Henry Holt.

Diani, M. 1997. Social Movements and Social Capital: A Network Perspective Movement Outcomes. *Mobilization* 2(2):129–147.

Dobbin, F. 1994. *Forging Industrial Policy: The United States, Britain, and France the Railway Age.* Cambridge: Cambridge University Press.

Doll, R., and A. B. Hill. 1952. A Study of the Etiology of Carcinoma of the Lung. *British Medical Journal* 2:1271–1286.

————. 1956. Lung Cancer and Other Causes of Death in Relation to Smoking: Second Report on Mortality of British Doctors. *British Medical Journal* 2:1071–1081.

Douglas, M. 1992. *Risk and Blame: Essays in Cultural Theory.* London: Routledge.

Douglas, M., and A. Wildavsky. 1982. *Risk and Culture: An Essay on the Selection of Technical and Environmental Dangers.* Berkeley: University of California Press.

Fingerhut, L. A., D. D. Ingram, and J. J. Feldman. 1992. Firearm Homicide among Black Teenage Males in Metropolitan Counties. *Journal of the American Medical Association* 267(22): 3054–3058.

Forster, J. L., D. M. Murray, M. Wolfson, T. M. Blaine, A. Wagenaar, and D. J. Hennrikus. 1998. The Effects of Community Policies to Reduce Youth Access to Tobacco. *American Journal of Public Health* 88(8):1193–1198.

Fox, R. C. 1979. The Medicalization and Demedicalization of American Society. In *Essays in Medical Sociology.* New York: Wiley.

Freeman, J., ed. 1983. *Societal Movements of the Sixties and Seventies.* New York: Longman.

Friedman, K. M. 1975. *Public Policy and the Smoking-Health Controversy.* Lexington, MA: Lexington Books.

Fritschler, A. L. 1989. *Smoking and Politics.* 4th ed. Englewood Cliffs, NJ: Prentice-Hall.

Gamson, W. 1990 *The Strategy of Social Protest.* 2d ed. Belmont, CA: Wadsworth.

Garfinkel, L. 1988. E. Cuyler Hammond. Sc.D. (1912–1986). *Ca—A Cancer Journal for Clintonians* 38(1):23–27.

Giovino, G. A., M. W. Schooley, B.-P. Zhu, J. H. Chrismon, S. L. Tomar, J. P. Peddicord, R. K. Merritt, C. G. Huston, and M. P. Erikson. 1994. Surveillance for Selected Tobacco Use Behaviors—United States, 1900–1994. *Morbidity and Mortality Weekly Report* 18 November, 1–43.

Glantz, S. A. 1996. Preventing Tobacco Use—The Youth Access Trap. *American Journal of Public Health* 86(2): 156–157.

Glantz, S. A., J. Slade, L. Bero, and P. Hanauer. 1996. *The Cigarette Papers.* Berkeley: University of California Press.

Glaser, B. G., and A. L. Strauss. 1967. *The Discovery of Grounded Theory.* New York: Aldine de Gruyter.

Glendon, M. A. 1991. *Rights Talk.* New York: Free Press.

Glick, S. 1998. "Smart Guns" Are a Dumb Idea. *Los Angeles Times,* 4 September, B9.

Gorovitz, E.1996. California Dreamin': The Myth of State Preemption of Local Firearm Regulation. *University of San Francisco Law Review* 30(2):395–426.

Gouin, C. L. 1975. Nonsmokers and Social Action. *Smoking and Health 2* (Proceedings of the 1975ACS/NCI Conference). DHEW Pub no (NIH)77-1413:353–356.

———. 1995. Interview by author. Baltimore, MD. 3 November.

Gusfield, J. R. 1963. *Symbolic Crusade: Status Politics and the American Temperance Movement.* Urbana: University of Illinois Press.

———. 1981. *The Culture of Public Problems: Drinking Driving and the Symbolic Order.* Chicago: University of Chicago Press.

———. 1993. The Social Symbolism of Smoking and Health. In *Smoking Policy: Law, Politics, and Culture,* ed. R. L. Rabin and S.D. Sugarman. New York: Oxford University Press.

Hammond, E. C., and D. Horn. 1954. The Relationship between Human Smoking Habits and Death Rates: A Follow-up Study of 187,766 Men. *Journal of the American Medical Association* 155(15):1316–1327.

Hanauer, P., G. Barr, and S. Glantz. 1986. *Legislative Approaches to a Smoke-Free Society.* Berkeley, CA: American Nonsmokers' Rights Foundation.

Hilts, P. J. 1996. *Smokescreen: The Truth behind the Tobacco-Industry Cover-up.* New York: Addison-Wesley.

Hunink, M. G. M., L. Goldman, A. Tosteson, M. A. M. Mittleman, P. A. Goodman, L. W.

Williams, J. Tsevat, and M. C. Weistein. 1997. The Recent Decline in Mortality from Coronary Heart Disease, 1980–1990: The Effect of Secular Trends in Risk Factors and Treatment. *Journal of the American Medical Association* 277(7):535–542.

Jacobson, P. D., J. Wasserman, and K. Raube. 1992. *The Political Evolution of Anti-smoking Legislation.* Santa Monica, CA: Rand.

Jenkins, C. C. 1983. Resource Mobilization Theory and the Study of Social Movements. *Annual Review of Sociology* 9:527–553.

Karlson, T. A., and S. W. Hargarten. 1997. *Reducing Firearm Injury and Death.* New Brunswick, NJ: Rutgers University Press.

Kellerman, A. L., and D. R. Reay. 1986. Protection or Peril? An Analysis of Firearm-Related Deaths in the Home. *New England Journal of Medicine* 314(24):1557–1560.

Kellerman, A. L., F. P. Rivera, G. Somes, D. T. Reay, J. Francisco, J. G. Banton, J. Prodzinski, C. Fligner, and B. B. Hackman. 1992. Suicide in the Home in Relation to Gun Ownership. *New England Journal of Medicine* 329(15):1084–1091.

Kellerman, A. L., F. P. Rivera, N. B. Rushforth, J. G. Blanton, D. T. Reay, J. T. Francisco, A. B. Locci, J. Prodzinski, B. B. Hackman, and G. Somes. 1993. Gun Ownership as a Risk Factor for Homicide in the Home. *New England Journal of Medicine* 329(15):1084–1091.

Kingdon, J. W. 1995. *Agendas, Alternatives, and Public Policies.* 2d ed. New York: HarperCollins.

Kleck, G. 1984. The Relationship between Gun Ownership Levels and Rates of Violence in the United States. In *Firearms and Violence: Issues of Public Policy,* ed. D. B. Kates Jr. Cambridge, MA: Ballinger.

Kluger, R. 1996. *Ashes to Ashes: America's Hundred-Year Cigarette War, the Public Health, and the Unabashed Triumph of Philip Morris.* New York: Knopf.

Knowles, J. H. 1977. The Responsibility of the Individual. *Daedalus* 106(1):57–80.

Koop, C. E. 1989. Preface. In *Reducing the Health Consequences of Smoking: Twenty-five Years of Progress.* A Report of the Surgeon General. DHHS Publication no. (CDC) 89-8411.

Koop, C. E., and G. C. Lundberg. 1992. Violence in America: A Public Health Emergency. *Journal of the American Medical Association* 267(22):3075–3076.

Kriesi, H., ed. 1995. *New Social Movements in Western Europe: A Comparative Analysis.* Minneapolis: University of Minnesota Press.

Kunreuther, H. C., and T. Linneruth, eds. 1983. *Risk Analysis and Decision Processes.* Berlin: Springer Verlag.

Lalonde, M. 1974. *A New Perspective on the Health of Canadians.* Ottawa: Ministry of National Health and Welfare.

LaPierre, W. 1994. *Guns, Crime, and Freedom.* Washington, DC: Regnery Press.

Legislation Works on Many Fronts to Restrict Children's Access to Guns. 1998. *Nation's Health* 47(7):1.

Lofland, J. 1996. *Social Movement Organizations: A Guide to Research on Insurgent Realities.* New York: Aldine de Gruyter.

Lott, J. R., and D. B. Mustard. 1997. Crime, Deterrence, and Right-to-Carry Concealed Handguns. *Journal of Legal Studies* 26:1–68.

McAdam, D. 1982. *Political Process and the Development of Black Insurgency, 1930–1970.* Chicago: University of Chicago Press.

———. 1994. Culture and Social Movement. In *New Social Movements,* ed. E. Larana, H. Johnston, and J. R. Gusfield. Philadelphia: Temple University Press.

McAdam, D., J. D. McCarthy, and M. N. Zald, eds. 1996. *Comparative Perspectives on Social Movements.* New York: Cambridge University Press.

McAneny, L. 1993. Americans Tell Congress: Pass Brady Bill, Other Tough Gun Laws. *Gallup Poll Monthly.* March, 2–5.

McCarthy, J. D. 1996. Constraints and Opportunities in Adopting, Adapting, and Inventing. In *Comparative Perspectives on Social Movements,* ed. D. McAdam, J. D. McCarthy, and M. N. Zald. New York: Cambridge University Press.

McCarthy, J. D., and M. N. Zald. 1977. Resource Mobilization and Social Movements: A Partial Theory. *American Journal of Sociology* 82(6):1212–1241.

McKenzie, M. N. 1998. Earning It: So Don't Even Think about Smoking Here. *New York Times,* 29 December, C13.

Mechanic, D. 1993. Social Research in Health and the American Sociopolitical Context: The Changing Fortunes of Medical Sociology. *Social Science and Medicine* 36(2):95–102.

Meier, B. 1998. Court Rules FDA Lacks Authority to Limit Tobacco. 1998. *New York Times,* 15 August, A1.

Meyer, D. S., and S. Staggenborg. 1996. Movements, Countermovements, and the Structure of Political Opportunity. *American Journal of Sociology* 101(6):1628–1660.

Moore, M. H., D. Prothrow-Stith, B. Guyer, and H. Spivak. 1994. Violence and Intentional Injuries: Criminal Justice and Public Health Perspectives on an Urgent National Problem. In *Understanding and Preventing Violence, Vol. 4, Consequences and Control,* ed. A. J. Reiss Jr. and J. A. Roth. Washington, DC: National Academy.

Nathanson, C. A. 1991. *Dangerous Passage: The Social Control of Sexuality in Women's Adolescence.* Philadelphia: Temple University Press.

———. 1996. Disease Prevention as Social Change: Toward a Theory of Public Health. *Population and Development Review* 22(6):609–637.

Nathanson, C. A., Y. J. Kim, and N.-Y. Weng. 1996. Hazards of Smoking: Smoking Cessation over Time among the Medical Elite. Poster presented at the annual meeting of the Population Association of America, 9 May, New Orleans.

National Opinion Research Center (NORC). 1997. *1996 Gun Policy Survey: Research Findings.* Chicago: University of Chicago Press.

Neuberger, M. B. 1963. *Smokescreen: Tobacco and the Public Welfare.* Englewood Cliffs, NJ: Prentice-Hall.

Newport, F., and L. Saad. 1993. Drugs Seen as Root Cause of Crime in the U.S. *Gallup Poll Monthly,* October, 33.

Norr, R. 1952. Cancer by the Carton. *Reader's Digest* 61 (December):7–8.

Oberschall, A. 1993. *Social Movements: Ideologies, Interests, and Identities.* New Brunswick, NJ: Transaction Publishers.

Pertschuk, M. 1986. *Giant Killers.* New York: Norton.

Pfeiffer, J. E. 1965. A Visit with Cuyler Hammond. *Think* 31 (March–April): 11–14.

Quadagno, J. 1992. Social Movements and State Transformation: Labor Unions and Racial Conflict in the War on Poverty. *American Sociological Review* 57(5):616–634.

Rigotti, N. A., J. R. DiFranza, Y. C. Chang, T. Tisdale, B. Kemp, and D. E. Singer. 1997. The Effect of Enforcing Tobacco-Sales Laws on Adolescents' Access to Tobacco and Smoking Behavior. *New England Journal of Medicine* 337(5):1044–1051.

Rosenbaum, D. E. 1998. Senate Drops Tobacco Bill with '98 Revival Unlikely; Clinton Lashes out at GOP. *New York Times,* 18 June, A1.

Royal College of Physicians of London. 1962. *Smoking and Health.* London: Pitman Medical.

Saltzman, L. E., J. A. Mercy, P. W. O'Carroll, M. L. Rosenberg, and P. Rhodes. 1992. Weapon Involvement and Injury Outcomes in Family and Intimate Assaults. *Journal of the American Medical Association* 267(22):3043–3047.

Schwartz, M., and S. Paul. 1992. Resource Mobilization versus the Mobilization of People: Why Consensus Movements Cannot Be Instruments of Social Change. In *Frontiers in Social Movement Theory,* ed. A. D. Morris and C. M. Mueller. New Haven, CT: Yale University Press.

Scott, W. R. 1994. Institutions and Organizations: Toward a Theoretical Synthesis. In *Institutional Environments and Organizations,* ed. W. R. Scott, J. Meyer, and Associates. Thousand Oaks, CA: Sage.

Seelye, K. Q. 1998. National Rifle Association Is Turning to World Stage to Fight Gun Control. *New York Times,* 2 April, A12.

Shapiro, T. M. 1985. Structure and Process in Social Movement Strategy: The Movement against Sterilization Abuse. *Research in Social Movements, Conflicts, and Change* 8:87–108.

Singer, E., and P. M. Endreny. 1993. *Reporting on Risk.* New York: Russell Sage Foundation.

Skinner, D. 1998. For Your Own Good. *The Public Interest,* summer, 117–121.

Slade, J., S. A. Glantz, D. E. Barnes, L. Bero, P. Hanauer, and J. Slade. 1995. Nicotine and Addiction: The Brown and Williamson Documents. *Journal of the American Medical Association* 274(3):225–233.

Snow, D. A., and R. D. Benford. 1992. Master Frames and Cycles of Protest. In *Frontiers in Social Movement Theory,* ed. A. D. Morris and C. M. Mueller. New Haven, CT: Yale University Press.

Spitzer, R. J. 1995. *The Politics of Gun Control.* Chatham, NJ: Chatham House.

Staggenborg, S. 1991. *The Pro-Choice Movement: Organization and Activism in the Abortion Conflict.* New York: Oxford University Press.

Starr, C. 1969. Social Benefit versus Technological Risk: What Is Our Society Willing to Pay? *Science* 165(3899):1232–1238.

Starr, P. 1982. *The Social Transformation of American Medicine: The Rise of a Sovereign Profession and the Making of a Vast Industry.* New York: Basic Books.

Steinfeld, J. L. 1983. Women and Children Last? Attitudes toward Cigarette Smoking and Nonsmokers' Rights, 1971. *New York State Journal of Medicine* 83(13):1257–1258.

Sugarmann, J. 1992. *National Rifle Association: Money, Firepower, and Fear.* Washington, DC: National Press Books.

———. 1997. The Politics of Gun Control (book review). *The New England Journal of Medicine* 336(1):74.

Tarrow, S. G. 1994. *Power in Management.* Cambridge: Cambridge University Press.

Taubes, G. 1995. Epidemiology Faces Its Limits. *Science* 269(5221):164.

Teret, S. P., and G. J. Wintermute. 1993. Policies to Prevent Firearm Injuries. *Health Affairs* 12(4):96–108.

Tilly, C. 1986. *The Contentious French.* Cambridge: Harvard University Press.

Tonso, W. R. 1984. Social Problems and Stagecraft: Gun Control as a Case in Point. In *Firearms and Violence: Issues of Public Policy,* ed. D. B. Kates Jr. Cambridge, MA: Ballinger.

Troyer, R. J., and G. E. Markle. 1983. *Cigarettes: The Battle over Smoking.* New Brunswick, NJ: Rutgers University Press.

U.S. Department of Agriculture (USDA). 1995–96. *National Agricultural Statistics Service: Agricultural Statistics, 1995–96.* Washington, DC: U.S. Government Printing Office. Table 129, p. 11–38.

———. 1998. *National Agricultural Statistics Service: Agricultural Statistics 1998.* Washington, DC: U.S. Government Printing Office. Table 2–50, p. 11–36.

U.S. Department of Commerce, Bureau of the Census. 1980. *Summary of Economic Characteristics.* Washington, DC: U.S. Government Printing Office.

U.S. Department of Health and Human Services (U.S. DHHS). 1988. *The Health Consequences of Smoking: Nicotine Addiction.* A Report of the Surgeon General. Rockville, MD: U.S. Department of Health and Human Services Publication no. (CDC) 88-8406.

———. 1989. *Reducing the Health Consequences of Smoking: Twenty-five years of Progress.* A Report of the Surgeon General. Rockville, MD: U.S. Department of Health and Human Services Publication no. (CDC) 89-8411.

———. 1990. *Smoking and Health: A National Status Report: A Report to Congress.* 2d ed. Rockville, MD: U.S. Department of Health and Human Services Publication no. (CDC) 87-8396, rev. 2/90.

———. 1991. *Strategies to Control Tobacco Use in the United States: A Blueprint for Public Health in the 1990s.* Rockville, MD: NIH Publication no. 92-3316 (October).

———. 1995. Analysis Regarding FDA's Jurisdiction over Nicotine-Containing Cigarettes and Smokeless Tobacco Products: Notice. *Federal Register* 60–454.

U.S. Department of Health and Human Services, National Institutes of Health (U.S. DHHS, NIH). 1993. *Major Local Tobacco Control Ordinances in the United States.* Bethesda, MD: NIH Publication no. 93-3532.

U.S. Department of Health, Education, and Welfare (U.S. DHEW). 1956. Tobacco Smoking Patterns in the United States. *Public Health Monograph No. 15.* Washington, DC: U.S. Government Printing Office.

———. 1964. *Smoking and Health: Report of the Advisory Committee to the Surgeon General of the Public Health Service.* Washington, DC: Public Health Service Publication no. 1103.

———. 1979. *Healthy People: The Surgeon General's Report on Health Promotion and Disease Prevention.* Washington, DC: U.S. Department of Health, Education, and Welfare, Office of the Assistant Secretary for Health, and the Surgeon General.

U.S. Occupational Safety and Health Administration (U.S. OSHA). 1995. *Public Hearing on the Proposed Standard for Indoor Air Quality, 20 January.* Washington, DC: U.S. Government Printing Office.

The Ventilator. 1971. March, 1.

Walker, J. L. Jr. 1991. *Mobilizing Interest Groups in America: Patrons, Professions, and Social Movements.* Ann Arbor: University of Michigan Press.

Warner, K. E. 1981. Cigarette Smoking in the 1970s: The Impact of the Antismoking Campaign. *Science* 211(4483):729–731.

Wayne, L. 1997. Gun Makers Learn from Tobacco Fight. *New York Times,* 18 December, A14.

Webster, D. W., J. S. Vernick, J. Ludwig, and K. J. Lester. 1997. Flawed Gun Policy Research Could Endanger Public Safety. *American Journal of Public Health* 87(6):918–921.

Wills, G. 1995. To Keep and Bear Arms. *New York Review of Books,* 21 September, 62–73.

———. 1995. To Keep and Bear Arms: An Exchange. *New York Review of Books,* 16 November, 61–63.

Wolinsky, H., and T. Brune. 1994. *The Serpent on the Staff.* New York: Putnam.

Wynder, E. L., and E. A. Graham. 1950. Tobacco Smoking as a Possible Etiologic Factor in Bronchiogenic Carcinoma. A Study of 684 Proved Cases. *Journal of the American Medical Association* 143(4):329–336.

Wynne, B. 1987. *Risk Management and Hazardous Waste: Implementation and the Dialectics of Credibility.* Berlin: Springer Verlag.

Zimring, F. E., and G. Hawkins. 1987. *The Citizen's Guide to Gun Control.* New York: Macmillan.

NOTES

Alan Brandt, Mayer Zald, Mark Peterson. and an anonymous reviewer read the manuscript in various stages and made extremely helpful comments; their important contributions are gratefully acknowledged as well. Finally, I would like to express particular thanks to Laury Oaks, currently assistant professor in the Women's Studies Program at the University of California–Santa Barbara, who carried out much of the research on the gun control movement reported in this article. Her assistance was, in every respect, invaluable.

1.   A detailed description of these sources is available from the author.

2.   A fully up-to-date chronology would include a fourth phase, "demonizing the tobacco industry," beginning arguably in 1988 when the industry was publicly attacked on national television by a representative of the American Cancer Society.

3.   An analysis of the timing of smoking decline among physicians during the period 1948–1993 demonstrates very clearly the impact of these publications on the behavior of their professional audience (Nathanson et al. 1996).

4.   While I have dated the struggle for regulation from the passage of the first national tobacco legislation in 1965, the effort to regulate cigarette advertising began well before 1965, as documented by a major protagonist—Senator Maurine B. Neuberger (D-OR)—in her book, *Smokescreen: Tobacco and the Public Welfare,* published in 1963.

5.   The Surgeon General was also required to issue legislative recommendations. There is little evidence of these recommendations in the reports. Kluger states that recommendations to ban smoking in enclosed public places inserted by Surgeon General Jesse Steinfeld were "regularly removed by Nixon's Office of Management and Budget" (1996: 366).

6.   For example, a major recent attempt at congressional regulation was defeated in June 1998 (Rosenbaum 1998).

7.   The FDA's authority to regulate nicotine was recently overturned by a federal appeals court, leaving the issue of its powers unsettled, for the time being at least (Meier 1998).

8.   The Interagency Council on Smoking and Health, formed in 1964, was a loose grouping of public and private organizations interested in the smoking and health issue.

9.   Interviews for this project were completed during the spring and summer of 1995, before and immediately after the Oklahoma City bombing. A recent review of Robert J. Spitzer's book, *The Politics of Gun Control,* by Josh Sugarmann, director of the Violence Policy Center, suggests that the Oklahoma City bombing was a major watershed event energizing the gun control movement (Sugarmann 1997). Recent schoolyard killings have led to the introduction in Congress of new regulatory legislation addressing children's access to guns (Legislation Works 1998; Butterfield 1998).

10.   As summarized by Spitzer, the bill "banned interstate shipment of firearms . . . and ammunition to private individuals; prohibited the sale of guns to minors, drug addicts, mental incompetents, and convicted felons; strengthened licensing and record-keeping requirements for gun dealers and collectors; extended federal regulation and taxation to 'destructive devices' such as land mines, bombs, hand grenades, and the like; increased penalties for those who used guns in the commission of a crime covered by federal law; and banned the importation of foreign-made surplus firearms, except those appropriate for sporting purposes" (Spitzer 1995: 145).

11.   The NRA's estimate is accepted by Spitzer and other authorities.

12.   The referendum fight was highly important in mobilizing antigun advocates in Maryland, including the police.

13.   These conflicts are colorfully described by Osha Gray Davidson (1993: 85–127).

14.   The problem of outcome measurement is particularly troublesome in the case of gun control for several reasons. First, there is disagreement among advocates about the

movement's goals; second, the involvement of the public health community is relatively recent; and third, the movement itself is a moving target, evolving in several directions simultaneously. In addition, measures of success have been selected, in part, for their comparability across the two movements. As a result, some measures that might work to the detriment of the smoking/tobacco control movement—for example, success in achieving tobacco tax increases or in curbing cigarette advertising—have not been used.

15.   Unfortunately, current smoking prevalence data are grouped by educational level rather than by occupation or income (with the exception of poverty level status, which is a fairly crude income index). Data on smoking prevalence by occupation in 1955 published by the National Center for Health Statistics show remarkably little variation in prevalence by occupation: among men, between 67 and 70 percent of white collar workers and between 69 and 74 percent of blue collar workers reported current, regular, smoking. A much smaller percentage of women smoked, but there was an equal absence of variation by occupation (U.S. DHEW 1956).

16.   These are not, of course, the only relevant attitudes and beliefs. They are, however, the ones for which data are available. In evaluating the data to be presented in this section, it is important to be aware that the exact wording of the questions about cigarettes varied in the different surveys carried out by different organizations. Some of the apparent variation in attitudes over time may be explained by these differences. The data on guns are from surveys conducted by the Gallup organization and NORC, using the same question wording.

17.   The NORC report from which these data are taken argues that the decline in household gun ownership "reflects the changing lifestyles of Americans. Traditional rural life in general and hunting in particular have declined during recent decades" (NORC 1997: 13). Consistent with this interpretation, the decline in household ownership is entirely attributable to the smaller percentage of households owning long guns; household ownership of handguns has increased slightly, from 20.3 percent in 1973 to 24.8 percent in 1996.

18.   Despite some claims to the contrary, there is no evidence of increased firearm ownership among women (NORC 1997: 14).

19.   My evaluation of public support for gun control is less positive than that of several recent books on this topic (Spitzer 1995; Davidson 1993). Spitzer opens his discussion of public opinion on gun control with the statement, "The initial and most important fact about public opinion on gun control has been its remarkable consistency in support of greater governmental control of guns" and comments extensively on the "opinion-policy gap" (i.e., the disjunction between popular support and the failure to enact stronger antigun laws) (1995: 118ff.). Although support for the Brady bill, assault weapons bans and permit and registration laws is extremely high, examination of a wider range of public opinion, in particular opinion about the dangers of guns, points to a far more ambivalent set of public beliefs about gun risks than about risks from tobacco.

20.   "The vast majority of gun laws exist at state and local levels," as Spitzer points out, but these laws are often more remarkable for what they allow than for what they prevent. Furthermore, "states and cities with tougher gun laws find them at least partly neutralized by the ease with which guns can be transported from areas with weak gun laws" (Spitzer 1995: 6). Restaurant and workplace cigarette smoking regulations are less easily evaded by crossing state lines.

21.   I have adopted Amenta and colleagues' argument (1994) that collective benefits are the best measure of movement success. Employing the acceptance criteria would give

mixed results for both movements. While the legitimacy of smoking/tobacco and gun control policy positions is recognized, few of the original movement organizers appear as current spokespersons for these positions. This is particularly true of smoking/tobacco control: attorneys general are not social movement representatives.

22.   The selection process and the background leading up to the committee's formation are described in many other sources and will not be repeated here (U.S. DHEW 1964; U.S. DHHS 1989; Brandt 1992; Kluger 1996).

23.   An important aspect of the Surgeon General's report, as Brandt points out, was that it marked the beginning of a new role for epidemiologists in the construction of risk (1992: 67).

24.   In July 1995, the journal *Science* published an article with the title, "Epidemiology Faces Its Limits," that began, "The news about health risks comes thick and fast these days, and it seems almost constitutionally contradictory" (Taubes 1995). *Science*'s primary concern was the public, not the scientific response to a deluge of "contradictory advice."

25.   The recent construction of cigarettes as an addictive drug has contributed to the federal government's assertion, through the FDA, of both ownership of and political responsibility for the smoking/tobacco control issue. Whether the FDA's authority will be sustained in court remains uncertain.

26.   The history and politics of police realignment are complex and beyond the scope of this article (see Davidson 1993 and Anderson 1996 for detailed accounts). However, I will refer to this realignment again in the section of the article discussing political opportunities.

27.   Social movement entrepreneurs (and other interested actors) portray risks in what they know to be culturally resonant terms, thereby reinforcing, in circular fashion, preexisting cultural preconceptions about the relevant dimensions of risk.

28.   Based on quantitative analysis of stories in a range of media (major newspapers, television, news magazines) in 1960 and 1984, Eleanor Singer and Phyllis M. Endreny report that "stories about alcohol and tobacco disproportionately blamed victims for risks associated with these hazards. In the case of tobacco, victims also appear to be disproportionately held responsible for prevention. . . . Thus, judging from the evidence of these stories, smoking was seen primarily as an activity within the individual's control, whereas prevention of the risks of drinking was seen, in the majority of stories, as requiring government intervention through the imposition of laws and the like" (1993: 117).

29.   A series of oral history interviews was conducted in 1990 with high-level staff and officials of the ACS. The ACS national office was generous in giving me access to these interviews. I quote from these interviews but do not identify the speakers by name.

30.   The civil rights movement is widely credited with providing an ideological template for the subsequent "cycle of protest" in the late 1960s and 1970s (Snow and Benford 1992: 133; McAdam 1994).

31.   Brandt comments perceptively on the social and cultural meanings attached to the different labels for other people's smoking: " 'Passive smoking' contrasted with active smoking; 'secondhand smoke' contained the ominous implication that someone else had used it first; 'involuntary smoking' indicated that the practice of smoking was indeed a voluntary act. And, of course, 'environmental tobacco smoke' or ETS . . . invited public concern as an 'environmental hazard' " (1995: 8).

32.   These fears were confirmed by a 1978 poll commissioned by the Tobacco Institute from the Roper Organization. Roper's report concluded that "the nonsmokers' rights movement was the single greatest threat to the viability of the tobacco industry" (cited in Hanauer, Barr, and Glantz 1986: 3). Shortly afterwards, industry counterpropaganda began to emphasize "smokers' rights."

33.   Calculations published in *Science* suggest that the threshold for public acceptance of "involuntary" risks is roughly 1,000 times less than the threshold for "voluntary" risks: "We are loathe to let others do unto us what we happily do to ourselves" (Starr 1969: 1235).

34.   Scientific controversy over the health effects of passive smoking is ongoing. In a recent article, Deborah Barnes and Lisa Bero report, based on an analysis of 106 review articles, that "the only factor associated with concluding that passive smoking is not harmful was whether an author was affiliated with the tobacco industry" (Barnes and Bero 1998: 1566).

35.   A favorite tactic of the early antismoking campaigners was to call attention to the hypocrisy of smoking by environmentalists, health crusaders (e.g., board members of groups such as the ACS and the ALA) and physicians.

36.   The underlying reasons for AFL-CIO opposition to federal regulation of smoking in the workplace are, of course, broader than this brief reference would suggest. I will refer to this opposition again when I discuss the political opportunities that have favored and impeded the movement for smoking/tobacco control.

37.   It is unclear to what extent this linkage is accepted by the general public. It is pervasive in public health circles, as evidenced, for example, by a marked increase over time in the number of articles in the *American Journal of Public Health* associating tobacco with alcohol and drugs and by the naming of an American Public Health Association (APHA) conference section "Alcohol, tobacco, and other drugs." It is popular in legal arguments against the tobacco industry (e.g., Brief for the State of Maryland at 52, *State of Maryland v. Philip Morris et al.*) and in antismoking messages focused on the industry's alleged targeting of children.

38.   The fact that medical and public health circles knew that nicotine was an addictive drug has clearly been far less powerful than the fact that the tobacco industries knew it as well. The companies' knowledge is critical to litigation against them, but the discovery of their knowledge had an impact beyond mere lawyerly concerns, perhaps akin to the discovery of Oedipus' parentage in Sophocles' play.

39.   "Protect our children from the tobacco companies" was a message sponsored by a public service announcement from the American Cancer Society broadcast on CNN in March 1996. This message is startling in evoking widespread fears in the early twentieth century of children being kidnapped into "white slavery" (Nathanson 1991:125).

40.   During 1996, antismoking advertising messages in the print and television media sponsored by private sources appeared to focus exclusively on the hazards of smoking to children. The recently established National Center for Tobacco-Free Kids, funded by the ACS and the Robert Wood Johnson Foundation, is a major source for these messages. Recent action at the federal level to require identification for cigarette purchasers under the age of twenty-seven is targeted at teenagers.

41.   The industry was almost invisible, but not quite. In the same year that *Healthy People* appeared, Secretary of HEW Joseph Califano referred in the Surgeon General's report on smoking and health to the millions of dollars spent on cigarette advertising

every year and to the existence of a "vested interest" in smoking. I have found no parallel references in subsequent Surgeon Generals' reports, however, and according to Richard Kluger, Secretary Califano was forced to resign as a result of his vigorous antitobacco campaign (Kluger 1996: 465).

42. Criminogenic circumstances were blamed by Mark H. Moore et al.: "Factors influencing individual incidents and aggregate levels of violence include (a) the availability and use of criminogenic commodities (such as guns, drugs, and alcohol); (b) the density of criminogenic situations (such as ongoing unresolved conflicts); and (c) a variety of cultural factors that help to justify and encourage violence" (1994: 170). These authors were careful to present their perspective as complementary to, not competitive with, the "criminal justice" perspective. The concept *criminogenic,* however, constructs causality in terms far removed from the world of offenders and perpetrators inhabited by police, prosecutors, and defense lawyers. Causes of crime become equivalent to causes of disease, implicitly beyond individual control and within the domain of medical (or at least public health) science. Gun design has been a particular focus of the Johns Hopkins Center for Gun Policy and Research, led by Steven Teret. Hazards of guns in the home have been examined in numbers of articles published by the *Journal of the American Medical Association* and the *New England Journal of Medicine* (e.g., Kellerman and Reay 1986; Kellerman et al. 1992; Kellerman et al. 1993; Saltzman et al. 1992).

43. This characterization has an exact parallel in advocacy literature on teenage pregnancy: mothers aged fifteen to nineteen are invariably described as "children having children."

44. Research results to date are conflicting (Rigotti et al. 1997; Forster et al. 1998), and the policy focus on children is controversial among tobacco control advocates (Glantz 1996).

45. Glendon evaluates rights discourse in negative terms, as being absolutist and inimical to reasoned dialogue. I would argue that rights discourse has been the principal strategy through which historically marginalized groups have obtained government protection against those who would deprive them of their rights. At issue is not the discourse but the uses to which it is put.

46. The statement that the gun control movement lacked a strong grass-roots base is based on interviews with gun control advocates during 1995 and was accurate at that time. There has been a very recent upsurge of local activism in California leading to local legislation. This activism follows the path pioneered by smoking/tobacco control activists in California and, indeed, is led by many of the same individuals, who have moved over from the smoking/tobacco control movement to the gun control movement.

47. The smoking/tobacco control scene shifted markedly in the last two years with the entry in force of state attorneys general to bring suit against the tobacco industry. These suits were settled in November 1998 by an agreement between individual states and the tobacco industry. Neither the federal government nor the smoking/tobacco control movement participated directly in this agreement. My story ends at the point when this major shift began. I have not included government as part of the movement core. I have already described the government's role in creating the scientific case for smoking as a credible threat. In the movement's early days, agencies of the government were more often targets than major players. The change, again, has been very recent.

48. Two groups that might have been expected to play major roles in the smoking/control drama but have not are the APHA and the AMA. While the relative inactivity of public health organizations has been noted by others (e.g., Jacobson, Wasserman,

and Raube 1992), no analyses of the APHA's role in the smoking/tobacco wars have been published, and I have not undertaken such an analysis beyond what is stated here. Consequently, it is unclear precisely why there was relatively little public health attention to what has now become a major public health issue. While Surgeon General Jesse Steinfeld played an important role in energizing and legitimizing the nonsmokers' rights movement, he appears to have had little impact on organized public health activities. Such activities are, of course, heavily dependent on federal, state, and local government funding, which may help account for this inactivity. A scathing analysis of the AMA's silence on smoking/tobacco control has been published by Wolinsky and Brune (1994).

49.   Ironically, a prime mover in this reorganization was Mary Lasker, whose husband, Albert Lasker, made at least some of his fortune in advertising from cigarettes (Kluger 1996: 76). As Kluger describes it, the Laskers brought in other prominent business leaders and, in addition, made use of their access to advertising talent and of their contacts in the media (e.g., *Reader's Digest*) to promote the American Cancer Society (renamed—originally the American Society for the Control of Cancer) both as an important humanitarian cause and as "smart business" (Kluger 1996: 143). In its volunteer recruitment policies immediately following the reorganization, the ACS very deliberately targeted "influential persons" (ACS 1948), and from this time forward influential business people played major roles in the ACS. By its constitution, the ACS board of directors is composed of half laypersons (primarily business) and half physicians (all volunteers): the society's leadership is divided between a physician and a layperson.

50.   By way of comparison, the total budget of the ALA during the same period never rose above $92 million, although in 1960 (the earliest date for which I have ALA data) the budgets of the two associations were close to equal.

51.   E. Cuyler Hammond, the study director and head of the ACS Department of Statistical Research, joined the ACS in 1946. Hammond was already a well-trained and experienced epidemiologist when he became the ACS's chief statistician. Evidence suggests that he played a major role in focusing the society's attention on the marked rise in lung cancer mortality rates (Garfinkel 1988; Kluger 1996).

52.   The comments by Peter Jacobson, Jeffrey Wasserman. and Kristiana Raube (1992), which refer to the late 1980s and early 1990s, suggest that the relatively conservative posture of the health voluntaries remains, despite their current more active involvement as lobbyists in Washington.

53.   Between 1960 and 1975 the lung cancer mortality rates of white males born between 1901 and 1910 quadrupled: the rates for white males born between 1911 and 1920 increased by a factor of eight (U.S. DHHS 1991: 92).

54.   Of the seven early (i.e., became active in the 1970s or, in one case, the early 1980s) nonsmokers' rights activists we interviewed, three had close relatives who died from causes the activists attributed to smoking, and two had previously been active in related social movement or public interest organizations.

55.   GASP's success was so great that in 1973 certain leaders of the Lung Association of Southern Maryland became concerned that the tail was wagging the dog and a report was generated recommending "disassociation" of GASP from the local association. The issue was resolved and dissociation did not occur (although relationships became more formalized), but the episode is evidence of the remarkable public response to GASP'S message.

56.   In 1981, California GASP became Californians for Nonsmokers' Rights and in 1986, Americans for Nonsmoker's Rights (ANR). In an anniversary issue, the ANR newsletter commented on the shift from state to local priorities: "The experience of having been burned twice at the state level while succeeding locally [in Berkeley in 1977 and in Los Altos in 1979] taught the nonsmokers' rights activists a great deal. They learned that the tobacco industry, while wealthier and more powerful at the state level, just wasn't able to thwart our efforts locally" (ANR 1996).

57.   Gouin was not alone in her perceptions either of the fact or of the nature of movement evolution. Her remarks were echoed by several other early activists we interviewed.

58.   The executive director of the Coalition to Stop Handgun Violence (CSGV) describes his constituency as follows: "It's still mostly older, college-educated people living in urban areas on the east coast, west coast, and Chicago. Primarily Jewish probably. I mean we just fit the standard profile in the direct mail [marketing]: college-educated, third generation, living in a suburb or urban area."

59.   My point is not that these individuals cannot be mobilized at all—Louis Farrakhan has clearly demonstrated otherwise—it is that they are unlikely to be mobilized by the gun control movement as presently constituted. This point is strikingly illustrated by the following comments from a gun control activist: "There's an organization in the city called 'Don't Smoke the Brothers—Cease Fire.' And they were founded by Farrakhan. Now they do good work. Yes, they do. But they also promote hate against certain organizations. I don't want that. And that was a very difficult decision because there are things that they do that are of value. But they were not willing to modify their language so that they weren't offending anybody other than Black."

60.   The "cycle" this activist describes appears clearly in data from our analysis of *New York Times* coverage of the gun control issue. The number of articles jumped from forty-two in 1980 to sixty-two in 1981 following the Reagan and other shootings; it dropped to between sixteen and thirty-nine in the period from 1982 to 1988, jumped again to seventy-six in 1989 following the Stockton, California schoolyard shooting, and dropped again to forty-six in 1990.

61.   Recently, however, the prospective tobacco settlement led to intense conflict within the smoking/tobacco control movement between proponents who believed it was the best deal they could get and opponents who believed it was a sellout.

62.   The consensus of observers, both scholarly and nonacademic, is that the 1965 cigarette labeling act was a victory for the tobacco industry and that health groups were weakened by "their failure to agree on a plan of action" (Fritschler 1989: 107; I infer that this is a reference to the nonparticipation of the AMA) and by other organizational limitations (Friedman 1975; Fritschler 1989; Pertschuk 1986). While I agree with the second point, I think the first point underestimates the role of even weak congressional action in legitimating subsequent antismoking protest.

63.   The complex and shifting relationships among actors in the smoking/tobacco arena do not fall readily into existing social movement taxonomies (see, e.g., McCarthy 1996). While the nonsmokers' rights movement clearly qualifies as a "mobilizing structure," it is less clear that the health voluntaries can be usefully so described; it is even less clear for the legal firms now engaged in large-scale litigation against the tobacco industry. Perhaps the concept of organizational field (defined by Scott [1994: 71] as "communities of organizations that participate in the same meaning system, are

defined by similar symbolic processes, and are subject to common regulatory processes" is applicable, particularly to the movement in its current configuration. Indeed, the movement's shift from mobilizing structure to organizational field is among the major changes I describe here.

64. In an interview published in September 1998, the *New York Times* describes a Kentucky tobacco grower as reserving his "deepest scorn . . . for the four big cigarette companies, whom he accused of profiteering and price manipulation. It is they 'who give the farmer a real licking, year in and year out' " (Apple 1998).

65. In the year prior to this writing (November 1998), events in the smoking/tobacco control arena moved at breakneck pace. Through mid-June, the tobacco industry appeared to be continuing its downward spiral: a strong antitobacco bill was introduced in Congress and the press regularly referred to the industry as a "pariah." In the second half of 1998, however the industry and its congressional allies defeated the tobacco bill, the industry received favorable treatment in the courts, and its lawsuits with the states were settled on better terms than the industry might have anticipated. Depending on one's perspective, the events of 1998 may be interpreted as evidence of the industry's continuing vulnerability (the glass is half full) or its continuing political clout (the glass is half empty).

66. It matters relatively little whether the NRA is as politically powerful as it is perceived to be as long as politicians, as well as potential gun control movement allies, perceive it to be all powerful. That which we perceive as real is real in its consequences.

67. This same point was made by a gun control activist we interviewed, who attributed the difference between the targets of the gun and the smoking/tobacco control movements to the gun industry's invisibility, compared with the visibility of tobacco manufacturers. A *New York Times* article suggests that not only gun control advocates but the gun industry has learned from the smoking/tobacco experience. A Washington lobbyist for the industry association is quoted as saying, "Everyone can vividly remember seeing those tobacco executives parade up to Capitol Hill and deny that tobacco was habit forming. . . . Everyone knew it was ridiculous. We are not going to go before Congress and say that guns are not dangerous and that kids are not killed with them" (Wayne 1997). This perspective led to a recent voluntary agreement, announced from the White House lawn, that gun manufacturers would install child safety locks on handguns.

68. The reviewer of a recent book on "the tyranny of public health" complains that "less dangerous alternatives" to cigarettes—cigars, pipes, and chewing tobacco—"have been rejected as distractions from the greater overall mission: advances in smokeless cigarettes and denicotined cigarettes have been dismissed" (Skinner 1998: 118–119).

69. I refer here to the oral history interviews in ACS files.

70. An article in the *New York Times* suggests that international disarmament groups, "once preoccupied with nuclear weapons, are focusing more on the proliferation of small arms and handguns as a major threat to individual health and safety" (Seelye 1998). The recently formed HELP (Handgun Epidemic Lowering Plan) network includes mainstream medical organizations such as the AMA and more activist groups such as Physicians for Social Responsibility.

71. In considering the relationship between social movements and social change, it is important to distinguish between conditions for movement emergence, conditions for movement endurance, and conditions for movement-effected social change. These conditions are clearly related, since movements must emerge and be sustained over some

period of time in order to produce change. But they are not the same. For example, a number of authors (e.g., Shapiro 1985; Schwartz, and Paul 1992) suggest that conflict is a condition for movement success: "it is very hard to work on an issue over a long period of time where all one is doing is education work. . . . What draws people in . . . is the contest over power" (movement activist cited in Shapiro 1985: 101). However, the conflict hypothesis refers to conditions for successful mobilization, not successful change. Meyer and Staggenborg hypothesize, to the contrary, that movements with strong opposition are "unable to take advantage of favorable political conditions after victories" (1996: 1652). In any case, the presence of "strong opposition" hardly distinguishes the smoking/tobacco and gun control movements. More important is the source and credibility of the opposition.

72.   Meyer and Staggenborg define a *countermovement* as "a movement that makes contrary claims simultaneously to those of the original movement" (1996: 1631). By this criteria, neither of our movements' principal antagonists qualify as countermovements, yet many of the propositions advanced by these authors apply to the relationships of the smoking/tobacco control movement with the tobacco industry and the gun control movement with the NRA. Thus, in both cases "the opposing movement (or organization in the present case) is a critical component of the structure of political opportunity the other side faces" (1633); "movements [organizations] often respond to a defeat in one venue by protesting in an alternative arena" (1645); movements thrive on threats, and so on. These parallels suggest that the critical dimension in these relationships is not that the parties are social movements but that they are engaged in ongoing political conflict.

<table>
<tr><td>

16

</td><td>

Genetic Privacy and Confidentiality: Why They Are So Hard to Protect

</td></tr>
</table>

Mark A. Rothstein

Genetic privacy and confidentiality have both intrinsic and consequential value. Although general agreement exists about the need to protect privacy and confidentiality in the abstract, most of the concern has focused on preventing the harmful uses of this sensitive information. I hope to demonstrate in this article that the reason why genetic privacy and confidentiality are so difficult to protect is that any effort to protect them inevitably implicates broader and extremely contentious issues, such as the right of access to health care.[1] Moreover, the tentative legislative and policy steps undertaken and proposed thus far have been, for the most part, misguided, simplistic, and ineffective.

DEFINING PRIVACY AND CONFIDENTIALITY

As I use the term privacy, I am referring to the limited access to a person, the right of an individual to be left alone, and the right to keep certain information from disclosure to other individuals.[2] Privacy would encompass an individual's right to decide whether to receive certain information about himself/herself from a third party. It would also involve the circumstances under which the individual shares information with others, such as family members, health care providers, or entities with a financial interest in the individual's current or future health, including an employer or an insurer.

By contrast, with confidentiality I am referring to the right of an individual to prevent the redisclosure of certain sensitive information that was disclosed

Reprinted from *Journal of Law, Medicine & Ethics*, 26, no. 3 (Fall 1998): 198–204. Copyright 1998. Reprinted with permission of the American Society of Law, Medicine & Ethics. All rights reserved.

originally in the confines of a confidential relationship.[3] The paradigmatic confidential relationship involves the patient and physician. With regard to genetics, the central question is: How can the confidentiality of genetic information be protected? In other words, is it possible to keep certain information a patient has given to a physician or a physician has developed from getting to a third party? Generally, most commentators and legislators have proposed erecting a barrier between the physician and the third party, limiting what, when, and how the physician may disclose genetic information about a patient to a third party. Accordingly, a variety of proposals have been put forward to limit access by computer, to impose requirements for express, written consent before the physician may disclose information, and to give the patient notice of each disclosure.[4] I believe that measures to protect against the unauthorized disclosure of genetic information are necessary but not sufficient to protect genetic privacy and confidentiality. Furthermore, this approach is fundamentally flawed if it is to be used as the primary method to protect against the involuntary disclosure of genetic information.

If a third party has enough leverage and economic power, it can go to an individual and require him/her to execute a release that authorizes a physician to release the medical records to the third party. Even if a law were enacted to prohibit physicians from ever disclosing the information (even with a release) to a third party, the law still would be ineffective. If the information were sufficiently important to a third party, that third party could require an individual to get a copy of his/her medical records, and to submit them directly to the third party along with the application for matters such as employment, insurance, or a mortgage. In addition, if a third party really wants the information, it may simply require an individual to provide a blood sample that the third party can test. With the emergence of multiplex and chip-based DNA tests, it will be increasingly quick and inexpensive for third parties to perform genetic testing themselves.

I believe less emphasis should be placed on regulating the procedures for disclosure of information by physicians and other holders of medical records and more detailed focus placed on the circumstances surrounding the acquisition of the information by third parties. Who are these third parties? What need do they have for the information? And what are they going to do with the information? In other words, what substantive rights of the individual are implicated by a third party's use of genetic information? It is apparent that a third party's needs and rights are going to vary tremendously depending on whether it is a health insurance company, a life insurance company, a disability or long-term care insurance company, an employer, a school, a mortgage company, a law enforcement agency, a court, or some other third party. That is why protecting genetic privacy and confidentiality is more complicated than some people have asserted, and these numerous applications cannot be resolved by a general procedural law.

HEALTH INSURANCE

As of 1998, laws have been enacted in over half the states to prohibit health insurance companies from requiring genetic tests as a condition of coverage or from denying or charging higher rates based on the results of a genetic test(s). A typical provision reads as follows:

No insurance company may require genetic testing or use the results of a genetic test to deny coverage or increase the rates for health insurance.

When these laws were enacted, many legislators and advocates believed that major strides had been made in eliminating genetic discrimination. Unfortunately, a closer examination reveals a problem. The laws only apply to individuals who are asymptomatic. Once the individual becomes symptomatic, the laws do not apply. For example, in a state with such a provision, an insurance company cannot use the positive result of a test to detect a genetic predisposition to breast cancer to deny coverage while the woman is asymptomatic. If she becomes symptomatic, however, then the insurance company can cancel the policy or increase the rates 100 percent or more, depending on the provisions of the state's general insurance laws.

To improve the effectiveness of the law, the following amendment would help:

No insurance company may use the results of a genetic test to deny coverage or increase the rates for health insurance for an individual who is asymptomatic or symptomatic.

This amendment would eliminate the problem of the woman who is asymptomatic when she applies for the coverage and then develops genetic-based breast cancer. The problem is that only a small percentage of breast cancers (about 5 percent) are known to be caused by genetic factors.[6] Why should the law treat women who have breast cancer caused by a genetic factor, 5 percent, different from the 95 percent of women whose breast cancer results from unknown causes?

The unfairness and illogic of such a law can be remedied by the following proviso:

An individual, who is symptomatic for a condition for which a particular genotype may increase the likelihood of getting the condition, shall not be denied coverage or assessed higher rates, whether or not the individual's condition can be shown to be caused by genetic factors.

The law now would protect women who are asymptomatic and carry one of the alleles predisposing them to breast cancer; it also would protect all women who get breast cancer, regardless of the cause.

This version of the law is better, but it still suffers from a major weakness. Is it logical to protect women with breast cancer from discrimination in health insurance, but not to protect the women (and men) who have infectious diseases, who are victims of assault, who have an occupational disease, who are injured in car accidents, or have other serious medical needs? Does it make any sense to draw a distinction between these classes of people who need health care coverage?

To remedy the problem of favoring one group of individuals in medical need over another in terms of access to health insurance, the following law could be enacted:

No insurance company may deny coverage or increase the rates for health insurance based on an individual's past, present, or predicted future health status.

Clever readers, no doubt, already have detected a problem with this version. This law can be classified as guaranteed issue, guaranteed renewal, community-rated health insurance. Under it, health insurance companies may not discriminate in policy issuance based on health status, they may not cancel coverage as long as the premiums are paid, and they must renew the policy without discrimination at the same rate.

The problem with this type of system stems from its optional nature. The essence of community rating is that low-risk people subsidize high-risk people. Over time, the low-risk people may become high-risk, but in those years they will be subsidized by someone else. In a community-rated system, the premiums of low-risk people will rise. Low-risk people tend to be younger and with lower incomes. They may not be able to afford the higher premiums or they may think that, because they are currently healthy, their discretionary dollars could be better spent. When low-risk people drop out of the pool, rates rise for the remaining individuals, which causes more low-risk people to drop out, and the pool increasingly is filled with older, sicker people. Eventually the system collapses.

To avoid the problem of people leaving the system, participation must be mandatory. The only logical solution, then, is a mandatory participation, guaranteed issue, guaranteed renewal, community-rated health care system. In theory, this would produce a fair health care system that would not discriminate against individuals based on genetic predisposition or other factors. Nevertheless, during 1993 and 1994, the U.S. Congress decided that any "universal access" health care system would not be in the best interests of the country.[7]

In light of the illogic at the starting point and the intransigence at the concluding point of this exercise, is it possible to prevent genetic-based discrimination in health insurance within a system that is unfair and illogical? Unfortunately, the answer is no, unless and until the United States is prepared to address in a comprehensive way the larger issue of who has access to health care. In the interim, we are left to decide what form of illogical, suboptimal health care tinkering makes us feel as if we have resolved the issue of genetic discrimination in health insurance.

The inability to solve a fundamentally flawed system through incremental approaches raises important issues of politics and advocacy. One wonders whether it is efficacious, tactically sound, or ethical for genetic advocacy groups to promote legislation prohibiting genetic discrimination in health insurance (or other areas) when the laws have so little value to those at risk of genetic disorders and no value to those who have illnesses from other causes. Indeed, such legislation may even result in further stigmatizing genetic conditions and fragmenting support for meaningful health care reform.

LIFE INSURANCE

The use of genetic information in other types of insurance also places genetic privacy and confidentiality in the context of substantive interests. For example, life insurance companies are in the business of assessing and classifying risks, primarily on an individual basis. Traditionally, life insurance companies either refused coverage or assessed higher premiums for individuals who were currently ill, had a history of serious illness, or who had risk factors, such as cigarette smoking, substance abuse, obesity, or hypertension, that negatively affected their life expectancy.

With the development of predictive genetic testing, individuals who are presymptomatic for late-onset, single-gene disorders can be identified, and the information can be used in medical underwriting. Furthermore, life insurance companies, fearing adverse selection, also use the results of genetic tests along with family health histories in applicants' medical records. Yet, the number of individuals with late-onset, single-gene disorders is quite small. The real challenge of genetics and life insurance involves more common multifactorial disorders, such as breast cancer, ovarian cancer, and colon cancer. Although mutations associated with an increased risk of these disorders have been identified only recently, some life insurers have begun using this predictive information in medical underwriting.

Two policy issues have been raised by insurers' use of predictive genetic information. The first concerns the accuracy of the predictions. Although some morbidity data have been developed for these predisposing mutations, it is still too early to develop any meaningful mortality data. For example, individuals with a genetic predisposition to colon cancer may undergo frequent colonoscopies, thereby detecting cancer in its earliest, treatable stages. It is not clear what the mortality risk for such a cohort would be. Thus, considerable risk exists that underwriting decisions could be based on incorrect data.

The second issue will arise with even greater force when predictive mortality data are better developed. It involves the role of life insurance in society. Is life insurance a purely commercial relationship, an estate-building investment vehicle, and an income-replacement arrangement? If so, it is reasonable to permit life insurers to have access to any information they want in underwriting, so long as their decisions are actuarially justified and medical information is kept confidential.[8] On the other hand, if life insurance has some other social value, such as preventing social disruption caused by the death of the primary wage-earner in a family, then it is reasonable to regulate the information on which underwriting is based and thereby the availability of the insurance product.[9]

State legislative activity dealing with genetic information and life insurance has increased in the last few years. Seven states have enacted laws requiring informed consent for using genetic information.[10] Eight states also have laws requiring that medical underwriting based on genetic factors be based on actuarial principles,[11] although actuarial determinations by insurance companies traditionally have been given great deference by state regulators. Proposed legislation in at least three states would prohibit the use of genetic information in life insurance for policies below a certain dollar amount[12] or altogether.[13]

As with health insurance, it is simplistic to say that restrictions on a life insurance company's access to genetic information will protect the privacy and confidentiality of genetic information. It is necessary to probe the underlying assumptions about the role of life insurance in contemporary American society.

LONG-TERM CARE INSURANCE

Private long-term care insurance is likely to become increasingly important over the next ten years. Currently, only about 25 percent of nursing home care is privately financed. Medicaid pays for a substantial portion of the care of individuals who have spent down their assets and meet eligibility standards. The combination of federal Medicaid cutbacks, growth in the elderly population, and the low ratio of potential caregivers to care-receivers means that private long-term care insurance will become increasingly important.

The profitability or solvency of insurance companies and long-term care institutions selling long-term care policies is threatened by the prospect of individuals needing skilled nursing services, but surviving for many years. Alzheimer's disease represents the biggest risk. Already, researchers have identified genetic factors with a link to Alzheimer's disease, and long-term care insurance companies will have a strong interest in obtaining the results of such tests or performing the tests themselves in advance of offering coverage.

Many states already prohibit nursing homes from discontinuing the treatment of patients with Alzheimer's disease or from discriminating in the treatment of such patients. Legislation in Colorado, however, goes a step farther by prohibiting any use of genetic information in long-term care insurance,[14] and other states are considering the issue.

The development of public policy on long-term care insurance depends to a large extent on whether long-term care is viewed more like health insurance or life (and disability) insurance. If the former, then more individuals would regard it as a necessity or a right to which all individuals, regardless of their medical histories or genetic predispositions, should have access. If the latter, then it is more likely to be considered an optional commercial transaction, and all parties may require access to any information deemed relevant. Again, the privacy and confidentiality interests of individuals depend on the substantive issues of entitlement or eligibility for insurance.

EMPLOYMENT

Employer coverage is extremely important in terms of how people get their health insurance. Employers may want to know the genetic make-up of employees to prevent occupational injury and illness or because of concerns about productivity, absenteeism, and turnover. But the number one reason why employers would want access to genetic information about applicants and employees is health insurance cost containment.

Employers often pay at least $5,000 per year per employee for health insurance. In some industries and in some companies, where the benefits are more generous, the cost may be much higher. In any given year, 5 percent of health care claimants consume 50 percent of health care resources, and 10 percent of claimants consume 70 percent of resources.[15] It quickly becomes clear to health benefits managers that if they can eliminate a class of very high cost users, they are going to save the company a lot of money. And those high-cost users do not even have to be employees; they can be the dependents of employees.

The primary federal law prohibiting discrimination in employment on the basis of health status is the Americans with Disabilities Act (ADA).[16] Medical examinations under the ADA may be divided into three parts, based on when they are performed. At the preemployment stage, when the employer considers the individual's background and qualifications, medical inquiries and examinations are not allowed. An employer is prohibited from performing a medical examination, asking about the use of prescription medications, asking about the use of sick leave, or similar matters. The employer is limited to asking whether the individual has the ability to perform essential job functions. For example, if essential to the job, the employer may ask whether the individual can climb telephone poles, has a driver's license, or is able to stand for long periods of time.

The key stage is the second. The ADA permits employers to make offers conditioned on a satisfactory report following a post-offer ("employment entrance" or "preplacement") medical examination. The medical examiner may be a company-paid, full-time employee or, more often the case, an independent consultant. The ADA places no limitation on the scope of this examination.

Except in the states where prohibited by a specific law, an employer may even require genetic testing.

Most significant, under the ADA, the employer may require, as a condition of employment, that a conditional offeree sign a blanket release, authorizing the disclosure of all of the individual's personal medical records to the company for review. My fear is not that employers are going to perform genetic tests themselves; it is currently not cost effective to do so. But employers can get access to the results of genetic tests performed in the clinical setting as well as family histories contained in personal medical files. This fact not only raises the prospect of discrimination, but it also discourages at-risk individuals from undergoing possibly beneficial genetic testing. Thus, a close nexus exists between the confidentiality of genetic information and public health objectives.

Even if a law were enacted making discrimination based on genetic information illegal, we have to assume that some employers that could lawfully get access to the information would then illegally use that information. In 1964, almost thirty-five years ago, Congress enacted Title VII of the Civil Rights Act of 1964,[17] which made it unlawful to discriminate in employment on the basis of race, color, religion, sex, and national origin. In 1967, the Age Discrimination in Employment Act[18] added age to the list of proscribed forms of discrimination. Despite these laws, it is obvious that discrimination based on these factors continues today. Yet, discrimination on the basis of criteria such as religion or national origin does not save employers any money. Discrimination on the basis of health status or perceived health status, however, could save hundreds of thousands of dollars on a single individual's health insurance claims. Therefore, we have to assume that at least some employers that would have access to genetic information would use it.

With regard to medical examinations and records of current employees, once the individual has started working, the employer may only require employees to undergo examinations that are job-related. Voluntary examinations and wellness programs of a broader scope are also permitted.

In March 1995, the Equal Employment Opportunity Commission (EEOC) issued an interpretation regarding the applicability of the ADA to genetic discrimination.[19] According to EEOC, covered entities (that is, employers) that discriminate against individuals on the basis of genetic predisposition are "regarding" the individuals as having a disability and therefore the individuals are covered by the third prong of the definition of individual with a disability under the ADA.[20]

EEOC's statement is of limited value for three reasons. First, EEOC interpretations are not binding on the courts, and the issue has not yet been addressed by any court.[21] Second, the interpretation does not apply to the unaffected carriers of recessive and X-linked disorders, who might be subject to discrimination by employers concerned about the health care costs of future dependents. Thus, it would not be unlawful for an employer to discriminate against an individual whose carrier state created a risk of having a child with Duchenne muscular dystrophy or cystic fibrosis. Third, and most important, EEOC's interpretation does not prohibit employers from requiring as a condition of employment that an individual sign a broad medical release, thereby giving the employer access to clinical records that could contain genetic information.

Nearly every state has considered legislation prohibiting genetic discrimination in employment. As of 1998, eighteen states have enacted laws providing that no employer may require genetic testing or may use the results of a genetic test or genetic information to discriminate in employment.[22] Unfortunately, these laws are inadequate. In general, they define "genetic discrimination" too narrowly. For example, Texas enacted a law in 1997 prohibiting employment discrimination based on genetic information, and genetic information is defined as the results of a DNA-based test.[23] Therefore, it would not violate the law for an employer to discriminate against an individual because his/her medical record contains a remark that "father died of Huntington disease."

A related, insurmountable problem, is defining genetic. Recent research has identified genetic associations with diabetes, epilepsy, hypercholesterolemia, hypertension, osteoporosis, and numerous common disorders. It is not clear whether information about such disorders is genetic information. From a medical standpoint, distinguishing genetic from other medical conditions is increasingly impossible, even though this significant fact has yet to be appreciated in the policy debates.

Another major limitation of these state laws is that they do not prohibit employers from compelling medical releases, thereby permitting employers to gain access to genetic information in medical records. Finally, the laws do not prohibit employers from getting genetic information through employee health insurance claims. Self-insured employers, in particular, may obtain a tremendous amount of individually identifiable information through health insurance claims, and little has been done thus far in the way of regulating that access.

Three main options are available to address the issue of genetic discrimination in employment. First, the ADA could be amended to prohibit employers from obtaining non-job-related medical information. It is doubtful, however, that this or any other amendment of the ADA would be given serious consideration by Congress, because the ADA's supporters (who would seem to be the likely sponsors of such an amendment) are afraid that, if the ADA were subject to amendment, ADA opponents would offer their own amendments to weaken the Act.

Another possibility is to enact a state law to prohibit access to non-job-related medical information. In 1983, Minnesota, enacted a law providing that all employee medical examinations, no matter when given, must be strictly job-related and consistent with business necessity.[24] Also, if an employer uses medical information from an applicant or employee in decision making, it must give the individual written notice within ten days.[25] In addition, anyone whose medical privacy rights have been violated has standing to bring an action for discrimination whether or not he/she has a condition that meets the definition of disability.[26] This approach is far superior to the other state laws dealing with genetic discrimination. Unfortunately, a widespread lack of knowledge about the law among Minnesota employers and employees means that there has been little or no compliance with it.[27]

The last option is to enact laws similar to the state laws enacted already. Although this model seems to be favored currently, as reflected by the legislation pending in Congress[28] and the states, it would merely perpetuate the status quo.

CONCLUSION

This review of insurance and employment demonstrates why it is so difficult to protect genetic privacy and confidentiality. Undoubtedly, procedural safeguards, such as strict application of informed consent and limits on disclosure by health care providers, are necessary. Nevertheless, clear substantive rights are also implicated by third-party access to and use of genetic information. What right do individuals have to health care? Is health insurance different from life insurance? What information does an employer legitimately need to have? These are only some of the questions that need to be answered.

The problem of genetic privacy and confidentiality cannot be solved by a single procedural law; resolution of the issues raises fundamental matters of equality of opportunity and allocation of resources. Only if we begin to understand the complexity and the difficulty of the challenge will we be able to develop comprehensive and thoughtful proposals to address genetic privacy and confidentiality.

REFERENCES

1. For further discussion, see M. A. Rothstein, "Genetic Secrets: A Policy Framework," in M. A. Rothstein, ed., Genetic Secrets: Protecting Privacy and Confidentiality in the Genetic Era (New Haven: Yale University Press, 1997): 451–95.

2. See A. L. Allen, "Genetic Privacy: Emerging Concepts and Values," in Rothstein, id. at 31–59.

3. See id.

4. See, for example, G. J. Annas, L. H. Glantz, and P.A. Roche, The Genetic Privacy Act and Commentary (Boston: Boston University School of Public Health, 1995).

5. For a listing of the state laws, see B. A. Trolin, ed., Mapping Public Policy for Genetic Technologies: A Legislator's Guide (Denver: National Conference of State Legislatures, 1998).

6. See P. Kahn, "Coming to Grips with Genes and Risk," Science, 274 (1996): 496.

7. See, for example, W. J. Thomas, "The Clinton Health Care Reform Plan: A Failed Dramatic Presentation," Stanford Law & Policy Review, 7 (1995–96): at 83; and see generally Symposium, "The Failure of Health Care Reform," Journal of Health Politics, Policy and Law, 20 (1995): 271–489.

8. See R. B. Meyer, "Justification for Permitting Life Insurers to Continue to Underwrite on the Basis of Genetic Information and Genetic Test Results," Suffolk University Law Review, 27 (1993): 1271–305.

9. See R. J. Pokorski, "Insurance Underwriting in the Genetic Era," American Journal of Human Genetics, 60 (1997): 205–16.

10. See Ariz. Rev. Stat. Ann. section 20-448.02 (West 1998); Cal. Ins. Code section 10148 (West 1998); Minn. Stat. section 72A. 139 (1998); N.J. Stat. Ann. section 10:5-45 (West 1998); N.M. Stat. Ann. sections 2421-3 to -4 (Michie 1998); N.Y. Ins. Law section 2612 (McKinney 1998); and Or. Rev. Stat. section 746.135 (1998).

11. See Ariz. Rev. Stat. Ann. section 20-448 (West 1998); Cal. Ins. Code section 10148; Me. Rev. Stat. Ann. tit. 24-A, section 2159-c (west 1998); Md. Code Ann., Ins. section 27-208(a)(2)(i) (1998); Mont. Code Ann. section 33-18-206(4) (1998); N.J. Stat. Ann. section 17B:3012(f) (West 1998); N.M. Stat. Ann. sections 24-21-3 to -4; and Wis. Stat. Ann. section 631.89(3)(b)(2) (West 1998).

12. See N.H.H.B. 241 (1997) (noting prohibition for policies below $500,000).

13. See Conn. H. B. 5053 (1997); and Haw. S. 112 (1998).

14. See Colo. Rev. Stat. Ann. section 10-3-1104.7(3)(b) (West 1998).

15. See D. W. Light, "The Practice and Ethics of Risk-Rated Health Insurance," JAMA, 267 (1992): at 2504.

16. Americans with Disabilities Act, 42 U.S.C. sections 12101–12213 (1994).

17. Civil Rights Act of 1964, 42 U.S.C. section 2000e (1994).

18. Age Discrimination in Employment Act, 29 U.S.C. sections 621-634 (1994).

19. See 2 EEOC Compliance Manual (CCH), sections 902-45 (Mar. 14, 1995), reprinted in Daily Labor Report (Mar. 16, 1995), E-1, E-23 (citing definition of disability).

20. See M. A. Rothstein, "Genetic Discrimination in Employment and the Americans with Disabilities Act," Houston Law Review, 29 (1992): 23–84.

21. In Bragdon v. Abbott, 118 S. Ct. 2196 (1998), the U.S. Supreme Court, ruling 5–4, held that a dental patient with asymptomatic human immunodeficiency virus (HIV) was covered under the public accommodation (Title III) provision of the Americans with Disabilities Act (ADA). Of potential relevance to genetic discrimination cases, the Court held that, at least as to this plaintiff, HIV infection was a substantial limitation of the major life activity of procreation. A similar argument is likely to be raised by an individual with a genetic predisposition to illness. For further discussion of Bragdon v. Abbott, see W.E. Parmet, "The Supreme Court Confronts HIV: Reflections on Bragdon v. Abbott," Journal of Law, Medicine & Ethics, 26 (1998): 22540.

22. See Ariz. Rev. Stat. 41-1463(B)(3) (West 1992 & Supp. 1997) (enacted 1997); Act of July 3, 1998, ch. 99, 1998 Cal. Legis. Serv. 468 (west) (enacted 1998); 1998 Conn. Legis. Serv. 98-180 (west) (enacted 1998); Del. Code Ann. tit. 18, section 2317 (1998) (enacted 1998); Iowa Code Ann. section 729.6 (1993) (enacted 1992); N.H. Rev.

Stat. Ann. section 141-H:3.I(b) (1997) (enacted 1995); 1998 N.M. Adv. Legis. Serv. ch. 77 (enacted 1998); N.Y. Exec. Law section 296(l)(a) (Consol. 1998) (enacted 1996); N.C. Gen. Stat. section 95-28.1A (1997) (enacted (1997); Okla. Stat. tit. 36, section 3614.1 (1998) (enacted 1998); R.I. Gen. Laws section 28-6.7-1 (1995) (enacted 1992); Tex. Lab. Code Ann. sections 21.410-.402 (West Supp. 1998) (enacted 1997); Vt. Stat. Ann. tit. 18, section 9333(a) (1998) (enacted 1998); and Wis. Stat. Ann. section 111.372 (West 1997) (enacted 1992).

23. See Tex. Lab. Code Ann. sections 21.410-.402.

24. See Minn. Stat. section 363.02, subdiv. 1, (9)(1) (West 1991).

25. See Minn. Stat. section 363.03, subdiv. 1a (West 1998). The ADA has no comparable provision. See generally M.A. Rothstein, "Legal and Ethical Aspects of Medical Screening," Occupational Medicine: State of the Art Reviews, 3, no. 1(1996): 31.

26. See Minn. Stat. section 363.03, subdiv. 1, (4)(c) (West Supp. 1998). Under the ADA, only qualified individuals with disabilities have standing to challenge unlawful preemployment inquiries. See Armstrong v. Turner Industries, Ltd., 141 F.3d 554 (5th Cir. 1998); and Griffin v. Steeltek, Inc., 964 F. Supp. 317 (N.D. Okla. 1997).

27. See M. A. Rothstein, B. D. Gelb, and S. G. Craig, "Protecting Genetic Privacy by Permitting Employer Access Only to Job-Related Employee Medical Information: Analysis of a Unique Minnesota Law," American Journal of Law & Medicine, XXIV (1998): 399–417.

28. See, for example, Genetic Employment Protection Act of 1997, H.R. 2275, 105th Cong. (1997) (Rep. Nita Lowey [D. N.Y.]); Genetic Nondiscrimination in the Workplace Act, H.R. 2215, 105th Cong. (1997) (Rep. Joseph Kennedy [D. Mass.]); Genetic Privacy and Nondiscrimination Act of 1997, H.R. 2198, 105th Cong. (1997) (Rep. Cliff Stearns [R. Fla.]); Genetic Justice Act, S. 1045, 105th Cong. (1997) (Sen. Tom Daschle [D. S.D.]); and Genetic Confidentiality and Nondiscrimination Act of 1997, S. 422, 105th Cong. (1997) (Sen. Pete Domenici [R. N.M.]).

<table>
<tr><td>17</td><td>

Antitrust Enforcement in the Healthcare Industry: The Expanding Scope of State Activity

Fred J. Hellinger

</td></tr>
</table>

This study describes the evolution of state antitrust activities and explores salient research and policy questions. Over the past five years, twenty states have passed laws that establish formal mechanisms for states to immunize collaborative activities among providers of healthcare services from state and federal prosecution. Moreover, in recent years, state attorneys general have issued numerous antitrust consent decrees that require ongoing oversight. In these decrees, merging entities have agreed to restrain price increases, pass on savings to consumers, and limit profits.

Although more than a dozen hospital mergers have been approved by state agencies, there is no information about their impact on the cost, content, and quality of care. In addition, there is no information about whether or not the stipulations imposed by state agencies have been satisfied. (Many of these stipulations require that the activities of the merged hospitals be supervised for five or more years.)

Most state laws that attempt to immunize collaborative arrangements from state and federal antitrust do not explicitly include hospital mergers. And often it is unclear whether or not hospital mergers are covered by these state laws.

Reprinted from *Health Services Research*, 33, no. 5 (December 1998, Part II): 1477–94, with permission, Health Administration Press.

Most of these laws refer to joint ventures, cooperative agreements, cooperative arrangements, or similar terminology, and in most instances it is ambiguous whether or not these terms encompass mergers.

Increased merger activity has accompanied the rise of managed care in the healthcare marketplace, and recent changes have transformed the healthcare marketplace from one dominated by solo physicians and single hospitals to one dominated by multispecialty group practices and networks of local hospitals. Some analysts have hailed this transformation as a necessary step toward the elimination of excess capacity and costly duplication ("Consolidation . . ." 1995). Others assert that the reduction in the number of competitors has limited consumer choice and reduced the quality of care (Magleby 1996).

Complex relationships among purchasers, plans, and providers pose significant problems for governmental entities entrusted with ensuring that new collaborative arrangements do not diminish the benefits of a competitive market. The task of weighing the benefits from enhanced efficiencies against the costs of reduced competition is considerably more demanding today than it was several years ago.

Whereas the primary responsibility for regulating health plans and insurers rests with state authorities, the responsibility to ensure that the market for health services remains competitive is shared by federal and state authorities. Although both federal and state authorities enforce antitrust policies, federal antitrust laws were not intended to be invoked against state regulatory schemes that fulfill the conditions specified in the "state action immunity" doctrine (Ross 1993).

THE FEDERAL ROLE

In 1992, for the first time, the Department of Justice (DOJ) and Federal Trade Commission (FTC) jointly issued merger guidelines (Department of Justice and Federal Trade Commission 1992). As these guidelines are usually implemented, they entail:

- Defining the market and assessing market concentration. Generally, the most attention is paid to defining the market in product and geographic terms. Both of these market dimensions require analysis of consumers' willingness to substitute alternative services and locations if faced with changes in price or quality. Measurement of concentration in a market generally has been uncomplicated. And:
- Assessing potential adverse effects of the merger. This exercise does not focus solely on concentration but also identifies characteristics of the market that facilitate or hinder unilateral or coordinated anticompetitive behavior.

In 1993, the DOJ and the FTC jointly issued a policy statement that addressed issues involving mergers (DOJ and FTC 1993). The *Department of Justice and Federal Trade Commission Antitrust Enforcement Policy Statements in the Health Area* is the first policy statement focused solely on antitrust issues in the healthcare industry.

The 1993 policy statement marks the first time that federal antitrust enforcement agencies issued guidance to providers in the form of "antitrust safety zones." These zones describe certain conditions under which mergers or other horizontal activities generally will not be carefully scrutinized.

In August 1996 the DOJ and FTC issued a statement that promulgated new guidelines that facilitate the formation of physician network joint ventures and multiprovider network joint ventures (DOJ and FTC 1996). The 1996 statement recognized that risk sharing may not be the only legitimate rationale for formulation of a physician or multiprovider joint venture that exceeds the safe harbor thresholds. In particular, the 1996 policy statement extended a rule of reason analysis to physician joint ventures that achieve sufficient clinical integration to generate significant efficiencies.

Relatively few hospital mergers have been challenged by federal authorities. In an analysis of 397 premerger notifications involving acute care hospitals from 1991 through 1993, the General Accounting Office (GAO) found that only 15 had been challenged by the DOJ or FTC (United States General Accounting Office 1994). This number may understate the full impact of antitrust legislation, however, because the terms of the proposed mergers were altered in some of the 68 proposed mergers for which federal agencies conducted a preliminary investigation, and the number of parties that would have merged but never filed an intent to do so due to anticipated antitrust problems can never be fully ascertained.

State Action Immunity

The "state action immunity doctrine" has evolved through case law over the past five decades and describes the conditions that must be satisfied in order for states to immunize collaborative arrangements from federal antitrust prosecution. Under this doctrine, anticompetitive activities authorized or invited by individual states are exempt from federal antitrust prosecution if the following two conditions are satisfied (*California . . .* 1980):

1. The activity is allowed by the state as evidenced by the promulgation of a clear and articulate policy permitting the activity (this articulation may be through the establishment of a state regulatory program or through the actions of the state attorneys general office).
2. The state actively supervises the anticompetitive activities of the private entities.

The genesis of the state action immunity doctrine may be traced to the *Parker v. Brown* case in 1943 (Parker 1940). In this case the plaintiff, Parker, alleged that the California Agricultural Prorate Act (Brown was the Director of the California Department of Agriculture), which authorized the establishment of a program to market agricultural commodities in the state in order to restrict competition among growers and maintain prices, violated Section One of the Sherman Antitrust Act.

The U.S. Supreme Court determined that the California Proration Act was not in conflict with the Sherman Antitrust Act, and it asserted that states have the right to regulate commerce within their borders even if this regulation entails activities that reduce or inhibit competition. This decision and its progeny establish the state action immunity doctrine.

STATE HEALTHCARE ANTITRUST EXEMPTION LAWS

The strict requirements for state action immunity led to efforts to pass state legislation establishing a mechanism to satisfy these requirements. In 1993, the American Hospital Association (AHA) sent a message to state hospital associations providing a prototype for state legislation to help guarantee that mergers approved by states would be safe from federal prosecution (United States General Accounting Office 1994, p. 1).

In general, regulatory programs established by state laws establish explicit application procedures, approval criteria, and a structural framework that ensure a comprehensive review and continued state supervision of approved activities. These laws provide applicants with written guidelines and a list of steps that must be completed in order to obtain approval for a collaborative venture. These efforts are designed to demonstrate that the state has endorsed a collaborative arrangement through the exercise of deliberate judgment and that the state has in place a means to provide continued supervision of the activity.

Each of the 20 state laws passed since 1992 initiates a voluntary state regulatory program to enable collaborative arrangements to be shielded from federal antitrust prosecution. Table 17.1 describes these laws using the language in each of the laws. Yet, because these laws rarely define what is meant by a "cooperative agreement," "cooperative arrangement," "joint venture," "merger," or "cooperative agreements and similar enterprises," their scope is open to interpretation by the state courts.

Although only 7 of the 20 state laws explicitly address hospital mergers (Georgia, Kansas, Maine, Minnesota, Montana, Nebraska, and North Carolina), it is unclear how mergers are categorized by each law. It also is unclear whether a merger-like partnership (i.e., a merger that does not involve the transfer of assets to a new entity) is viewed as a merger or a cooperative arrangement. For example, South Carolina's law applies to "cooperative agreements" that are defined to include an "acquisition or merger of assets among or by two or more health providers" (South Carolina Code, § 1, Ch. 7 of Title 44).

TABLE 17.1

State Healthcare Antitrust Exemptions Laws

State	Scope	Approval Agency
Colorado	Cooperative healthcare agreements involving hospitals	Cooperative Health Care Agreements Board
Florida	Providers who are members of certified rural health networks seeking to consolidate services or technologies or to enter into cooperative arrangements	Agency for Health Care Administration
Georgia	Mergers among specified hospitals within a county	County Hospital Authority
Idaho	Cooperative agreements among healthcare providers	Attorney General
Kansas	Mergers and joint ventures among hospitals, physicians, and other healthcare providers	Secretary of the Department of Health and the Environment
Maine	Cooperative agreements among hospitals and mergers among hospitals	Department of Human Services
Minnesota	Cooperative arrangements involving healthcare providers and purchasers	Commissioner of Health
Montana	Mergers and joint ventures among hospitals, physicians, and other healthcare providers	Health Care Authority
Nebraska	Joint ventures and consolidations among hospitals, physicians, and other healthcare providers	Department of Health
New York	Joint ventures among hospitals, physicians, and other healthcare providers in rural healthcare networks	Department of Public Health
North Carolina	Cooperative agreements and mergers among physicians, hospitals, and other healthcare providers	Department of Human Resources
North Dakota	Joint ventures among hospitals, physicians, and other healthcare providers	Department of Human Resources
Ohio	Cooperative actions among hospitals	Department of Health

continued

TABLE 17.1 *continued*

State	Scope	Approval Agency
Oregon	Joint ventures among hospitals involving heart and kidney services	Department of Human Resources
South Carolina	Cooperative agreements among healthcare providers including hospitals	Department of Health and Environmental Control
Tennessee	Joint ventures among hospitals	Department of Health
Texas	Joint ventures among hospitals	Department of Human Resources
Washington State	Joint ventures among hospitals, physicians, and other healthcare providers	Health Services Commission
Wisconsin	Joint ventures among hospitals, physicians, and other healthcare providers	Department of Health and Social Services
Wyoming	Cooperative arrangements including joint ventures and similar enterprises among healthcare providers and purchasers	Department of Health

Sources: United States General Accounting Office, *Federal and State Antitrust Actions Concerning the Health Care Industry,* Washington, DC: Government Printing Office, GAO/HEHS-94-220, August 1994.
Each of the state statutes that defines the state's healthcare antitrust exemption law.

In April 1992, Maine passed the first state law attempting to provide immunity from federal and state antitrust prosecution. The wording in this act is typical of others (Maine Revised Statutes, Title 22, Subtitle 2, Part 4, Ch. 405-D):

> The Department shall issue a certificate of public advantage for a cooperative agreement if it determines that the applicants have demonstrated by clear and convincing evidence that the likely benefits resulting from the agreements outweigh any disadvantages attributable to a reduction in competition that may result from the agreement.

In evaluating applications for a certificate of public advantage (COPA), the Maine Department of Human Services must consider the following potential benefits:

1. Enhancement of quality;
2. Preservation of geographic proximity to communities being served by an operating facility that might not continue to operate in the absence of the collaborative arrangement; and
3. Gains in cost efficiency through reductions in duplication and the attainment of greater economies of scale.

In turn, the Department must consider the following potential costs:

1. Reduction in the ability of purchasers to negotiate optimal payment and service arrangements;
2. Any reduction in competition among providers;
3. Increases in the price and decreases in the quality of care that affect patients; and
4. The availability of alternative arrangements that are less restrictive but enable the collaborating entities to achieve the same benefits.

Proponents of these laws often assert that they are necessary because federal and state antitrust enforcement in the health sector has prevented beneficial collaborative arrangements. For example, the Minnesota law states (Minnesota Statutes, Ch. 62J, Art. 6, § 26):

> The legislature finds that the goals of controlling health care costs and improving the quality of and access to health care services will be significantly enhanced by some cooperative agreements involving providers or purchasers that may be prohibited by state and federal antitrust laws if undertaken without governmental involvement.

The Colorado law states (Colorado Revised Statutes, Title 25.5, Art. 1, Part 5):

> Federal and state antitrust laws have inhibited the formation of cooperative health care arrangements involving hospitals. However, such cooperative arrangements are likely to foster improvements in the delivery, quality, or cost effectiveness of health care, improve access to needed services, enhance the likelihood that rural hospitals in Colorado will remain open to serve their communities, and provide flexibility for local communities to design, foster, and develop programs to meet their specific health care needs.

And the South Carolina law states (South Carolina Code, § 1, Ch. 7 of Title 44):

> Competition as currently mandated by federal and state antitrust laws should be supplanted by a regulatory program to permit and encourage cooperative agreements between hospitals, health care purchasers, or other health care providers when the benefits outweigh the disadvantages caused by their potential adverse effects on competition.

Hospitals are more likely to approach states for antitrust clearance in situations where their proposed collaboration constitutes a high market share. In such situations, the hospitals may expect to be challenged by a federal agency if they do not obtain state approval.

In perhaps the first application of a state antitrust exemption law, the Minnesota Department of Health approved the merger of the Health One and LifeSpan hospital systems in July 1994. The Minnesota Department of Health concluded that the merger would save $31 million, and the new system, HealthSpan Health System Corporation, agreed to abide by revenue limits to be set by the Minnesota Department of Health ("Minnesota . . ." 1994).

The review of the Health One and LifeSpan merger by the Minnesota Department of Health under Minnesota's law was mandated by a consent decree (Kempainen 1996). Minnesota's attorney general had filed suit against the proposed merger of Health One and LifeSpan, arguing that the postmerger market share resulting from the proposed merger was unacceptably high and that the proposed merger violated Section One of the Sherman Antitrust Act and Section Seven of the Clayton Antitrust Act. The Minnesota attorney general and the defendants settled the suit by agreeing to a consent decree that shifted the decision to the Minnesota Department of Health.

In December 1995, a merger-like partnership between hospitals was approved under North Carolina's law (Burda 1996a). The merger was between Memorial Mission Medical Center and St. Joseph's Hospital, the only two acute care facilities in Asheville, North Carolina (Gurley 1995). The two hospitals maintain separate identities, assets, and ownership, but are controlled by a 17-member governing board that oversees almost all of their operations including strategic, operational, and financial planning.

In March 1994, Memorial Mission and St. Joseph's Hospital had elected to apprise the DOJ of their intention to pursue a merger-like partnership, and the DOJ responded with a civil investigative demand for documents associated with the planned deal. The hospitals did not submit formal premerger notification documents with DOJ because this would have precipitated a formal ruling. Instead, they lobbied to have the law in North Carolina expanded to include hospital mergers. They were successful, and in June 1995 the state law was expanded to include hospitals. Shortly thereafter, the hospitals applied for a COPA under the expanded law.

North Carolina's attorney general approved the deal four months later and issued a COPA that outlined numerous requirements. The COPA requires the two hospitals to generate $74.2 million of savings between 1996 and 2001, and to limit their operating profit margin to the average profit margin of similar North Carolina hospitals. Furthermore, it requires that the two hospitals refrain from employing or exclusively contracting with 20 percent or more of the primary care physicians in their service area.

The state assures compliance with the COPA by requiring quarterly and annual reports, and through firsthand inspection of hospital records, and the new hospital system, the Mission–St. Joseph's Health System, has established a COPA monitoring committee composed of departmental directors and other administrative officials in order to assure compliance with the COPA.

The law in North Carolina spurred a series of collaborative activities among hospitals, physicians, and outpatient care facilities. A recent article in an Asheville, North Carolina, newspaper states that "the trend all across the state is to form alliances made possible with certificates of public advantage authorized by the General Assembly last year"("Holding . . ." 1996).

A similar situation arose in Montana (Bellinghausen 1995). In November 1994, the only two hospitals in Great Falls, Montana (Montana Deaconess Medical Center and Columbus Hospital) announced plans for a full-asset merger but were deterred due to a potential antitrust suit from the FTC (Burda 1996c). Subsequently, the two hospitals lobbied successfully for an extension of Montana's law to include hospitals, and in October 1995 they applied for an exemption under the expanded law.

In March 1996, Montana's attorney general approved the exemption subject to several conditions. The most important condition requires the hospitals to limit future price increases for patient care services. The FTC subsequently indicated that it would not challenge the merger because Montana's attorney general had been intimately involved in the merger process and there was strong evidence that the state would closely monitor the activities of the merged entities to ensure compliance. In July 1996, these hospitals consummated a full-asset merger.

OTHER STATE ACTIVITIES

Entities in states with laws attempting to provide antitrust immunity to approved activities may bypass the voluntary program established by these laws and seek approval from their state attorney general. In this situation, approval from the state attorney general would shield the collaborating entities from federal antitrust prosecution only if the actions of the state attorney general satisfied the conditions required by the state action immunity doctrine.

In 1995, four Maine hospitals sought protection under the state's antitrust immunity law in order to integrate their respective physician-hospital organizations (PHOs) into a single network (Burda 1996b; Austin 1995). Three of the four Maine hospitals were solo community providers and the fourth was located in a two-hospital town. The approval agency for the antitrust immunity law in Maine is the Department of Human Services.

These four hospitals simultaneously sought protection from the state attorney general, and in January 1996 an agreement was signed between the four hospitals and the Maine attorney general. The agreement required the four PHOs to integrate their financial operations into a single organization in order to absolve them of price-fixing charges (a single entity is incapable of conspiring with itself). The newly formed "super PHO" also agreed to accept capitated contracts from payers and other payment arrangements such as fee-for-service with a substantial withhold in order to forge a single economic unit.

Presumably, approval from the state attorney general obviates the need for approval from the Maine Department of Human Service. However, it is unclear whether the consent decree issued by Maine's attorney general will deter federal prosecution (Pristave, Becker, and Gutierrez 1995).

There have been a few instances where state and federal antitrust authorities have acted jointly. In the first joint action, Florida's attorney general and the DOJ in June 1994 agreed to permit two hospitals in North Pinellas County, Florida (Mease Health System and Morton Plant Hospital) to consolidate certain highly specialized services such as open-heart surgery and some administrative functions such as accounting, billing, medical records, and procurement (Magleby 1996). It is important to note that the Mease–Morton Plant joint action by the Florida attorney general and the DOJ did involve a consent decree. Therefore, even though the federal government was involved, the solution resembled a state action.

In another joint action, Virginia's attorney general and the FTC acted to dissolve a physician network in Danville, Virginia in May 1995 (McCormick 1995). The state and federal antitrust officials alleged that PGI Inc. conspired to prevent managed care plans from entering the market and to fix prices. PGI Inc. included fewer than 20 percent of the physicians in its market, but it was an independent practice association (IPA) and it did not involve any sharing of financial risk. In order to avoid costly and lengthy litigation, members of PGI Inc. agreed to dissolve the corporation.

Some state attorneys general not only actively review proposed collaborative activities among healthcare entities in their state; they also exercise considerable creativity. In an unusual antitrust consent decree, Maine's attorney general recently approved the merger of the practices of nine of the ten cardiothoracic surgeons practicing in Portland, Maine (Goad 1996). One of the conditions of the settlement was that the new corporation, the Maine Heart Surgical Associates, agree to limit their charges to those of similar physicians in Boston, Massachusetts. Presumably, the competitive market that restrains price increases of cardiothoracic surgeons in Boston will act to restrain price increases in the near-monopoly market in Portland, Maine.

In at least eight instances, state antitrust officials have approved agreements with merging hospitals that include the promise to constrain future price increases (Burda and Jaklevic 1996). In two instances, the promise to constrain future price increases has been included as part of an agreement to obtain approval under a state antitrust immunity law. In the merger in Great Falls, Montana, the hospitals agreed to freeze prices for one year and to limit price increases to the rate of increase of the hospital component of the U.S. Labor Department's Producer Price Index for the succeeding five years. Earlier, the two health systems that merged to form HealthSpan in Minnesota agreed to limit their price increases to levels that would ensure that their revenue growth was below limits set by the Minnesota Department of Health.

In the first merger to trade state antitrust clearance for price concessions (1989), the only two hospitals in Bellingham, Washington agreed to limit their price increases to the rate of increase in the hospital marketbasket index published by the Health Care Financing Administration. In another instance (1994), the only three hospitals in Williamsport, Pennsylvania received antitrust clearance from Pennsylvania's attorney general after promising not to raise prices faster than the hospital marketbasket index as calculated by the American Hospital Association.

Similarly, the parent companies of two of the three hospitals in Harrisburg, Pennsylvania approached the state's attorney general with a merger proposal that included a promise to limit price increases to the rate of growth of the general inflation as measured in the Consumer Price Index (CPI) plus 2 percent. The two hospitals, Polyclinic Medical Center and Harrisburg Hospital, contained almost 90 percent of the licensed beds in the city. Yet the Pennsylvania attorney general issued an antitrust consent decree approving the merger, and the two hospitals consummated their merger on January 1, 1996.

The only two hospitals in Everett, Washington received antitrust clearance for a merger from Washington's attorney general in December 1993 after agreeing to limit price increases to the rate of increase in the hospital component of the Producer Price Index (PPI) until the year 2000. The PPI measures the rate of increase in wholesale prices. The rate of increase in the hospital component of the PPI almost always exceeds the overall rate of increase of the PPI and usually exceeds the rate of increase in the overall CPI.

In a consent decree sanctioned by the Massachusetts attorney general in early 1996, a hospital in Fall River (Charleton Memorial Hospital) and a hospital in New Bedford (St. Luke's Hospital) were granted permission to merge (Czurak 1996). The seven-page consent decree included a requirement that the merged entity restrain its price increase to the rate of inflation.

DISCUSSION

All hospitals that have received state antitrust consent decrees for mergers in exchange for price concessions have been located in small markets, and in five of the eight mergers the hospitals involved were the only two hospitals in the city. In each of these instances, the proposed merger probably would have provoked a reaction from federal antitrust officials because the postmerger concentration rates were so high.

Mergers may enhance operational efficiency, and mergers may reduce costs by combining operations or by eliminating expensive technologies at one or more of the merging entities (e.g., two hospitals with transplantation units might consolidate this function at one of the hospitals). Moreover, a merger might enable a provider to purchase vital equipment. Thus, mergers have the potential both to lower costs and enhance quality.

Mergers also have the potential to raise prices. Mergers enhance the concentration rate among providers and enhance economic power. In towns where the only two hospitals combine operations, the potential for the exercise of economic power is considerable.

To enable hospitals to achieve efficiencies while precluding their injudicious use of market power, some state attorneys general have entered into consent decrees that permit hospitals to merge in exchange for a promise not to increase prices at a rate faster than an established price index (e.g., the hospital market-basket index as calculated by the American Hospital Association) for a specific time period (usually three to seven years). Through consent decrees, state attorneys general have attempted to maximize the positive effects of hospital mergers while minimizing their negative effects.

One of the major differences between state and federal antitrust regulators in their approach to healthcare mergers involves the willingness to approve mergers in exchange for price concessions and other promises by the merging entities. Federal antitrust officials contend that they do not have the resources to monitor future performance and that a merger should be judged solely on its likely effects on market performance (Grulley and McGinley 1996).

Federal officials have been unwilling to exchange promises to restrain future price increases for the permission to merge in situations where they believe that a merger will substantially increase the economic power of the merging providers. Federal officials maintain that promises to restrain prices for a specified time period do not protect consumers after that time period and that it is unclear how well state authorities will be able to monitor hospital performance and hold merged hospitals to their promises. For instance, a hospital that is part of a larger system may transfer services to the larger system (e.g., it may reschedule tests, normally provided on admittance, to a related outpatient facility) in an attempt to avoid the force of a price agreement.

State authorities, however, may be better suited than federal authorities to ensure that hospitals abide by the stipulations in consent decrees. Numerous states require hospitals to provide uniform patient abstracts and cost reports. Moreover, all states regulate many aspects of a hospital's operations as part of their licensure function. Thus, it may be difficult for hospitals to avoid complying with price agreements with states by altering their accounting practices or reorganizing their operations. In any case, regulators must continually scrutinize the operation of merged entities to ensure that they meet all of the requirements of consent decrees.

It is uncertain, too, how merged entities will behave after the price agreement expires. If hospitals raise prices immediately after their price agreement expires, then consent decrees may simply postpone the increase in prices.

Nonprofit hospitals have argued that they will not exercise economic power injudiciously because they are governed by boards of trustees that are composed of community representatives. Often these representatives are executives from local businesses that would bear the consequences of higher hospital prices.

This argument has been buttressed by recent empirical work showing that higher concentration rates among nonprofit hospitals in a market are not related to higher prices (Lynk 1995). However, the evidence available regarding the relationship between ownership status and prices in the hospital industry is limited, and more research is needed for a definitive assessment of this relationship.

FINAL REMARKS

Current research about the impact of hospital concentration is almost entirely limited to hospitals in California (Zwanziger and Melnick 1988; Melnick and Zwanziger 1988; Melnick, Zwanziger, and Bradley 1989; Melnick, Bamezai, and Pattison 1992). This research indicates that increases in the concentration of hospitals are related to higher prices.

Yet this research does not indicate how mergers have affected market performance outside of California, and it does not indicate how mergers approved under COPAs and consent decrees issued by state attorneys general have affected market performance. (California has not passed a law that attempts to confer immunity from state and federal antitrust prosecution, and its attorney general has not entered into any consent decrees with merging hospitals.)

In addition, these findings do not differentiate between increases in concentration in markets that are already highly concentrated from increases in markets that were initially quite competitive. The models used to assess the impact of increased concentration in these studies have not been flexible enough to permit the effect of increased concentration to vary according to the initial level of concentration.

The communities where states have approved mergers have been relatively small, and even before the approved mergers took place they included few competitors. Research is needed to determine whether or not hospital mergers in such communities are likely to produce unwanted consequences. In order to do this researchers must estimate models that are flexible enough to permit the impact of concentration levels to vary according to the initial level of concentration as well as by the change in concentration.

More importantly, researchers should examine market performance (e.g., the hospital cost per day, the hospital cost per stay, the per capita cost of hospital care, and the per capita cost of healthcare) in communities where states have approved hospital mergers. Economists predict that enhanced economic power will result in higher prices and a reduction in the quantity of services available. Yet many COPAs and consent decrees prohibit newly formed entities from increasing their prices for many years.

Researchers also should examine how the remaining competitors in these markets (if any) have reacted to the merger. The reduction in the number of competitors in a market facilitates the opportunity for informal collusion, and remaining competitors may increase prices and reduce output (the remaining competitors are not subject to restrictions in a COPA or consent decree).

Moreover, some COPAs and consent decrees limit the profitability of newly formed entities. The remaining competitors are not constrained, and researchers should compare the profitability of the remaining competitors before and after the merger.

Hospitals attempting to merge often argue that consolidation will convey efficiencies attributable to economies of scale and the elimination of duplicative facilities. They also often assert that consolidation will increase the quality of care because physicians at the hospital where the services are consolidated will acquire more experience and expertise.

Researchers should examine whether these efficiencies have been realized and whether the quality of care has improved. Efficiency may be measured by changes in the cost of care at the hospital and at the departmental levels. Quality of care may be measured by changes in the adjusted mortality rates, changes in the complication and readmission rates, and changes in patient satisfaction.

There is considerable skepticism about the ability of states to effectively enforce the stipulations of COPAs and consent decrees. Research should be conducted to determine whether or not the merged entities are abiding by the stipulations of their COPA or consent decree. Evidently, the ability of states to enforce the stipulations of COPAs and consent decrees varies based on the resources available to the enforcement agency (e.g., the availability of skilled personnel), the adequacy of the data provided by the merged entity (some states require little data), and the sanctions available to the enforcement agency. Furthermore, political considerations are likely to play a role in the vigilance displayed by state agencies in enforcing COPAs and consent decrees.

In sum, the consequences of state-approved mergers on healthcare providers, markets, and consumers are unknown. Supporters of these mergers argue that consent decrees and COPAs guarantee that mergers will not result in higher prices and profitability, and that they will increase efficiency and the quality of care. Opponents argue that states are incapable of enforcing the complex requirements of consent decrees and COPAs, and that when agreements expire merged entities will increase prices. Research that examines the impact of state-approved mergers on market performance may provide valuable information to policymakers and thus help shape future decisions regarding proposed mergers.

REFERENCES

Austin, P. 1995. "The Managed Care Bandwagon." *Maine Times* 27 (31 August): 6–8.

Bellinghausen, P. 1995. "Billings Hospitals: No Merger in Sight." *Billings Gazette* (6 November): A6–A7.

Bergstrom, R. W., and R. W. Olsen. 1985. "Trade Associations and Other Associations of Competitors." In *Antitrust Advisor, 3d ed.,* edited by C. Anderson, pp. 479–514. Colorado Springs, CO: Shepard's/McGraw-Hill.

Burda, D. 1996a. "North Carolina Hospitals' Antitrust Victory Looks Hollow." *Modern Healthcare* 26 (1): 6, 14.

———. 1996b. "Maine Hospitals' Antitrust Deal OKs Joint Contracting." *Modern Healthcare* 26 (7): 7.

———. 1996c. "Montana Antitrust Trade-Off Key to Hospital Merger." *Modern Healthcare* 26 (12): 5, 12, 18.

Burda, D., and M. C. Jaklevic. 1996. "Promises, Promises: Hospitals Are Using Price-Control Pledges to Win Antitrust Clearance from States, But the Feds Are Wary." *Modern Healthcare* 26 (8): 26–29.

California Retail Liquor Dealers Association v. *Midcal Aluminum.* 1994. Department of Justice and Federal Trade Commission, Statements of Enforcement Policy and Analytical Principles Relating to Health Care and Antitrust. Washington, DC: Government Printing Office. Inc. et al., 445 U.S. 97 (U.S. Supreme Court, 1980).

"Consolidation in the Health Care Marketplace and Antitrust Policy." 1995. Issue Brief, No. 600, National Health Policy Forum, The George Washington University, p. 2.

Czurak, D. 1996. "Health-Merger Similarities Noted in Massachusetts Case." *Grand Rapids Business Journal* 14 (30): 3–4.

Department of Justice and Federal Trade Commission. 1993. *Statements of Antitrust Enforcement Policy in the Health Care Area.* Washington, DC: Government Printing Office.

———. 1992. *Horizontal Merger Guidelines.* Washington, DC: Government Printing Office.

———. 1996. *Statements of Antitrust Enforcement Policy in Health Care.* Washington, DC: Government Printing Office, August.

Goad, M. 1996. "Surgeons Agree to Price Limits: The Antitrust Agreement Between the Portland Surgeons Is Aimed at Assuring Fair and Competitive Prices." *Portland Press Herald* (Portland, ME, 24 July): 3B–4B.

Grulley, B., and L. McGinley. 1996. "Antitrust Lawyers Fail to Stop Hospital Deal, with Big Consequences." *Wall Street Journal* (4 January): A1.

Gurley, M. L. 1995. "How to Stop Losing Your Patients: Special Report—Health Care." *Business North Carolina* 15 (8): 8–11.

Hittinger, C. W., and D. E. Brehm. 1996. "How Other States Handle Touchy Hospital Mergers." *The Legal Intelligencer* (16 May): 9–11.

"Holding Down Region's Cost for Health Care." 1996. *Asheville Citizen-Times* (Asheville, NC, 16 August): A8.

Institute of Medicine. 1993. *Employment and Health Benefits: A Connection at Risk,* edited by M. J. Field and H. T. Shapiro, p. 109. Washington, DC: National Academy Press.

Kempainen, P. R. (Assistant Attorney General, Antitrust Division, Minnesota Attorney General's Office). 1996. "Summary and Analysis of Minnesota's Antitrust Actions Affecting the Health Care Industry." Paper presented at a meeting of the National Academy for State Health Policy, Minneapolis, MN, 11 August.

Lynk, W. 1995. "Nonprofit Hospital Mergers and the Exercise of Market Power." *The Journal of Law and Economics* 38 (2): 437–61.

Magleby, J. E. 1996. "Hospital Mergers and Antitrust Policy: Arguments Against a Modification of Current Antitrust Law." *Antitrust Bulletin* 41 (1): 137–49.

McCormick, B. 1995. "Physician Network Broken Up: Antitrust Violations Alleged." *American Medical News* 38 (19): 7–8.

Melnick, G. A., A. Bamezai, and R. Pattison. 1992. "The Effects of Market Structure and Bargaining Position on Hospital Prices." *Journal of Health Economics* 11 (2): 217–33.

Melnick, G. A., and J. Zwanziger. 1988. "Hospital Behavior Under Competition and Cost-Containment Policies: The California Experience, 1980 to 1985." *Journal of the American Medical Association* 260 (18): 2669–75.

Melnick, G. A., J. Zwanziger, and T. Bradley. 1989. "Competition and Cost Containment in California: 1980–1987." *Health Affairs* 8 (2): 129–36.

"Minnesota OKs Merger of HealthSpan Hospitals." 1994. *Health Care Competition Week* 11, no. 16 (5 August): 2.

Page, L. 1995. "Market Spawns Doctor-Patient Alliances." *American Medical News* (13 November): 3, 24.

Parker, Director of Agriculture, et al. v. Brown, 317 U.S. 341 (U.S. Supreme Court, 1940).

Pristave, R. J., S. Becker, and L. Gutierrez. 1995. "Development of Provider Networks for Specific Diseases." *Journal of Health Care Finance* 22 (2): 27–33.

Prospective Payment Assessment Commission. 1996. *Medicare and the American Health Care System: Report to the Congress.* Washington, DC: Government Printing Office, June.

Ross, S. F. 1993. *Principles of Antitrust Law.* Westbury, NY: The Foundation Press, Inc.

United States General Accounting Office. 1994. *Federal and State Antitrust Actions Concerning the Health Care Industry.* Pub. No. GAO/HEHS-94-220. Washington, DC: Government Printing Office.

Zwanziger, J., and G. A. Melnick. 1988 "The Effects of Hospital Competition and the Medicare PPS Program on Hospital Cost Behavior in California." *Journal of Health Economics* 7 (3): 301–20.

Part III

The Contemporary American Healthcare System

18 | Expenditures

John K. Iglehart

The United States operates a health care system that is unique among nations. It is the most expensive of systems, outstripping by over half again the health care expenditures of any other country.[1] The number of people without insurance continues to increase, however, reaching 43.4 million, or 16.1 percent of the population, in 1997—the highest level in a decade.[2] By many technical standards, U.S. medical care is the best in the world,[3] but leaders in the field declared recently at a national round table that there is an "urgent need to improve health care quality."[4] The stringency of managed care and a low inflation rate have slowed the growth of medical spending appreciably, but a new government study projects that health care expenditures will soon begin escalating again and will double over the next decade.[5] In short, the American system is a work in progress, driven by a disparate array of interests with two goals that are often in conflict: providing health care to the sick, and generating income for the persons and organizations that assume the financial risk. In this report, I will take stock of this dynamic sector, which now represents one seventh of the economy, by tracking it in the most American of ways—following the money from its collection to its expenditure.

Almost five years has elapsed since the ambitious efforts of the Clinton administration to reform the health care system fell to defeat without even reaching the floor of the House or Senate for a vote. Since then, with the enthusiastic approval of the Republican-controlled Congress and the acceptance of the Clinton administration, large numbers of private-sector employees and beneficiaries of publicly financed insurance programs have enrolled in managed-care plans. Those covered by such plans now make up an estimated 75 percent of all persons with private health insurance.

In strictly monetary terms, two trends dominate. One is the decline in the growth of health care expenditures in the past five years. In 1997, the growth rate was the slowest in the more than 35 years for which there are data on medical spending.[6] The second trend is the growth in the government's share of the nation's health care bill. Spending by federal, state, and local governments rose in 1997 to $507 billion, or 46 percent of the total, an increase from 40 percent in 1990. Private resources financed 54 percent of personal health services ($585 billion) in 1997, down from 60 percent in 1990.[6]

The magnitude of public expenditures in any health care system is important because it indicates the amount of attention governments are likely to pay to the system and thus the influence they bring to bear on its configuration. Rhetoric notwithstanding, the government's role in the financing and regulation of health care has grown inexorably under both Republicans and Democrats ever since the enactment of Medicare and Medicaid in 1965. As the health economist Victor Fuchs puts it, "No matter how committed the country is in general to the idea of free markets and capitalism, government plays a substantial role in health care."[7]

THE ROLE OF ECONOMIC SYSTEMS

Nevertheless, the U.S. economy is driven primarily by market-based capitalism. A market-based system consists of a collection of decision-making units called households and another collection of businesses and other larger organizations. This structure is important to recognize because, as Fuchs asserts, "The households own all the productive resources in the society."[8] Thus, although funds for personal health services flow from three basic sources—employers, governments, and individuals—all of these resources are initially extracted from households as payroll deductions from the wages of working adults, as taxes and other surcharges, and as direct payments to providers and suppliers. In reality, government and employers are only intermediaries in the process. A fourth source is, as Uwe Reinhardt has described it, "an informal, albeit unreliable, catastrophic health insurance program operated by hospitals and many physicians . . . who extract the premium for that insurance through higher charges to paying patients."[9]

THE ROLE OF EMPLOYERS

Collectively, private employers and employees are the most important purchasers of health care through the insurance premiums they pay together for coverage. Of the $585 billion that private payers expended for medical services in 1997, about 60 percent ($348 billion) was spent by employers and employees to purchase health insurance.[6] The premiums that finance coverage are paid in part by the employee through the explicit deduction of regular (usually weekly or monthly) amounts from the gross wages stated on the employee's paycheck. The remainder (usually 80 percent or more) is ostensibly paid by employers and not deducted from the employee's pay. There is a sharp division of opinion over who actually foots the bill for the employer-paid portion. The question is important because as employers steer their workers into insurance arrangements that employers select, very few employees (17 percent in the most recent estimate[10]) have a choice of plans.

Most employees have long believed that the employer's portion comes out of the employer's profits. Most employers share that view, believing that their premium payments are a cost of doing business and, as such, cut into the profitability of the firm. Economists and the Congressional Budget Office, on the other hand, are convinced by theory and empirical evidence that this portion, too, is actually shifted back to employees in the form of lower take-home pay.[11,12] In a recent book, the economist Mark Pauly asserted that "higher medical costs do not harm employers or owners but do reduce money wages for workers. . . . Lower costs benefit workers, not employers; they add to take-home pay, not profits."[13]

By exempting from federal and state taxes the income earned by employees that is used to pay insurance premiums, the government encourages employers to provide coverage to workers. Employers' costs are treated as a deductible business expense. The exclusion from income taxes and Social Security payroll deductions creates a substantial tax subsidy for employment-based insurance. In 1999, according to the Clinton administration, this exemption will reduce federal revenues by an estimated $76 billion. If this were a federal health program, it would be the third most expensive one after Medicare and Medicaid.[14] Families with higher incomes benefit disproportionately because they are in higher tax brackets. This subsidy provides little or no benefit to people who are uninsured or who purchase their own health insurance. This regressive tax structure was an unintended consequence of the policy, but employers strongly oppose its elimination. Recently, Congress extended the tax benefit to self-employed people in a phased-in provision that will take full effect in 2003.

THE ROLE OF GOVERNMENT

One of the key characteristics of all modern economies is that as they prosper, they spend more money for health care. For example, high-income countries (those with per capita annual incomes above $8,500) accounted for 89 percent of global health expenditures in 1994, even though they comprised only 16 percent of the global population and represented just 7 percent of the estimated number of disability-adjusted years of life worldwide (1.4 trillion) that were lost to disease.[15] Although all nations purchase more health care as they prosper— so that about 80 percent of the variation among countries in per capita health care spending is explained by the per capita income of a country—the United States is once again an exception. Its annual bill for personal health services ($3,925 per person in 1997) is about $1,000 per person above the level that its per capita income would seemingly predict. Three reasons are that physicians in the United States are paid more than those in other countries for each unit of service,[16] a day in the hospital for similar patients is considerably more expensive in the United States, and medical technology diffuses more rapidly and is generally used to treat more patients than in other countries. In a survey of 50 health economists in 1995, 81 percent agreed with the following statement: "The primary reason for the increase in the health sector's share of [the gross domestic product] over the past 30 years is technological change in medicine."[17]

Federal and state expenditures for medical care are collected as taxes of one type or another and redistributed as income to providers and suppliers, who bill for services rendered and goods delivered. The dynamics of this system have begun to change, however, as more payments for health care are fixed and set prospectively. The federal government pays the physicians it employs and other employees of publicly operated health care facilities. States also employ physicians directly and operate public health care facilities. Public monies are allocated for health care through a variety of agencies after being appropriated by federal and state legislative bodies or collected in earmarked accounts such as social-insurance trust funds (e.g., Medicare).

One important component of national health care spending is the transfer of money from the federal to the state governments. Such transfers evolved after World War II, and their total value tripled during the 1960s. By 1995, the number of intergovernmental grants for education, health, transportation, and other purposes had risen to 633, with outlays totaling $226 billion.[18] Democrats and Republicans differ about how federal aid to states should be structured. In general, Republicans favor block grants to states—that is, grants with few strings attached—because their party supports shifting power from Washington, D.C., to the states. Democrats generally prefer categorical grants—that is, those that stipulate with greater specificity how the money should be spent.

The largest program involving the intergovernmental transfer of funds is Medicaid, which accounted for 39 percent of all federal grant outlays in 1995. In 1997, Medicaid financed acute care and long-term care services for 41.3 million aged, blind, and disabled people with low incomes, as well as poor mothers and children, at a cost of $160 billion.[6] Of that amount, the federal share was $95 billion and the state and local share $65 billion. The federal funds are appropriated annually, with the amounts determined by a formula based on each state's per capita income. Medicaid spending grew by only 3.8 percent in 1997, the smallest annual increase in the history of the program. In large part, Medicaid's slow growth stemmed from the effects of welfare-reform legislation (the Personal Responsibility and Work Opportunity Reconciliation Act of 1996), which led to an unprecedented decline in welfare caseloads[19,20] and low unemployment rates.

The largest federal health program, Medicare, is funded from four different sources: mandatory contributions by employers and employees, general tax revenues, beneficiaries' premiums, and deductibles and copayments paid by patients (or supplemental health insurance). Medicare beneficiaries include people over 65 years of age, the disabled, and those with end-stage renal disease. Medicare's Hospital Insurance Trust Fund (Part A of the program) is grounded in the principle of social insurance. That is, workers make mandatory contributions to a dedicated trust fund during their working years, with the promise of receiving benefits after they retire. By law, the nation's employers and some 151 million employees are required to pay equal amounts of a payroll tax that totals 2.9 percent of earned income. Self employed workers pay the entire 2.9 percent of their net income into the trust fund. In 1997, these payroll taxes totaled $115 billion and made up 88 percent of the income of the trust fund; the remainder came from interest earned on the monies in the trust fund and miscellaneous sources. Approximately 22 percent of the 38 million people who are eligible for Medicare hospital insurance received hospital services in 1997.

Medicare Part B finances care by physicians and outpatient, home health, and other services; it is called the Supplementary Medical Insurance Program. The funds come largely from general tax revenues appropriated by Congress ($60 billion, or about 73 percent of the total Part B income, in 1997), rather than from a mandatory tax collected for that specific purpose. Part B funds are often erroneously called a "trust fund." Medicare beneficiaries who enroll in Part B are required to pay monthly premiums (in 1998, the premium was $43.80). Enrollment is voluntary, but virtually all people who are eligible sign up. Premiums are not related to income. Thus, in Medicare, unlike Medicaid, the rich and the poor are treated the same. In 1997, premiums accounted for $19 billion, or about 24 percent of Part B income. The remainder of its funding came from interest income on revenues.

Medicare has low administrative costs, as compared with those of managed-care companies or private insurers. Benefit payments represent 99 percent of outlays for Medicare Part A; administrative expenses, including funds to support fiscal intermediaries (generally private insurance companies), make up only 1 percent of the total.[21] More than 98 percent of the Part B outlays are for benefit payments; less than 2 percent are for administration.

THE CONTRIBUTIONS OF INDIVIDUAL CITIZENS

The share of national health expenditures paid for directly by individual citizens declined for 11 straight years until 1997, when it grew markedly faster than private health insurance premiums.[6] Out-of-pocket spending is generally defined as including expenditures for coinsurance and deductibles required by insurers, as well as direct payments for services not covered by a third party. Premium amounts contributed by employees are generally not considered as out-of-pocket expenditures. Out-of-pocket spending amounted to $188 billion in 1997, or 17.2 percent of all national health expenditures. The general decline in direct consumer spending has been attributed in large part to the growth in health maintenance organizations (HMOs), which traditionally offer broad benefits with only modest out-of-pocket payments. In the past few years, however, most HMO enrollees have had increased cost-sharing requirements, as employers and health plan managers have sought to constrain spending even further.[22] In general, out-of-pocket payments are still considerably less in an HMO than with indemnity insurance.

The overall declines in per capita out-of-pocket spending mask the financial difficulties of many poor people and families.[23] A recent study estimated that Medicare beneficiaries over 65 years of age with incomes below the federal poverty level (in 1997 the level was $7,755 for individuals and $9,780 for couples) who were also eligible for Medicaid assistance (which usually covers the monthly Part B premium) still spent 35 percent of their incomes on out-of-pocket health care costs.[24] Medicare beneficiaries with incomes below the federal poverty level who did not receive Medicaid assistance spent, on average, half their incomes on out-of-pocket health care costs.

THE FLOW OF HEALTH CARE EXPENDITURES

In 1997, national health expenditures totaled $1,092 billion, according to the Health Care Financing Administration (HCFA), which tracks expenditures (Table 18.1).[6] Health care spending consumed 13.5 percent of the gross domestic product in 1997, which was a slight drop from the previous year. Health care spending increased only 4.8 percent in 1997—the slowest annual growth rate in more than 35 years. Personal health expenditures accounted for 89 percent of health care spending, or $969 billion. HCFA's analysts recently projected that, beginning in 1998, national health spending would again begin to grow faster than the rest of the economy. By 2002, the agency projected that national health expenditures would total $2.1 trillion (Table 18.2)—an estimated 16.6 percent of the gross domestic product.[5] This analysis was based on two assumptions that are certain to be challenged by employers and the managed-care industry: that "the higher anticipated growth in real per capita national health spending will be driven almost entirely by rising expenditures in the private rather than the public sector," and that savings from managed care will be a one-time phenomenon, rather than a long-term trend.

Before the emergence of managed care, it was largely physicians, acting individually on behalf of their patients, who decided how most health care dollars were spent. They billed for their services, and third-party insurers usually reimbursed them without asking any questions, because the ultimate payers—

TABLE 18.1

National Health Expenditures for Selected Years from 1960 through 1997*

Spending Category	1960	1970	1980	1990	1994	1995	1996	1997
Total national expenditures (billions of dollars)	26.9	73.2	247.3	699.4	947.7	993.7	1,042.5	1,092.4
Expenditures for health services and supplies (billions of dollars)	25.2	67.9	235.6	674.8	917.2	963.1	1,010.6	1,057.5
Personal health care	23.6	63.8	217.0	614.7	834.0	879.3	924.0	969.0
Hospital care	9.3	28.0	102.7	256.4	335.7	347.2	360.8	371.1
Physicians' services	5.3	13.6	45.2	146.3	193.0	201.9	208.5	217.6
Dental services	2.0	4.7	13.3	31.6	42.4	45.0	47.5	50.6
Other professional services	0.6	1.4	6.4	34.7	49.6	53.6	57.5	61.9
Home health care†	0.1	0.2	2.4	13.1	26.2	29.1	31.2	32.3
Drugs and other nondurable medical products	4.2	8.8	21.6	59.9	81.6	88.9	98.3	108.9
Prescription drugs	2.7	5.5	12.0	37.7	55.2	61.1	69.1	78.9
Vision products and other durable medical products	0.6	1.6	3.8	10.5	12.5	13.1	13.4	13.9
Nursing home care†	0.8	4.2	17.6	50.9	71.1	75.5	79.4	82.8
Other personal health care	0.7	1.3	4.0	11.2	21.9	25.1	27.4	29.9
Program administration and net cost of private health insurance	1.2	2.7	11.9	40.5	55.1	53.3	52.5	50.0
Government public health activities	0.4	1.3	6.7	19.6	28.2	30.4	34.0	38.5
Expenditures for research and construction (billions of dollars)	1.7	5.3	11.6	24.5	30.5	30.6	32.0	34.9
Research‡	0.7	2.0	5.5	12.2	15.9	16.7	17.2	18.0
Construction	1.0	3.4	6.2	12.3	14.6	13.9	14.8	16.9
National expenditures per capita (dollars)	141	341	1,052	2,690	3,500	3,637	3,781	3,925
Population (millions)	190	215	235	260	271	273	276	278
GDP (billions of dollars)	527	1,036	2,784	5,744	6,947	7,270	7,662	8,111
National expenditures as percentage of GDP	5.1	7.1	8.9	12.2	13.6	13.7	13.6	13.5

*Major revisions were recently introduced into expenditure estimates, including a new data source (IMS) for estimating spending on prescription drugs in 1993 through 1997 and revised Census Bureau Services Annual Survey data for 1993 through 1996 for physician services. Numbers may not add to totals because of rounding. GDP denotes gross domestic product. Data are from the Health Care Financing Administration, Office of the Actuary, National Health Statistics Group; the Department of Commerce, Bureau of Economic Analysis; and the Social Security Administration.
†This category includes free-standing facilities only. Additional services of this type are provided in hospital-based facilities and counted as hospital care.
‡Research-and-development expenditures of drug companies and other manufacturers and providers of medical equipment and supplies are excluded from this category and instead are included in the category in which the product falls.

TABLE 18.2

Actual and Projected National Health Expenditures for Selected Calendar Years from 1970 through 2007*

Spending Category	Billions of Dollars (percent)				
	1970	1980	1990	1998	2007
Total national expenditures	73.2 (100.0)	247.3 (100.0)	699.5 (100.0)	1,146.8 (100.0)	2,133.3 (100.0)
Expenditures for health services and supplies	67.9 (92.8)	235.6 (95.3)	775.0 (96.5)	1,113.2 (97.1)	2,085.3 (97.8)
Personal health care	63.8 (87.2)	217.0 (87.8)	614.7 (87.9)	998.2 (87.0)	1,859.2 (87.2)
Hospital care	28.0 (38.2)	102.7 (41.5)	256.4 (36.7)	383.2 (33.4)	649.4 (30.4)
Physicians' services	13.6 (18.6)	45.2 (18.3)	146.3 (20.9)	221.4 (19.3)	427.3 (20.0)
Dental services	4.7 (6.4)	13.3 (5.4)	31.6 (4.5)	53.7 (4.7)	95.2 (4.5)
Other professional services	1.4 (1.9)	6.4 (2.6)	34.7 (5.0)	66.8 (5.8)	134.5 (6.3)
Home health care†	0.2 (0.3)	2.4 (1.0)	13.1 (1.9)	33.2 (2.9)	66.1 (3.1)
Drugs and other nondurable medical products	8.8 (12.0)	21.6 (8.7)	59.9 (8.6)	106.1 (9.3)	223.6 (10.5)
Prescription drugs	5.5 (7.5)	12.0 (4.9)	37.7 (5.4)	74.3 (6.5)	171.1 (8.0)
Vision products and other durable medical products	1.6 (2.2)	3.8 (1.5)	10.5 (1.5)	14.3 (1.2)	23.3 (1.1)
Nursing home care†	4.2 (5.7)	17.6 (7.1)	50.9 (7.3)	87.3 (7.6)	148.3 (7.0)
Other personal health care	1.3 (1.8)	4.0 (1.6)	11.2 (1.6)	32.4 (2.8)	91.4 (4.3)
Program administration and net cost	2.7 (3.7)	11.9 (4.8)	40.7 (5.8)	74.1 (6.5)	151.3 (7.1)
Government public health activities	1.3 (1.8)	6.7 (2.7)	19.6 (2.8)	40.9 (3.6)	74.9 (3.5)
Expenditures for research and construction	5.3 (7.2)	11.6 (4.7)	24.5 (3.5)	33.5 (2.9)	48.0 (2.3)
Research‡	2.0 (2.7)	5.5 (2.2)	12.2 (1.7)	18.4 (1.6)	27.5 (1.3)
Construction	3.4 (4.6)	6.2 (2.5)	12.3 (1.8)	15.1 (1.3)	20.5 (1.0)

*Figures for 1998 and 2007 are projections. Numbers may not add to totals because of rounding. Data are from the Health Care Financing Administration, Office of the Actuary, National Health Statistics Group.
†This category includes free-standing facilities only. Additional services of this type are provided in hospital-based facilities and counted as hospital care.
‡Research-and-development expenditures of drug companies and other manufacturers and providers of medical equipment and supplies are excluded from this category and instead are included in the category in which the product falls.

employers—demanded no greater accounting. Now, many employers have changed from passive payers[25,26] to aggressive purchasers[27] and are exerting more influence on payment rates, on where patients are cared for, and on the content of care. Through selective contracting with physicians, stringent review of the use of services, practice protocols, and payment on a fixed, per capita basis, managed-care plans have pressured doctors to furnish fewer services and to improve the coordination and management of care, thereby altering the way in which many physicians treat patients.[28] In striving to balance the conflicts that arise in caring for patients within these constraints, physicians have become "double agents."[29,30] The ideological tie that long linked many physicians and private executives—a belief in capitalism and free enterprise—has been weakened by the aggressive intervention of business into the practice of medicine through managed care.

THE SHIFTING PATTERN OF EXPENDITURES

Hospital spending continues to consume the largest portion of the health care dollar ($371 billion in 1997, or 38 percent of spending on personal health services), but in large part as a consequence of the pressure applied by managed-care plans, growth in such spending has slowed appreciably.[31] The mix of services offered by most hospitals has shifted away from inpatient stays toward greater use of outpatient and postdischarge services (such as home health care and skilled-nursing facilities). Medicare and Medicaid funded half of all hospital expenditures in 1997, private insurance paid for another third, and consumers paid directly for only 3 percent of all hospital services.[6] The remainder was funded by the Departments of Defense and Veterans Affairs, state and local subsidies to hospitals, and private philanthropy.

The number of hospital days per 1000 HMO enrollees has declined steadily since 1985. Occupancy rates in community hospitals fell from 64 percent in 1990 to 60 percent in 1997; relatively few hospitals have closed, but many have merged. Hospital spending grew by only 2.9 percent in 1997, making it the slowest-growing component in HCFA's expenditure survey. Nonetheless, most hospitals maintained profit margins that were greater than in almost any earlier period.[32] Many hospitals increased their profit margins by reducing their expenses, expanding their capacity to provide outpatient services, and diversifying into postdischarge care.

Expenditures for physicians' services represented another 19.9 percent of the health care dollar in 1997, or $217.6 billion. This figure represented an increase in spending of 4.4 percent over 1996, continuing a trend of single-digit growth that began in 1992. Largely as a result of the efforts of managed-care organizations to constrain medical spending, the annual growth in mean net income for all physicians declined from an average of 7.2 percent during the period from 1986 through 1992 to 1.7 percent in 1993 through 1996.[6]

According to a new analysis of data collected by the National Institutes of Health (NIH), spending on research and development has increased steadily in recent years, both in absolute terms and as a percentage of total health care spending.[33] In 1995, the total was $35.8 billion. This represented 3.5 percent of total health expenditures, as compared with 3.2 percent in 1986. Over the decade from 1986 through 1995, the share of health-related research and development supported by private industry increased from 42 percent to 52 percent, largely as a consequence of increased spending by pharmaceutical companies.

Recently, Congress has indicated that it is prepared to double the NIH's annual appropriation over the next 5 to 10 years; the only question is how fast. Congress approved an appropriation of $15.6 billion for the NIH for fiscal 1999, an increase of almost $2 billion over the previous year and almost double the increase sought by the Clinton administration. The current situation is a far cry from the bleak assessment of the agency's future provided by the NIH director, Dr. Harold Varmus, in his Shattuck Lecture of 1995.[34]

Congress supports medical research not only because legislators are enthusiastic about its potential, but also because funding research is far less expensive than providing health care coverage for the uninsured.[35] In addition, NIH research benefits the thriving biotechnology industry by providing its raw material. Congress has taken a far different view of research on health services, as reflected in the budget of the Agency for Health Care Policy and Research (AHCPR). Several years ago, in response to a small but vocal group of spinal surgeons who opposed the results of a study of low-back pain sponsored by the AHCPR, the Republican-controlled Congress flirted with the idea of abolishing the agency.[36] Having survived that near-death experience, the AHCPR received an appropriation of $171 million in fiscal 1999, an increase of $24 million over the previous year, but considerably less than the funds provided for only one small component of the NIH—the National Human Genome Research Institute, which received $237 million.

Prescription drugs are the fastest-growing component of personal health expenditures, amounting to $78.9 billion in 1997.[6] This trend is troubling to employers, health plans, physicians, and policy makers alike.[37,38] In recent years, spending for prescription drugs has increased at double-digit rates: 10.6 percent in 1995, 13.2 percent in 1996, and 14.1 percent in 1997.[6] The federal Office of Personnel Management announced recently that in 1999 insurance premiums will increase by an average of 10.2 percent for the 8.7 million federal employees, retirees, dependents, and others covered by the Federal Employees Health Benefits Program, the largest premium hike in a decade.[39] The Office of Personnel Management attributed the increase in part to the rising costs of prescription drugs (which have increased 17 percent annually in recent years). There are several explanations for this acceleration in costs, including broader insurance coverage of prescription drugs, growth in the number of drugs dispensed, more approvals of expensive new drugs by the Food and Drug Administration, and direct advertising of pharmaceutical products to consumers. The use of some new drugs reduces hospital costs, but not enough to offset the increase in expenditures for drugs.

CONCLUSIONS

America's trillion-dollar health care system is vast—indeed, larger than the budgets of most nations—and it serves as a perpetual job-creating enterprise, providing employment to some 9 million people. Expenditures for health care are perceived in a variety of ways by different interest groups. Many health care purchasers view them as one of the few uncontrollable costs and have taken unprecedented steps to rein in costs through the constraints imposed by managed-care companies. Patients with employer-sponsored health insurance, who want the best medical care but are fearful of the costs, have sought refuge in managed-care plans, sometimes with mixed results. Physicians may also see health care expenditures as the means to earn a living, or, as Reinhardt has put it, "the allocation of lifestyles to providers."[40] But in spite of all the money spent for medical care, education, and research, no one—whether patient, provider, or purchaser—seems satisfied with the status quo.

REFERENCES

1. OECD health data 1998: a comparative analysis of 29 countries. Paris: Organisation for Economic Cooperation and Development, 1998 (CD-ROM).

2. Bureau of the Census. Current population reports. Health insurance coverage, 1997 and 1998. Washington, D.C.: Government Printing Office, 1997,1998.

3. Berwick DM. As good as it should get: making health care better in the new millennium. Washington, D.C.: National Coalition on Health Care, 1998.

4. Chassin MR, Galvin RW. The urgent need to improve health care quality. JAMA 1998;280:1000–5.

5. Smith S, Freeland M, Heffler S, McKusick D, Health Expenditures Projection Team. The next ten years of health spending: what does the future hold? Health Aff (Millwood) 1998;17(5):128–40.

6. Levit K, Cowan C, Braden B, Stiller J, Sensenig A, Lazenby H. National health expenditures in 1997: more slow growth. Health Aff (Millwood) 1998;17(6):99–110.

7. Fuchs VR. The challenges to health policy in modern economies. The 1997 syarahan perdana. (The Prime Minister of Malaysia Fellowship Exchange Program Lecture.) Kuala Lumpur, Malaysia, September 23,1997.

8. Fuchs VR. Health care and the United States economic system: an essay in abnormal physiology. Milbank Mem Fund Q 1972;50(2):211–44.

9. Reinhardt UE. Wanted: a clearly articulated social ethic for American health care. JAMA 1997;278:1446–7.

10.   Long SH, Marquis SM. How widespread is managed competition? Data bulletin results from community tracking study. Washington, D.C.: Center for Studying Health System Change, 1998:12.

11.   Krueger AB, Reinhardt UE. The economics of employer versus individual mandates. Health Aff (Millwood) 1994;13(2):34–53.

12.   Congressional Budget Office, Hamilton DR. Economic implications of rising health care costs. Washington, D.C.: Government Printing Office, 1992.

13.   Pauly MV. Health benefits at work: an economic and political analysis of employment-based health insurance. Ann Arbor: University of Michigan Press, 1997.

14.   Budget of the United States Government: analytical perspectives of the United States: fiscal 1999. Washington, D.C.: Executive Office of the President, 1998.

15.   Schieber G, Maeda A. A curmudgeon's guide to financing health care in developing countries. In: Innovations in health care financing: proceedings of a World Bank conference. World Bank discussion paper no. 365. Washington, D.C.: World Bank, 1997.

16.   Fuchs VR, Hahn JS. How does Canada do it? A comparison of expenditures for physicians' services in the United States and Canada. N Engl J Med 1990;323:884–90.

17.   Fuchs VR. Economics, values and health care reform. Am Econ Rev 1996; 86(1):1–24.

18.   Advisory Commission on Intergovernmental Relations. Characteristics of federal grant-in-aid programs to state and local governments: grants funded FY 1995. Washington, D.C.: Advisory Commission on Intergovernmental Relations.

19.   Ellwood ML, Ku L. Welfare and immigration reforms: unintended side effects for Medicaid. Health Aff (Millwood) 1998;17(3):137–51.

20.   The Kaiser Commission on Medicaid and the Uninsured. The decline in Medicaid spending growth in 1996: why did it happen? Menlo Park, Calif.: Henry J. Kaiser Family Foundation, 1998.

21.   Federal Hospital Insurance Trust Fund. 1998 Annual report of the Board of Trustees. U.S. House Document 105-245, 105th Congress, 2d session. Washington, D.C.: Government Printing Office, 1998.

22.   Gabel J. Ten ways HMOs have changed during the 1990s. Health Aff (Millwood) 1997;16(1):134–45.

23.   Shearer G. Hidden from view: the growing burden of health care costs. Washington, D.C.: Consumers Union, 1998.

24.   Gross DJ, Gibson MJ, Caplan CF, et al. Out of pocket health spending by Medicare beneficiaries age 65 and older: 1997 projections. Washington, D.C.: AARP Public Policy Institute, 1997.

25.   Iglehart JK. Health care and American business. N Engl J Med 1982; 306: 120–4.

26.   Sapolsky HM, Altman D, Greene K, Moore JD. Corporate attitudes toward health case costs. Milbank Mem Fund Q 1981;59:561–85.

27.   Bodenheimer T, Sullivan K. How large employers are shaping the health care marketplace. N Engl J Med 1998;338:1003–7.

28. Report to the Congress: context for a changing Medicare program. Washington, D.C.: Medicare Payment Advisory Commission, 1998.

29. Angell M. The doctor as double agent. Kennedy Inst Ethics J 1993;3:279–86.

30. Shortell SM, Waters TM, Clarke KW, Budetti PP. Physicians as double agents: maintaining trust in an era of multiple accountabilities. JAMA 1998;280:1102–8.

31. Robinson JC. HMO market penetration and hospital cost inflation in California. JAMA 1991;266:2719–23.

32. Guterman S. The Balanced Budget Act of 1997: will hospitals take a hit on their PPS margins? Health Aff (Millwood) 1998;17(1):159–66.

33. Neumann PJ, Sandberg EA. Trends in health care R & D and technology innovation. Health Aff (Millwood) 1998;17(6):111–9.

34. Varmus H. Biomedical research enters the steady state. N Engl J Med 1995; 333:811–5.

35. Greenberg DS. Fighting cancer in the wrong arena. Washington Post. October 12, 1998: A21.

36. Iglehart JK. Politics and public health. N Engl J Med 1996;334:203–7.

37. Tanouye E. Drug dependency: U.S. has developed an expensive habit; now, how to pay for it. Wall Street Journal. November 16,1998:Al.

38. Lagnado L. The uncovered: drug costs can leave elderly a grim choice: pills or other needs. Wall Street Journal. November 17, 1998:A1.

39. Barr S. Federal workers face largest health insurance hike since 1989. Washington Post. September 13, 1998: A2.

40. Reinhardt UE. Resource allocation in health care: the allocation of lifestyles to providers. Milbank Q 1987;65(2):153–76.

19 | Health Insurance Coverage

Robert Kuttner

The most prominent feature of American health insurance coverage is its slow erosion, even as the government seeks to plug the gaps in coverage through such new programs as Medicare+Choice, the Health Insurance Portability and Accountability Act (HIPAA), expansions of state Medicaid programs, and the $24 billion Children's Health Insurance Program of 1997. Despite these efforts, the proportion of Americans without insurance increased from 14.2 percent in 1995 to 15.3 percent in 1996 and to 16.1 percent in 1997, when 43.4 million people were uninsured. Not as well appreciated is the fact that the number of people who are underinsured, and thus must either pay out of pocket or forgo medical care, is growing even faster.

This report addresses several trends that account for the erosion of health insurance coverage. The most important trend is the deterioration of employer-provided coverage, the source of health insurance for nearly two in three Americans.[1] I will discuss this cause in detail in the next article in this series. To summarize briefly for now, a few employers have eliminated coverage entirely because of the escalating costs of premiums. Most employers have narrowed the choice of plans and shifted costs to employees by capping the employer's contribution, choosing plans with higher out-of-pocket payments, or both. These changes, in turn, have caused some employees to forgo coverage for themselves and their families and have also led to underinsurance, since many employees, especially those who receive low wages, cannot afford the out-of-pocket charges.

The following trends are also eroding insurance coverage of all types.

Rising premium costs, both for persons who have access to insurance through their employers and for those who buy insurance individually.

Reprinted from *New England Journal of Medicine*, 340, no. 2 (January 14, 1999): 163–68, with permission. Copyright 1999, Massachusetts Medical Society. All rights reserved.

Costs will rise in 1999 for both groups, but more sharply for persons with individual coverage.[2,3]

The trend toward temporary and part-time work, which seldom includes health care coverage.   In 1997, about 29 percent of working Americans held "non-standard" jobs, a category that includes temporary, part-time, contract, and day-labor positions.[4]

A reduction in explicit coverage, most notably pharmaceutical benefits. Most plans cap outpatient pharmaceutical benefits. Prescription drugs now constitute the largest category of out-of-pocket payments for the elderly, and the costs are rapidly rising.

Greater de facto limitations on covered care, especially by health maintenance organizations (HMOs).   More stringent utilization reviews and economic disincentives for physicians and hospitals are resulting in denial of care and shifting of costs to patients.

A broad shift from traditional HMOs requiring very low out-of-pocket payments to point-of-service plans and preferred-provider organizations (PPOs) requiring higher payments by patients.   Ostensibly, the rationale for this shift is to provide greater choice for consumers, but consumers often enroll in a PPO or a point-of-service plan not because HMOs restrict choice but because they are perceived as restricting care. By 1997, there were more than twice as many Americans enrolled in point-of-service plans or PPOs as there were in HMOs.[1]

Loss of Medicaid coverage due to welfare reform.   The 1996 welfare-reform law separates Medicaid eligibility from eligibility for public assistance, but it also pushes many former welfare recipients into low-wage employment that does not provide health insurance. Although the termination of welfare benefits does not necessarily entail loss of Medicaid coverage, preliminary reports suggest that in practice the added administrative complexity is leading to reduced enrollment in Medicaid.[5]

The rising cost of "Medigap" coverage for the elderly, which leads to substantial underinsurance.   In some states, such as Massachusetts, comprehensive Medigap policies are now in a death spiral: only a small number of persons with high medical expenses find it cost effective to buy such policies, and low enrollment, in turn, leads to even higher premiums and lower enrollment.

The crackdown on illegal immigrants and the reduction in services to legal immigrants.   These policies are forcing many immigrants to forgo Medicaid and other forms of health coverage that are legally available to their children who are citizens.

The trend away from community rating of individual insurance premiums, which results in rising costs and, hence, reduced rates of coverage for middle-aged persons. For the 8.7 million Americans who buy insurance individually, premiums are partly adjusted for age and are also adjusted for prior medical conditions.

As a result of these trends, lack of insurance and underinsurance are becoming more widespread problems. Not surprisingly, it is lower-income Americans who bear the disproportionate costs, since as compared with higher-income Americans, they are more likely to work for employers who do not provide health care coverage or who require employees to make sizable contributions to insurance premiums, they are more likely to have part-time or temporary jobs with no health care coverage, and they are less able to afford individual insurance or high out-of-pocket payments.

Surprisingly, unemployment is scarcely implicated in these trends. Indeed, all of them have occurred while unemployment rates have been declining. Other things being equal, a decline in the unemployment rate should bring an increase in health insurance coverage, given the prevalence of employer-provided coverage. But the low unemployment rates of the late 1990s have not been sufficient to offset the above-mentioned trends. Today, the vast majority of uninsured persons are employed.

THE UNINSURED

The number of uninsured persons rose from 41.7 million (15.6 percent) in 1996 to 43.4 million (16.1 percent) in 1997, according to a September 1998 Census Bureau report (Tables 19.1 and 19.2).[6] This widely publicized increase tends to understate the extent of the problem, however. The Census Bureau also calculated that a much larger number of Americans, about 71.5 million, lacked insurance for at least part of the year. The latter figure was based on a study conducted from 1993 through 1995.[7] Poor and low-income persons, as well as members of minority groups, were most likely to have periods without coverage. Twenty-five percent of non-Hispanic whites had at least one month without coverage, as compared with 37 percent of blacks and 50 percent of Hispanics.

Lack of insurance is very closely correlated with low income. Whereas 8 percent of Americans with incomes over $75,000 and 16.1 percent of all Americans lacked health insurance in 1997, 24 percent of those with incomes of less than $25,000 had no coverage. Fifty percent of persons with incomes below the poverty line had at least one month without insurance, as compared with 27 percent of those with higher incomes. Despite Medicaid, 11.2 million

TABLE 19.1

Type of Health Insurance and Coverage Status, 1997*

Status and Type of Coverage	Thousands of Persons	(%)
All persons		
Total	269,094	(100.0)
Covered	225,646	(33.9)
Private	188,533	(70.1)
Employment-based	165,092	(61.4)
Government	66,685	(24.8)
Medicare	35,590	(13.2)
Medicaid	28,956	(10.8)
Military	8,527	(3.2)
Not covered	43,448	(16.1)
Poor persons		
Total	35,574	(100.0)
Covered	24,336	(68.4)
Private	8,264	(23.2)
Employment-based	5,521	(15.5)
Government	18,585	(52.2)
Medicare	4,637	(13.0)
Medicaid	15,386	(43.3)
Not covered	11,238	(31.6)

*Data are from the U.S. Census Bureau.[6] Percentages add up to more than 100 because some people had more than one type of coverage.

persons with incomes below the poverty line, or 31.6 percent of all the poor, had no health insurance at all in 1997.

The high cost of health insurance relative to income is the main reason for high rates of uninsurance among poor and low-income persons. A study conducted by KMPG Peat Marwick for the Commonwealth Fund found that a person with an annual income at the poverty threshold would need to pay 26 percent of that income to purchase health insurance. In more expensive markets, this cost rises to 40 percent of income for a family of four.[8] Since such families are barely able to pay for food and shelter, these figures suggest that for poor and low-income persons, health insurance is effectively unaffordable unless it is provided by employers or the government.

Lack of insurance is also correlated with loss of employment. According to the Census Bureau, during the period from 1993 to 1995, 44 percent of persons who lost their jobs also reported loss of insurance coverage. At the same time, however, almost half (49 percent) of fully employed people with incomes below

TABLE 19.2

**Persons Without Health Insurance for the Entire
Year, According to Selected Characteristics, 1997***

Characteristic	Thousands of Persons		(%)
	All Persons	Uninsured Persons	
Total	269,094	43,448	(16.1)
Sex			
Male	131,705	23,130	(17.6)
Female	137,390	20,319	(14.8)
Age (yr)			
<18	71,682	10,743	(15.0)
18–24	25,201	7,582	(30.1)
25–34	39,354	9,162	(23.3)
35–44	44,462	7,699	(17.3)
45–64	56,313	7,928	(14.1)
≥ 65	32,082	333	(1.0)
Race or ethnic group			
White	221,651	33,242	(15.0)
Non-Hispanic white	192,179	23,135	(12.0)
Black	34,598	7,432	(21.5)
Asian or Pacific Islander	10,492	2,172	(20.7)
Hispanic	30,773	10,534	(34.2)

*Data are from the U.S Census Bureau.[6]

the poverty line had no insurance.[7] The figure was even higher in 1996, when 52 percent of poor full-time workers had no insurance. This study was conducted before the enactment in 1996 of the HIPAA, which makes it easier for persons who have lost employer-provided insurance to qualify for other coverage.

However, to the extent that loss of insurance coverage is the result of lost purchasing power due to job loss, HIPAA is of no help, because it provides no subsidy and does not regulate price. The 1985 Consolidated Omnibus Budget Reconciliation Act (COBRA), which allows people leaving employment to pay insurance premiums out of pocket for up to 18 months in order to retain their coverage, likewise fails to address economic barriers to coverage. Moreover, although HIPAA prohibits outright denial of insurance because of previous medical conditions, it allows insurers to charge people with previous conditions substantially higher premiums, thus sharply limiting effective coverage.[9] Although in principle HIPAA protects as many as 25 million people from loss of insurance, in practice it benefits only a few hundred thousand.[10]

A 1997 national survey of health insurance conducted by Louis Harris Associates for the Henry J. Kaiser Family Foundation and the Commonwealth Fund confirms these trends. According to the survey, one in three adults between the ages of 18 and 64 years had been without insurance at some point in the previous two years. The survey confirmed that persons with low incomes were most likely to lack coverage: 59 percent of adults with incomes below $20,000 had been without coverage, as compared with 8 percent of adults with incomes above $60,000.[11] The survey also confirmed that lack of insurance was more often due to the high cost of coverage (reported by 51 percent of respondents) than to job loss or the employer's failure to provide access to coverage (reported by 25 percent). Fifty-seven percent of respondents without insurance were employed full time.[12] The survey also showed considerable discontinuity of coverage, with one third of insured adults reporting that they had been enrolled in their current health plan for less than two years.[13]

CHILDREN WITHOUT INSURANCE

Several reports have documented high and rising rates of uninsurance among children. According to a March 1997 Families USA report based on Census data, approximately one child in three had no insurance coverage for one or more months during 1995 and 1996.[14] Almost half these children (47 percent) were uninsured for a year or more. Unemployment of the family breadwinner was not the main reason, since 91 percent of the children who lacked health coverage for the entire two years lived in households where the breadwinners were employed all or part of the 24-month period. Lack of insurance was more closely correlated with low income. Fifty percent of children with family incomes between $15,000 and $25,000 had no health care coverage. For the very poor, Medicaid in principle provides coverage. According to the General Accounting Office, however, nearly 3 million children who are eligible for Medicaid are not enrolled in the program[15] because of inadequate outreach, fears on the part of immigrants that enrollment will lead to problems with the authorities, and other barriers.

On the basis of a survey of health care coverage for children, the Census Bureau reported that the proportion of children lacking insurance rose from 12 percent in 1989 to 15 percent in 1996,[16] a period of increasing prosperity in general, decreasing unemployment, and nominal expansion of eligibility for Medicaid. Noting that the number of poor children covered by Medicaid fell from 16.5 million to 15.5 million between 1995 and 1996, the Census Bureau observed, "The growth in the number of children lacking health insurance is largely attributable to the fall-off in Medicaid coverage."[16] Some 34 percent of the survey respondents whose children did not receive regular medical care reported that the reason was that they had no insurance and could not afford visits to doctors.[17] Approximately 800,000 children were taken to emergency rooms for all their care.[18]

In 10 jurisdictions, at least 37 percent of children went without insurance for some portion of the period from 1995 through 1996: Texas (46 percent), New Mexico (43 percent), Louisiana (43 percent), Arkansas (42 percent), Mississippi (41 percent), the District of Columbia (39 percent), Alabama (38 percent), Arizona (38 percent), Nevada (37 percent), and California (37 percent).[19]

Not surprisingly, several studies confirm that children without health insurance receive less care in the form of diagnostic, screening, and immunization services than children with coverage. Uninsured children have fewer checkups, are less likely to be treated for chronic conditions such as asthma and recurrent ear infections, are less likely to be treated by doctors for injuries, and are more likely to go without eyeglasses or prescribed drugs.[20]

THE UNDERINSURED

The increasing prevalence of underinsurance may well be the more serious trend. Underinsurance here refers to medical needs that either are not covered by health plans at all or are covered but with high copayments that force beneficiaries to forgo treatment. Stringent "management" of care that results in denial of medically necessary treatment may also be considered a form of underinsurance.

Studies by the Employee Benefit Research Institute, several private consultants, and Consumers Union all document substantial cost shifting and rising rates of underinsurance. A January 1998 study conducted by the Lewin Group for Consumers Union found that 11 million families without elderly members (1 in 8 families) spend on average more than 10 percent of their income on out-of-pocket health care costs and health insurance premiums not paid for by employers.[21] This figure rises to 20 percent for families with members who are 55 to 64 years old, and to 50 percent for families with members who are 65 or older. Among all age groups, the 10 percent of people with the most serious health problems spend an average of $21,000 a year in premium and out-of-pocket payments.[21]

In addition, recent trends in both employment and health insurance have made ties between patients and doctors less stable. The Kaiser–Commonwealth survey found that 34 percent of insured adults under the age of 65 had been enrolled in their current health plan for less than two years.[22] Only 36 percent had had the same primary care doctor for five years or more.[23] Respondents with conventional Medicare or Medicaid coverage actually had more stable relationships with providers than those in managed-care plans, a finding that is largely due to the fragmentation and turbulence of the managed-care industry.

PHARMACEUTICAL COVERAGE

The costs of prescription drugs continue to rise faster than the costs of other components of health care, and they are increasingly less likely to be covered by insurance. Total expenditures for prescription drugs increased by 85 percent between 1993 and 1998, with an estimated 17 percent increase from 1997 to 1998 alone, or more than four times the rate of increase for all health care expenditures in that period.[24] In 1995, more than half of all pharmaceutical costs were paid out of pocket,[25] and the proportion is almost certainly higher now.

The elderly are most dependent on prescription drugs, which Medicare does not cover. More than 19 million elderly persons, or about half of all Medicare enrollees, have no drug coverage. Press reports indicate that countless prescriptions go unfilled because elderly patients cannot afford to pay for them.[26] Expenditures for prescription drugs account for 34 percent of medical expenditures by the elderly, representing a larger proportion of expenditures than that for either hospital charges or physicians' services, according to the American Association of Retired Persons.

In 1995, elderly people with some pharmaceutical benefits received them through HMOs (12 percent), Medicaid (6 percent), employer-provided supplemental polities for retirees (26 percent), or privately purchased Medigap politics (9 percent).[27] Each of these sources, however, is being cut back, either in diminished coverage or in diminished enrollment. In 1998, some Medicare HMOs quit the business and others capped or dropped drug coverage. In the case of Medigap plans, only 3 of the 10 standard plans mandated by the 1990 federal Medigap legislation provided any prescription-drug coverage, and only a small minority of people who bought Medigap coverage purchased these plans. According to the Lewin Group, the proportion of employer-provided supplemental plans for retirees that included prescription-drug coverage declined from 90 percent in 1989 to 81 percent in 1995.[28] And the proportion of employers offering retirees supplemental health coverage declined from over 60 percent in the 1980s to less than 40 percent today, according to the General Accounting Office.[29]

Virtually all supplemental plans for the elderly require copayments for prescription drugs. In 1998, only 9 percent of Medicare beneficiaries who were enrolled in HMO plans had unlimited prescription-drug benefits; 43 percent were in plans that had no annual dollar cap but that limited coverage to generic drugs or drugs on an approved formulary. In the case of plans that provided coverage for brand-name drugs, more than half of enrollees had an annual cap of $1,000 or less.[30]

McCormack et al.[31] reported in 1996 that 84 percent of Medigap policies in six states provided no drug coverage at all, and only 7 percent provided "high-option" coverage (Plan I), with an annual benefit cap of $3,000. Such plans cost over $200 per month, which few elderly people can afford. The lower-option policies (Plans H and I) required a $250 annual deductible for drug costs, a 50 percent copayment, and a $1,250 annual cap. The Lewin Group, using a different method, found that 28 percent of persons with Medigap policies had some pharmaceutical benefits but confirmed that most did not have the high-option plan. Medigap policies paid for only 3 percent of all prescription-drug costs for the elderly. The largest source of insurance coverage, accounting for 21 percent of the costs, was employer-provided supplemental plans; 52 percent of drug costs were paid out of pocket.[32] Obviously, as drug prices keep rising, the relative value of the covered benefit declines. The drug industry continues to resist efforts by Representative Pete Stark (D-Calif.) and others to add drug coverage to Medicare by using federal purchasing power to buy discounted drugs, and such measures currently have little chance of enactment.

THE OUTLOOK

Few of these trends toward increasing numbers of uninsured and underinsured Americans show signs of abatement or reversal. Although managed care dramatically reduced the inflation in health insurance costs for employers in the mid-1990s, this seems to have been a one-time savings. The underlying demographic and technological trends are unchanged, and employers and benefit consultants report sharply rising premium costs in 1999.[3] Employers, facing little resistance from unions or public policy, are continuing both to reduce the options for coverage and to shift costs to employees, leading to both lack of insurance and underinsurance.

Likewise, despite the early promise of Medicare HMOs, the gaps in Medicare coverage are growing larger. Even before the implementation of Medicare+Choice (which allows the insurance industry to market a wider variety of point-of-service plans and PPOs), private insurers had already begun to reduce benefits or withdraw from selected markets. In October 1998, insurers announced they were dropping coverage for some 400,000 of the approximately 6 million enrollees in Medicare HMOs.[33,34]

With premium costs continuing to rise, more employers are dropping or reducing coverage than are expanding it. Health care coverage is seen as a particular burden by smaller businesses, which represent the fastest-growing sector of American employers.[35] And as the shift from full-time to part-time and temporary jobs continues, more employees are likely to find themselves with no benefits.

Congress, in several budget resolutions beginning in 1989, has extended Medicaid eligibility, especially to children who are living in poverty but are not on welfare. Some states, such as Oregon and Tennessee, have sought to turn Medicaid into a nearly universal health insurance program for the working poor as well as the indigent. However, these programs entail a degree of rationing, which is either explicit, as in the Oregon program, or implicit, as in Tennessee's stringent approach to managed care. Rationing, in turn, gives people the "choice" of paying for uncovered services out of pocket or doing without them. The shift to Medicaid managed care suggests that although more people will be nominally covered, many will in effect have less coverage.

The expansions in Medicaid are also offset by the 1996 welfare-reform law, Temporary Assistance for Needy Families, which limits the duration of welfare benefits. As the welfare limits gradually become effective in most states during 1999, millions of people will lose their eligibility for Medicaid along with their welfare benefits. Many heads of households will take relatively low-paid jobs, most of which do not offer health insurance; even those that do tend to require high premium payments by employees.

One small bright spot is the likelihood that the number of uninsured children will decline, thanks to the new Children's Health Insurance Program. Enacted as part of the 1997 Balanced Budget Act, the program provides the states with $24 billion over a period of five years. Some states are using these funds to expand Medicaid, and others are setting up new, parallel children's programs.

However, the interactions among Medicaid, the welfare-reform law, and the Children's Health Insurance Program are highly complex and confusing. For example, most children whose mothers will lose Medicaid coverage under welfare reform may retain their eligibility for Medicaid, but coverage is not automatic. Moreover, press reports indicate that immigrants, both legal and illegal, are reluctant to obtain coverage for their children for fear that enrollment will bring investigations by the immigration authorities. As of November 1998, California, which has a complex 28-page application for coverage that includes several questions about immigration status, had enrolled only 4 percent of 580,000 eligible children,[36] despite a payment of $25 to $50 to insurance vendors for every child they enroll. The Congressional Budget Office estimates that the net effect of the welfare-reform law, the Children's Health Insurance Program, and Medicaid expansions will be to extend coverage to some 2 million of the 10.6 million children who were uninsured as of 1997.[37]

With unemployment rates approaching a 30-year low, the overall trend in declining health insurance coverage is, if anything, understated. In the next recession, when the unemployment rate increases, loss of coverage is likely to increase apace. Because all sources of coverage are eroding, the long-term trend is toward a continued decline in both nominal and effective rates of coverage, unless there is a dramatic change in national policy.

REFERENCES

1.   Fronstin P. Features of employment based health plans. Washington, D.C.: Employee Benefit Research Institute, 1998.

2. Kilborn P. Premiums rising for individuals. New York Times. December 5, 1998:A7.

3. Freudenheim M. Employees facing steep increases in health care. New York Times. November 27, 1998:A1.

4. Mishel L, Bernstein J, Schmitt J. The state of working America, 1998–99. Washington, D.C.: Economic Policy Institute, 1998:243.

5. Greenberg M. Participation in welfare and Medicaid enrollment. Menlo Park, Calif.: Kaiser Family Foundation, September 1998.

6. Bureau of the Census. Health insurance coverage, 1997. Washington, D.C.: Government Printing Office, September 1998 (P60–202).

7. *Idem.* Dynamics of economic well-being: health insurance, 1993–1995. Washington, D.C.: Government Printing Office, September 1993 (P70–64).

8. Gabel J, Hunt K, Kim J. The financial burden of self-paid health insurance on the poor and near-poor. New York: Commonwealth Fund, 1998.

9. Kuttner R. The Kassebaum-Kennedy bill—the limits of incrementalism. N Engl J Med 1997;337:64–7.

10. Department of Health and Human Services, Department of Labor, Department of the Treasury. Rulemaking package implementing HIPAA. Washington, D.C.: Government Printing Office, April 1,1997:72.

11. Schoen C, Hoffman C, Rowland D, Davis K, Altman D. Working families at risk: coverage, access, cost and worries. New York: Commonwealth Fund, 1998.

12. *Idem.* Working families at risk: coverage, access, cost and worries. New York: Commonwealth Fund, 1998:12.

13. *Idem.* Working families at risk: coverage, access, cost and worries. New York: Commonwealth Fund, 1998:6.

14. One out of three: kids without health insurance, 1995–1996. Washington, D.C.: Families USA, 1997.

15. General Accounting Office. Health insurance for children: private insurance coverage continues to deteriorate. Washington, D.C.: Government Printing Office, 1996. (GAO/HEHS 96-129.)

16. Bureau of the Census. Census brief: children without health insurance. Washington, D.C.: Government Printing Office, 1998.

17. *Idem.* Census brief: children without health insurance. Washington, D.C.: Government Printing Office, 1998:5.

18. *Idem.* Census brief: children without health insurance. Washington, D.C.: Government Printing Office, 1998:6.

19. One out of three: kids without health insurance. Washington, DC: Families USA, 1997:5.

20. One out of three: kids without health insurance. Washington, D.C.: Families USA, 1997:9.

21. Shearer G. Hidden from view: the growing burden of health care costs. Washington, D.C.: Consumers Union, 1998:3.

22.   Schoen C, Hoffman C, Rowland D, Davis K, Altman D. Working families at risk: coverage, access, cost and worries. New York: Commonwealth Fund, 1998:25.

23.   *Idem.*. Working families at risk: coverage, access, cost and worries. New York: Commonwealth Fund, 1998:51.

24.   Tanouye E. U.S. has developed an expensive drug habit; now, how to pay far it? Wall Street Journal. November 16, 1998:A1.

25.   Current knowledge of third party outpatient drug coverage for Medicare beneficiaries. Fairfax, Va.: Lewin Group, 1998.

26.   Lagnado L. Drug costs can leave elderly a grim choice: pills or other needs. Wall Street Journal. November 17, 1998:A1.

27.   Current knowledge of third party outpatient drug coverage for Medicare beneficiaries. Fairfax, Va.: Lewin Group, November 9,1998:4.

28.   Current knowledge of third party outpatient drug coverage for Medicare beneficiaries. Fairfax, Va.: Lewin Group, 1998:7.

29.   Closing the huge hole in Medicare's benefits package. Remarks by Congressman Pete Stark, U.S. House of Representatives, Washington, D.C., October 9,1998.

30.   Current knowledge of third party outpatient drug coverage for Medicare beneficiaries. Fairfax, Va.: Lewin Group, 1998:19.

31.   McCormack LA, Fox PD, Rice T, Graham ML. Medigap reform legislation of 1990: have the objectives been met.? Health Care Financ Rev 1996;18(1):157–74.

32.   Current knowledge of third party outpatient drug coverage for Medicare beneficiaries. Fairfax, Va.: Lewin Group, 1998:13.

33.   Pear R. HMOs are retreating from Medicare, citing high costs. New York Times. October 2, 1998:A17.

34.   *Idem.* Clinton to announce help as HMOs leave Medicare. New York Times. October 3, 1998:A20.

35.   National survey of small business executives on health care. Menlo Park, Calif.: Henry J. Kaiser Family Foundation, June 1988.

36.   Healthy Families Program subscribers enrolled by county. Sacramento: California Managed Risk Medical Insurance Board, November 24, 1998.

37.   Congressional Budget Office memorandum: budgetary implications of the Balanced Budget Act of 1997. Washington, D.C.: Congressional Budget Office, December 1997:54.

20 | Medicare

John K. Iglehart

When Medicare was enacted in 1965 as the health care linchpin of President Lyndon Johnson's Great Society, its architects considered this insurance program for the elderly only an interim step toward the broader goal of universal health care coverage.[1] That goal has never been achieved, although Medicare is the nation's single largest source of payment for medical care, insuring 39 million beneficiaries against the financial consequences of acute illness. Since Congress established the program, the benefits covered by Medicare have remained largely unchanged, with the exception of a few added preventive services, and they are certainly inadequate by current medical standards. Medicare expended $214.6 billion in 1997 in two large funding streams: Part A, for hospital services, and Part B, for physicians' services. These two types of care are financed from four different sources, the most important of which is mandatory contributions by employers and employees. The other three are general tax revenues, premiums paid by beneficiaries, and deductibles and copayments.

Medicare is the subject of this report, the fourth in the current series on the American health care system.[2-4] Medicare's hospital-financing scheme, like that of the Social Security program, is grounded in the principle of social insurance, which requires all employers and employees to make payments to a trust fund. Some 151 million employees make mandatory contributions to Medicare's Part A Hospital Insurance Trust Fund during their working years, with the promise of receiving benefits after they retire. The money contributed by employees that finances Medicare's Hospital Insurance Trust Fund is not set aside to meet their own future health expenses. Rather, it is used to cover the medical bills of the people who are currently covered by Medicare. All eligible beneficiaries are automatically enrolled in Part A, which finances inpatient hospital services, continued treatment or rehabilitation in a skilled-nursing facility, and hospice care for the terminally ill.

Medicare's other major component, supplemental medical insurance (Part B), was modeled after traditional indemnity coverage and was initially created to win the support of Republicans for the program. Enrollment in Part B is voluntary, although the vast majority of beneficiaries sign on. Part B pays for physicians' services and outpatient hospital services, including emergency room visits, ambulatory surgery, diagnostic tests, laboratory services, and durable medical equipment. Under Part B, Medicare pays 80 percent of the approved amount (according to a fee schedule) for covered services in excess of an annual deductible of $100. Overall, 89 percent of Medicare's annual revenue now comes primarily from people who are less than 65 years old, through payroll taxes, income taxes, and interest on the trust fund, and 11 percent comes from the monthly premiums contributed by elderly beneficiaries.

THE CHALLENGE FACED BY THE HEALTH CARE FINANCING ADMINISTRATION

Medicare and Medicaid (which I will discuss in my next report) are administered by the Health Care Financing Administration (HCFA), a beleaguered federal agency that is criticized by observers on all sides as bureaucratic, rigid, and at times, overwhelmed by its administrative responsibilities, which have grown exponentially in the 1990s. In contrast to its vast charge, HCFA is a remarkably small agency, primarily as a consequence of "downsizing" that occurred during the administration of President Ronald Reagan. Since HCFA's creation, its spending on behalf of Medicare beneficiaries has increased by a factor of almost 10 (from $21.5 billion in 1977 to $214.6 billion in 1997) and the population eligible for Medicare has grown from 26 million to 38.6 million. But the full-time–equivalent staff of the agency has remained about the same, at roughly 4000 people. The performance of HCFA will come under closer scrutiny this year because the Republican-controlled Congress plans to conduct hearings on its performance. But in the view of 14 distinguished people from different parts of the political spectrum, including three former HCFA administrators (Dr. William L. Rope, Leonard D. Schaeffer, and Gail R. Wilensky), the agency's problems are not all of its own making. The 14 recently urged Congress and the administration to reexamine what they consider the inadequate resources at HCFA's command: "The signatories to this statement believe that many of the difficulties that threaten to cripple HCFA stem from an unwillingness of both Congress and the Clinton administration to provide the agency the resources and administrative flexibility necessary to carry out its mammoth assignment."[5]

Despite HCFA's problems, Medicare is a highly popular federal program, particularly among its beneficiaries, many of whom could not afford health insurance coverage if they had to pay its entire cost. Medicare beneficiaries include 34 million persons over the age of 65, 5 million of all ages who are permanently disabled, and 284,000 with end-stage renal disease.[6] In 1993, almost three quarters of elderly people reported annual household incomes of less than $25,000, at a time when per capita Medicare expenditures averaged $4,083. In the estimation of a recently departed HCFA administrator, Bruce C. Vladeck, Medicare is "an extremely powerful weapon for reducing poverty for the elderly and disabled."[7] But not all its beneficiaries support the program's role as a redistributor of income. On July 1, 1988, when President Reagan signed into law the Medicare Catastrophic Coverage Act, its financing mechanism represented a formal acknowledgment by Congress of the disparities in economic status among the elderly. The law called for "an enormous increase in beneficiary contributions"[8] by elderly people with greater means to help finance the care of people with lower incomes. Less than two years later, on November 22, 1989, Congress repealed the law after coming under pressure from a vocal minority of relatively affluent elderly people, who resented paying higher premiums, and from the pharmaceutical industry, which was concerned that a new outpatient drug benefit would lead to federal price controls. Since the law's repeal, there has been no cap on beneficiaries' out-of-pocket liability.

Public-opinion polls show strong and consistent support for Medicare[9] and its intergenerational social compact; most beneficiaries who require medical care receive far more from the program than they contributed in payroll taxes, and far more than members of the baby-boom generation, the first of whom will turn 65 in 2010, are likely to receive. For example, a couple retiring in 1998, with one wage earner who paid average Medicare taxes since 1966, would have contributed a total of $16,790, with interest, not including the employer's equal contribution. The present value of future Part A benefits for such a couple is estimated at $109,000, more than six times the amount they paid into the trust fund (Foster RS, HCFA: personal communication).

Medicare is so popular that politicians who are seen as threatening it put themselves in jeopardy, as Republicans learned to their regret in 1995. After newly elected Republican majorities took control of the House and Senate and set out to cut the budget by trimming Medicare, their plan was vetoed by President Bill Clinton as too draconian and was strongly opposed by the elderly, who helped Clinton win reelection the next year. Whereas many billions of dollars separated what Republicans and Democrats were prepared in 1995 to excise from Medicare's future growth, Clinton focused on a figure that ordinary Americans could comprehend: the additional $264 that Republicans wanted an elderly couple to pay in annual Medicare premiums. As Charles N. Kahn III, a former Republican congressional staff member who was centrally involved in the issue, wrote recently, "President Clinton used the Part B premium issue to transform the debate."[10]

MEDICARE'S FINANCIAL PROBLEMS

In 1992, I reported that Medicare's trustees estimated that the program's Hospital Insurance Trust Fund would run out of money by 2001.[11] With bankruptcy looming, I concluded that Congress would have to soon decide how to close the gap between the program's income and its expenses. Its options were further paring payments to providers, raising taxes, reducing benefits, asking beneficiaries to pay more of the costs, or some combination of these options. Five years later, Congress followed a formula that it has applied consistently over the past two decades. In the Balanced Budget Act of 1997,[12] Congress extracted the vast bulk of savings to the Medicare program ($116.6 billion over the period from 1998 through 2002) from future payments to providers. To balance the budget and extend the solvency of the hospital trust fund to 2007, Congress took 56.5 percent of the government-wide savings contained in the Balanced Budget Act from Medicare's estimated future expenditures, although the program represents only 12 percent of federal spending.

In the process of shaping the Balanced Budget Act, Congress largely insulated beneficiaries from greater financial liability, but legislators also got a taste of the dilemma that looms ahead when the baby-boom population transforms Medicare's demographic characteristics[13] and health care costs nearly double over the next decade, as HCFA projects.[14] The Senate, whose members stand for election every six years, as compared with every two years for House members, showed a greater willingness to ask beneficiaries to shoulder more of the financial burden. The Senate voted to raise the age of initial eligibility for Medicare from 65 to 67 years,[15,16] to adjust a beneficiary's Part B premium on the basis of his or her income, and to require copayments for home health services. House members, always running for reelection and therefore more sensitive to the concerns of elderly voters, rejected all three of these ideas, relying instead on reductions in payments to providers.

RESTRUCTURING MEDICARE

With the enactment of the Balanced Budget Act of 1997, Congress and the Clinton administration approved the most far-reaching reforms in the 34-year history of Medicare—some 300 provisions that are certain to add more complexity to the program. In the process, Congress greatly expanded the responsibilities of HCFA and the Medicare Payment Advisory Commission, which Congress created to monitor the administration of the program.[17] The reforms were intended to expand the choices among private health plans that beneficiaries may select by creating the new Medicare+Choice program and to strengthen Medicare's finances by including policies further constraining payments to providers in the traditional fee-for-service program and in managed-care plans.

Although news reports have focused on problems in the early implementation of Medicare+Choice, most beneficiaries are still covered under the program's traditional component—that is, indemnity insurance combined with fee-for-service payments to physicians, the model that prevailed when Medicare began. The program's original structure remains intact except for the imposition of administered prices through the prospective payment system for hospitals and the Medicare fee schedule for physicians' services. Under Medicare's traditional insurance program, all physicians and hospitals that meet Medicare's conditions of participation take part in the program without regard to whether they are affiliated with health plans or aggregated in medical groups. In 1997, 33 million Medicare beneficiaries were still in the traditional program, which cost an estimated $183 billion, representing 88 percent of total Medicare spending that year.

Most of the provisions of the Balanced Budget Act of 1997 that applied to traditional Medicare coverage reduced its growth instead of moving to upgrade it, as called for in a recent study by the National Academy of Social Insurance.[18] Congress directed HCFA to replace Medicare's cost-based reimbursement method with more restrictive prospective payment approaches that would apply to postdischarge services, the fastest-growing component of Medicare in the 1990s.[19] These services include care in skilled-nursing facilities, hospital outpatient services, inpatient rehabilitation services, and home health care. The growth of home health services, one of two major Medicare benefits for which there is no cost sharing by the beneficiary (the other is clinical laboratory services), has been particularly explosive; total expenditures increased from $2 billion in 1988 to more than $17 billion in 1997, largely because of increased rates of use. In 1988, about 5 percent of beneficiaries received home health care services, with the average user receiving 23 visits. In 1997, 1 in 10 beneficiaries received home care, and the average number of visits exceeded 80.[17]

MEDICARE+CHOICE

The Medicare-related provisions of the 1997 Balanced Budget Act to which Republicans attached the greatest ideological importance were those that expanded the array of insurance plan choices beyond fee-for-service indemnity coverage and health maintenance organizations (HMOs). Congress directed HCFA to offer options involving provider-sponsored organizations, preferred-provider organizations, private fee-for-service plans, and on a limited basis, medical savings accounts that combine high deductibles with a tax benefit. Congress also required the agency to develop a method of adjusting its payments to health plans so as to reflect more accurately the actual health status or recent medical experience of patients.[20–22] In the 18 months since the enactment of the law, the policy Congress designed and HCFA has set about implementing to broaden participation in the Medicare+Choice program has been fraught with problems.

As of last November, the date when HMOs in which Medicare beneficiaries were already enrolled were required to inform HCFA whether they planned to continue their participation in the program, 43 of the 347 plans announced their intention not to renew their contracts with Medicare for 1999, citing financial losses and other problems as the main reasons. Another 54 HMOs announced plans to reduce the number of geographic areas in which they were prepared to enroll Medicare beneficiaries. These changes affect the coverage of some 406,000 beneficiaries. Because almost all these enrollees live in areas where other HMOs operate, they have the option of switching to another such plan. Beneficiaries who do not live in areas with other HMOs will have to return to Medicare's traditional insurance program and, in all likelihood, to purchase supplemental coverage to pay for the additional benefits that HMOs offered elderly enrollees (coverage of outpatient prescription drugs is the most expensive of these). The plans cited several reasons for withdrawing from Medicare or from selected services areas. They considered HCFA's payment rates as reduced by the Balanced Budget Act too low and the law's new regulatory strictures as implemented by the agency too burdensome. An estimated 87 percent of all beneficiaries affected by the withdrawals of insurance plans were enrolled in for-profit plans (as compared with 68 percent of all Medicare beneficiaries enrolled in HMOs).[23]

Dr. Robert A. Berenson, director of HCFA's Center for Health Plans and Providers, said in an interview that Medicare had been overpaying health plans that operate in markets with high per capita rates and that HCFA had no plans to support rate increases, as sought by the industry:

> In 1999 payment rates will vary from almost $800 in Staten Island, New York, to about $380 in many rural areas . . . What we are witnessing is that HMOs are eager to enroll Medicare beneficiaries in high-payment areas, but they are dropping out of marginal-payment areas. . . . Each decision to pull out of a service area makes sense as a narrow business decision. But when you add up all of these decisions, the HMO industry is losing a reputation for reliability and stability. And that is a very unfortunate trend for the industry and the Medicare population. Indeed, it casts in some doubt that a competitive market might be a solution to Medicare's long-term financial problems.

CONFLICTS AMONG PHYSICIANS

Medicare's schedule of physicians' fees, like the prospective payment system that pits different kinds of hospitals against each other, provokes conflict between medical generalists and specialists. These disputes have grown in prominence ever since 1989, when Congress directed HCFA to develop a schedule of physicians' fees.[24] In search of savings and greater equality in Medicare payments to generalists and specialists, Congress said the schedule should be based on a resource-based relative-value scale that would take into consideration three distinct types of cost that doctors incur: their time, energy, and skill (referred to as physicians' work); practice expenses such as medical equipment and office space; and premiums for malpractice insurance.[25] In 1992, the Physician Payment Review Commission estimated that by 1996, when the new payment schedule was due to be fully implemented, fees paid to generalist physicians would be 39 percent higher than they would have been under the previous payment method, whereas those paid to cardiothoracic surgeons and ophthalmologists would be 35 percent and 25 percent lower, respectively.[11]

How accurate was the commission's 1992 estimate? As Table 20.1 shows, family and general practitioners saw a cumulative increase of 36.1 percent in their average payments from Medicare between 1991 and 1997. But because Congress required separate but unequal relative-value–scale conversion factors for surgical and nonsurgical services, many specialist physicians fared better during this period than the commission had earlier estimated. For example, the cumulative reduction in Medicare payments from 1991 to 1997 for cardiothoracic surgeons was 9.3 percent and that for ophthalmologists was 18.4 percent. As Table 20.2 shows, Medicare has reduced payments for many of the procedures performed by cardiologists, gastroenterologists, and ophthalmologists. The Balanced Budget Act of 1997 directed HCFA to cease to apply different conversion factors and established a single conversion factor (payments to physicians are the product of the number of relative-value units established for each service in the fee schedule and the conversion factor). HCFA set this factor at $34.73 for 1999, a change that will most likely lead to further reductions in Medicare payments to surgeons.

Recently, what has provoked the most controversy among medical organizations in regard to Medicare's fee schedule is the way in which HCFA plans to phase practice expenses into the payment formula, as required by the Balanced Budget Act. The agency, believing it was following congressional intent, proposed to phase in practice expenses in a way that had the effect of granting generalist physicians higher payments and specialists lower payments. The dispute prompted 11 specialty societies (representing cardiologists, gastroenterologists, ophthalmologists, and different types of surgeons) to file suit last November 4 in U.S. District Court to halt the implementarion of what they called HCFA's "unlawful transition formula."[26] The plan, scheduled to take effect January 1, 1999, would cost members of the 11 societies $495 million in Medicare payments over the next three years, the suit asserted. But a coalition of primary care medical groups, which formed the Practice Expense Fairness Coalition, disagreed, saying in a letter to HCFA, congressional committees, and others that if the plaintiffs won their court case, it would undo a compromise

TABLE 20.1

Change in Average Medicare Payment Rates, According to Area of Practice, from 1991 to 1997*

	Percent	
Group of Physicians and Area of Practice	Annual Change	Cumulative Change
Generalist physicians		
Family and general practice	5.3	36.1
Internal medicine	2.6	16.5
Medical subspecialists		
Cardiology	−2.7	−15.0
Gastroenterology	−2.6	−14.4
Other	2.4	15.3
Surgeons		
General surgery	0.0	0.1
Dermatology	1.5	9.0
Ophthalmology	−3.3	−18.4
Orthopedic surgery	−0.3	−1.7
Cardiothoracic surgery	−1.6	−9.3
Urology	1.9	12.2
Other	0.7	4.1

*Data are from the analysis by the Medicare Payment Advisory Commission of claims for a sample consisting of 5 percent of beneficiaries in 1991 through 1997 (Hayes KJ, Medicare Payment Advisory Commission: personal communication). Values shown are average percent changes in payment rates.

fashioned in the Balanced Budget Act that had settled a divisive debate within the medical profession.[26]

The American Medical Association (AMA) has remained neutral on this matter, recognizing that its physician members are divided by it. But, on other matters related to Medicare, the association has carved out a unique relation with HCFA that holds both pluses and minuses for it. The AMA helped develop Medicare's fee schedule and also publishes *Current Procedural Terminology,* the widely used manual for coding physicians' services. Moreover, according to Vladeck, the agency has "largely delegated to [the AMA] responsibility for maintaining many of the system's technical aspects. This requires the increasingly disputatious specialty societies to go through an AMA process to achieve some of their objectives."[7] On the other hand, the AMA came in for sharp criticism over its role in the development of draft guidelines for documenting cognitive services (evaluation and management) in the medical record.[27,28] On balance, Vladeck said, the relation between HCFA and the AMA is "functional for both parties, although the extent to which it protects the

TABLE 20.2

**Average Medicare Payments for Selected High-Volume
Procedures, According to Specialty, in 1991 and 1997***

	Dollars		*%*
Specialty and Procedure	*1991*	*1997*	*Change*
Cardiology			
Echocardiography of heart	215.60	202.66	−6.00
Heart image (3D) multiple	531.91	469.16	−11.80
Cardiovascular stress test	131.43	109.56	−16.64
Complete electrocardiography	29.70	27.44	−7.60
Doppler color-flow ultrasonography	94.45	107.78	14.10
Report on electrocardiography	12.28	11.04	−10.10
Doppler echocardiography of heart	104.89	91.24	−13.01
Coronary-artery dilation	1,517.42	833.14	−45.10
Gastroenterology			
Colonscopy and removal of lesion	567.40	406.67	−28.33
Diagnostic colonoscopy	352.01	264.64	−24.82
Upper gastrointestinal endoscopy and biopsy	347.45	207.36	−40.32
Ophthalmology			
Removal of cataract and insertion of lens	1,358.63	912.67	−32.81
Eye examination and treatment	44.06	53.10	20.54
Eye examination for established patient	35.00	36.39	3.96
Treatment of localized retinal lesion	702.75	740.98	5.44
Eye examination for new patient	50.33	74.51	48.05
Treatment of extensive or progressive retinopathy	733.29	868.88	18.49
Follow-up care after laser cataract surgery	517.50	247.00	−52.27
Ultrasound examination of eye	66.35	67.99	2.47

*Data are from the analysis by the Medicare Payment Advisory Commission of claims for a
sample consisting of 5 percent of beneficiaries in 1991 through 1997 (Hayes KJ, Medicare
Payment Advisory Commission: personal communication).

interests of practicing physicians, even that fraction that belong to the AMA,
is subject to increasing question."[7]

GRADUATE MEDICAL EDUCATION

Underscoring the increasingly precarious nature of Medicare's status as the
largest explicit financing source for graduate medical education, Congress
took a first step in the Balanced Budget Act toward changing this policy by
reducing the program's funding for this purpose.[29] Of the federal programs and

agencies that support graduate medical education (Medicare, Medicaid, and the departments of Defense and Veterans Affairs), Medicare is by far the largest single source of such funds. Medicare recognizes the costs of education in two ways. It provides direct medical-education payments to hospitals that cover a share of residents' stipends, faculty salaries, and administrative expense, and it provides an indirect medical-education adjustment that reflects the added costs of patient care associated with the operation of teaching programs.[30]

In 1997, Medicare's indirect medical-education adjustment totaled $4.6 billion. In the Balanced Budget Act, Congress reduced Medicare's indirect support for medical education by $5.6 billion over the next four years by changing the formula to make the payments less generous. Medicare's direct payments for graduate medical education totaled $2.2 billion in fiscal 1997. The budget legislation reduced Medicare's direct payments over the next five years by an estimated $700 million. The reductions in payments to teaching hospitals were partially offset by returning to the hospitals a portion of the premiums Medicare pays to managed-care plans. These funds, earmarked for education and amounting to some $4 billion, will be returned in annual installments of 20 percent over the five-year period from 1998 through 2002.

Although the Balanced Budget Act signaled the intention of Congress to cut back Medicare's commitment to financial support for teaching, several members of the National Bipartisan Commission on the Future of Medicare have urged more fundamental changes in federal policy as it applies to graduate medical education. Congress created the commission, a body whose deliberations have been contentious because some of its 17 members were appointed by Republicans and some by the Clinton administration. Its report to Congress is due March 1. Senator Phil Gramm (R-Tex.), who is a member of both the bipartisan commission and the Senate Finance Committee, which has jurisdiction over Medicare, has proposed that support for graduate medical education be subject to the greater scrutiny of the annual appropriations process rather than take the form of assistance to which teaching facilities are entitled according to a fixed payment formula. The Association of American Medical Colleges (AAMC) strongly opposes this proposal. With the departure of New York's two senators—the defeat last November of Republican Alfonse M. D'Amato and announcement by Democrat Daniel Patrick Moynihan that he will retire when his term expires in 2001—proposed changes in federal policy on graduate medical education that are opposed by the AAMC must be taken more seriously. For many years, D'Amato and Moynihan used their positions on the Finance Committee essentially to veto any changes in Medicare's policy on support for teaching.

FUTURE DIRECTIONS

As the 21st century nears and the baby-boom population heads closer to retirement, the changes included in the Balanced Budget Act are strictly a down payment in terms of closing Medicare's funding gap. Economist Victor Fuchs estimates that "if the trends of the past decade or two continue until 2020, the elderly's health care consumption in that year will be approximately $25,000 per person (in 1995 dollars), compared with $9200 in 1995."[31] In the short term, provoked by President Clinton's insistence that the current federal budget surplus be used to shore up the financial base of Social Security, Congress plans to consider replenishing the coffers of the Social Security program even though Medicare is slated to run out of money first. When it does focus on Medicare again, one proposal that may be considered seriously would make the government's financial obligation more predictable and shift more of the risk to beneficiaries. It has gained the support of Senator John B. Breaux (D-La.), chair of the National Bipartisan Commission on the Future of Medicare, a number of commission members,[32] and prominent economists of various persuasions.[33,34] The proposal would replace Medicare's commitment to provide a defined set of benefits to all eligible beneficiaries with a "premium support" system. All beneficiaries would receive a predetermined amount to be applied to the purchase of a health plan providing defined benefits. The amount would vary according to the beneficiary's age, sex, geographic area, health-risk status, income and assets, and use of services. If a beneficiary wanted benefits that went beyond those that could be purchased with the voucher, the amount of which would probably be related to income, he or she would be responsible for the additional cost. In many respects, the proposal resembles the Federal Employee Health Benefits Plan.

Beyond financial questions, Congress must consider how to improve Medicare's benefits package, which is based on a model of acute care that is wholly inadequate for the many elderly beneficiaries who have chronic illnesses.[35,36] A critical shortcoming is Medicare's failure to cover outpatient prescription drugs, particularly because most Medicare HMO enrollees do have such coverage.[37,38] Congress has taken note of this disparity and may well examine it this year. In any event, balancing the health care needs of the population eligible for Medicare with the available resources will be a continuing challenge well into the new millennium.

REFERENCES

1. Ball RM. What Medicare's architects had in mind. Health Aff (Millwood) 1995;14(4):62–72.

2. Iglehart JK. The American health care system—expenditures. N Engl J Med 1999;340:70–6.

3. Kuttner R. The American health care system—health insurance coverage. N Engl J Med 1999;340:163–8.

4. *Idem.* The American health care system—employer-sponsored health coverage. N Engl J Med 1999;340:248–52.

5.   Butler SM, Danzon PM, Gradison B. Open letter to Congress & the Executive: crisis facing HCFA & millions of Americans. Health Aff (Millwood) 1999;18(1):8–10.

6.   Nissenson AR, Rettig RA. Medicare's end-stage renal disease program: current status and future prospects. Health Aff (Mlllwood) 1999;18(1):161–79.

7.   Vladeck BC. The political economy of Medicare. Health Aff (Millwood) 1999; 18(1):22–36.

8.   Moon M. Medicare now and in the future. Washington, D.C.: Urban Institute Press, 1993.

9.   Bernstein J, Stevens RA. Pubic opinion, knowledge, and Medicare reform. Health Aff (Millwood) 1999;18(1):180–93.

10.   Kahn CN III, Kutner H. Budget bills and Medicare policy: the politics of the BBA. Health Aff (Millwood) 1999;18(1):37–47.

11.   Iglehart JK. The American health care system: Medicare. N Engl J Med 1992;327:1467–72.

12.   Balanced Budget Act of 1997, P.L. 105-33,105th Congress, August 5, 1997.

13.   McKusick D. Demographic issues in Medicare reform. Health Aff (Millwood) 1999;18(1):194–207.

14.   Smith S, Freeland M, Heffler S, McKussick D, Health Expenditures Projection Team. The next ten years of health spending: what does the future hold? Health Aff (Millwood) 1998;17(5):128–40.

15.   Waidmann TA. Potential effects of raising Medicare's eligibility age. Health Aff (Millwood) 1998;17(2):156–64.

16.   Shells J, Stapleton D, Graus J, Fishman A. Rethinking the Medicare eligibility age. Washington, D.C.: National Coalition on Health Care, 1998.

17.   Medicare Payment Advisory Commission. Report to the Congress: context for a changing Medicare program. Washington, D.C.: Medicare Payment Advisory Commission, 1998.

18.   Study Panel on Capitation and Choice. Structuring Medicare choices. Washington, D.C.: National Academy of Social Insurance, 1998.

19.   Welch HG, Wennberg DE, Welch WP. The use of Medicare home health care services. N Engl J Med 1996;335:324–9.

20.   Kassirer JP, Angel M. Risk adjustment or risk avoidance? N Engl J Med 1998;339:1925–6.

21.   Iezzoni LI, Ayanian JZ, Bates DW, Burstin HR. Paying more fairly for Medicare capitated care. N Engl J Med 1998;339:1933–8.

22.   Kuttner R. The risk-adjustment debate. N Engl J Med 1998;339:1952–6.

23.   Neuman P, Langwell KM. Medicare's choice explosion? Implications for beneficiaries. Health Aff (Millwood) 1999;18(1):150–60.

24.   Iglehart JK. The new law on Medicare's payments to physicians. N Engl J Med 1990;322:1247–52.

25.   Hsiao WC, Braun P, Yntema D, Becker ER. Estimating physicians' work for a resource-based relative-value scale. N Engl J Med 1988;319:835–41.

26. Aaron G. Specialists sue over practice expense rule. American Medical News. November 23–30, 1998:1.

27. Kassirer JP, Angell M. Evaluation and management guidelines—fatally flawed. N Engl J Med 1998;339:1697–8.

28. Brett AS. New guidelines for coding physicians' services—a step backward. N Engl J Med 1998;339:1705–8.

29. Iglehatt JK. Medicare and graduate medical education. N Engl J Med 1998; 338:402–7.

30. Fishman LE. Medicare payment with an educational label: fundamentals and the future. Washington, D.C.: Association of American Medical Colleges, 1996.

31. Fuchs VR. Health care for the elderly: how much? Who will pay for it? Health Aff (Millwood) 1998;18(1)1–11.

32. Serafini MW. Now, the hard part. National Journal. November 21, 1998:2774–80.

33. Aaron HJ, Reischauer RD. The Medicare reform debate: what is the next step? Health Aff (Millwood) 1995;14(4):8–30.

34. Wilensky GR, Newhouse JP. Medicare: what's right? What's wrong? What's next? Health Aff (Millwood) 1999;18(1):92–106.

35. Cassel CK, Besdine RW, Siegel LC. Restructuring Medicare for the next century: what will beneficiaries really need? Health Aff (Millwood) 1999;18(1):118–31.

36. Whitelaw NA, Warden GL. Reexamining the delivery system as part of Medicare reform. Health Aff (Millwood) 1999;18(1):132–43.

37. Davis M, Poisal J, Chulis G, et al. Prescription drug coverage, utilization, and spending among Medicare beneficiaries. Health Aff (Millwood) 1999;18(1):231–43.

38. McBride TD. Disparities in access to Medicare managed care plans and their benefits. Health Aff (Millwood) 1998;17(6):170–80.

21 | Medicaid

John K. Iglehart

Medicaid is the largest health insurer in the United States, in terms of eligible beneficiaries, covering medical services and long-term care for some 41.3 million people. In 1997, Medicaid expended $159.9 billion (12.4 percent of total national health care expenditures) to pay for covered services for low-income people who were elderly, blind, disabled, receiving public assistance, or among the working poor. The vast majority of such persons fall outside the employment-based insurance system, the mainstay of coverage for the working population. This fifth report in the series on the American health care system[1–4] examines the federal and state roles in Medicaid, program expenditures, eligibility for coverage, and Medicaid managed-care plans.

In recent years, Medicaid has changed in important ways. The change that has affected the greatest number of people is the expansion of the population eligible for Medicaid, from 28.3 million in 1993, when I last wrote about the program[5] in a series similar to this one, to 41.3 million today. The Republican-controlled Congress enacted legislation to shift most of the responsibility for Medicaid to state governments, but President Bill Clinton vetoed the measure in 1995. The growth in Medicaid expenditures, which almost tripled over the past decade, has slowed in recent years, with the smallest annual increase ever in 1997. An increasing number of eligible beneficiaries have enrolled in or are being required to join managed-care plans as a result of policies that no longer give them a choice of providers. However, none of these changes have made the program any more attractive to physicians, most of whom do not provide care for Medicaid beneficiaries because the payments to providers are low, and the associated administrative burden can be quite large.

Although Medicaid and Medicare were the key elements of historic legislation enacted in 1965 as part of President Lyndon Johnson's Great Society, Medicaid was essentially a creature of Congress. After Johnson's landslide victory in 1964, the enactment of Medicare seemed almost a foregone conclusion,

Reprinted from *New England Journal of Medicine*, 340, no. 5 (February 4, 1999): 403–408, with permission. Copyright 1999, Massachusetts Medical Society. All rights reserved.

although its final design reflected countless compromises. Medicaid, however, was largely a product of the House Ways and Means Committee and its powerful chairman, Representative Wilbur Mills (D-Ark.), who favored the expansion of earlier federal efforts (embodied in the Kerr-Mills Act) to provide medical assistance to elderly and disabled people. During the congressional debate over the two programs, conservative legislators and the American Medical Association promoted a federal-state model for Medicare, but Mills instead chose this model for Medicaid.[6] Wilbur Cohen, who worked closely with Mills in crafting the Medicaid legislation and later became secretary of the Department of Health, Education, and Welfare, wrote: "Many people, since 1965, have called Medicaid the 'sleeper' in the legislation. Most people did not pay attention to that part of the bill. . . . [It] was not a secret, but neither the press nor the health policy community paid any attention to it."[7]

The structures of Medicare and Medicaid have little in common, except that both are now administered at the federal level by the same agency, the Health Care Financing Administration (HCFA). Congress made it clear in 1965 that providing health insurance to the elderly through Medicare was a federal responsibility. But the division of authority over Medicaid between the federal and state governments resulted in a persistent struggle over how to apportion payment of the bill. In 1997, of the total expenditures of $159.9 billion, the federal share was $95.4 billion, and the states' contribution (combined in some jurisdictions with local expenditures) was $64.5 billion. The federal share of expenditures is determined by a formula based on each state's per capita income, with a legislatively set minimum of 50 percent and a maximum of 83 percent. States with relatively low per capita incomes receive proportionately more federal funding. Medicaid expenditures represent about 40 percent of all federal funds received by the states.

STATE MEDICAID PROGRAMS

Following broad national guidelines established by Congress and monitored by HCFA, the states set their own standards of eligibility; determine the type, amount, duration, and scope of covered services; establish the rate of payment for services; and administer their own programs. At first, a guiding principle was to provide mainstream medical services to the poor. But Medicaid was grafted administratively onto state welfare programs, largely because the only social-service agency operating in every state at the time was the welfare authority, and its clients were recipients of public assistance.[8] Thus, the seeds of Medicaid as a welfare program were sown at the beginning, and ever since, it has been treated as a political stepchild by HCFA, the executive branch, and Congress.

Nevertheless, Medicaid is the main public insurance program for many people of limited means. Studies have found that poor persons enrolled in

Medicaid are more likely to have a usual source of care, have a higher number of annual ambulatory care visits, and have a higher rate of hospitalization than poor persons with no public or private health care coverage.[9] Medicaid's eligible population comprises 21.3 million children, 9.2 million adults in families, 4.1 million elderly persons, and 6.7 million blind or disabled persons. Over the past decade, the national expansion in Medicaid's eligible population was driven by federal requirements to increase health care coverage for pregnant women and children, state efforts to cover more uninsured people of low income, and court-ordered expansions in coverage for the disabled. On average, Medicaid beneficiaries account for about 11 percent of a state's population, but some jurisdictions have substantially higher percentages, including Tennessee (21.7 percent), the District of Columbia (17.8 percent), Vermont (17.4 percent), New Mexico (16.1 percent), New York (15.1 percent), West Virginia (14.1 percent), California (13.6 percent), Michigan (13.6 percent), Washington (12.9 percent), Georgia (12.8 percent), Kentucky (12.8 percent), Mississippi (12.3 percent), and Hawaii (11.4 percent).[10]

Being poor does not automatically make a person eligible for Medicaid. Indeed, in 1997, Medicaid covered only 44.4 percent of nonelderly persons with an income of less than $13,330 for a family of three (Salganicoff A, Henry J. Kaiser Family Foundation: personal communication). Most people become eligible by meeting a federally defined criterion (i.e., advanced age, blindness, disability, or membership in a single-parent family with dependent children). Within the federal guidelines, the states set their own criteria for eligibility with respect to income and assets, resulting in large variations in coverage from state to state. Indeed, it is no exaggeration to say that there are actually more than 50 Medicaid programs—one in each state, plus the program in the District of Columbia and those in the U.S. territories—because the rules under which they operate vary so enormously.

THE CONCENTRATION OF MEDICAID SPENDING

Although adults and children in low-income families account for nearly three fourths of Medicaid beneficiaries, their medical care accounts for less than 30 percent of program expenditures (Fig. 21.1). Elderly and blind or disabled persons account for most of the expenditures because of their greater use of acute and long-term care services. In 1997, Medicaid's costs per beneficiary were $9,539 for elderly persons, $8,832 for blind or disabled beneficiaries, $1,810 for adults in low-income families, and $1,027 for children (Hoffman D, HCFA: personal communication). The figures for elderly and blind or disabled persons do not include Medicare payments. Payments to physicians represented only 5.9 percent of Medicaid's total expenditures in 1996, less than the program paid out for home health services or prescription drugs (Table 21.1). By comparison,

FIGURE 21.1

Medicaid Beneficiaries and Expenditures in 1996, According to Enrollment Group

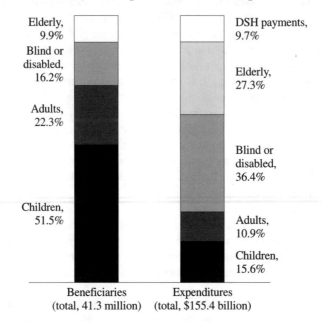

Beneficiaries   Expenditures
(total, 41.3 million)   (total, $155.4 billion)

Total expenditures exclude administrative expenses. DSH payments denotes disproportionate-share hospital payments. Percentages do not sum to 100, because of rounding. Data provided by the Kaiser Commission on Medicaid and the Uninsured.

payments to physicians made up 25.4 percent of Medicare expenditures in 1996. According to the most recent study of Medicaid's payments to physicians, in 1993 average payments were about 73 percent of Medicare payments and about 47 percent of private fees.[11]

Medicaid covers a broad range of services with nominal cost-sharing requirements because of the limited financial resources of beneficiaries. The benefit package extends well beyond the services covered by Medicare and most employer-sponsored plans. By federal law, states must cover inpatient and outpatient hospital services; care provided by physicians, midwives, and certified nurse practitioners; laboratory and radiographic services; nursing home care and home health care; early and periodic screening, diagnosis, and treatment for persons under 21 years of age; family planning; and care provided by rural

TABLE 21.1

Medicaid Payments for Selected Fiscal
Years, According to Type of Service*

	Payment — Millions of Dollars				% Distribution
Category	1985	1994	1995	1996	in 1996
Total	37,508	108,270	120,141	121,685	100.0
Inpatient services	10,645	28,237	28,842	27,216	22.4
General hospitals	9,453	26,180	26,331	25,176	20.7
Mental hospitals	1,192	2,057	2,511	2,040	1.7
Nursing facilities‡	5,071	27,095	29,052	29,630	24.3
Intermediate-care facilities‡	11,245	8,347	10,383	9,555	7.9
For mentally retarded persons	4,719	8,347	10,383	9,555	7.9
For all other persons	6,526	0	0	0	0
Physicians' services	2,346	7,189	7,360	7,238	5.9
Dental services	458	969	1,019	1,028	0.8
Other practitioners' services	251	1,040	986	1,094	0.9
Outpatient hospital services	1,789	6,342	6,627	6,504	5.3
Clinic services	714	3,747	4,280	4,222	3.5
Laboratory and radiologic services	337	1,176	1,180	1,208	1.0
Home health services	1,120	7,042	9,406	10,868	8.9
Prescription drugs	2,315	8,875	9,791	10,697	8.8
Family-planning services	195	516	514	474	0.4
Early and periodic screening	85	980	1,169	1,399	1.1
Rural health clinics	7	188	215	302	0.2
Other care	928	6,522	9,214	10,247	8.4

*Data are from the Health Care Financing Administration.
†Payments exclude premiums and capitation amounts. Total payments include payments for unknown services, which are not shown in this table. The percent distribution is based on rounded numbers.
‡Beginning in 1991, nursing facilities included skilled nursing facilities and intermediate-care facilities for all persons other than the mentally retarded.

health clinics and federally qualified community health centers. Medicaid also acts as a supplementary insurance program for elderly and disabled Medicare beneficiaries of low income, paying their Medicare premiums and cost-sharing requirements and covering additional services, most notably prescription drugs. The states have the option to cover additional services for Medicaid recipients and receive matching federal funds for them. Items commonly covered by the states include prescription drugs, clinic services, prosthetic devices, hearing aids, dental care, and services provided by intermediate-care facilities for the mentally retarded.

THE DEVOLUTION OF FEDERAL AUTHORITY

When Republicans took control of the Congress in 1995, one of their overriding policy goals was to devolve federal authority and money to state governments, particularly in the realm of social welfare. A year late, Republicans were successful in reforming welfare policies, many of which had been enacted in 1935 as part of President Franklin D. Roosevelt's New Deal. The debate in Congress included "a massive reexamination of who 'deserves' public assistance?"[12] The main decisions were that the states should decide who is needy, welfare should be linked to work,[13] cash assistance should be temporary, and immigrants who arrive in this country after the law's enactment should not receive full Medicaid benefits.[12] Congress scrapped the federal guarantee of cash assistance for the nation's poorest children and granted states the authority to operate their own welfare and work programs, largely with federal resources. These changes were incorporated into the Personal Responsibility and Work Opportunity Reconciliation Act of 1996, which President Clinton signed into law over the vigorous protest of the liberal wing of the Democratic Party.

Congress also enacted legislation in 1995 to recast Medicaid as it had welfare, converting the program from an open-ended entitlement program for eligible beneficiaries to essentially a state-operated program funded largely by a capped federal block grant. Clinton vetoed this measure and offered his own counter-proposal, which the Republicans rejected. Two years later, in the Balanced Budget Act of 1997, Congress and the administration finally agreed on a new federal-state division of authority for Medicaid, although the debate on this subject continues.[14-16] Among various provisions, all of which granted the states more authority, the budget law repealed the Boren amendment (named after the Oklahoma senator who initially sponsored it),[17] which stipulated that the states must provide payments for services at levels that meet the costs incurred by "efficiently and economically operated" hospitals and nursing homes.

THE ELIGIBILITY MAZE

Medicaid's complex eligibility policy, which "both states and the federal government have relied on . . . as a tool for limiting their financial exposure for the cost of covered benefits,"[18] makes the program difficult for its beneficiaries to understand and for the states to administer. Before welfare reform was enacted, adults and children in low-income families that qualified for public assistance were automatically eligible for Medicaid. The new welfare law severed this link between Medicaid and public assistance, with the goal of preserving Medicaid coverage for poor families facing possible cutbacks in public assistance, but now one must apply to the program in order to be declared eligible for medical coverage. This policy has had an unintended consequence. As welfare caseloads have declined nationally, by about 42 percent since 1994, there have been unexpected reductions in the number of people seeking Medicaid coverage. In recent meetings involving administrators of state human-service agencies and specialists in Medicaid eligibility, sponsored by the Kaiser Commission on Medicaid and the Uninsured, the participants concluded that because many people now view public cash assistance as a temporary benefit, "even when Medicaid enrollment would be in the economic interest of the beneficiary, fewer potential recipients are likely to apply for coverage or to maintain Medicaid enrollment."[19] If the decline in Medicaid enrollment were explained by the transition from welfare assistance to jobs that offered health insurance, neither HCFA nor the states would be concerned, but most former welfare recipients who have found employment are in low-paying positions that do not provide health care coverage.

The number of people who are not taking advantage of Medicaid coverage is quite large, and the problem speaks to the obstacles that many poor people face in trying to navigate publicly run systems. State governments, in turn, have only limited success in persuading parents to enroll their children in the Medicaid program, almost regardless of the specific circumstance. One recent federal study estimated that 4.7 million children were uninsured despite their eligibility for Medicaid, representing about 2 of every 5 uninsured children in the United States.[20] A similar problem faces the new State Children's Health Insurance Program, which authorizes the expenditure of $24 billion over a period of five years to extend coverage to low-income children who are not already eligible for Medicaid.[21,22] Congress gave the states the option of using this money to expand their existing Medicaid programs, create new programs, or implement combined approaches. Recognizing the challenge of actually signing up children, federal and state governments and private foundations are investing hundreds of millions of dollars in outreach efforts to identify eligible children and enroll them in Medicaid or the State Children's Health Insurance Program.[23]

THE STATES' BOOMING ECONOMIES

Although the states are grappling with the multiple challenges of welfare reform, the State Children's Health Insurance Program, and Medicaid, they have more room to maneuver because the costs of Medicaid have been brought under strict control and the economies of most states are booming. Total Medicaid expenditures increased by only 3.8 percent in 1997, the slowest annual rate of growth since the program's inception. In its latest report on national health care expenditures, HCFA's Office of the Actuary stated:

> Average annual growth in Medicaid spending decelerated to 5.9 percent over the 1994–1997 period, compared with 12.7 percent for 1991–1994 and 19.5 percent for 1988–1991. The rapid growth over the 1988–1994 period is attributable to

three basic factors: (1) an increase in the number of Medicaid enrollees, (2) an increase in nominal (not adjusted for inflation) spending per recipient, and (3) explosive growth in disproportionate-share hospital payments, a substantial portion of which states used to supplement their state treasuries in ways that Congress has now outlawed.[24]

(Disproportionate-share payments, which totaled $15 billion in 1996, are made to compensate hospitals for the higher operating costs they incur by treating disproportionately large numbers of low-income and Medicaid patients.[25])

At the start of 1999, despite five straight years of tax cuts and moderate increases in expenditures, all the states except Alaska and Hawaii had healthy budget surpluses that collectively are estimated to total $31 billion. As a percentage of the overall budget for all the states, this surplus is twice that of the federal budget, according to a report issued by the National Governors' Association.[26,27] Nevertheless, many governors have adopted social policies designed to slow, if not prevent, further expansion of publicly financed insurance programs. For example, California made an explicit decision under its former Republican governor, Pete Wilson, not to accept the full federal allotment of funds from the State Children's Health Insurance Program. Such policies reflect the concern that federal funding for Medicaid will eventually decline, forcing the states to make up the shortfall. In addition, Republicans see little political gain in creating new publicly financed programs in this era of limited government. Only Kentucky, Massachusetts, Nevada, and Vermont have said that they plan to spend their full allotment of funds from the State Children's Health Insurance Program this year. Many other states are in earlier stages of implementing the program and may not be able to spend all the available program funds in 1999.

MEDICAID MANAGED CARE

Since the 1980s, many states have experimented with managed care, largely as a means of limiting Medicaid expenditures, but they had no authority to require eligible beneficiaries to enroll in managed-care plans. Moreover, the beneficiaries had no incentive for enrollment, such as the extra benefits that elderly persons could obtain if they signed up with health maintenance organizations (HMOs) under Medicare. To make managed care mandatory, the states had to receive a waiver from HCFA. Under President Clinton, a former governor, HCFA adopted a liberal policy of issuing such waivers, which enabled some 40 states to make managed care mandatory in whole or in part for certain groups of beneficiaries. The Balanced Budget Act of 1997 eliminated the waiver requirement altogether, except for persons who are eligible for both Medicare and Medicaid (disabled and elderly poor people), children with special needs, and Native Americans. The budget law also eliminated the requirement that in HMOs with Medicaid beneficiaries, at least 25 percent of the members must receive coverage from third parties other than Medicaid. Congress had imposed this stricture as a proxy for ensuring that the plans would provide high-quality care.

Forty-nine states (all except Alaska) now rely on some form of managed care to serve their Medicaid populations. The proportion of Medicaid beneficiaries enrolled in managed-care plans increased from 9.5 percent (2.7 million people) in 1991 to 48 percent (15.3 million) in 1997. The states use one of three forms of Medicaid managed care: arrangements with primary care physicians to act as gatekeepers, approving and monitoring the provision of services to individual beneficiaries in return for a fixed fee; enrollment of beneficiaries in HMOs that assume the full financial risk of providing a comprehensive package of services; and contracts with medical clinics or large group practices, which provide services but do not assume the full financial risk for them. In areas where HMOs are prepared to assume the full financial risk of enrolling Medicaid beneficiaries, the states are choosing this approach and turning away from the other two.

The most comprehensive examination of the effect of Medicaid's growing relationship with managed care is being conducted by researchers at the Urban Institute as part of an ambitious project called Assessing the New Federalism.[28] The project, funded by private foundations, is a major new effort to understand changes in health care and social programs at the stare level.[29-37] Researchers have examined the effect of Medicaid managed care in 13 states (Alabama, California, Colorado, Florida, Massachusetts, Michigan, Minnesota, Mississippi, New Jersey, New York, Texas, Washington, and Wisconsin). Their preliminary conclusions, reached three years after the start of the study, which will continue for another three years or more, are as follows:

> The Medicaid managed care revolution has been more of a skirmish than a revolution. The goals of Medicaid managed care were to expand access to mainstream providers and to save money, but success on both fronts has been limited. Medicaid managed care is predominantly limited to children and younger adults; few states have extended enrollment to more expensive elderly and disabled enrollees, limiting potential savings. States are also finding that managed care savings are modest because traditionally low Medicaid fee-for-service payment rates make it difficult for states to substantially slash capitation levels or for HMOs to negotiate further discounts. In addition, safety net providers that need Medicaid revenues to survive have received special protections from states, which has both reduced potential savings and steered Medicaid beneficiaries to traditional providers of charity care. The combination of low capitation rates and protections for safety net providers have limited the willingness of commercial HMOs in several states to contract with states, thus restricting the expansion of access to maintain providers.[38]

A number of commercial HMOs that were enrolling Medicaid beneficiaries have withdrawn from the program in the past year, citing multiple reasons for their dissatisfaction.[39,40] In interviews conducted recently by Hurley and McCue at the Medical College of Virginia, state policy makers, health-plan executives, venture capitalists, and stock analysts expressed little optimism that commercial HMOs would continue to enroll Medicaid beneficiaries, particularly in states with very low per capita payment rates. Citing the views of stock analysts, Hurley and McCue note:

> The early promises of profitable market opportunities were overshadowed by un-expected rate rollbacks, contracting volatility, and administrative burdens which soured analysts and investors on the Medicaid market. . . . Given this history, stock analysts see limited opportunities for success in Medicaid and view the exodus from the Medicaid market as evidence of management's desire to enhance stockholder wealth.[41]

CONCLUSIONS

Medicaid underscores the ambivalence of a society that continually struggles with the question of which citizens deserve access to publicly financed medical care and under what conditions. On a more positive note, Medicaid now provides health insurance to a larger population of poor persons than ever before, reflecting the strength of a bullish economy and expanded criteria for eligibility. Yet, nationally, the number of uninsured people grew to 16.1 percent of the population in 1997, the largest level in a decade, because employer-sponsored coverage has eroded.[2,3] This divergence prompts a question: What potential does Medicaid have for further expanding its eligible population so that poor families with incomes that minimally exceed the federal poverty level could be insured through this program? Some states (Massachusetts, Minnesota, Oregon, Tennessee, and Wisconsin are examples) have used public funds to broaden private coverage through managed care, and the welfare-reform law permits the states to raise the threshold for income and assets so that more beneficiaries will be eligible for Medicaid. But many states have shifted to managed care without expanding coverage for the working poor, a population that constitutes the bulk of the uninsured population, and rates of payment to providers remain woefully low.

Medicaid's architects envisioned a program that would provide poor people with mainstream medical care in a fashion similar to that of private insurance. As the decades have passed, that vision has largely faded, and several tiers of care have emerged. Mainstream medical care is provided to people covered by private insurance or Medicare. For the most part, poor people continue to rely on providers that make up the nation's medical safety net: public and some private not-for-profit hospitals and clinics and their medical staffs that, by virtue of their location or their social calling, provide a disproportionate amount of care to the poor. These providers are increasingly stressed as Medicaid diverts funds to managed-care plans. The United States remains the only industrialized nation that has never settled on a social policy that, however policy makers choose to accomplish it, offers a basic set of health care benefits to all residents regardless of their ability to pay—certainly a regrettable failure in a nation blessed with so many resources.

REFERENCES

1. Iglehart JK. The American health care system—expenditures. N Engl J Med 1999;340:70–6.

2. Kuttner R. The American health care system—health insurance coverage. N Engl J Med 1999;340:163–8.

3. *Idem.* The American health care system—employer-sponsored health coverage. N Engl J Med 1999;340:248–52.

4. Iglehart JK. The American health care system — Medicare. N Engl J Med 1999;340:327–32.

5. *Idem.* The American health care system — Medicaid. N Engl J Med 1993;328: 896–900.

6. Tallon JR, Brown LD. Who gets what? Devolution of eligibility and benefits in Medicaid. In: Thompson FJ, Dilulio JJ Jr, eds. Medicaid and devolution: a view from the states. Washington, D.C.: Brookings Institution Press, 1998.

7. Cohen W. Reflections on the enactment of Medicare and Medicaid. Health Care Financ Rev 1985;Suppl.

8. Friedman E. The little engine that could: Medicaid at the Millennium. Front Health Serv Manage 1998;14(4):3–24.

9. Berk ML, Schur CL. Access to care: how much difference does Medicaid make? Health Aff (Millwood) 1998;17(3):169–80.

10. Frontsin P. Sources of health insurance and characteristics of the uninsured: analysis of the March 1998 current population survey. EBRI issue brief no. 204. Washington, D.C.: Employee Benefit Research Institute, 1998.

11. Colby DC. Medicaid physician fees, 1993. Health Aff (Millwood) 1994,13(2): 255–63.

12. Ellwood MR, Ku L. Welfare and immigration reforms: unintended side effects for Medicaid. Health Aff (Millwood) 1998;17(3):137–51.

13. Pear R. Most states meet work requirement of welfare law. New York Times. December 30, 1998:A1.

14. Spitz B. The elusive New Federalism. Health Aff (Millwood) 1998; 17(6):150–61.

15. Weil A, Wiener JM, Holahan J. 'Assessing the New Federalism' and state health policy. Health Aff (Millwood) 1998;17(6):162–4.

16. Bartels PL, Boroniec P. BadgerCare: a case study of the elusive New Federalism. Health Aff (Millwood) 1998;17(6):165–9.

17.   Wiener JM, Stevenson DG. Repeal of the "Boren Amendment": implications for quality of care in nursing homes. Series A, no. A-30. Washington, D.C.: Urban institute, 1998.

18.   Schneider A, Fennel K, Long P. Medicaid eligibility for families and children. Washington, DC.: Henry J. Kaiser Family Foundation, 1998.

19.   Smith VK, Lovell RG, Peterson KA, O'Brien MJ. The dynamics of current Medicaid enrollment changes: insights from focus groups of state human service administrators, Medicaid eligibility specialists and welfare agency analysts. Washington, D.C.: Henry J, Kaiser Family Foundation, 1998.

20.   Selden TM, Banthin JS, Cohen JW. Medicaid's problem children: eligible but not enrolled. Health Aff (Millwood) 1998;17(3):192–200.

21.   Budetti PP. Health insurance for children—a model for incremental health reform? N Engl J Med 1998;338:541–2.

22.   Newacheck PW, Stoddard JJ, Hughes DC, Pearl M. Health insurance and access to primary care for children. N Engl J Med 1998:338:513–9.

23.   Kenesson MS. Medicaid managed care: outreach and enrollment for special populations. Princeton, N.J.: Center for Health Care Strategies, 1998.

24.   Levit K, Cowan C, Braden B, Stiller J, Sensenig A, Lazenby H. National health expenditures in 1997: more slow growth. Health Aff (Millwood) 1998;17(6):66–110.

25.   Coughlin TA. Changing state and federal payment policies for Medicaid disproportionate-share hospitals. Health Aff (Millwood) 1998;17(3):118–36.

26.   Broder DS. States pass their fiscals: they're trimming taxes, beefing up 'rainy day' funds. Washington Post. December 31, 1998: A25.

27.   Broder DS. Golden years for governors. Washington Post. January 3, 1999:C7.

28.   Kondratas A. Weil A, Goldstein N. Assessing the new federalism: an introduction. Health Aff (Millwood) 1998;17(3):43–63.

29.   Holahan J, Zuckerman S, Evans A, Rangarajan S. Medicaid managed care in thirteen states. Health Aff (Millwood) 1998;17(3):43–63.

30.   Nichols LM, Blumberg JL. A different kind of 'new federalism'? The Health Insurance Portability and Accountability Act of 1996. Health Aff (Millwood) 1998;17(3): 25–42.

31.   Wall S. Transformations in public health systems. Health Aff (Millwood) 1998;17(3):64–80.

32.   Wiener JM, Stevenson DG. State policy on long-term care for the elderly. Health Aff (Millwood) 1998;17(3):81–100.

33.   Rajan S. Publicly subsidized health insurance: a typology of state approaches. Health Aff (Millwood) 1998;17(3):101–17.

34.   Norton SA, Lipson DJ. Portraits of the safety net: the market, policy environment, and safety net response. Occasional paper no. 19. Washington, D.C.: Urban institute, 1998.

35.   Bovbjerg RR, Marsteller JA. Health care market competition in six states: implications for the poor. Occasional paper no. 17. Washington, D.C.: Urban Institute, 1998.

36. Wiener TM, Stevenson DG. Long-term care for the elderly: profiles of thirteen states. Occasional paper no. 12. Washington, D.C.: Urban Institute, 1998.

37. *Idem.* Controlling the supply of long-term care providers at the state level. Occasional paper no. 22. Washington, D.C.: Urban Institute, 1998.

38. Holahan J, Wiener J, Wallin S. Health policy for the low-income population: major findings from the Assessing the New Federalism case studies. Occasional paper no. 18. Washington, D.C.: Urban Institute, 1998.

39. Aston G. Widespread HMO defections starting to hit Medicaid, too. American Medical News. December 14,1998:5.

40. McCue MJ, Hurley RE, Draper DA, Jurgensen M. Reversal of fortune: commercial HMOs in the Medicaid market. Health Aff (Millwood) 1999;18(1):223–30.

41. Huxley RE, McCue MA. Medicaid and commercial HMOs: an at-risk relationship. Princeton, N.J.: Center for Health Care Strategies, 1998.

Index

About the Editor

Beaufort B. Longest, Jr., Ph.D., FACHE, is Professor of Health Policy and Management in the Graduate School of Public Health, University of Pittsburgh. He holds a secondary appointment as Professor of Business Administration in the University's Katz Graduate School of Business. He also is Director of the University of Pittsburgh's Health Policy Institute.

He received an undergraduate education at Davidson College and received the Master's of Health Administration (MHA) and doctorate degrees from Georgia State University. He is a Fellow of the American College of Healthcare Executives and holds memberships in the Academy of Health Services Research and Health Policy, the Academy of Management, Beta Gamma Sigma Honor Society in Business, and Delta Omega Honor Society in Public Health.

His research on issues of health policy and management has generated substantial grant support and has led to the publication of numerous peer-reviewed articles. In addition, he has authored or co-authored nine books. Two of his books, *Managing Health Services Organizations and Systems* and *Health Policymaking in the United States* are widely used in graduate health policy and management programs. He consults with healthcare organizations and systems, universities, associations, and government agencies on health policy and management issues.